S E C O N

HANDBOOK OF PATHOPHYSIOLOGY

SECOND EDITION

HANDBOOK OF PATHOPHYSIOLOGY

ELIZABETH J. CORWIN, MSN, PhD, FNP

School of Nursing and the Department of Physiology

The Pennsylvania State University

University Park, Pennsylvania

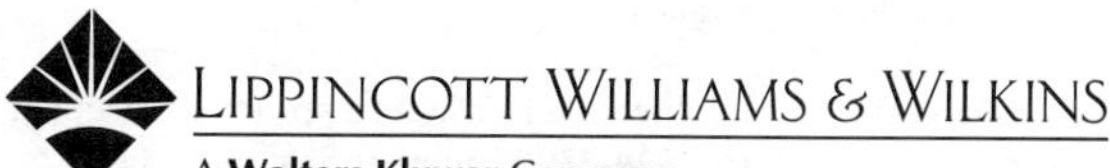

A Wolters Kluwer Company

Philadelphia • Baltimore • New York • London
Buenos Aires • Hong Kong • Sydney • Tokyo

Editor: Lisa Stead
Managing Editor: Claudia Vaughn
Production Editor: Lisa JC Franko
Marketing Manager: Jean Rodenberger
Design Coordinator: Mario Fernandez

351 West Camden Street
Baltimore, Maryland 21201-2436 USA

530 Walnut St.
Philadelphia, Pennsylvania 19106 USA

Printed in the United States of America.

First edition, 1996.

Library of Congress Cataloging-in-Publication Data

Corwin, Elizabeth J.
Handbook of pathophysiology / Elizabeth J. Corwin.–2nd ed.
p. cm.
Includes bibliographical references and index.
ISBN 0-7817-1938-0
1. Physiology, Pathological Handbooks, manuals, etc. I. Title.
[DNLM: 1. Pathology Handbooks. 2. Physiology Handbooks. QZ 39 C832h 1999]
RB113.C785 1999
616.07–dc21
DNLM/DLC
for Library of Congress 99-37060
CIP

To purchase additional copies of this book call our customer service department at (800) 638-3030 or fax orders to (301) 824-7390. International customers should call (301) 714-2324.

00 01 02
2 3 4 5 6 7 8 9 10

To my father, who gave to me a great love of books,
and to Bob, who believed all along I could write one.

PREFACE

Many classes in the health sciences revolve around the basic questions of how the body works, and what happens when something goes wrong. These two concepts are the focus of physiology and pathophysiology, and their mastery is essential for anyone planning a career in a health care profession. As in the first edition of this book, the second edition of the *Handbook of Pathophysiology* has been designed to provide a clear, accurate, and understandable description of health and disease. It is meant to be succinct and readable, and to be useful to students and practitioners at a variety of levels.

As a physiologist, I have taught physiology and pathophysiology to biology, physical therapy, and pharmacy undergraduates and to many different groups of graduate and medical students. As a nurse and a nurse practitioner, I also have taught pathophysiology to undergraduate and graduate-level nurses. I believe this text can be used as a reference and a resource for students at all these levels. For health care providers and students in the classroom, in the laboratory, or in practice, this text is designed to keep you informed, answer your questions, and help you to be the best health care provider you can possibly be. Finally, this text has been written with the goal of sharing with all students and practitioners the same wonder and excitement for physiology and the human body that I have enjoyed since undergraduate school and that I appreciate more and more each year that I practice as a health care provider.

Content Organization

The format of this edition of the *Handbook of Pathophysiology* has continued to follow the same outline as in the previous book, with section headings of "Physiologic Concepts," "Pathophysiologic Concepts," and "Conditions of Disease or Injury." The text is organized this way because I believe that a solid understanding of physiology is essential to understanding pathophysiology, and likewise, understanding both physiology and pathophysiology is required in order for a description of any disease to make sense.

The text has been expanded from 19 chapters to 21, to include a presentation of health and disease (Chapter 4) and a highly focused and up-to-date description of the interaction of the nervous and immune systems. This latter chapter (Chapter 10) was written by Dr. Joseph Cannon, a world-renowned expert in the field of neuroimmunobiology. These two additional chapters bring to the forefront the concept that good health represents an intricate balance between all systems of the body, as well as an individual's genetic predisposition, the environment, and his or her behavior.

The rest of the chapters in this edition have also been expanded, in three primary ways. First, all information presented has been updated where appropriate. For example, the information presented in the chapters on cancer (Chapter 5) and the immune system (Chapter 3) includes the most recent and cutting-edge scientific studies. For all other chapters as well, the most recent advances in concepts or treatment strategies have been added. Second, under the "Conditions of Disease or Injury," the "Clinical Manifestations," "Diagnostic Techniques," "Complications," and "Treatment Outlines" have been markedly expanded. Undoubtedly, this is a result of my personal growth as a nurse practitioner: Although I still believe that physiology is the foundation of pathophysiology, I am immersed as well in the excitement of diagnosis and treatment. The third main change in the text is the addition of many more visual tools. Figures and tables have been added to the chapters, to offer the reader another view of the material.

As in the previous edition, "Pediatric and Geriatric Considerations" are included where appropriate to alert the reader to variations in both normal and pathophysiologic processes in children and older adults. Many of these too have been expanded to include pearls gleaned from practice.

Many of the additions were incorporated as the result of extensive reviews both by students and subject specialists. I thank each of them for their time and expertise.

Special Features

Each chapter includes teaching aids designed to assist the reader's understanding of pathophysiology.

KEY WORDS are indicated in boldface type and are defined in the text in order to help readers quickly master what can sometimes be a difficult vocabulary.

FIGURES, especially chosen or created for the Handbook, are used throughout the text to visually explain concepts that are not easily grasped by words alone.

GERIATRIC CONSIDERATIONS appear throughout the Handbook to alert readers to the important differences in the physiologic and pathophysiologic systems, and conditions of disease or injury in the older adult.

PEDIATRIC CONSIDERATIONS highlight developmental, physiologic, and pathophysiolgic differences in both wellness and illness in children.

ACKNOWLEDGMENTS

I again thank the faculty in the Department of Physiology at the University of Michigan for providing me with the foundation of knowledge to write this textbook. They also are responsible for teaching me to teach, to enjoy teaching, and to respect my students. In this light, I thank all my former and current students who have offered suggestions and ideas, and have expanded my horizons with their enthusiasm and high standards. At Lippincott Williams & Wilkins, I thank Lisa Stead and Claudia Vaughn for their excellent guidance, support, and patience.

CONTRIBUTOR AND REVIEWERS

Contributor

Joseph Cannon, MS, PhD
The Noll Physiological Laboratory
Departments of Kinesiology and Physiology
The Pennsylvania State University
University Park, Pennsylvania

Reviewers

Maxine Adegbloa, RN, MSN
Associate Degree Nursing Instructor
El Centro College
Dallas, Texas

Catherine Azubuike, RN, BSHA, MSN
Nursing Instructor
Department of Nursing
LA Southwest Community College
Los Angeles, California

Judith Bryan, MSN, EdD, RN
Associate Professor
School of Nursing, BSN Program
University of Indianapolis
Indianapolis, Indiana

Christine Cannon, RN, BSN, MSN, PhD
Associate Professor
College of Health and Nursing Sciences
University of Delaware
Newark, Delaware

Lois Doane, MSN, RN, AOCN
Oncology Clinical Nurse Specialist
University of Tennessee Medical Center
Faculty
University of Tennessee College of Nursing
Knoxville, Tennessee

Janet L. Gysi, RN, MA, CCN
Instructor, Division of Nursing
Iowa Wesleyan College
Staff RN
Emergency Treatment Center
Burlington Medical Center
Burlington, Iowa

Jetta Hogenmiller, RN, MC, cFNP
Assistant Professor
Graduate Nurse Practitioner Program
Creighton University School of Nursing
Omaha, Nebraska

Karen C. Johnson-Brennan, EdD, RN
Professor ad Associate Director
BSN Program
San Francisco State University School of Nursing
San Francisco, California

Marjorie Knox, RN, MA, MPA
Professor, Nursing Program
Community College of Rhode Island
Warwick, Rhode Island

Kathy Lauer, RN, PhD
Associate Chairperson
Department of Adult Health Nursing
Rush University College of Nursing
Chicago, Illinois

Dorothy B. Liddel, MSN, RN, ONC
Assistant Professor
Department of Nursing
Columbia Union College
Columbia, Maryland

Dorothy Obester, BSNE, MSN, PhD
Professor of Nursing
St. Francis College
Loretto, Pennsylvania

Jane C. Shivnan, RN, MSN
Nurse Manager
Bone Marrow Transplant
Johns Hopkins Oncology Center
Baltimore, Maryland

CONTENTS

1 CELL STRUCTURE AND FUNCTION

The cell is the building block of each living organism. Each cell is a self-contained system that undergoes the functions of energy production and usage, respiration, reproduction, and excretion. Cells join together to form tissues, tissues join to form organs, and organs form body systems. To understand how the organs and systems of the body work, one must first understand the cell.

● ● ●

PHYSIOLOGIC CONCEPTS

Cell Structure

A cell is made up of internal structures separated from each other by semipermeable membranes. These internal structures are bound together inside one cell membrane to form a single unit. Although cells differ as to their function in the body, all cells contain the same internal structures (Fig. 1-1). The inside of each cell can be divided into two main compartments—the cytoplasm and the nucleus. All internal structures reside in the cytoplasm or the nucleus.

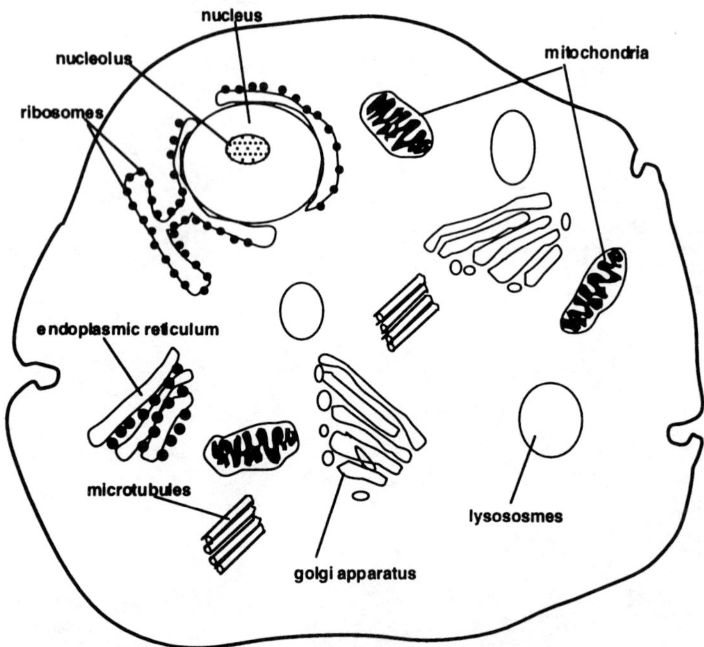

Figure 1-1. The internal structure of the cell.

CYTOPLASM

The cytoplasm includes everything inside the cell but outside the nucleus. The **mitochondria** are the energy sources of the cell, and the **endoplasmic reticulum** and **ribosomes** are cytoplasmic structures (organelles) necessary for protein synthesis. The **Golgi apparatus** is a complex of membranes and vesicles responsible for the secretion of proteins synthesized on the ribosomes. Intracellular **lysosomes** are vesicles that contain potent digestive enzymes. The internal skeleton, called the cytoskeleton, consists of **microtubules** and **microfilaments.** The cytoskeleton supports the cell from the inside and allows for the movement of substances inside the cell. The cytoskeleton also supports the movement of projections on the outside of cells, such as the hairlike projections called **cilia.** The microtubules play an important role in chromosome separation during cell division.

THE NUCLEUS

The nucleus of the cell is a large, membrane-bound organelle that contains **deoxyribonucleic acid** (DNA), the genetic material of the cell. To protect itself from breakage, the DNA is folded up inside the **nucleus.** Proteins responsible for folding and protecting the DNA are called histones. Histones and DNA are found in a part of the nucleus called the nucleolus. It is inside the nucleolus that DNA replication, cell division, and DNA transcription occur.

CELL MEMBRANE

A cell membrane encircles each cell. The cell membrane is a semipermeable barrier composed of a floating bilayer of phospholipids, with interspersed, freely moving, protein molecules. The protein molecules extend totally or partially through the membrane.

PHOSPHOLIPID BILAYER

The phospholipid molecules consist of a polar (charged) phosphate molecule joined with a nonpolar fat or lipid extension. The polar head, containing the phosphate, points inside or outside the cell, where it interacts with other polar molecules including water. The nonpolar extension makes up the body of the membrane layer itself (Fig. 1-2). Because there are two layers of lipid in the membrane, it is called a lipid bilayer. Diffusion through the lipid bilayer is limited to lipid soluble substances. For non-lipid substances to enter the cell, they must take advantage of the interspersed integral proteins.

INTEGRAL PROTEINS

Proteins that extend completely through the membrane are called integral proteins. Integral proteins are usually glycosylated (glucose

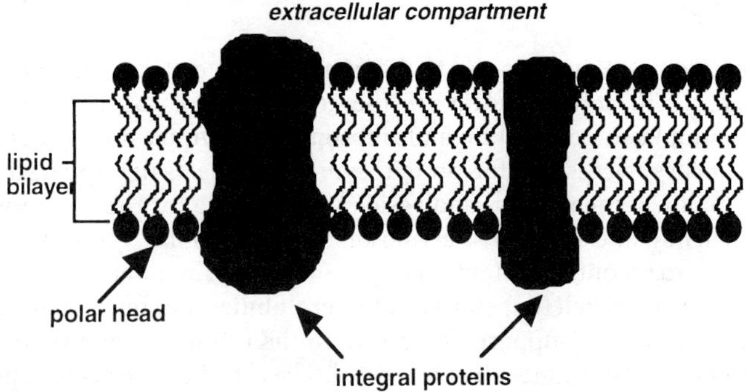

Figure 1-2. A schematic diagram of the cell membrane showing the lipid bilayer and integral proteins.

bound) or are bound by lipids on the extracellular side (Fig. 1-3). These protein-carbohydrate or lipid complexes often act as receptor molecules for protein hormones, or function in ways that allow cells to communicate with each other. Integral proteins may also act as channels in the membrane to provide pores for the movement of small ions into the cell, or as carriers for polar substances too large to move through the pores. Some integral proteins are membrane-bound enzymes needed to catalyze reactions.

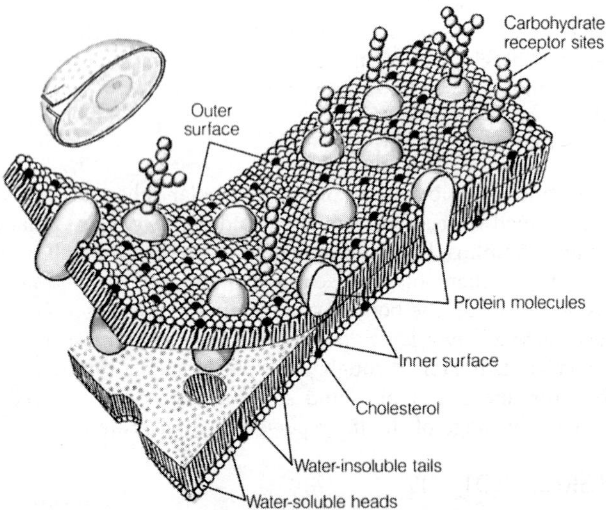

Figure 1-3. Cell membrane. The right end is intact, but the left end has been split along the plane of the lipid tails.

Movement Through the Membrane

Lipid-soluble substances, such as oxygen, carbon dioxide, neutral fats, cholesterol, alcohol, and urea, move across the lipid bilayer by simple diffusion. Other substances that are not lipid soluble, such as most small ions, glucose, amino acids, and proteins, move between the extracellular fluid and the intracellular compartments through pores provided by the integral proteins or through carrier-mediated transport systems. Carrier-mediated transport also originates in the integral proteins. The extracellular fluid consists of the fluid between the cells, called the **interstitial fluid**, and the blood. The fluid inside the cell is called the **intracellular fluid.**

SIMPLE DIFFUSION THROUGH THE CELL MEMBRANE

Simple diffusion through the cell membrane occurs through random movement of molecules. This process does not require energy, but can result in the movement of a substance across a membrane. However, the substance cannot accumulate in higher concentration on one side of the membrane compared to the other. Therefore, a substance that is permeable across the cell membrane will diffuse into or out of the cell until its concentration is equal on both sides (Fig. 1-4).

OSMOSIS

The diffusion of water into the cell is called osmosis. Osmosis occurs continually between intracellular and extracellular compartments, as water moves down its concentration gradient (i.e., from high concentration to low). The drive for water to move in one direction or the other is described as the **osmotic pressure.** The osmotic pressure of a solution depends on the number of particles or ions present in the water solution. The more ions that are present in the solution, the less the water concentration, and the greater the osmotic pressure (i.e., the pressure for water to diffuse into).

A cell also has osmotic pressure. A dehydrated cell has high osmotic pressure: low water concentration and high particle concentration. Water would diffuse *into* this cell if possible. An overhydrated cell has low osmotic pressure: high water concentration and low particle concentration. Water would diffuse *out* of this cell if possible.

SIMPLE DIFFUSION THROUGH PROTEIN PORES

Small ions, such as hydrogen, sodium, potassium, and calcium, are too electrically charged to diffuse through the lipid membrane of the cell. Instead, small ions diffuse through the pores provided by the integral proteins. These protein channels are usually selective about which ions they allow to pass. Selectivity is based on the shape and size of the channel and the electrical nature of the ion.

Many protein channels are gated; they can be open or closed to an

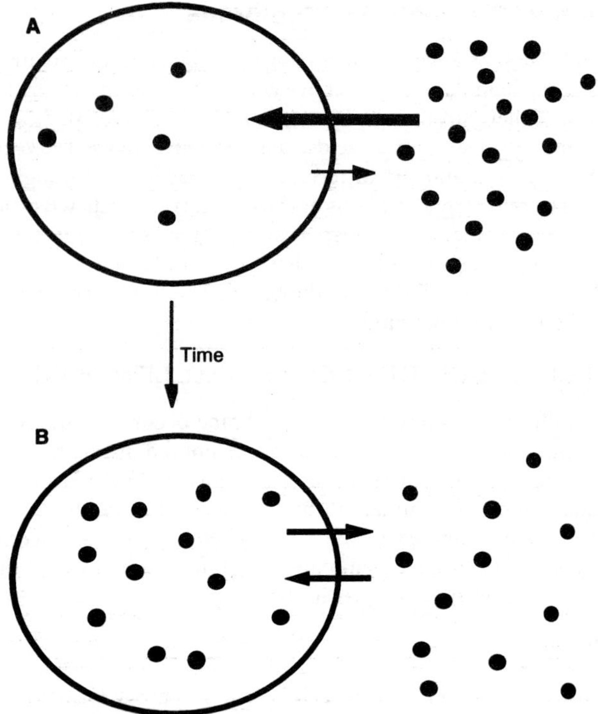

Figure 1-4. Simple diffusion across a membrane. Permeable substances randomly diffuse from an area of high concentration to an area of low concentration (**A**) until the concentrations are equal (**B**).

ion. Whether the gate is open or closed usually depends on the electrical potential across the gate (i.e., the sodium gate), or on binding to the gate by a ligand that causes it to open or close. An example of ligand gating is when acetylcholine binds to proteins on the neuromuscular junction, thereby opening gates to many small molecules, including sodium and calcium ions. Like all types of simple diffusion, diffusion through a gate continues until the concentrations on either side of the membrane are equal or the gate is shut.

MEDIATED TRANSPORT

For many substances like glucose and amino acids, simple diffusion is impossible. These molecules are too charged to pass through the lipid portion of the membrane or too large to pass through a pore. Instead, these substances, called substrates, are transported across the membrane with the assistance of a **carrier**. This type of movement is called mediated transport and may require energy derived from the splitting of adenosine triphosphate (ATP) (see Energy Production later).

Active transport is mediated transport that requires energy (Fig. 1-5A). With active transport, energy is used by the cell to maintain a substance at higher concentration on one side of the membrane than the other. Examples of substances moved by active transport include sodium, potassium, calcium, and the amino acids. Each of these substances is actively transported, with the assistance of a carrier, in one direction against a concentration gradient. It then moves down its concentration gradient by simple diffusion in the opposite direction.

Facilitated diffusion is mediated transport that does not require energy. Facilitated diffusion is similar to simple diffusion in that no energy is used by the cell to transport a substance; therefore, no concentration gradient across a membrane can be maintained for that substance. Facilitated diffusion differs from simple diffusion in that, with facilitated diffusion, a molecule that is unable to cross the cell membrane is assisted (facilitated) by a carrier and so can cross the membrane. Glucose moves into most cells by facilitated diffusion.

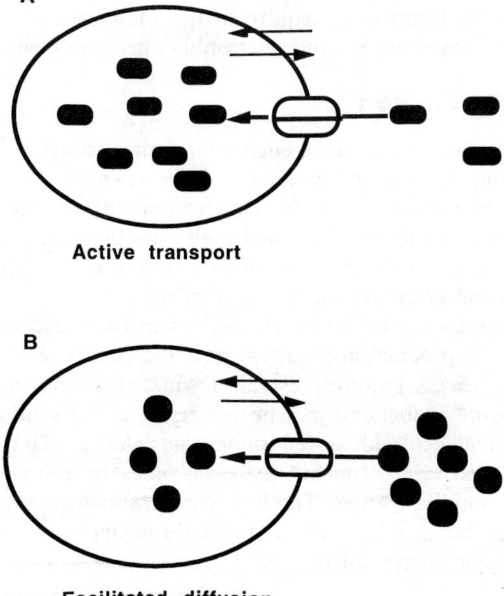

Figure 1-5. Transport of a substrate using a carrier. Active transport (**A**) requires energy to provide a final difference in concentration and facilitated diffusion (**B**) transports substrates without requiring energy, but cannot concentrate a substance. Simple diffusion continues at some level in all carrier-mediated systems.

CHARACTERISTICS OF CARRIERS

Active transport and facilitated diffusion require carriers. All carriers are affected by the properties of specificity, saturation, and competition.

Specificity of carriers means that only certain substrates will be transported by any one carrier. It appears that the carrier and its specific substrate fit together like a lock and a key.

Saturation of carriers means that at a certain concentration of substrate, all carriers will be filled and transport will level off. Additional substrate will not increase transport across the membrane.

Competition of carriers occurs when there is more than one substrate transported by the same carrier. The multiple substrates compete with each other for the limited number of carrier sites available. Many drugs, naturally occurring and synthetic, compete with endogenous hormones and neurotransmitters for various carrier molecules.

ENDOCYTOSIS

When large substances cannot enter the cell by diffusion or mediated transport, endocytosis (engulfment) of the substance by the cell membrane occurs. **Pinocytosis** is the engulfment of macromolecules, such as protein, by vesicles. **Phagocytosis** is the engulfment of dead cells or bacteria. Both processes require energy. Only cells of the immune system (i.e., macrophages and neutrophils) perform phagocytosis.

Energy Production

Cells are required to produce energy for their own use. Cells do this by extracting the energy contained in the chemical bonds of food molecules by combining the food molecules with oxygen inside the mitochondria of the cell. The food molecules used are glucose from carbohydrate metabolism, amino acids from protein metabolism, and fatty acids and glycerol from fat metabolism.

The process whereby the food molecules are combined with oxygen, leading to the production of energy, is called oxidative phosphorylation. This process requires several enzymes, working in sequential fashion in the mitochondria. The net result is the synthesis of the energy-rich molecule adenosine triphosphate (ATP). ATP is composed of the nitrogen base adenosine, the sugar ribose, and three phosphate molecules bound together. The last two phosphates are joined by a high-energy bond, which when split releases approximately 7 kcal/mole of usable energy for the cell.

OXIDATIVE PHOSPHORYLATION OF GLUCOSE

Although the **oxidative phosphorylation** of glucose occurs in the mitochondria, an initial step in the handling of glucose must occur before oxidative phosphorylation is initiated. This step is called **glycolysis** and occurs in the cytoplasm outside the mitochondria. It is anaerobic, meaning it occurs without requiring oxygen. During glycolysis, cytoplasmic enzymes convert glucose into pyruvic acid. This process requires two molecules of ATP and produces four molecules of ATP: a result of two net molecules. In times of oxygen deprivation, glycolysis plays a limited but important role in supplying the cell with ATP (see Anaerobic Glycolysis section).

If oxygen is present (aerobic), the molecules of pyruvic acid move into the mitochondria where they enter the citric acid cycle, also called the Krebs' cycle, and are converted by enzymes present there into a compound called acetyl coenzyme A (acetyl CoA). This process produces two more ATP molecules. Acetyl CoA is then enzymatically converted to carbon dioxide and hydrogen. The carbon dioxide diffuses out of the mitochondria and out of the cell, where it is picked up by the blood supplying that cell. It is then carried to the lungs and exhaled from the body. The hydrogen atoms remaining in the mitochondria begin the process of oxidative phosphorylation during which they are combined with molecules of oxygen through an elaborate electron transport chain present in the mitochondrial membrane. The result of this process is to produce a tremendous amount of energy, in the form of 36 ATP molecules. From the metabolism of one molecule of glucose, therefore, a total of 38 net ATP molecules are formed (36 from oxidative phosphorylation and 2 from glycolysis).

OXIDATIVE PHOSPHORYLATION OF FATTY ACIDS AND GLYCEROL

The cell also uses free fatty acids and glycerol in oxidative phosphorylation to produce ATP. Glycerol is a three-carbon carbohydrate, which undergoes glycolysis in the cytoplasm and enters the Krebs' cycle as acetyl CoA. Free fatty acids diffuse directly into the mitochondria where they are acted on by enzymes and transformed into acetyl CoA. This acetyl CoA also enters the Krebs' cycle. The breakdown of one molecule of fat results in 463 molecules of ATP. Fat has a five times greater weight per mole than glucose. Thus, gram for gram, the metabolism of fat provides about three times as much ATP as glucose metabolism. Therefore, fat is a more efficient form of energy storage than carbohydrate is.

OXIDATIVE PHOSPHORYLATION OF AMINO ACIDS

Amino acids enter the mitochondria after removal of the nitrogen molecule (deamination). After deamination, amino acids enter the Krebs' cycle at various points. Some, such as alanine, enter as pyruvic acid; others enter as later intermediates. Where they enter the Krebs' cycle determines how many hydrogen atoms they add to the electron transfer chain and thus how many ATP molecules are synthesized.

ANAEROBIC GLYCOLYSIS

If oxygen is unavailable, the pyruvic acid produced by glycolysis does not enter the Krebs' cycle, but combines with hydrogen in the cytoplasm to form lactic acid. Although the two molecules of ATP produced in the breakdown of one molecule of glucose to pyruvic acid are available to keep the cell alive, this is a wasteful use of glucose because it results in the loss of the other 36 molecules of ATP that would have been produced had pyruvic acid entered the Krebs' cycle. This process can only continue a short while before glucose is depleted.

The lactic acid produced by anaerobic glycolysis diffuses out of the cell and into the bloodstream. This can create a decrease in plasma pH (an increase in plasma acidity). With the return of oxygen, lactic acid will be reconverted to pyruvic acid, primarily in the liver, and the Krebs' cycle will resume.

USE OF ATP AS AN ENERGY SOURCE

ATP formed in the mitochondria moves into the cytoplasm by a combination of simple and facilitated diffusion. When needed by the cell, ATP can be broken down rapidly into adenosine diphosphate (ADP) by enzymatic splitting of the bond between the last two phosphates. This results in the release of energy, which is used by the cell to perform its duties of solute transport, protein synthesis, reproduction, and movement.

Although it is through ATP synthesis and breakdown that energy is transferred in the cell, very little ATP is stored in the cell. Instead, energy is stored in the form of substrates for ATP—carbohydrates, fats, proteins, and their metabolic products. The other essential component for ATP production, oxygen, is continually delivered to all cells by combined efforts of the cardiovascular and respiratory systems.

THE SODIUM-POTASSIUM PUMP

An important example of active transport is the pumping of sodium and potassium across cell membranes. This transport depends on an integral carrier protein known as the sodium-potassium pump. Associated with the pump is an enzyme that splits ATP and provides the energy needed for the pump to function. This enzyme is known as the sodium-potassium ATPase.

The sodium-potassium pump transports sodium ions out of and potassium into the cell. This causes greater sodium concentration in the extracellular fluid (142 mEq/L) compared to the intracellular fluid (14 mEq/L), and greater potassium concentration in the intracellular fluid (140 mEq/L) compared to the extracellular fluid (4 mEq/L).

The sodium-potassium pump carries three sodium molecules out of the cell for every two potassium molecules it carries in.

THE EFFECTS OF PUMPING SODIUM AND POTASSIUM

Because sodium and potassium are cations (carrying a positive charge), the transport of three sodium ions out of the cell and only two potassium ions into the cell creates an electrical gradient across the cell membrane. It is this electrical **membrane potential** that allows nerve function and action potentials to occur (Chapter 6).

The sodium-potassium pump also is essential in controlling cell volume. The presence of intracellular proteins and other organic substances that cannot cross the cell membrane increases intracellular osmotic pressure, and creates a tendency for water to diffuse into the cell. This diffusion of water, if unlimited, would cause the cell to swell and eventually burst. However, with the active transport of three sodium ions out of the cell, the osmotic pressure inside the cell is reduced and the diffusion of water into the cell is contained.

COUPLED TRANSPORT

Many substances are transported coupled to the active transport of sodium. These substances include glucose, amino acids, hydrogen ions, and calcium. The energy required for the transport of these other substances is indirectly supplied through the splitting of ATP by the sodium-potassium ATPase. This type of transport is called secondary active transport.

Coupled transport can be in the same direction as sodium transport (out of the cell—cotransport) or it may occur in the opposite direction as sodium transport (into the cell—countertransport) (Fig. 1-6). Both types of transport depend on the diffusion of sodium down its concen-

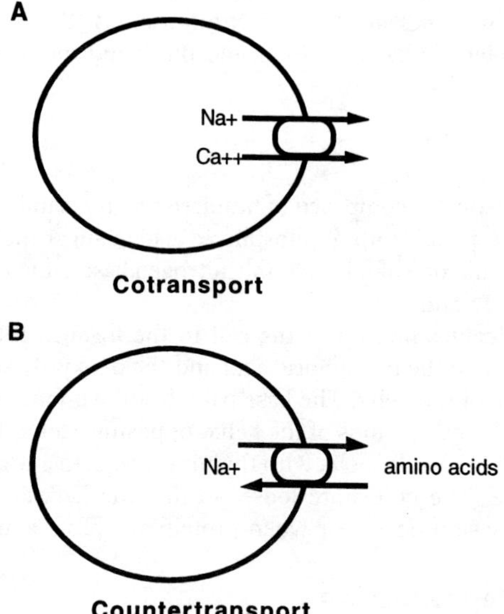

Figure 1-6. Cotransport (**A**) and countertransport (**B**) across the cell membrane.

tration gradient, which in turn depends on the active transport of sodium by the sodium-potassium pump. In cotransport, sodium pulls the coupled substance out of the cell. In countertransport, the coupled substance binds to the sodium carrier on the outside of the membrane with sodium on the inside. Therefore, when sodium is delivered to the outside of the cell, the other substance is delivered to the inside.

CALCIUM TRANSPORT

Calcium can be transported by coupled transport with sodium or moved by primary active transport through a calcium pump. There are two known calcium pumps. One is part of an integral protein present in the cell membrane, which moves calcium out of the cell. The other is an intracellular pump, which pumps calcium out of the cytoplasm into intracellular compartments such as the sarcoplasmic reticulum. This results in sequestering calcium inside the cell. Both pumps keep free intracellular calcium concentration low. The calcium pumps serve as ATPases, which derive energy needed to pump the calcium against its concentration gradient by the splitting of ATP.

CELLULAR GENETICS

In humans, the genetic material of each cell is contained in 23 pairs of chromosomes (1 pair from each parent) for a total of 46 chromosomes. Each cell of the body has the same 46 chromosomes. Of the 23 pairs of chromosomes, 22 are the same in both sexes. The 23rd pair of chromosomes are the sex chromosomes, the X or the Y. In humans, the female has two X chromosomes and the male has one X and one Y.

DNA

Each chromosome is composed of hundreds of thousands of molecules of DNA. DNA is made up of phosphoric acid, a sugar molecule called deoxyribose, and one of four possible nitrogen bases: adenine, guanine, cytosine, or thymine.

DNA molecules line up in the cell in the form of a double helix (Fig. 1-7), where the phosphoric acid and the deoxyribose sugar form the backbone of the helix. The base pairs from two molecules of DNA lie between the two strands of the helix, opposing each other. Adenine always bonds across the helix with thymine, and cytosine always bonds with guanine. The bonds are loose, so that the helixes can separate when cell division occurs or when protein synthesis is initiated.

Cellular Reproduction

Many cells of the body reproduce and make copies of themselves throughout a lifetime. To reproduce, a cell has to replicate its genetic

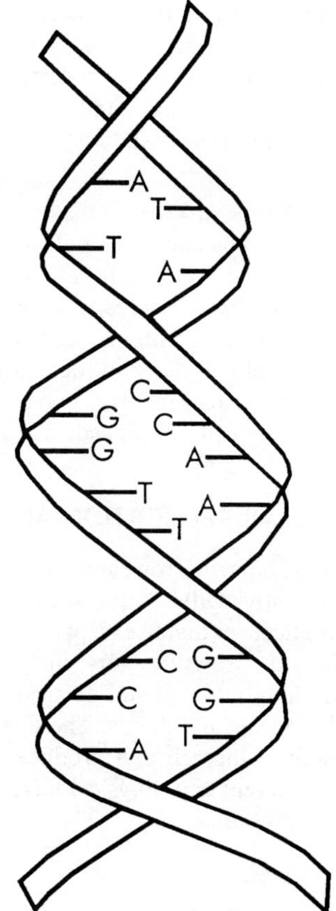

Figure 1-7. The DNA double helix.

material and then split in two. Replication and division of a cell occurs during the cell cycle (Chapter 2).

REPLICATION

To replicate, the DNA double helix uncoils and each strand of DNA serves as a template for a new strand. In the formation of a new strand of DNA, each adenine will only bind with a thymine and each cytosine will only pair with guanine. Therefore, only one strand, acting as a mirror-image template for the other, is needed to replicate the entire double helix.

Replication of the chromosome pairs and the DNA occurs in the nucleus of the cell. Various enzymes participate in DNA replication, which results in each chromosome being exactly copied or duplicated.

To be exact, the duplication is checked and double-checked by several "proofreading" enzymes to ensure no mistakes are made. If a mistake is identified, proofreading or other enzymes remove the error and correct it, or the cell may initiate its own death, in a process called **apoptosis.** If a mistake is not repaired, and the cell does not undergo apoptosis, a mutation in the DNA will exist.

CELL DIVISION

Once duplicated, the chromosome pairs pull apart and the original cell splits into two cells. Each new cell contains the entire genetic information in 23 pairs of chromosomes. The process whereby a cell divides to produce two identical daughter cells is called **mitosis.**

Meiosis, another type of cell division, occurs in the reproductive cells—the egg and sperm. Meiosis involves two cell divisions resulting in a total of four daughter cells produced. Meiosis and mitosis are described in Chapter 2.

CONTROL OF CELLULAR REPLICATION AND DIVISION

Some cells, such as liver, bone marrow, and gut cells, undergo replication and mitosis frequently. Other cells, such as nerve and cardiac muscle cells, do not replicate or divide except during fetal development or in the neonatal period. Growth factors, hormones, and other cell products turn cell division on or off and determine whether and how frequently a cell will replicate and divide. These factors may affect the replication and division of the cell that produces them, or they may circulate and affect a different cell. Physical factors such as crowding can also influence cell division.

Protein Synthesis

Protein synthesis is ongoing in all cells. Protein synthesis occurs when sections of DNA are turned on, which causes the cell to begin making a certain protein. Although each cell contains identical DNA on the 46 chromosomes, some cells have different sections of DNA turned on at a given time compared to other cells. Sections of DNA that turn on and off in different cells are called genes. There are approximately 50,000 to 100,000 genes in the human body distributed among the 46 chromosomes. Each gene contains 90 to 3,000 DNA molecules. Each gene codes for a particular protein or enzyme. Turning on or off different genes causes a cell to make different proteins compared to other cells.

Although genes controlling protein synthesis are in the nucleus, proteins are made in the cytoplasm on specialized structures called ribosomes. The message from the activated gene in the nucleus must be carried to the ribosomes. This is accomplished by making a copy of the gene in the nucleus and transporting the copy to the ribosomes, where it is then translated into a protein.

TRANSCRIPTION OF DNA INTO MESSENGER RNA

To transcribe or make a copy of a gene, the area of the double helix on the chromosome where that gene is contained must unravel. Once unraveled, a special enzyme, called an RNA polymerase, attaches to a certain section at the start of the gene, called the promoter or controlling sequence. When the RNA polymerase attaches to this site, the gene is copied, as a mirror image, in a manner similar to that described for DNA replication. The new copy is not another piece of DNA, but is a similar molecule called ribonucleic acid (RNA). RNA, like DNA, contains phosphoric acid, but unlike DNA, it contains the sugar ribose instead of deoxyribose and the base uracil instead of thymine. When the gene is copied as RNA, each cytosine base in the gene becomes a guanine in the copy, each guanine becomes a cytosine, each thymine becomes an adenine, and each adenine becomes a uracil. The entire gene is transcribed by this procedure. After the gene is copied, the RNA polymerase will reach a special sequence on the DNA (called the termination sequence) and the process will stop. The RNA copy is then released from the gene and moves into the cytoplasm. The RNA copy that carries the DNA message out of the nucleus is called the **messenger RNA** (mRNA). The mRNA then moves through the cytoplasm to the ribosomes.

Adenine, guanine, cytosine, or uracil are carried as mRNA to the ribosomes in groups of three, called triplets or codons. Each triplet codes for one amino acid. There are 20 amino acids used in the human body that combine in various ways to make up all the proteins of the body. The long strand of mRNA triplets can be snipped at any point before the molecule leaves the nucleus, allowing different proteins to be made from one original gene.

TRANSFER RNA

Before the ribosomes make the protein from the mRNA template, another type of RNA, called **transfer RNA** (tRNA), binds to the mRNA by connecting mirror-image bases (called the anticodon) to each triplet of mRNA bases. At the opposite end of the anticodon is the amino acid coded for by those three bases. There are at least 20 types of tRNA, each one carrying a certain amino acid on one end and the anticodon for that amino acid on the other end.

THE TRANSLATION OF MESSENGER RNA INTO PROTEIN

When the mRNA has found its matching tRNA, both molecules bind onto the ribosome, which is composed partly of a third type of RNA—**ribosomal RNA.** The amino acid carried by the tRNA is added to a chain of amino acids growing on the ribosome until the ribosome is signaled to stop adding to the chain by a special codon known as a stop signal. The protein is then complete and is freed from the ribosome. This process is called translation.

The processes of transcription and translation are shown in Figure 1-8.

CONTROL OF PROTEIN SYNTHESIS

Regulatory proteins block or activate the promoter section of each gene in the cell, determining which genes will be turned on, transcribed

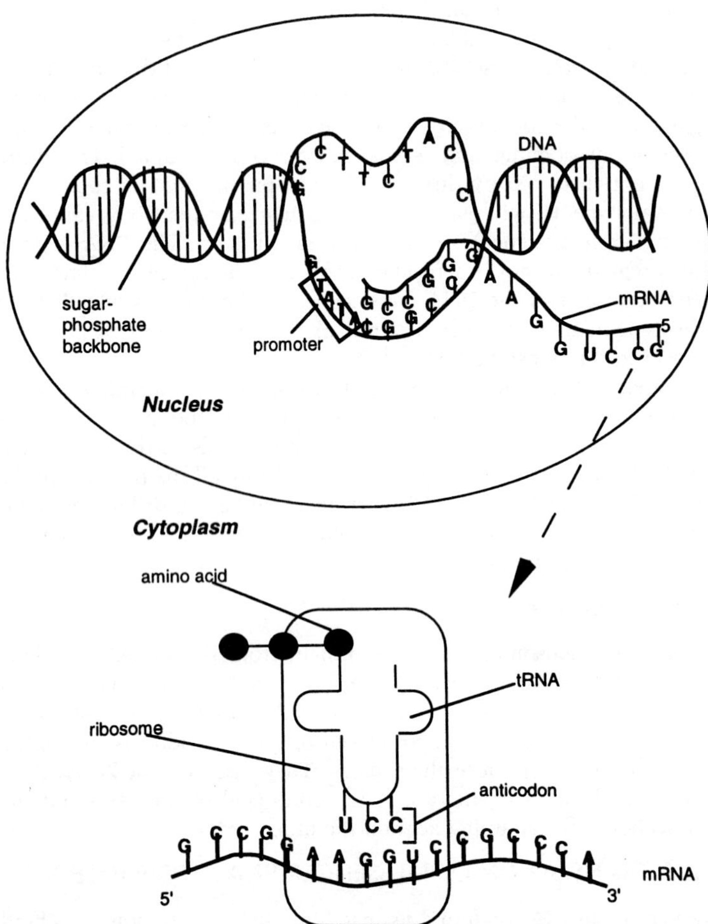

Figure 1-8. Transcription (copying) of DNA into mRNA occurs in the nucleus. The mRNA moves into the cytoplasm and attaches to the ribosome. On the ribosomes, the matching anticodon is carried on one end of tRNA and the corresponding amino acid on the other end. The amino acid chain grows as the ribosome moves along the mRNA.

into mRNA, and made into a protein. If a regulatory protein blocks the promoter region of a gene, protein synthesis will not occur from that gene. If a regulatory protein binds to or near the promoter area in such a way that it makes the area accessible to the RNA polymerase, it will activate the gene's transcription into mRNA.

Production of regulatory proteins appears to be linked to other genes responding to feedback signals, chemical cues, and hormones such as thyroid hormone and growth hormone. These signals result in the production of proteins with repressor or activator functions. Other factors that alter the function of the histones responsible for folding and exposing different portions of the DNA may also affect DNA transcription.

Cell Types

EPITHELIAL CELLS

Epithelial cells make up the tissue that lines most internal and external structures of the body. These cells are packed together, providing support for overlying structures. Epithelial tissue also acts as a protective barrier and a medium for absorption and secretion.

Examples of epithelial tissue include the skin (epidermis), the covering on all internal organs and tubules, the microvilli of the intestine, and the cilia lining the respiratory passageways. Glandular cells that secrete substances into ducts (exocrine glands) or into the bloodstream (endocrine glands) are made of epithelial tissue. Sensory organs also contain epithelial cells. Epithelial layers are usually one to two cells thick.

CONNECTIVE TISSUE CELLS

Connective tissue is composed of many different cell types, including fibroblasts, adipose (fat) cells, mast cells, and vascular endothelial cells.

Connective tissue holds different tissues together by the accumulation of protein and gel-like substances secreted from the fibroblasts into the spaces surrounding the cells. Protein substances include collagen, a thick, white fiber that acts to provide structural support; elastin, a stretchy protein that allows tissues to "give" when stretched; and reticular fibers, thin flexible strands that allow organs to accommodate increases in volume. Tissue gel is primarily hyaluronic acid, which intersperses throughout the interstitial spaces to retain water and provide support and protection.

Adipose tissue and endothelial cells provide nourishment and support for the fibroblasts. Mast cells contain granules filled with histamine and other vasoactive substances. Mast cell degranulation is an important step in initiating an inflammatory reaction.

Hematopoietic tissue is considered connective tissue. Hematopoietic tissue includes bone marrow, blood cells, and lymphatic tissue. The basement membrane found along the interface between connective tissue and an adjacent tissue is also considered a connective tissue layer. This membrane bonds, supports, and allows for tissue repair.

MUSCLE CELLS

Muscle cells are highly differentiated (specialized) cells that have the ability to contract and cause movement or increased tension. Groups of muscle cells form one of three types of muscle tissue: skeletal, smooth, or cardiac.

Muscle cells are composed of the proteins actin and myosin. Cross-bridges located between the actin and myosin connect and swing when stimulated in the proper sequence (Chapter 10). This causes the muscle as a whole to contract and do work or produce tension. All types of muscle require an increase in intracellular calcium to contract. Different muscles may use different sources of calcium and thus have slightly different methods of contraction stimulation.

Skeletal muscle is attached to bones by tendons. Skeletal muscle voluntarily contracts when stimulated by motor neuron impulses. Skeletal muscle uses calcium released from intracellular compartments to initiate contraction. Mature skeletal muscle does not undergo further cell division. Cardiac muscle, found in the heart, contracts spontaneously because of an intrinsic ability to depolarize and fire action potentials. Cardiac muscle is innervated by the nerves of the autonomic nervous system: the sympathetic and parasympathetic nerves. These inputs can increase or decrease the inherent rate or strength of cardiac contraction. Cardiac contraction involves calcium entry into the muscle cell from the extracellular fluid and from intracellular compartments. Cardiac muscle cells become highly differentiated during embryogenesis and do not undergo further cell division.

Smooth muscle is found throughout the body, including the vascular system, the genitourinary tract, and all the parts of the gut. Its function is often considered involuntary. Smooth muscle is innervated by the autonomic nervous system, which can increase or decrease the rate of contraction. When stretched, smooth muscle responds with an increase in contraction. Smooth muscle relies primarily on calcium entry from the extracellular fluid toinitiate contraction. Mature smooth muscle cells can undergo celldivision.

PATHOPHYSIOLOGIC CONCEPTS

Cells are continually exposed to changing conditions and potentially damaging stimuli. If these changes and stimuli are minor or brief, the cell easily adapts to them. More prolonged or intense stimuli can cause cell injury or death.

Atrophy

Atrophy is a decrease in the size of a cell or tissue. Atrophy can be an adaptive response that occurs when there is a decrease in the workload of a cell or tissue. With decreased work, the oxygen and nutrient requirements of a cell decrease. This causes most of intracellular structures, including the mitochondria, the endoplasmic reticulum, the intracellular vesicles, and the contractile proteins, to shrink.

EXAMPLES OF CELLULAR ATROPHY

Atrophy can occur as a result of disuse, for instance, as seen in the muscles of an individual who is immobilized or in a weightless (zero gravity) state. Atrophy also can occur as a result of decreased hormonal or neural stimulation of a cell or tissue, which is seen in the breasts of women after menopause or in skeletal muscle after spinal cord transection. Atrophy of fat and muscle occurs in response to a nutritional deficiency and is seen in malnourished or starving people. Atrophy also may occur as a result of insufficient blood supply to cells, which cuts off vital nutrient and oxygen supply.

Hypertrophy

Hypertrophy is the increase in the size of a cell or tissue. Hypertrophy is an adaptive response that occurs when there is an increase in the workload of a cell. The demand of the cell for oxygen and nutrients increases, causing growth of most intracellular structures, including the mitochondria, the endoplasmic reticulum, intracellular vesicles, and the contractile proteins. Protein synthesis increases.

EXAMPLES OF CELLULAR HYPERTROPHY

Hypertrophy is primarily seen in cells that cannot adapt to increased work by increasing their numbers through mitosis. Examples of cells that cannot undergo mitosis, but experience hypertrophy, are cardiac and skeletal muscle cells. Smooth muscle may undergo hypertrophy and hyperplasia. There are three main types of hypertrophy.

Physiologic hypertrophy occurs as a result of a healthy increase in the workload of a cell (i.e., increased muscle bulk through exercise).

Pathologic hypertrophy occurs in response to a disease state, for example, hypertrophy of the left ventricle in response to longstanding hypertension and an increase in the workload of the heart.

Compensatory hypertrophy occurs when cells grow to take over the role of other cells that have died. For example, the loss of one kidney causes the cells of the remaining kidney to undergo hypertrophy, resulting in a substantial increase in the size of the remaining kidney.

Hyperplasia

Hyperplasia is the increase in cell number occurring in an organ as a result of increased mitosis.

EXAMPLES OF HYPERPLASIA

Hyperplasia is seen in cells stimulated by an increased workload, hormonal signals, or signals produced locally in response to a decrease in tissue crowding. It can only occur in cells that undergo mitosis, such as liver, kidney, and connective tissue cells. Hyperplasia may be physiologic, pathologic, or may occur as a compensation to tissue loss or injury.

Physiologic hyperplasia occurs monthly in uterine endometrial cells during the follicular stage of the menstrual cycle.

Pathophysiologic hyperplasia can occur with excessive hormonal stimulation, which is seen in acromegaly, a connective tissue disease characterized by growth hormone excess.

Compensatory hyperplasia occurs when cells of a tissue reproduce to make up for a previous decrease in cells. An example of compensatory hyperplasia is that which occurs in liver cells after surgical removal of sections of liver tissue. The compensation is striking in its rapidity.

Metaplasia

Metaplasia is the change in a cell from one subtype to another. It usually occurs in response to some continual irritation or injury that results in chronic inflammation of the tissue. By undergoing metaplasia, cells that are better able to withstand chronic irritation and inflammation replace the original tissue. Although metaplastic cells are not cancer cells, the irritants that caused the initial change may be carcinogenic, and metaplasia is a sign of significant cellular irritation.

EXAMPLES OF METAPLASIA

The most common example of metaplasia is the change in the cells of the respiratory passages from ciliated columnar epithelial cells to stratified squamous epithelial cells in response to years of cigarette smoking. The ciliated cells, essential for the removal of dirt, microorganisms, and toxins in the respiratory passages, are easily injured by cigarette smoke. Stratified epithelial cells are better able to survive smoke damage. Unfortunately they do not assume the vital protective role of ciliated cells. Squamous cell carcinoma is the most common type of lung cancer in the United States.

Dysplasia

Dysplasia is a derangement in cell growth that results in cells that differ in shape, size, and appearance from their predecessors. Dysplasia appears to occur in cells exposed to chronic irritation and inflammation. Although this cell change is not cancerous, dysplasia indicates a dangerous situation and the possibility that a cancerous condition may occur.

EXAMPLES OF DYSPLASIA

The most common sites of dysplasia are the respiratory tract (especially the squamous cells present as a result of metaplasia) and the cervix in women. Cervical dysplasia usually results from infection of the cells with the human papilloma virus (HPV). Dysplasia is usually rated on a scale to reflect its degree, from minor to severe.

Cell Injury

Cell injury occurs when a cell can no longer adapt to stimuli. This can occur if the stimuli are too long in duration or too severe in nature. Whether a cell recovers from an injury or dies depends on the cell and on the extent and type of injury.

CAUSES OF CELL INJURY

Hypoxia (oxygen deprivation), microorganism infection, temperature extremes, physical trauma, radiation, and free radical exposure cause cell injury. When a cell is injured, it may demonstrate alterations in shape, size, protein synthesis, genetic makeup, and transport properties.

Cell Death

There are two main categories of cell death. The first category is necrotic cell death, which occurs when injurious stimuli to a cell are too intense or prolonged. Necrotic cell death is characterized by cell swelling and rupture of internal organelles, most obviously the mitochondria. Necrotic cell death is characterized by marked stimulation of the inflammatory response. The second category of cell death is apoptosis, which is programmed cell death, a process in which an orderly sequence of molecular steps occurs, leading to cellular disintegration. Apoptosis is not characterized by swelling or inflammation, but rather the dying cell shrinks on itself and then is engulfed by neighboring cells. Apoptosis is responsible for keeping cell numbers relatively constant and is a mechanism by which unwanted cells, aged cells, dangerous cells, or cells carrying a mistake in DNA transcription can be eliminated. It is an active process, in which the cell itself participates, and draws its name from a Greek word referring to "a dropping off" as in petals off a flower.

CAUSES OF NECROTIC CELL DEATH

Common causes of necrotic cell death include prolonged hypoxia, infection leading to the production of toxins and free radicals, and disruption in membrane integrity; the ultimate result of which is cellular bursting. Typically the immune and inflammatory responses often stimulated by necrosis lead to further injury and death of neighboring cells. Necrotic cell death can be widespread in the body without causing death of the individual.

CAUSES OF APOPTOSIS

Programmed cell death begins during embryogenesis and continues throughout the lifetime of an organism. Stimuli that initiate apoptosis include hormonal cues, antigen stimulation, immune peptides, and genetically programmed signals that identify aging cells. Viral infection of a cell will often turn on apoptosis, ultimately leading to the death of the virus and the host cell. This is one way living organisms have evolved to fight viral infection. Certain viruses (i.e., the Epstein-Barr virus responsible for mononucleosis) have in turn evolved to produce specialized proteins that deactivate the apoptosis response. Deficiencies in apoptosis have been implicated in the development of cancer, and in neurodegenerative diseases of unknown origin, including Alzheimer's disease and amyotrophic lateral sclerosis (Lou Gehrig's disease). Antigen-stimulated apoptosis of immune cells (T and B cells) is essential for the development and maintenance of immune self-tolerance.

RESULTS OF CELL DEATH

Dead cells liquefy or coagulate and are removed from the area or isolated from the rest of the tissue by immune cells in the process of phagocytosis. If mitosis is possible and the area of necrosis is not too large, new cells of the same type fill in the empty space. Scar tissue will form in the vacated space if cell division is impossible or if the area of necrosis is extensive.

Gangrene refers to the death of a large mass of cells. Gangrene may be classified as dry or wet. Dry gangrene spreads slowly with few symptoms and is frequently seen in the extremities, often as a result of prolonged hypoxia. Wet gangrene is a rapidly spreading area of dead tissue, often of internal organs, and is associated with bacterial invasion of the dead tissue. It exudes a strong odor and is usually accompanied by systemic manifestations. Wet gangrene may develop from dry gangrene. Gas gangrene is a special type of gangrene that occurs in response to an infection of the tissue by a type of anaerobic bacteria called clostridium. It is seen most often after significant trauma. Gas gangrene rapidly spreads to neighboring tissue as the bacteria release deadly toxins that kill neighboring cells. Muscle cells are especially susceptible and release characteristic hydrogen sulfide gas when affected. This type of gangrene may prove fatal.

Wound Repair

Destroyed or injured tissues must be repaired by regeneration of the cells or the formation of scar tissue. The goal of both types of repair is to fill in the areas of damage in order to return structural integrity to the tissue.

Tissue regeneration and scar formation begin with inflammatory reactions (Chapter 3). Platelets control bleeding and white blood cells digest and remove dead tissue in the area. Growth factors and immune peptides (cytokines) (Chapter 3) are released that draw healing cells to the area. Other factors are produced to stimulate mitosis or scar tissue formation.

TYPES OF WOUND REPAIR

Tissues that heal cleanly and quickly are said to heal by primary intention. Large wounds that heal slowly and with a great deal of scar tissue heal by secondary intention.

DELAYED HEALING AND REPAIR

Tissue repair can be delayed if the host is compromised in any way by malnutrition, systemic disease, or a poorly functioning immune system. If there is reduced blood flow to the injured tissue or an infection develops, healing also can be poor or delayed.

Geriatric Consideration

The elderly may have delayed healing caused by reduced blood flow and tissue oxygenation caused by systemic diseases such as diabetes mellitus or atherosclerosis. Immune function also appears to be reduced in the elderly and nutrition may be poor.

CONDITIONS OF DISEASE OR INJURY

Hypoxia

Hypoxia is the decreased concentration of oxygen in the blood. The concentration of oxygen in the blood depends on the amount brought in by the lungs and the amount carried in the blood, either dissolved or bound to hemoglobin.

Although a small amount of oxygen is carried in a dissolved state in the blood, most oxygen is carried bound to an iron-based protein called hemoglobin, present in the red blood cell. Cells and tissues become hypoxic when there is inadequate intake of oxygen by the respiratory system, inadequate delivery of oxygen by the cardiovascular system, or a lack of hemoglobin.

Oxygen is required by the mitochondria for oxidative phosphorylation and the production of ATP. Without oxygen, this process cannot occur. Although some ATP will be produced through anaerobic glycolysis, this is an inefficient source of ATP and cannot support the cellular energy requirements if there is a prolonged period of hypoxia.

CONSEQUENCES OF HYPOXIA

When cells are deprived of ATP, they can no longer maintain cellular functions, including the transport of sodium and potassium through the sodium-potassium pump. Without sodium-potassium pumping, cells begin to accumulate sodium as it diffuses into the cell down its concentration and electrical gradients. The electrical potential across the membrane begins to decrease as intracellular sodium—a positive ion—accumulates. Osmotic pressure inside the cell increases, drawing water into the cell. Ischemic cells (those deprived of oxygen) begin to swell, resulting in dilation of the endoplasmic reticulum, decreased mitochondrial function, and increased permeability of intracellular membranes.

Another consequence of hypoxia is the production of lactic acid, which occurs during anaerobic glycolysis. Increased lactic acid causes cellular and blood pH levels to decrease. Decreased intra-cellular pH (increased acidity) causes damage to the nuclear structures, the cellular membranes, and the microfilaments. An alteration in pH can also affect the electrical potential across the membrane.

The effects of hypoxia are reversible if oxygen is returned within a certain period of time, the amount of which varies and depends on the tissue. However, cell swelling can lead to bursting of lysosomal vesicles, release of their enzymes, and lysis (bursting) of the cell. Cell death is marked by higher than normal levels of intracellular enzymes in the general circulation.

CAUSES OF HYPOXIA

Causes of hypoxia include respiratory diseases and anything that affects blood flow. Examples include myocardial infarct, hemorrhagic shock, blood clots, various poisons, and some toxins released from microorganisms.

Cyanide poisoning occurs as a result of the chemical reaction between cyanide and the final substrate in the electron transport chain. Without this final step, oxidative phosphorylation ceases and ATP is not produced in the mitochondria. Cyanide is present in the seeds of many fruits such as apricots and some apple seeds. Laetrile, an unproven therapy for cancer, is made from the pits of apricots and contains enough cyanide to be fatal.

Carbon monoxide poisoning occurs when carbon monoxide is inhaled and binds to oxygen sites on the hemoglobin molecule. The affinity of hemoglobin for carbon monoxide is 300 times greater than for oxygen. Therefore, exposure to carbon monoxide decreases the binding and transport of oxygen in the blood, causing cellular and tissue hypoxia. Carbon monoxide is a product of cigarette smoke, some heating systems, and automobile exhaust.

Lead poisoning can occur from ingesting lead-based paint. Although lead affects many organ systems, including the brain, it also is known to inhibit hemoglobin synthesis and thus causes hypoxia. Large doses of lead also cause red blood cell lysis with resultant severe hypoxia.

CLINICAL MANIFESTATIONS

- Decreased cell functioning. If the source of hypoxia is respiratory failure or myocardial infarct, all tissues will be affected. Cell death may occur.
- Increased heart rate.
- Increased respiratory rate.
- Muscle weakness.
- Decreased level of consciousness.
- Cyanide poisoning: a choking sensation with accelerated respirations, then gasping.
- Carbon monoxide poisoning: accelerated respirations followed by ringing in the ears, drowsiness, and confusion. Respirations quickly cease and unconsciousness develops.
- Lead poisoning: abdominal cramping, hyperactivity, anorexia, lead line on gums, and muscle cramps.

COMPLICATIONS

- Altered consciousness progressing to coma and death if prolonged cerebral (brain) hypoxia occurs.
- Organ failure, including adult respiratory distress syndrome, cardiac failure, or kidney failure, may occur if hypoxia is prolonged.

TREATMENT

- Increase oxygen in inspired air through a mask or mechanical ventilation.
- For cyanide poisoning, nitrates and sodium thiosulfate therapy.
- For carbon monoxide poisoning, hyperbaric (high pressure) oxygen treatments.
- For lead poisoning, emetics to induce vomiting if acute poisoning. For chronic conditions, various chelating agents (to take the lead out of the circulation).

Pediatric Consideration

Children are at an increased risk of suffering lead poisoning because lead is absorbed more rapidly through their intestine and they are attracted to lead's sweet taste in paint. Children are also closer to and more frequently sitting on the ground where lead tends to accumulate in soil and dust. Pediatric lead exposure may lead to learning disabilities and behavioral problems.

Temperature Extremes

Too hot or too cold temperatures may injure or kill cells. Exposure to very high temperatures can cause burn injuries, which directly kill cells or indirectly injure or kill cells by causing coagulation of blood vessels or the breakdown of cell membranes (see Chapter 18). Exposure to very cold temperatures injures cells in two ways. First, cold exposure causes constriction of the blood vessels that deliver nutrients and oxygen to the extremities. This occurs as the body attempts to preserve its core (central) temperature, initially at the expense of the fingers, toes, ears, and nose. Decreased blood flow causes cellular and tissue ischemia. Sluggish blood flow also increases the risk of clot formation, which further blocks tissue oxygenation. The second effect of exposure to very cold temperature is the formation of ice crystals in the cells. These directly damage the cells and can lead to cell lysis (bursting). Prolonged exposure to the cold can lead to hypothermia.

CLINICAL MANIFESTATIONS OF COLD EXPOSURE AND HYPOTHERMIA

- Numbness or tingling of the skin or extremities.
- Pale or blue skin that is cool to the touch.
- Shivering early on, then lack of shivering as condition worsens.
- Decreased level of consciousness, drowsiness, and confusion.

COMPLICATIONS

- Blood clotting, characterized by pain and a decrease in pulse downstream from the clot. If blood flow is inadequate for an extended time, gangrene may result.
- Frostbite.
- Ventricular dysrhythmia.

TREATMENT

- Transport immediately to a hospital for active rewarming. Any individual who appears dead who may have suffered hypothermia needs to be evaluated at a medical facility and rewarmed to 32°C before being confirmed dead.
- During transport to a clinical facility, wet clothing should be removed and the patient covered with blankets. Active rewarming is discouraged until the patient reaches the treatment facility. Warm humidified air or oxygen may be administered during transport.
- For a blood clot, drugs to dissolve the clot may be necessary.
- For gangrene, antibiotics and possible amputation are required.
- Cardiopulmonary resuscitation may be necessary if the patient is in ventricular fibrillation.

Radiation Injury

Radiation is the transmission of energy through the emission of rays or waves. Radiation energy may be in the visible range of light, or it may be higher or lower energy than visible light. High-energy radiation (including ultraviolet radiation) is called ionizing radiation because it has the capability of knocking electrons off atoms or molecules, thereby ionizing them. Low-energy radiation is called nonionizing radiation because it cannot displace electrons off atoms or molecules.

EFFECTS OF IONIZING RADIATION

Ionizing radiation may injure or kill cells directly by destroying the cell membrane and causing intracellular swelling, leading to cell lysis. It may also act indirectly by damaging the bonds between the base pairs of the DNA molecules, leading to mistakes in DNA replication or transcription. These mistakes may be repaired: if not, damage may cause programmed cell death or subsequent cancer as a result of the loss of genetic control over cell division.

Ionizing radiation can cause the production of free radicals. A free radical is a highly reactive atom or molecule with an unpaired electron. The free radical seeks out reactions whereby it may gain back an electron. Sequential reactions may occur, where a series of free radicals are produced. Once produced, a free radical can engage in an energy-rich collision with another molecule, destroying intramolecular bonds. This may ultimately damage the cell membrane, the endoplasmic reticulum, or the DNA of a susceptible cell. It is thought that DNA errors resulting from free radical damage may be involved in the development of some cancers. It is also hypothesized that the free radical production that occurs during the normal metabolism of lipids may damage the endothelial cells lining the blood vessels, leading to atherosclerosis.

Free radicals also accumulate in response to infectious agents and hypoxia. For example, during a period of reduced blood flow, lack of oxygen causes cellular injury or death. If blood flow is restored, free radical production is stimulated by the white blood cells that swarm to the area as part of the inflammatory response; this accumulation of free radicals leads to serious "reperfusion injury" and a worsening of tissue damage. Free radicals also are produced with exposure to cigarette smoke and are present in many pesticides.

Normally, cells have in place mechanisms to eradicate free radicals or to minimize their effects. Vitamins E, C, and beta-carotene are known as free radical scavengers and are believed to protect cells against the damaging effects of free radicals.

CELLS SUSCEPTIBLE TO IONIZING RADIATION

Cells most susceptible to damage by ionizing radiation are cells that undergo frequent divisions, including cells of the gastrointestinal (GI) tract, the integument (skin and hair), and the blood-forming cells of the bone marrow.

Ionizing radiation is emitted by the sun, in x-rays, and in substances undergoing radioactive decay, including substances found in the soil and rocks and those produced by nuclear weapons and reactors. Ionizing radiation is also emitted by substances used in medical diagnosis and treatment.

EFFECTS OF NONIONIZING RADIATION

Nonionizing radiation includes microwave and ultrasound radiation. The energy of this radiation is too low to break DNA bonds or damage the cell membrane, but may increase the temperature of a system, causing alterations in transport functions. Nonionizing radiation does not appear to cause health hazards, but research in this area is ongoing.

CLINICAL MANIFESTATIONS OF IONIZING RADIATION

- Skin redness or breakdown.
- With high doses, vomiting and nausea caused by GI damage.
- Anemia if the bone marrow is destroyed.
- Cancer may develop years after the exposure as a result of the production of chromosomal breaks, deletions, or translocations.

TREATMENT

- Damage caused by low doses will be repaired by the cells and does not require treatment.
- Cancers should be treated with radiation therapy, chemotherapy, immunotherapy, or surgery.

Pediatric Consideration

Fetal cells rapidly undergo cellular replication and division and are highly susceptible to the damaging effects of ionizing radiation. Infants and young children also experience periods of rapid cellular growth and proliferation and are at risk of genetic damage from ionizing radiation. Recent studies suggest that there are no apparent health risks to fetuses exposed to nonionizing radiation (i.e., when a pregnant woman uses an electric blanket or video display terminal) at least in moderation.

Injury Caused by Microorganisms

Microorganisms infectious to humans include bacteria, viruses, mycoplasmas, rickettsiae, chlamydiae, fungi, and protozoa. Some of these organisms infect humans through direct access, such as inhalation, whereas others infect through transmission by an intermediate vector, such as from an insect bite.

Cells of the body may be destroyed directly by the microorganism or by a toxin released from the microorganism, or may be indirectly injured as a result of the immune and inflammatory reactions stimulated in response to the microorganism (Chapter 3). In addition, as described earlier, infection of a cell by a microorganism may so destabilize the cell that it undergoes apoptosis.

BACTERIA

Bacteria are free-living, one-celled organisms that reproduce on their own, but use animal hosts for nutrient access. Bacteria contain no nucleus. They consist of cytoplasm surrounded by a rigid cell wall made out of a specific substance called peptidoglycan. Inside the cytoplasm is the genetic material, both DNA and RNA, and the intracellular structures needed for energy metabolism. Bacteria reproduce asexually by DNA replication and simple cell division. Some bacteria synthesize a capsule that surrounds the cell wall, making it less susceptible to the host's immune system. Other bacteria secrete proteins that reduce their susceptibility to standard antibiotics. Bacteria can be aerobic or anaerobic. Bacteria often release toxins specifically damaging to the host.

Laboratories frequently classify bacteria as gram-positive or negative. Gram-positive bacteria release toxins (exotoxins) that damage host cells. Gram-negative bacteria contain in their cell walls proteins that stimulate the inflammatory response (endotoxins). Gram-positive bacteria stain purple with a standard laboratory dye. Gram-negative bacteria stain red with a second laboratory dye.

Examples of human disease caused by bacteria include staphylococcal and streptococcal infections, gonorrhea, syphilis, cholera, plague, salmonellosis, shigellosis, typhoid fever, Legionnaire's disease, diphtheria, Haemophilus influenzae, pertussis, tetanus, and Lyme disease. A subset of especially difficult-to-treat bacteria are the mycobacteria. These microorganisms cause tuberculosis and leprosy.

VIRUSES

Viruses, unlike bacteria, require a host to reproduce. Viruses consist of a single strand of DNA or RNA that is contained within a protein coat called a capsid. Viruses must bind to the host cell membrane, enter the cell, and then move into the host cell nucleus to reproduce. Once inside the nucleus, viral DNA becomes incorporated into the host cell DNA, thus ensuring that viral genes will be passed to each daughter cell during mitosis. Once in the DNA, the virus begins to take over the functions of the cell. RNA viruses also begin to control cell function after their translation into proteins.

Examples of human disease caused by viruses include encephalitis, yellow fever, German measles, rubella, mumps, poliomyelitis, hepatitis, and many viral respiratory infections. Certain types of viruses can enter the host DNA and remain latent for years, producing infections occasionally or not at all. Viruses that remain latent include all those of the herpes family, including the herpes viruses responsible for varicella (chickenpox), zoster (shingles), cytomegalovirus, mononucleosis, and the herpes simplex viruses 1 and 2, which produce oral cold sores and genital herpes.

RETROVIRUSES

A unique type of virus is the retrovirus. These viruses are RNA viruses that can incorporate into the host DNA as a result of the action of the enzyme reverse transcriptase that changes the viral RNA into DNA. Retroviruses appear to carry reverse transcriptase as part of their structure.

Examples of human disease caused by retroviruses include acquired immunodeficiency syndrome (AIDS), caused by the human immunodeficiency virus (HIV), and a form of leukemia, HTLV-I. Retroviruses also may remain dormant for long periods of time.

MYCOPLASMAS

Mycoplasmas are unicellular microorganisms similar in action to bacteria except much smaller and without the peptidoglycan cell wall. Because many antibiotics (i.e., the penicillins) act by destroying the peptidoglycan cell wall, mycoplasmas are insensitive to these antibiotics.

Examples of human disease caused by mycoplasmas include mycoplasma pneumonia, upper respiratory tract infections, and some genital infections.

RICKETTSIA

Rickettsia require a host to asexually reproduce. They contain RNA and DNA inside a rigid peptidoglycan cell wall. Rickettsia are transmitted to humans through the bite of the flea, tick, or lice. Examples of human disease caused by rickettsia include typhus and Rocky Mountain spotted fever.

CHLAMYDIAE

Chlamydiae are unicellular organisms that reproduce asexually inside a host cell. They transmit directly to humans and undergo cycles of replication. Human diseases caused by chlamydia include a sexually transmitted urogenital infection and pneumonia.

FUNGI

Fungi include yeast and molds. Fungi contain a nucleus and are surrounded by a rigid cell wall. Fungi usually do not cause disease in healthy humans, and some fungi are considered normal human flora. Most fungal infections are superficial, but some may be deep, causing infection of vital organs and tissues.

Superficial fungal infections in humans include oral (thrush) and vaginal candidiasis (yeast infections) and infections of the skin such as ringworm (tinea corporus), athlete's foot (tinea pedis), and jock itch. Onychomycosis refers to fungal infection of the toenails and fingernails.

Deep, opportunistic fungal infections in humans include the respiratory infections histoplasmosis and coccidiomycosis, which are common in individuals with AIDS. Systemic and brain fungal infections may also occur. Deep fungal infections are common in individuals who are immunocompromised. These infections are considered to be opportunistic (produced by organisms that only proliferate if the immune response is poor).

PARASITES

The term parasite refers to protozoa, helminths, and arthropods.

Protozoans are unicellular organisms capable of causing infections. Infection is passed directly between individuals through contaminated food or water, or through an insect vector. Examples of human disease caused by protozoans include malaria and the intestinal disease giardiasis.

Helminths are "worms" that require a host to sexually reproduce. Transmission to humans occurs through ingestion or penetration of the skin. Examples of human disease caused by helminths include roundworm (nematodes) and tapeworm (cestodes). Helminths are a significant problem in developing countries.

Arthropods are ticks and mosquitoes that act as vectors to carry diseases to humans. Examples of human disease carried by arthropods include bubonic plague (caused by a bacillus) and typhus (caused by a rickettsia). Other arthropods infect and damage body surfaces by their bite or burrowing. Arthropods that infect body surfaces include lice, scabies, chiggers, and fleas.

CLINICAL MANIFESTATIONS

Clinical manifestations of infection depend on the specific agent involved, the site of the infection, and the initial state of health of the host.

- Infection by bacteria, viruses, and mycoplasmas often results in:
  - regional lymph node enlargement
  - fever (usually low-grade with a viral infection)
  - body aches
  - skin rash or eruption, especially with viral infections
  - site-specific responses, such as pharyngitis, cough, otitis media
- Infection by chlamydia often results in:
  - urethritis (inflammation of the urethra) in males
  - cervicitis (inflammation of the cervix) in females, often with a mucopurulent discharge and itching or burning during urination
- Infection by rickettsia often results in:
  - skin rash
  - fever and chills
  - headache
  - myalgia (muscle aches)

  - thrombus formation in any organ
- Infection by fungi often results in:
  - itching and redness of skin or scalp with superficial infections
  - discoloration and thickening with superficial nail infections
  - creamy white vaginal discharge with a yeast infection
  - white plaques on inside of mouth with oral thrush
  - signs of pneumonia with deep infections or in an immunocompromised host
- Infection with parasites often results in:
  - diarrhea with intestinal parasites
  - fever with malaria
  - itching and rash with skin infections

TREATMENT

- Bacteria and mycoplasms are treated with antibiotics, preferably after culturing the infection to determine what the infecting microorganism is and to what antibiotic it is sensitive.
- Certain viral infections may be treated with antiviral agents. Other viral infections usually are left to resolve on their own, with care taken that a subsequent bacterial infection does not infect the original site or elsewhere.
- Rickettsiae are usually treated with the antibiotic tetracycline.
- Fungi are treated with topical antifungals, such as nystatin for superficial skin infections, and amphotericin B for systemic infections. New oral antifungals are available for treating nail infections, which previously were stubborn to treatment. These new therapies, including terbinafine and itraconazole, have a high cure rate, even with sporadic dosing regimens. Pentamidine is used for *Pneumocystis carinii.*
- Parasitic infections of the GI tract are treated with specific agents, including metronidazole (Flagyl) for giardiasis. Malaria is treated with various antimalarial drugs. Prophylactic (preventative) therapy is recommended for individuals traveling to areas where malaria is common. Plague is treated with various antibiotics, including tetracycline. Skin infections are treated with various topical agents.

Selected Bibliography

Arvidson, C. R. & Cooledge, P. (1996). Lead screening in children: the role of the school nurse. *Journal of School Nursing* 12, 8–13.

Brent, G. A., Moore, D. D., & Larsen, P. R. (1991). Thyroid hormone regulation of gene expression. *Annual Review of Physiology* 53, 17–35.

Bracken, M. B., Belanger, K., Hellenbrand, K., Dlugosz, L., Holford, T. R., McSharry, J. E., Addesso, K., & Leaderer, B. (1995). Exposure to electromagnetic fields during pregnancy with emphasis on electrically heated beds: association with birthweight and intrauterine growth retardation. *Epidemiology* 6, 263–270.

Duke, R. C., Ojcius, D. M., & Young, J. D. (1996). Cell suicide in health and disease. *Scientific American* 275, 80–87.

Fedoroff, N., & Botstein, D., ed. (1992). The dynamic genome: Barbara McClintock's ideas in the century of genetics. Cold Spring Harbor Laboratory Press. Plainview, N.Y.

Guyton, A. C., & Hall, J. E. (1996). Textbook of medical physiology (9th ed). Philadelphia: W.B. Saunders.

Harruff, R. C. (1994). Pathology facts. Philadelphia: J.B. Lippincott Company.

Ho, G., Bierman, R., Beardsley, L., Chang, C., & Burk, R. D. (1998). Natural history of cervicovaginal papillomavirus infection in young women. *New England Journal of Medicine* 338, 423–428.

Kadham, M. A., MacDonald, D. A., Goodhead, D. T., Lorimore, S. A., Marsden, S. J., & Wright, E. (1992). Transmission of chromosomal instability after plutonium alpha-particle irradiation. *Nature* 355, 738–740.

Mazarakis, N. D., Edwards, A. D., & Mehmet, H. (1997). Apoptosis in neural development and disease. *Archives of Disease in Childhood: Fetal and Neonatal Edition* 77, F165–F170.

Porth, C. M. (1998). Pathophysiology concepts of altered health states (5th ed.). Philadelphia: J.B. Lippincott Company.

Rennie, J. (1993). DNA's new twists. *Scientific American* March, 122–132.

Repacholi, M. H. (1998). Low-level exposure to radiofrequency electromagnetic fields: health effects and research needs. *Bioelectromagnetics* 19, 1–19.

Rosenthal, N. (1994). Regulation of gene expression. *New England Journal of Medicine* 331, 931–933.

Silbergeld, E. K. (1997). Preventing lead poisoning in children. *Annual Review of Public Health* 18, 187–210.

Tynes, T. & Haldorsen, T. (1997). Electromagnetic fields and cancer in children residing near Norwegian high-voltage power lines. *American Journal of Epidemiology* 145, 219–226.

Vander, A., Sherman, J., & Luciano, D. (1998). Human physiology (7th ed.). Boston: McGraw-Hill.

Wittmers, L. E. (1996). Cold. In: Noble, J. (ed). Textbook of primary care medicine (2nd ed.) St. Louis: Mosby, pp. 77–83.

Wong, B., Park, C. G., & Choi, Y. (1997). Identifying the molecular control of T-cell death; on the hunt for killer genes. *Seminars in Immunology* 9, 7–16.

2 GENETICS

Genetics is the study of genes. Genes are pieces of DNA passed from parent to offspring that determine who we are and how we function at the most basic cellular level. Transmission of genetic information is a balance between ensuring that genes are passed error-free between the generations and allowing enough diversity for the adaptation and survival of the species. Sometimes mistakes (mutations) are made that advance the species; other times mutations cause significant disability or death.

● ● ●

PHYSIOLOGIC CONCEPTS

Chromosomes

Chromosomes contain the genetic blueprint of an individual. All nonsex (somatic) cells of the body contain 23 pairs of chromosomes, one pair from each parent, for a total of 46. Each sex cell, the egg and sperm, contain 23 unpaired chromosomes. Each chromosome is nearly identical (approximately 99.9%) across the human species in the genetic information it contains. The remaining variations are subtle but enough to make each one of us unique.

The Genes

The 46 chromosomes are made up of millions of molecules of DNA, twisted into a double helix and complexed with proteins called histones. The DNA is divided into sections called genes. There are approximately 50,000 to 100,000 genes, distributed on the 46 chromosomes, with each gene containing a hundred to a few thousand molecules of DNA. Each gene codes for a particular protein, often an enzyme. Enzymes and other proteins control the synthesis and function of each and every cell or tissue of the body. The function of the rest of the millions of molecules of DNA is unclear.

GENE ACTIVATION

Although each somatic cell contains the same 23 pairs of chromosomes, only certain genes are activated in any given cell; therefore, only certain proteins or enzymes are produced by that cell. Which genes are activated in which cell is determined during embryologic development and throughout life by circulating growth factors, hormones, and chemical cues produced by a given cell and its neighboring cells. Cells that express similar genes perform similar functions and group together as tissues.

Cellular Reproduction

All cells reproduce during embryonic development, which allows for growth of the embryo and differentiation (specialization) of the cells making up tissues and organs. After birth and throughout adulthood, many cells continue to reproduce. Cells that reproduce throughout a lifetime include cells of the bone marrow, skin, and digestive tract. Special cells, called stem cells, may reproduce indefinitely. Liver and kidney cells reproduce when replacement of lost or destroyed cells is required. Other cells, including nerve, skeletal muscle, and cardiac muscle cells, do not reproduce significantly after the first few months after birth. Damage to these tissues generally cannot be repaired by growth of new cells (although nearby stem cells may differentiate into replacement cells).

THE CELL CYCLE

The cell cycle refers to a sequence of stages a cell goes through during its lifetime (Fig. 2-1). During embryogenesis, all cells go through all stages, as do adult cells that continue to reproduce. The rate that a cell goes through its cell cycle depends on the given cell and the growth factors and hormones to which it is exposed. Cells that do not continue to reproduce after embryogenesis remain in a resting stage and do not cycle through the other stages. The cell cycle is divided into two parts: interphase and mitosis.

INTERPHASE

When not actively dividing, a cell is said to be in interphase. There are three standard stages of interphase; G1, S, and G2. A fourth stage, Go, is a specialized resting stage. In these designations, the "G" stands

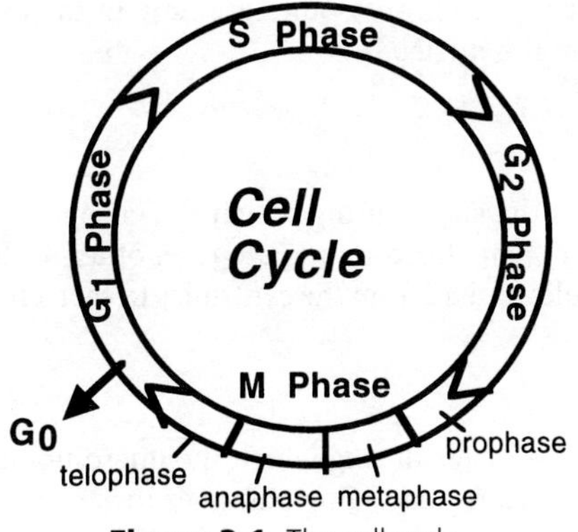

Figure 2-1. The cell cycle.

for "gap"; referring to a time period the cell uses to check and recheck the preceding steps.

G1 is the stage during which a cell prepares for DNA replication by synthesizing new proteins and activating cytoskeletal components. During this stage, the cell monitors its environment to determine if the time is right for DNA replication. This stage is considered a checkpoint for the cell because if conditions are not right, the cell will not progress further through its cycle. **S** is the stage during which replication (copying) of the DNA occurs; DNA replication is described in Chapter 1. **G2** is the stage before cell division, during which the cell again undergoes protein synthesis, this time in preparation for division. This stage is also a checkpoint because if the DNA has not been copied correctly, the cell can again stop the cycle before mitosis occurs.

Go is a resting stage in which a cell in G1 that has not committed itself to DNA replication, may pause. A cell may stay in Go indefinitely, but once a cell is stimulated to leave the Go stage, it will progress through the other stages, unless its progress is restricted at a subsequent checkpoint. The progression through interphase is a lengthy 10- to 22-hour process.

MITOSIS

Mitosis (the **M** stage) is the stage of cell division. Mitosis is a shorter event than is interphase and lasts approximately 1 hour. During mitosis, the cell that has duplicated during interphase splits into two daughter cells that each contain the 23 pairs of chromosomes. Mitosis consists of the substages of prophase, metaphase, anaphase, and telophase.

Prophase

Prophase is the stage in which protein structures (centrioles) present in the cytoplasm of the cell begin to move toward opposite sides or poles of the cell. This stretches the nuclear membrane and causes it to break apart. The chromosomes are now in the cytoplasm rather than isolated in the nucleus.

Metaphase

Metaphase is the stage during which the chromosomes visibly become two sets of pairs lined up next to each other in the center of the cell. Microtubules extend from the centrioles to each chromosome pair.

Anaphase

Anaphase is the stage during which the microtubules begin to pull the chromosome pairs apart. One pair goes toward one centriole pole and one pair goes toward the other centriole pole.

Telophase

Telophase is the stage during which the cell splits down the middle and a new nuclear membrane develops surrounding each of the two new cells including the 23 pairs of chromosomes (46 total) present in each cell.

CONTROL OF THE CELL CYCLE

Cells that continually go through the cell cycle (i.e., cells of the gut and bone marrow) do so at an intrinsic rate that can be increased or decreased by internal and external cues. External cues that turn on the cell cycle may include neural or hormonal stimulation, or may come from cell products released in response to tissue injury and activation of the inflammatory and immune systems. Brakes on the cell cycle may also include neural and hormonal stimulation and proteins synthesized by cells in response to activation of regulator genes (see Chapter 4). Uncontrollable cell growth and cancer may occur with the destruction or inactivation of regulator genes or by excessive hormonal stimulation.

Another recently recognized mechanism that serves to limit cell replication involves structures present on the chromosomes themselves, known as telomeres. A **telomere** is the end region of a chromosome that shortens with each replication. When the telomere shortens to a threshold length, after a certain number of cell cycles, it shuts off cellular replication. This results in replicative senescence, the characteristic that ensures normal somatic cells do not divide indefinitely. However, a few cells, including cancer cells and germ line cells, contain the enzyme telomerase: telomerase adds telomere sections back onto the chromosome. Telomerase stabilizes telomere length, functioning to immortalize these cells.

Meiosis

Meiosis is the process during which germ cells of the ovary (primary oocytes) or testicle (primary spermatocytes) give rise to mature eggs or sperm (Fig. 2-2). Meiosis involves DNA replication in the germ cell, followed by two cell divisions rather than one, which results in four daughter cells, each with 23 (unpaired) chromosomes. In males, all four daughter cells are viable and continue to differentiate into mature sperm. In females, only one viable daughter cell (egg) is formed; the other three cells become nonfunctional polar bodies. During fertilization, genetic information contained in the 23 chromosomes of the egg joins with genetic information contained in the 23 chromosomes of the sperm. This results in an embryo with 46 total chromosomes (two pairs of 23).

An interesting phenomenon occurs during DNA replication in the first meiotic stage. At this time, pieces of DNA may shift between

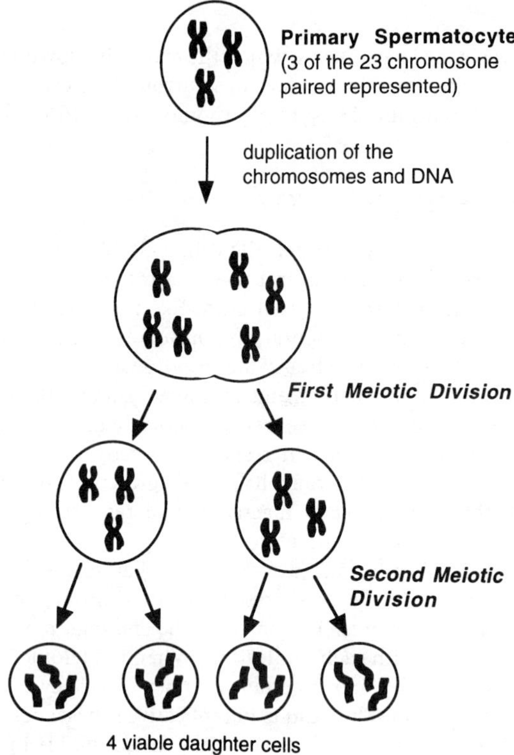

Figure 2-2. A schematic representation of meiosis in a male germ cell, leading to four daughter cells, called spermatids. Each spermatid will develop further to become mature sperm, as described in Chapter 21.

the matched chromosome pairs, in a process called crossing-over. Crossing-over increases the genetic variability of offspring, and is one reason why siblings within a family may vary considerably in genotype and phenotype.

Genotype and Phenotype

Precise genetic information carried in the chromosomes of the offspring is termed the genotype. Physical presentation of genetic information (tall or short, dark or light) is called the phenotype.

SINGLE-GENE INHERITANCE

Some traits of the phenotype (i.e., eye color) are determined by a single gene. A gene that determines a specific trait is called an **allele.**

For each single-gene trait, there are two controlling alleles: one on the chromosome delivered from the mother and one on the chromosome delivered from the father.

HETEROZYGOUS AND HOMOZYGOUS ALLELES

If an individual has two identical alleles (i.e., two alleles coding for brown eyes), that individual is said to be homozygous for the trait. If an individual has different alleles coding for a trait (i.e., one allele for brown eyes and one for blue), the individual is said to be heterozygous for the trait. One allele is usually dominant over the other, for instance, brown eyes over blue, but alleles are occasionally codominant (equally expressed). If a person is heterozygous for a single-gene trait, the phenotype will depend on which, if either, of the alleles is dominant. If the alleles are codominant, for example, those coding for the A and B red blood cell antigens, the individual will express both alleles (i.e., AB blood type).

MULTIFACTORIAL INHERITANCE

Most phenotypic characteristics are influenced by several genes. Height, intelligence, and personality characteristics are among those traits termed multifactorial. They are inherited in a more complicated manner and usually involve many contributing genes present on the same or different chromosomes. The expression of these genes is influenced by nongenetic factors such as nutrition, family support, culture, and exposure to various toxins or microorganisms.

Genetic Testing

Genetic testing, called cytogenetics, involves looking at the overall structure and number of the chromosomes. Genetic testing can be performed on any cell of the body, but is usually done by withdrawing white blood cells in a venous blood sample.

In cytogenetics, chemicals are added to cultured blood cells to arrest the chromosomes in metaphase. The chromosomes are spread out with members of a pair lined up together. The chromosomes are counted and the structures of the chromosomes under study are compared to control samples. The spread of 23 chromosome pairs is called the **karyotype**; the process is called karyotyping. The 23rd chromosome pair in males will show two chromosomes dissimilar in shape, the X and the Y. Females have two X chromosomes. An example of a normal male karyotype is shown in Figure 2-3.

Although genetic testing can be performed on anyone, prenatal testing of the fetal chromosomes accounts for a large percentage of all tests. Fetal cells may be gathered during the processes of amniocentesis or chorionic villi sampling.

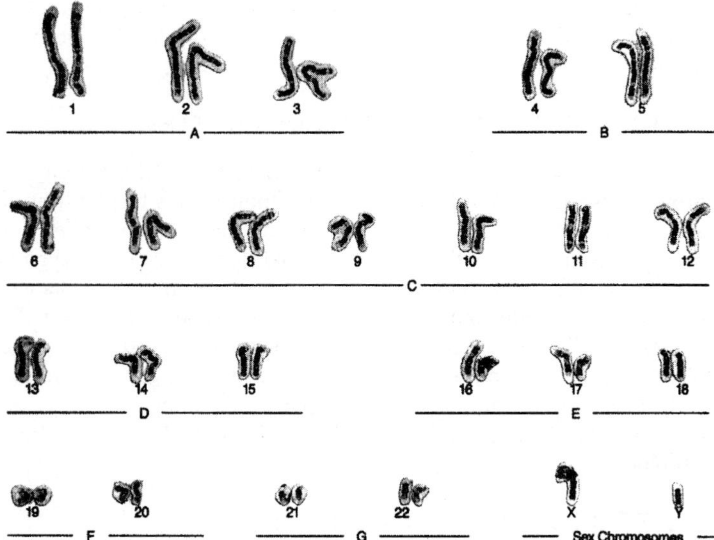

Figure 2-3. Karyotype of normal human boy. (Courtesy of the Prenatal Diagnostic and Imaging Center, Sacramento, CA. Frederick W. Hansen, MD, Medical Director). (Porth, C., (1998). Pathophysiology: Concepts of Altered Health States. Philadelphia: Lippincott-Raven Publishers).

AMNIOCENTESIS

Amniocentesis is performed by inserting a needle through the abdominal wall of a pregnant woman into the amniotic sac that surrounds the fetus. Amniotic fluid, into which fetal cells have been shed, is withdrawn. Chromosomes present in the fluid sample are then cultured and fixed, and their number and shape are evaluated. This test is usually done at approximately 16 weeks' gestation and results are available in approximately 2 weeks. Performance of amniocentesis earlier in gestation has been attempted with mixed results.

CHORIONIC VILLI SAMPLING

Chorionic villi sampling involves gathering cells of the chorion, the outer border of the fetal membranes. The cells are gathered through the woman's cervix between 8 and 12 weeks of pregnancy. The cells do not need to be cultured, so the chromosomal analysis is available in approximately 1 to 2 days. Chorionic villi sampling earlier than 8 to 12 weeks' gestation is possible, although sporadic reports of associated limb abnormalities have resulted in discontinuation of early sampling.

Genetic Engineering

Genetic engineering refers to experimental manipulation of the genome to produce certain characteristics. One technique of genetic engineering is gene splicing. This involves snipping a certain gene out of one cell and inserting it into another cell or into an attenuated (nonvirulent) virus. The cell or virus may then be administered to an individual who suffers from a lack of that particular gene. This has been performed in clinical trials involving the gene for cystic fibrosis. The goal of gene splicing is that the genetically engineered gene will insert into the host's DNA, allowing the host to produce the missing protein or enzyme coded for by that gene.

Another procedure that takes advantage of the ability to manipulate genes is recombinant DNA technology. With this technology, a piece of DNA extracted from one organism can be inserted into another organism such as a single-celled bacterium. If the DNA incorporates into the bacterium's own genome, it will start directing the bacterium to produce large amounts of a specific protein. In this way, valuable proteins can be produced for mass distribution. Examples of substances produced by recombinant DNA include growth hormone, insulin, clotting factors, and various vaccines.

The Human Genome Project

Several advanced techniques to identify the DNA code of specific genes have been developed in the last few decades. In 1990 a major national initiative, the Human Genome Project, was inaugurated in the United States, with joint funding from the National Institutes of Health and the Department of Energy. The goal of this initiative is to perform DNA mapping for each of the 80,000 or so genes of the human genome and to identify each gene's coded protein by the year 2005. This initiative has enormous significance for revealing the gene or genes responsible for thousands of genetic diseases and for synthesizing proteins or enzymes absent or deficient in each disease. Specific genes for many diseases, including cystic fibrosis, Huntington's disease, and some inheritable types of breast and colon cancer, have already been identified. The Project is moving forward more rapidly than predicted in fulfilling its spectacular goal.

ETHICAL IMPLICATIONS

Results of the Human Genome Project will have enormous ethical implications for prenatal testing and selective abortion of defective embryos. Ethical implications are also involved in testing concerned adults who seek to know the likelihood of their developing a specific disease in the future. This is especially troubling if the identified disease is one for which there is no treatment or cure, or if testing involves children. For adults and children with disease-causing mutations, future childbearing choices, the ability to purchase health insurance or life insurance, and the ability to find future employment are important considerations. The Human Genome Project has dedicated funding and time to explore the ethical factors involved in gene mapping.

PATHOPHYSIOLOGIC CONCEPTS

Mutation

A mutation is a mistake in the DNA sequence. Mutations can occur spontaneously, or after the exposure of a cell to radiation, certain chemicals, or various viral agents.

Most mutations will be identified and repaired by enzymes working in the cell. Other times, a mutation may lead to apoptosis. If a mutation is not identified or repaired, or if the cell does not undergo programmed death, that mutation will be passed on in all subsequent cell divisions. Mutations may result in a cell becoming cancerous. Mutations in the gametes (the egg or sperm) may lead to congenital defects in an offspring.

CONGENITAL DEFECTS

Congenital defects, also called birth defects, include genotypic and phenotypic errors occurring during embryogenesis and fetal development. Some congenital defects, such as cleft palate and limb abnormalities, may be apparent at birth, whereas other congenital defects, such as an abnormal or absent kidney and certain types of heart disease, may not be recognized immediately. Congenital defects may result from genetic mistakes made during meiosis of the sperm or egg, or from environmental insults experienced by the fetus during gestation. Examples of genetic mistakes include chromosomal breaks, unstable DNA, and mistakes in chromosome number. Environmental insults during gestation that are known to increase the likelihood of a congenital defect include maternal exposure to alcohol, certain drugs, and viruses. Environmental insults may lead to a genotypic or phenotypic error.

CHROMOSOMAL BREAKS

During mitosis and meiosis, pieces of chromosomes may break off, may be added inappropriately to other chromosomes, or may be deleted entirely. If deletions or additions occur during meiosis in the egg or sperm, a congenital defect or death of a resulting embryo results. During fetal development and throughout the life of an individual, mistakes may occur during mitosis in somatic (body) cells. If deletions or additions of chromosomes occur during mitosis, the affected cell line usually dies out.

HEREDITARY UNSTABLE DNA

Inheritance patterns of some genetic disorders are not easily explained. Recent evidence suggests that occasionally genes coding for a certain trait may not be passed down in a stable fashion from parents to offspring, but instead may have their effect magnified in succeeding generations of offspring. Other genes may be expressed only in certain members of a family, even though all members of the family may carry the gene. Whether an individual in the family expresses the trait coded for by these genes may depend on the individual's sex, the sex of the parent donating the unstable gene, or environmental conditions.

Fragile X Syndrome

A particularly striking finding concerning hereditary unstable DNA is that some diseases occur when a certain group of repeating codons (a set of three DNA bases grouped together) expands. For instance, the genetic disorder known as Fragile X syndrome is the most common cause of inherited mental retardation. Fragile X syndrome results when the codon CCG, normally repeated approximately 40 times in a gene near the top of the long arm of the X chromosome, begins to expand and is repeated excessively. Carriers of the disorder show 70 to 200 repeats on the chromosome, but are mentally normal. However, offspring of the carriers can show the region expanding to greater than 200 repeats of the codon. The degree of mental retardation corresponds to the length of the repeated codon. The degree to which the syndrome is expressed in any one family member depends on whether the expanded codon is inherited from the mother or the father, and whether the offspring is male or female, with male offspring being more likely affected. The tendency for the pattern to repeat is caused by a fragility of the chromosome.

ERRORS IN CHROMOSOME NUMBER

Any change from the normal human chromosome number of 46 chromosomes is called aneuploidy. An aneuploidy in which there are only 45 chromosomes is called a monosomy. An aneuploidy in which there are 47 chromosomes is called a triploidy. More than 47 chromosomes is possible but rare.

Monosomy

If any chromosome other than the X or Y is lost, the embryo will spontaneously abort. However, the loss of one of the sex chromosomes may result in a viable offspring. Usually the Y chromosome is lost, resulting in 44 somatic chromosomes and one sex chromosome, for a total of 45 chromosomes (often expressed 45 X/O, to indicate no Y chromosome). The resulting disorder is called Turner's syndrome.

Monosomy of any chromosome is a major cause of spontaneous abortion in the first trimester.

Trisomy

A trisomy occurs when somatic or sex chromosomes do not separate properly during meiosis. This is called nondisjunction. Most trisomies cause spontaneous abortion of the embryo, but rarely live births may result. Trisomies that may result in live births include trisomies of the sex chromosomes and trisomies of chromosomes 8, 13, 18, and 21. Trisomy 21 is called Down syndrome.

TERATOGENESIS

Teratogenesis is an error in fetal development that results in a structural or functional deficit (e.g., brain functioning). Environmental stimuli that cause congenital defects are called **teratogenic agents.** Teratogenic agents can lead to genetic mutations or errors in phenotype. Common manifestations of teratogenic exposure include congenital heart disease, abnormal limb development, mental retardation, blindness, hearing loss, and abnormalities in growth. Some teratogenic agents, including x-rays and some viruses, are known to cause chromosomal breakage, additions, and deletions. Many drugs, including the anticoagulant coumadin (Panwarfin) and the anti-acne medication isotretinoin (Accutane), can also be teratogenic.

Alcohol

The most common teratogenic drug used in the United States is alcohol. Alcohol at any dose is capable of causing neurologic deficits and facial deformities ranging from mild to severe. Alcohol can adversely affect several cellular functions associated with fetal development, including DNA synthesis, protein synthesis, glucose uptake, and the development of neural signaling pathways. Human infants who experience a complex group of congenital effects as a result of exposure to alcohol may be diagnosed as suffering from fetal alcohol syndrome.

Pediatric Consideration

Alcohol is the number 1 cause of birth defects in certain parts of the United States and is the leading cause of mental retardation in this country. Each year, approximately 4,000 children are born in the United States with fetal alcohol syndrome and at least twice that number will have various forms of the disorder in absence of the full syndrome. Fetal alcohol syndrome is 100% preventable.

THE TORCH GROUP OF TERATOGENS

Several different microorganisms are known to be teratogenic in humans. Many of these are described under the acronym TORCH, in which each letter stands for a particular microorganism that may infect the embryo or fetus. T stands for toxoplasmosis, R for rubella, C for cytomegalovirus, and H for the herpes simplex virus 2. The letter O stands for all other infections, especially syphilis, hepatitis B, mumps, gonorrhea, and varicella (chickenpox or shingles).

Effects of Teratogenic Agents

A newborn infected during gestation with any of the TORCH group of microorganisms may show microcephaly, hydrocephaly, mental retardation, or loss of hearing or sight. Congenital heart defects are common, especially with rubella. Radiation exposure may increase the risk that the child will later develop cancer. Certain drugs (i.e., thalidomide, sedatives, and sleeping pills) may affect the growth of the embryo or fetus. Angiotensin converting enzyme inhibitors, used to treat hypertension, may cause the embryo not to develop normal kidneys. Whether an embryo or fetus will be affected by any teratogenic agent depends on several factors, which include the timing and dose of exposure, maternal and paternal health, and nutritional status.

Timing of Exposure to a Teratogen

Because most organs and tissues are formed during the first trimester, teratogenic agents are most likely to cause structural defects at this time. This is especially true of rubella infection and exposure to drugs that interfere with development. However, the nervous system is always susceptible to a teratogen because it continues to develop even after birth. Infants exposed to an infectious agent in the third trimester or during the birth process, are at increased risk of developing the disease. This is true for neonatal infection by the hepatitis B virus and the HIV that causes AIDS. Primary maternal infection with the herpes simplex virus near the time of labor is associated with the occurrence of neonatal herpes and increased neonatal morbidity and mortality.

Dose of a Teratogen

The dose of exposure is important in determining the likelihood that a teratogenic agent will cause a congenital defect. Levels of radiation used in most diagnostic techniques or low concentrations of a drug may not produce any discernible effect on the fetus. Higher doses of radiation or a drug may adversely affect the fetus.

Maternal Health and Nutritional Status

Maternal health and nutritional status also play a role in determining teratogen effect. Maternal diets low in folic acid have been associated with development of neural tube defects such as spina bifida. Because most adults do not ingest adequate amounts of folic acid, folic acid supplementation (usually found in a One-A-Day or prenatal vitamin) is recommended for all women at least 3 months before conception. Folic acid is required for full functioning of the DNA proofreading enzymes responsible for checking and rechecking DNA replication, which may explain its protective effect against certain congenital malformations.

Paternal Health and Chemical Exposures

Studies on the effect of diet, chemical exposure, or drug usage in fathers suggest that teratogenic effects may also be passed through damaged sperm. Some studies suggest paternal (and maternal) cigarette smoking may be associated with increased risk of childhood leukemia in offspring. Paternal occupational hazards, such as exposure to paint fumes, may increase the risk of spontaneous abortion.

CONDITIONS OF DISEASE OR INJURY

Single-Gene Disorders

Single-gene disorders are caused by a single gene mistake on the DNA strand. There are approximately 4,500 known single-gene disorders, some of which are identified in Table 2-1.

CAUSES OF SINGLE-GENE DISORDERS

Single-gene disorders may result from a mistake in the copying of a single code letter. For example, the codon CCG can be transcribed incorrectly to CGG during DNA replication. Because each codon codes for a specific amino acid in a protein, these mistakes make the gene incapable of correctly directing the production of its protein.

The enormity of how important it is to transcribe exactly each letter of each codon is apparent when one considers that although there are approximately three billion code letters used in the human genome, a mistake in the copying of a single codon is what causes several of the disorders in Table 2-1. For example, sickle cell disease results when one A (adenine) in one gene is replaced by a T (thymine). The fatal neurologic disorder Huntington's chorea, the congenital bone disease osteogenesis imperfecta, and the metabolic disorders phenylketonuria and Tay-Sachs disease also occur as a result of miscopying a single codon.

Codon meanings also will be destroyed and single-gene disorders may result if DNA bases are added or deleted inadvertently. Other single-gene disorders may result from a codon being repeated excessively, as described earlier for the X-linked disorder fragile X syndrome.

Table 2-1. Some Disorders of Mendelian of Single-Gene Inheritance and Their Significance

DISORDER	SIGNIFICANCE
Autosomal dominant	
Achondroplasia	Short-limb dwarfism
Adult polycystic kidney disease	Kidney failure
Huntington's chorea	Neurodegenerative disorder
Familial hypercholesterolemia	Premature atherosclerosis
Marfan syndrome	Connective tissue disorder with abnormalities of skeletal, ocular, and cardiovascular systems
Neurofibromatosis (NF)	Neurogenic tumors: fibromatous skin tumors, pigmented skin lesions, and ocular nodules in NF-1; bilateral acoustic neuromas in NF-2
Osteogenesis imperfecta	Molecular defect of collagen
Spherocytosis	Disorder of red blood cells
von Willebrand disease	Bleeding disorder
Autosomal recessive	
Color blindness	Color blindness
Cystic fibrosis	Disorder of membrane transport of ions in exocrine glands, causing lung and pancreatic disease
Glycogen storage diseases	Excess accumulation of glycogen in the liver and hypoglycemia (von Gierke's disease); glycogen accumulation in striated muscle in myopathic forms
Oculocutaneous albinism	Hypopigmentation of skin, hair, and eyes as the result of inability to synthesize melanin
Phenylketonuria (PKU)	Lack of phenylalanine hydroxylase with hyperphenylalaninemia and impaired brain development
Sickle cell disease	Red blood cell defect
Tay-Sachs disease	Deficiency of hexosaminidase A; severe mental and physical deterioration beginning in infancy
X-linked recessive	
Burton-type hypogammaglobulinemia	Immunodeficiency
Hemophilia A	Bleeding disorder
Duchenne's dystrophy	Muscular dystrophy
Fragile X syndrome	Mental retardation

THE INHERITANCE PATTERN OF SINGLE-GENE DISORDERS

Single-gene disorders may be passed on as dominant or recessive genes. For a disease passed by a dominant gene to be expressed phenotypically, only one gene for the disease is required. For a disease passed by a recessive gene to be expressed phenotypically, the maternal and paternal chromosomes must carry the recessive gene. Individuals who carry one defective recessive gene causing a particular disease are called carriers for the disease. Although they will not usually express the disease clinically, the gene may pass to their offspring. If their offspring receive a second defective gene from the other parent, they will be homozygous for the recessive gene and will express the disease as shown in Figure 2-4. The capital "D" is normal, and the small "d" is the defective gene.

SEX-LINKED SINGLE-GENE DISORDERS

Some single-gene disorders are considered sex-linked disorders because they are passed on the X or Y sex chromosomes. Most sex-linked disorders are passed on the X chromosome and are recessive traits. These disorders are usually seen in males because any woman carrying the defective gene on one X chromosome will most likely carry the healthy gene on her other X chromosome. A male has a 50% chance of inheriting the defective X chromosome if his mother is a carrier. Because his other sex chromosome is a Y, the recessive gene would be expressed as shown in Figure 2-5. In Figure 2-5, the X chromosome carrying the defective gene is shown in bold letters. Rarely, a female may inherit a defective X chromosome from her mother and father. She would then be homozygous for the defective gene and express the disorder.

CLINICAL MANIFESTATIONS

- Clinical manifestations depend on the specific altered or missing gene.

DIAGNOSTIC TOOLS

- Prenatal amniocentesis or chorionic villi sampling may identify a single-gene defect.

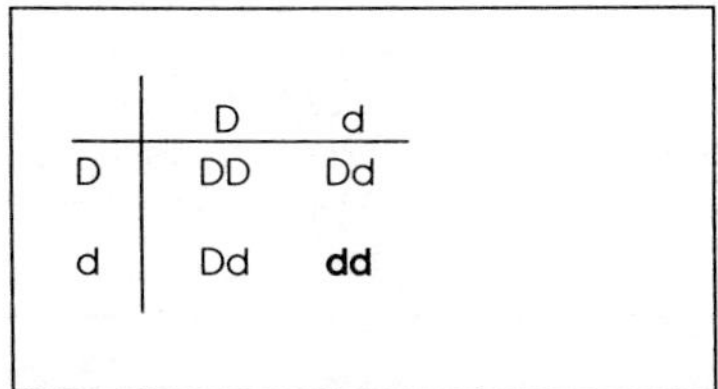

	D	d
D	DD	Dd
d	Dd	**dd**

Figure 2-4. The inheritance of a single-gene recessive trait, identified as "d."

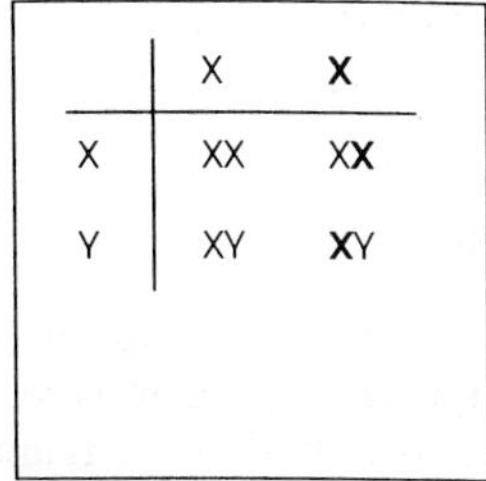

Figure 2-5. The inheritance of a sex-linked recessive gene on the X chromosome. Note that 50% of the daughters are carriers of the defect and 50% of the sons express the defect.

- Karyotyping of cells from an adult or child may confirm a clinical diagnosis of a single-gene defect.

TREATMENT

- Treatment for each disease may be supportive if no cure is available as is the case for Huntington's chorea, phenylketonuria, fragile X syndrome, or sickle cell disease.
- Treatment may involve replacing the missing protein or enzyme if possible. This has been tried for persons with hemophilia A.
- Gene splicing may allow insertion of a correct copy of a defective gene into the host genome. Gene splicing has been tried in individuals suffering from cystic fibrosis and muscular dystrophy.

Multifactorial Disorders

Multifactorial disorders are polygenic in nature; they are caused by multiple genes, each having a small, additive effect. If the additive effects reach a threshold level, the disorder will be expressed. The severity of any combination of genetic errors in any one person cannot be predicted.

Some multifactorial disorders may be apparent at birth; others may develop during adulthood. Examples of multifactorial diseases apparent at birth include cleft palate, congenital heart disease, anencephaly, and club foot. Multifactorial disorders expressed in later childhood or adulthood include hypertension, hyperlipidemia, diabetes mellitus, most autoimmune diseases, many cancers, and schizophrenia. Multifactorial disorders that develop during adulthood are usually strongly influenced by environmental factors.

CAUSES OF MULTIFACTORIAL DISORDERS

Multifactorial disorders result from additive effects of many gene errors. Multifactorial disorders also may result from less-than-optimum expression of many different genes and not from any particular error.

Environmental influences may increase or decrease the likelihood of a multifactorial disorder being expressed and to what degree.

PREDICTING THE OCCURRENCE OF A MULTIFACTORIAL DISEASE

Whether an individual will develop a multifactorial disease cannot be accurately predicted. However, with complete mapping of the genome it may become possible to identify who is most likely to develop a disease. This would influence risk behavior and preventive screening measures.

For example, individuals with type II diabetes mellitus, also called adult-onset diabetes mellitus, often have a strong family history of the disease, but not every member of the family will develop the disease. A strong predictor of developing type II diabetes is obesity, a clear example of the interdependency of genetics and environment. Similarly, various genes have been shown to contribute to the risk of developing cancer. However, whether an individual will develop cancer depends on a variety of personal behaviors, including exercise, smoking, and diet.

Ethical concerns abound for individuals at risk of developing certain multifactorial disorders. For example, certain high-paying jobs that expose workers to potential carcinogens may not be offered to an individual with a high risk of developing cancer.

CLINICAL MANIFESTATIONS

- Each disorder has unique clinical manifestations ranging from nonexistent, to mild, to severe.

DIAGNOSTIC TOOLS

- In families at high risk for a multifactorial disease, genetic mapping may indicate which members of the family are likely to develop the disease and which are not.

TREATMENT

- An individual at known risk for developing a multifactorial disorder based on genetic mapping or family history may modify his or her diet, toxin exposure, and exercise level to reduce additive environmental factors.
- An individual at known risk for developing a multifactorial disorder based on genetic mapping or family history may consider not having children of his or her own.

Down Syndrome

Down syndrome is a genetic disorder caused by a trisomy of chromosome 21. It is the most common chromosomal disorder seen in live births. In most cases, Down syndrome is caused by nondisjunction of maternal chromosome number 21 during meiosis. The incidence of Down syndrome increases with maternal age. Down occurs in 1 in 1,350 infants born to mothers younger than 24 years of age, but in 1 in 65 infants born to mothers 41 to 45 years old. Only 5% of Down cases can be traced to an extra paternal chromosome. Children with Down syndrome have variable levels of mental retardation and can often be positively influenced by early child intervention programs. A karyotype of a male with Down syndrome is shown in Figure 2-6.

CLINICAL MANIFESTATIONS

- Variable level of mental retardation
- Upward slanting of the eyes, short hands that have only one crease on the palm (a simian crease), and low-set ears.
- Short stature.
- Protruding tongue.

DIAGNOSTIC TOOLS

- Prenatal genetic testing (amniocentesis or chorionic villi sampling) can identify fetuses with Down syndrome.
- Maternal blood tests are available that can identify fetuses at increased risk of having Down syndrome. One test, called the triple test, is commonly used during the second trimester of pregnancy.

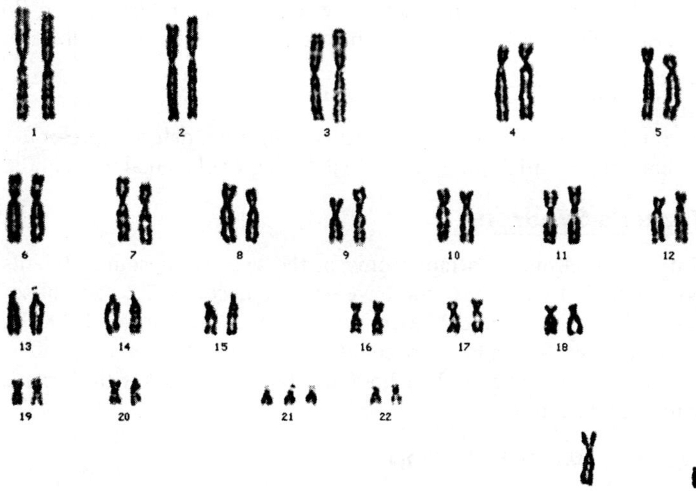

Figure 2-6. Trisomy 21 in the karyotype of a child with Down syndrome. All other chromosomes are normal. (Rubin, E., and Farber, J. L. (1999). Pathology, 3rd ed. Philadelphia: Lippincott Williams & Wilkins.)

In the triple test, the ratio of three circulating maternal substances are measured: estriol, human chorionic gonadotropin (hCG), and alpha-fetoprotein. Levels of estriol and alpha-fetoprotein are reported to be lower in fetuses with Down syndrome, whereas hCG is abnormally high. More recently, another maternal protein, pregnancy-associated protein A, has also been shown to be lower in fetuses with Down syndrome. Early indications suggest that measurement of pregnancy-associated protein A, together with hCG, in the first trimester, is predictive of Down syndrome.

- Ultrasound screening in the prenatal period may demonstrate physical suggestions of Down syndrome, especially involving abnormalities in nuchal thickness.
- Genetic karyotyping after birth can confirm a clinical diagnosis of Down syndrome.

COMPLICATIONS

- Congenital heart or other organ defects frequently occur in association with Down syndrome.
- Risk of childhood leukemia may be increased in children with Down syndrome. This is related to the observation that some forms of leukemia may be related to defects on chromosome 21.
- Development of Alzheimer's disease in the fourth or fifth decade of life is common in individuals with Down syndrome. This is related to the observation that Alzheimer's disease may occur partially as a result of a defect on chromosome 21.
- Approximately 20% of fetuses with Down syndrome are spontaneously aborted between 10 and 16 weeks' gestation. Many others do not implant or are miscarried before 6 to 8 weeks' gestation.

TREATMENT

- Surgery may be required if another congenital defect is present.
- Early intervention programs may limit degree of mental retardation.

Turner's Syndrome

Turner's syndrome is a monosomy of the sex chromosomes. Infants born with Turner's syndrome have 45 chromosomes: 22 pairs of somatic chromosomes and 1 sex chromosome, usually the X (45, X/O). This disorder is common in spontaneously aborted fetuses, and is present in approximately 1 in 2,500 live births. Females with Turner's syndrome lack ovaries.

CLINICAL MANIFESTATIONS

Clinical manifestations may be nonexistent, mild, or moderate and include:

- Short stature and webbing of the neck.

- Lack of secondary sex characteristics and amenorrhea (no menstrual cycles) with associated sterility.

DIAGNOSTIC TOOLS

- Prenatal genetic testing can identify fetuses afflicted with Turner's syndrome.
- Genetic karyotyping after birth can confirm the clinical diagnosis.

COMPLICATIONS

- Congenital heart defects may accompany the sex chromosome monosomy.
- Some individuals may demonstrate signs of mental retardation.

TREATMENT

- Surgery may be required if a congenital heart defect is present.
- Estrogen replacement for a female may increase growth and allow development of secondary sex characteristics. Growth hormone replacement may also stimulate skeletal growth.
- Counseling to assist with the issue of infertility may be desired. There are incidents of successful pregnancies after in vitro fertilization.

Klinefelter's Syndrome

Klinefelter's syndrome is a polysomic disorder characterized by one or more extra X chromosomes in a genotypic male (47, X/X/Y; 47, X/X/X/Y). Klinefelter's syndrome occurs in approximately 1 in 600 live births. Klinefelter's syndrome may result from nondisjunction of the male or female X chromosome during the first meiotic division, at approximately equal rates.

CLINICAL MANIFESTATIONS

- Although the infant may appear normal at birth, he may show a decrease in male secondary sex characteristics during puberty.
- Gynecomastia (breast enlargement) and other female patterns of fat deposit.
- Infertility and sexual dysfunction.
- Tall stature in adult life because decreased levels of testosterone do not contribute to epiphyseal bone plate closure.
- Individuals may demonstrate reduced mental functioning, especially with increasing number of X chromosomes.

TREATMENT

- Testosterone replacement.
- Counseling may be required.

Selected Bibliography

Alberts, B., Bray, D., Lewis, J., Raff, M., Roberts, K., & Watson, J. (1997). The cell-division cycle. In: *Molecular biology of the cell (3rd ed.)* New York: Garland Publishing Company.

Beardsley, T. (1996). Vital data; trends in human genetics. *Scientific American* 274, 100–105.

Brown, A. A., Selke, S., Zeh, J., et al. (1997). The acquisition of herpes simplex virus during pregnancy. *New England Journal of Medicine* 337, 509–515.

Campisi, J. (1997). Aging and cancer: the double-edged sword of replicative senescence. *Journal of Geriatrics Society* 45, 482–488.

Chiu, C. P. & Harley, C. B. (1997). Replicative senescence and cell immortality: the role of telomeres and telomerase. *Proceedings of the Society for Experimental Biology and Medicine* 214, 99–106.

Collins, F. S. (1997). Sequencing the human genome. *Hospital Practice* 32, 35–43.

Guyton, A. C. & Hall, J. E. (1996). *Textbook of medical physiology (9th ed.)* Philadelphia: W.B. Saunders.

Haddow, J. E., Palomaki, G. E., Knight, G. J., Williams, J., Miller, W. A., & Johnson, A. (1998). Screening of maternal serum for fetal Down's syndrome in the first trimester. *New England Journal of Medicine* 338, 955–961.

Koren, G., Pastuszak, A., & Ito, S. (1998). Drugs in pregnancy. *New England Journal of Medicine* 338, 1128–1137.

Nicklas, R. B. (1997). How cells get the right chromosomes. *Science* 275, 632–637.

Rennie, J. (1993). DNA's new twists. *Scientific American* March, 122–132.

Shibley, I. A. Jr. & Pennington, S. N. (1997). Metabolic and mitotic changes asociated with the fetal alcohol syndrome. *Alcohol and Alcoholism* 32, 423–434.

Stranc, L. C., Evans, J. A., & Hamerton, J. L. (1997). Chorionic villus sampling and amniocentesis for prenatal diagnosis. *Lancet* 349, 711–714.

Sutherland, G. R. & Richards, R. I. (1994). DNA repeats—a treasury of human variation. *New England Journal of Medicine* 331, 191–193.

Warren, S. T. (1997). Trinucleotide repetition and fragile X Syndrome. *Hospital Practice* 32, 73–76, 81–85, 90–92.

3 THE IMMUNE AND INFLAMMATORY SYSTEMS

The immune and inflammatory systems work together to protect the body from infection by microorganisms, and to help the body heal if an infection or injury occurs. The immune system also identifies self from non-self: the cells, tissues, and organs of the host versus the cells and tissues of foreign origin. Likewise, the immune system recognizes and eliminates host cells that have been changed by injury or disease, such as cancer. Alterations in the immune or inflammatory response can result in attack against the body's own cells, the development of cancer, or an inability to respond and heal from infection.

● ● ●

PHYSIOLOGIC CONCEPTS

Characteristics of the Immune and Inflammatory Systems

Any molecule that can stimulate an immune response against itself or the cell that bears it is called an **antigen.** An antigen is usually a protein or large carbohydrate that is foreign to the host, although occasionally the immune system will also attack host cells. The immune system can respond with specificity and precision to virtually any antigen an individual may encounter in a lifetime. Once the original response is made, the memory of that antigen will remain in the immune system. If a second encounter with the antigen occurs, the immune response will be swifter than before.

Although the inflammatory system is not characterized by specificity or memory, it is fast and effective. Like the immune response, the inflammatory response occurs after tissue injury or infection. The goal of the inflammatory response is to deliver white blood cells and platelets to the tissues to limit damage and promote healing.

WHITE BLOOD CELLS

White blood cells function to protect the body from infection and cancer and to assist in healing. White blood cells include the cells of inflammation: neutrophils, eosinophils, basophils, monocytes, and macrophages; and the cells of the immune response: the lymphocytes. Platelets are fragments of cells that also play a role in healing. All white blood cells and platelets derive from a basic stem (originator) cell, called the pluripotential stem cell, in the bone marrow. From this cell, succeeding generations of stem cells differentiate and commit to producing one type of cell. White blood cells and their differentiation are discussed in Chapter 5.

NEUTROPHILS, EOSINOPHILS, AND BASOPHILS

Neutrophils, eosinophils, and basophils are called granulocytes because of the cytoplasmic granules that dominate their appearance under the microscope. The granulocytes remain in the bone marrow or circulation until they are drawn to an area of inflammation by substances released from damaged tissues, by microorganisms, or by activation of the immune cells. The intracellular granules contain enzymes that when released serve to break down and destroy microorganisms and digest cellular debris. Once granulocytes complete their function, they die. In a serious infection, granulocytes may only survive a few hours.

Neutrophils are the first white blood cells to arrive at an area of inflammation. They begin phagocytizing cells and debris immediately. Neutrophils arriving on the scene release chemicals that attract other white blood cells to the area, in a process called **chemotaxis**. They also participate in initiating the inflammatory responses of vasodilation and increased capillary permeability. Clinically, neutrophils are often referred to as polymorphonuclear cells (PMNs) or segmented neutrophils ("segs") because of the segmented appearance of their multilobed nuclei. In adults, approximately 50% of circulating white blood cells are neutrophils.

Eosinophils have several functions. First, they are involved in the allergic response (Type I hypersensitivity reaction). Second, they are important in the defense against parasitic infections. They also appear to perform a protective role for the host by helping to end the inflammatory reaction. The eosinophils phagocytize cell debris, although to a lesser degree than do neutrophils. Eosinophils normally account for only 1% to 3% of circulating white blood cells. The level of eosinophils is tightly regulated but may become elevated during an allergic response or in response to helminthic infection.

Basophils circulate in the bloodstream and, when activated by injury or infection, release histamine, bradykinin, and serotonin. These substances increase capillary permeability and blood flow to the area. Basophils secrete the natural anticlotting substance heparin, which ensures that clotting and coagulation pathways do not continue without check. Basophils are also involved in producing allergic responses. They are similar in function to important initiators of tissue inflammation, the mast cells, but unlike mast cells, basophils circulate in the blood. Basophils account for approximately 0 % to 1% of circulating white blood cells.

MONOCYTES AND MACROPHAGES

Monocytes circulate in the blood and enter injured tissue across capillary membranes that become permeable as a part of the inflammatory reaction. Monocytes are not phagocytic, but after several hours in the tissue area they mature into macrophages. Macrophages are large cells capable of ingesting large quantities of cell debris and bacteria. Macrophages can phagocytize lysed red blood cells and other white blood cells. Some macrophage cells colonize tissues, such as skin, lymph nodes, and lungs, for months or years. These cells are readily available to scavenge microorganisms that may enter the body through those routes. The monocyte-macrophage cell system is called the reticuloendothelial system. Circulating monocytes account for approximately 3% to 7% of white blood cells in the adult.

LYMPHOCYTES

Lymphocytes include the B and T cells, and a type of cell called the natural killer (NK) cell. Lymphocytes are produced in the bone marrow and mature there or in other lymphoid tissues. B and T cells circulate in the blood or migrate to the lymph nodes, thymus, or tonsils, where they remain until activated by an antigen. The B and T cells respond with specificity and memory to prevent infection. The NK cells also react to antigens, but do not demonstrate antigenic specificity. The natural history of NK cell origin and maturation is unclear. Circulating lymphocytes account for approximately 30% of white blood cells in the adult.

B lymphocytes, also called B cells, mature in the bone marrow. After maturation, a B cell circulates in the blood in an inactive state and becomes active only after exposure to a specific antigen to which it has been genetically programmed during development to respond. When activated, the B cell matures to become a specialized cell that orchestrates the immune and inflammatory responses against the substance that caused its activation. B lymphocytes comprise the humoral immune system, meaning they circulate in the blood (the humor).

T cells comprise the cellular immune system. T-cell maturation occurs during passage through the thymus gland. When a T cell encounters a microorganism (or other protein) to which it has been programmed during development to respond, it can directly attack and destroy the substance. It also releases chemicals that alert the B cells to the invader and stimulate an inflammatory reaction. T cells are important for recognizing and destroying parasites and viruses that hide intracellularly, where the B cells are unable to encounter them.

PLATELETS

Platelets are not cells, but cytoplasmic fragments of special white blood cells from the bone marrow. Like white blood cells, they are drawn to an area of inflammation. Platelets release serotonin, which increases blood flow and capillary permeability. Platelets are important in initiating blood clotting. Blood clotting isolates and contains infection and prevents blood loss.

The Immune Response

The immune response begins when a B or T cell encounters and binds with an antigen that the B or T cell identifies as foreign. Billions of B and T cells are produced during fetal development with the potential to bind to at least 100 million distinct antigens (there is some duplication). Antigens that can bind to a T or B cell include those present on the cell wall of a bacterium or mycoplasm, the coat of a virus, or on certain pollens, dusts, or foods. Every cell of a person has surface proteins that would be recognized as foreign by a B or T cell from another person. If an antigen causes the B or T cell to become activated and to multiply or differentiate further, it is an immunogenic antigen.

B-CELL RESPONSE TO AN ANTIGEN

When a B cell binds its specific antigen, it undergoes a final maturation step and becomes a **plasma cell**. The plasma cell in turn begins to secrete millions of molecules of **antibody** made specifically against that antigen. It is estimated that there are more than 100 billion B cells, each of which is capable of becoming a plasma cell and producing antibody that is different from most of the others. Once produced by a plasma cell, the antibodies circulate throughout the bloodstream seeking to eliminate the antigen that stimulated their production. Antibody-mediated responses are important for defense against bacteria and circulating viruses, and toxins released from bacteria.

MEMORY CELLS

Some B cells do not become plasma cells after antigenic stimulation, but rather become **memory cells**. Memory cells circulate indefinitely in the blood and become active immediately on any repeat exposure to the antigen.

Production of antibodies after primary exposure of B cells to an antigen can take 2 weeks to more than 1 year, but normally antibodies to an antigen are detectable in the blood within 3 to 6 months. Because of memory cells, the next time that antigen is encountered, the antibody response occurs almost immediately (Fig. 3-1).

IMMUNOGLOBULINS

Antibodies are also called immunoglobulins. There are at least five specific immunoglobulins produced in response to an antigen.

IgG is the most common antibody and represents approximately 80% of all circulating immunoglobulin. IgG is the main antibody that crosses the placenta from the mother to the fetus during pregnancy. IgG levels increase slowly during the primary response to an antigen, but increase immediately and to a much greater extent with a second exposure (Fig. 3-1).

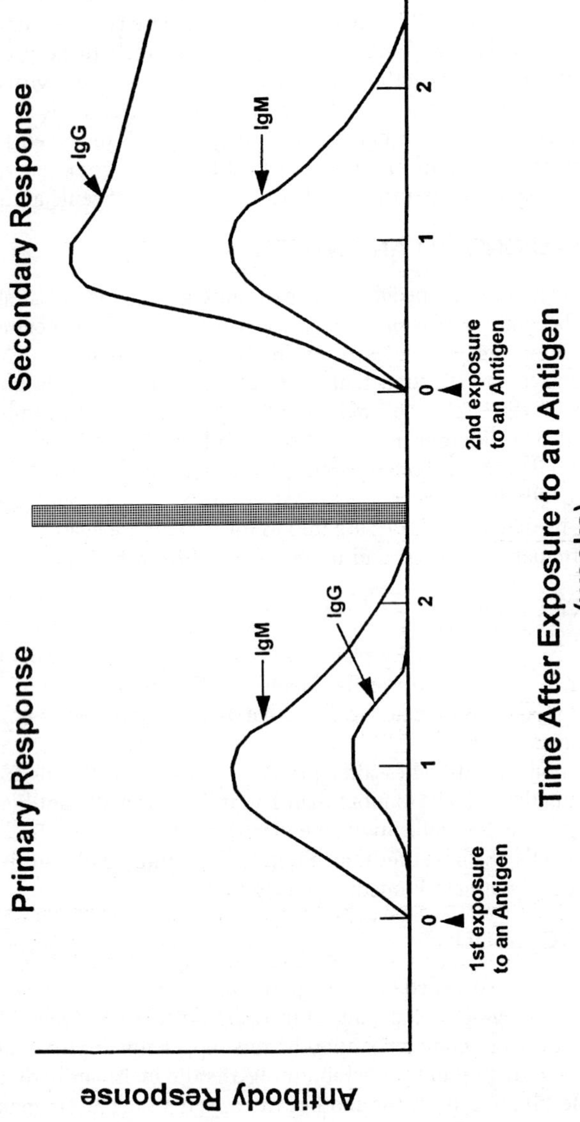

Figure 3-1. Primary and secondary antibody responses to an antigen.

IgM is produced first and in highest concentration during primary exposure to an antigen. IgM is the largest antibody. It is the antibody responsible for natural immunity in a species.

IgA is most concentrated in secretions such as saliva, vaginal mucus, breast milk, gastrointestinal (GI) and lung secretions, and semen. IgA acts locally rather than through the systemic circulation. Maternal IgA passes to an infant during breastfeeding (as do IgG and IgM to a lesser extent).

IgE is responsible for allergic reactions. It is also the antibody most stimulated during a parasitic infection.

IgD is in low concentration in the plasma. Its role in the immune response is not completely clear, although it appears to be important for the maturation and differentiation of all B cells.

ANTIBODY STRUCTURE

All antibodies are similar in appearance. They consist of two long heavy chains called the Fc portion, and two small heads called the Fab portion. The Fc portion is identical for all antibodies of a single class (i.e., IgG, IgM). The Fab portion is specific for each antibody and contains the specific binding site for an antigen. Binding of antigen to the Fab portion of the antibody activates the Fc portion, leading to destruction of the microorganism or other antigen-bearing cell. An antibody is shown in Figure 3-2.

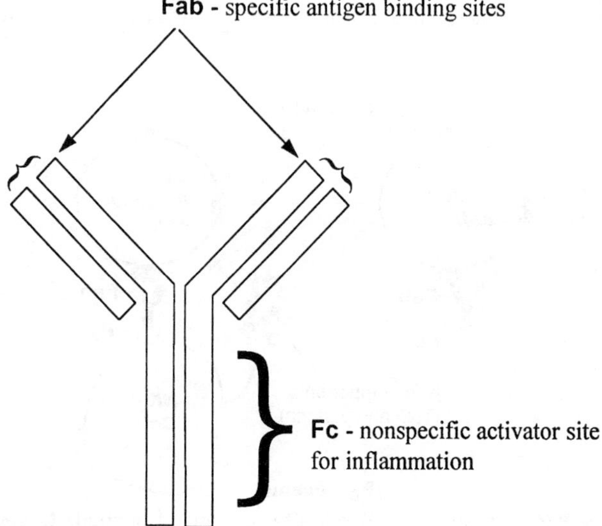

Figure 3-2. Diagrammatic representation of an antibody, showing sites for antigen binding and inflammatory activation.

ANTIBODY DESTRUCTION OF A MICROORGANISM

Antibodies cause the destruction of bound antigen by a variety of mechanisms. Usually, the antibody does not kill the cell (i.e., a bacteria) but instead functions to coordinate the attack by turning on NK cells, activating complement, and enhancing phagocytosis. Under some circumstances, an antibody may directly inactivate an antigen.

NK cell activation occurs when binding of the antigen to the Fab (specific) portion of the antibody allows an NK cell to bind to the Fc (nonspecific) portion, thus linking up the NK cell with the antigen (Fig. 3-3). The NK cell then releases toxic chemicals that directly kill the antigen target.

Complement activation is described more fully later. In short, complement is a series of molecules that when activated lead to the initiation of an inflammatory response and the killing of the antigen-bearing cell. Like NK cell activation, binding of the antigen to the Fab portion of the antibody allows the first molecule in the complement chain (C1) to bind nonspecifically to the Fc portion. This hooks up the antigen-bearing cell with complement, ultimately leading to the destruction of the antigen-bearing cell.

Phagocytic stimulation occurs similarly; when the antigen binds to the Fab portion of the antibody, this allows a phagocytic cell (usually a macrophage or neutrophil) to bind to the nonspecific Fc portion, stimulating phagocytosis of the linked antigen and the cell that bears it.

Direct effects of an antibody may occur if, for example, an antibody binds to a virus at the same site the virus uses to bind to and enter a susceptible cell. This would inactivate the virus. Similarly, the antibody may bind to a bacterial toxin at the same site that the toxin would

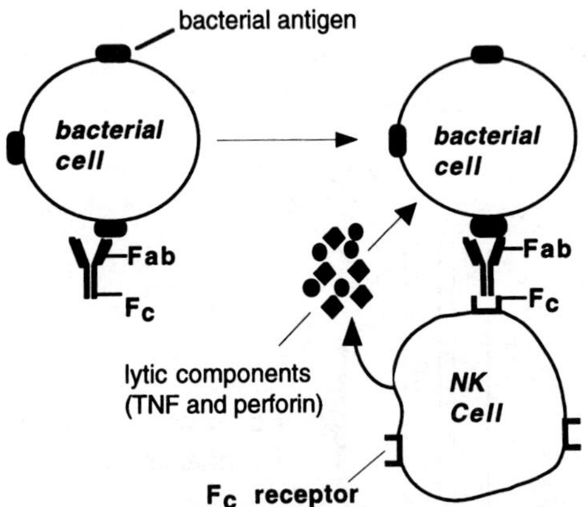

Figure 3-3. Activation of NK cell after binding of antibody to bacterial antigen. Activated NK cell secretes lytic components that lyse the bacterial cell. Similar patterns occur after binding of complement or phagocyte.

use to interact with susceptible cells. This would eliminate the effect of the toxin.

OPSONIZATION

Binding of an antibody to an antigen on a bacterium causes **opsonization** of the bacterium. Opsonization refers to a change in a bacterial cell wall that renders an otherwise impenetrable bacterium susceptible to phagocytosis. Complement also serves as an opsonin (an agent that can cause opsonization).

THE ROLE OF THE T CELL IN B-CELL RESPONSE TO AN ANTIGEN

To mount an antibody attack against a microorganism, T-cell support is almost always required. The T cells release chemicals, called cytokines, which are necessary to trigger B-cell proliferation and differentiation into plasma cells.

T-CELL RESPONSE TO AN ANTIGEN

When a T cell binds to an immunogenic antigen, it is stimulated to mature and reproduce. This results in at least three subtypes of T cells capable of acting in response to the antigen; cytotoxic T cells, helper T cells, and memory cells. The T-cell response to antigen is called a cell-mediated response, because the T cells respond directly; they do not need to become plasma cells and secrete antibody to destroy the antigen.

Cytotic T cells directly destroy the antigen by releasing toxic chemicals. These chemicals punch holes into the cells carrying the antigen. Cytotoxic T cells also are called CD8+ cells because of a specific protein present on their plasma membrane.

Helper T cells secrete chemicals, called cytokines, essential in stimulating the response of the cytotoxic T cells and in stimulating B-cell activation. Various cytokines released by helper cells also stimulate macrophage phagocytosis, and act as chemotaxic substances to draw other white blood cells to the area. Macrophages also secrete cytokines that increase responsiveness of the T helper cells, which results in a positive feedback cycle designed to amplify the defense response. Helper T cells are essential for successful destruction of most microorganisms. These cells are called CD4+ cells because of the presence of a specific protein on their membranes.

Memory cells circulate in the bloodstream until the specific antigen that stimulated their production is encountered again. Subsequent responses to that antigen occur immediately.

Geriatric Consideration

As an individual ages, the number and function of immune cells decrease, which results in an increased prevalence of infection and malignancy in the elderly. Some studies suggest that moderate exercise may be able to improve immunocompetence in the elderly by increasing NK and cytotoxic T-cell number.

THE ROLE OF THE T CELL IN RECOGNITION OF SELF VERSUS FOREIGN ANTIGENS

Cell-mediated immunity is important for combating intracellular invaders such as viruses. In addition, cell-mediated immunity, through the T-helper cells, has the important role of turning on the antibody response. It is essential that T cells recognize self-antigens, and only initiate attack against non-self or damaged cells. To ensure only appropriate T-cell responses, potential antigens are always presented to the T cell in combination with self-antigens, called major histocompatibility complex (MHC) proteins.

SELF-ANTIGENS

Each individual possesses cell surface antigens that are unique to that individual. These antigens, the MHC proteins, serve as a sort of cellular fingerprint. (In humans, these proteins are sometimes called histocompatibility antigens.) There are two groups of MHC proteins, **MHC I** and **MHC II**. The MHC I proteins are found on nearly all cells of the body except the red blood cells. The MHC II proteins are found only on the surface of macrophages and B cells. MHC proteins have two functions: 1) they present self-antigens to T cells, and 2) they bind foreign antigens and present these to T cells. The MHC I molecules bind and present antigens only to cytotoxic T cells. The MHC II molecules bind and present antigens only to helper T cells.

THE MHC GENES

The MHC proteins are inherited as four closely linked loci (group of genes) on chromosome 6. This group of genes, called the major histocompatibility complex, are usually inherited together, with one set of loci received from each parent. There are many different possible alleles for each loci, resulting in more than one trillion possible antigen combinations. Therefore, it is virtually impossible for two unrelated individuals to match MHC proteins. Identical twins will have the same proteins, and an individual's siblings and offspring will likely have MHC proteins more similar than unrelated individuals.

THE ROLE OF THE MHC PROTEINS IN STIMULATING CELL-MEDIATED IMMUNITY

A T-helper (CD4+) cell recognizes a cell antigen as foreign after the cell has been phagocytized by macrophages or has encountered its matching B cell. The MHC II molecules found on a macrophage or B cell bind the antigen and present it to the passing helper cells at the same time that they present their MHC II antigens (Fig. 3-4). This allows the helper cell, which may respond to the antigen, to compare the foreign antigen to host tissue before becoming activated to secrete essential cytokines. If the antigen presented is too similar to the MHC II proteins, the helper T cells will not become activated so the antigen will not be attacked.

To activate cytotoxic (CD8+) cells, MHC I proteins must be presented. All cells express MHC I proteins; therefore, any cell can present foreign proteins to CD8+ cells for comparison. Cells infected with a virus begin to make abnormal proteins, as do cancerous cells. These abnormal proteins are presented to CD8+ cells along with the MHC I proteins. When the cytotoxic T cells identify abnormal proteins compared to the MHC I proteins, the T cells initiate killing of the cells.

GRAFT REJECTION AND MHC PROTEINS

A poor match of MHC proteins is the major cause of graft rejection. Not all cellular antigens need to match; however, the closer the MHC profile match between donor and host, the greater the chance a graft will be accepted. Graft rejection is an example of cell-mediated immunity.

SUMMARY OF B-CELL AND T-CELL RESPONSE TO A FOREIGN ANTIGEN

In a **B-cell response**, B cells bind a foreign antigen. T-helper cells are presented pieces of the antigen, either by the B cell directly or by macrophages that have begun phagocytizing the antigen. If the antigen is different enough from the MHC II proteins expressed by the B cell or macrophage, the helper T cell will release cytokines that activate the B cell and cause it to become an antibody-secreting plasma cell. The antibody binds the antigen throughout the body and orchestrates

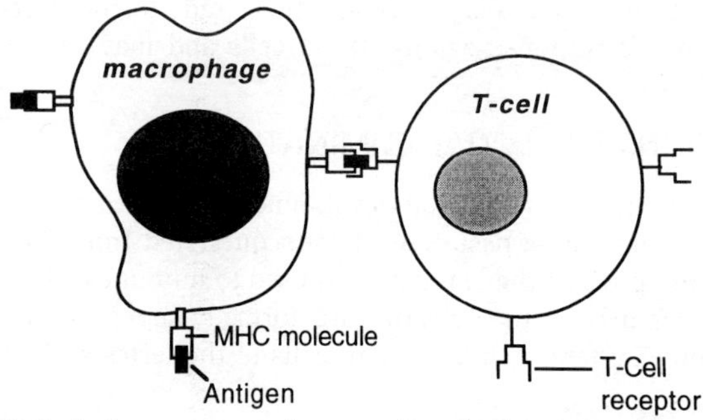

Figure 3-4. Antigen presentation to a T cell. The macrophage presents processed antigen with the MHC self molecule on its membrane to the T cell, which becomes activated against the antigen.

its destruction. The T cells also stimulate the macrophage to increase phagocytosis of the organism and activates other white blood cells to assist in the defense response.

In a **T-cell response**, cells of any type infected with an intracellular microorganism or cells that have become cancerous, present foreign proteins to cytotoxic T cells along with their own MHC I proteins. This activates cytotoxic cells and NK cells to destroy organisms carrying the foreign protein.

DEVELOPMENT OF SELF-TOLERANCE

During gestation, hundreds of thousands of T and B cells are formed. Some of these T and B cells are complimentary to, and therefore capable of reacting against, host antigens. To eliminate the potential of attack against host cells, T cells residing in the thymus and B cells in the bone marrow are exposed during a critical period of embryogenesis, to a multitude of host antigens. If during this time, a B or T cell encounters an antigen to which it matches, the B or T cell is programmed to undergo apoptosis and self-destruct. This leaves behind only cells tolerant to host antigens. This theory of tolerance is called the **clonal deletion** because it explains the elimination of clones of immune cells that react with self-antigens.

A second method also exists to ensure the elimination of cells with the potential to attack host antigens. This theory, called **clonal inactivation**, occurs outside the thymus, also during fetal development and throughout life. In this scenario, MHC II antigens are presented to T-helper cells. If a T-helper cell encounters the specific antigen against which it matches among the MHC proteins, the helper cell undergoes apoptosis.

Because T-helper cells are essential in activating B cells to become plasma cells, clonal deletion and clonal inactivation of T cells can eliminate humoral and cellular immunity against self-antigens. In clonal deletion and clonal inactivation, tolerance is recognized as an active process, essential for the survival of the host. Occasionally, tolerance to host cells may be lost, which leads to the development of an immune response against those cells and may cause autoimmune disease.

EXCEPTIONS TO CLONAL ELIMINATION

Some tissues grow during fetal development without exposure to immature T cells. These tissues are kept sequestered from the immune system after birth. If they are later exposed to immune cells, an attack against them may occur. Cells that are normally kept sequestered from the immune system include certain cells of the testes and eye.

Red Blood Cell Antigens

There are at least 80 different antigens present on the red blood cells. The most important of these are the ABO antigens and the Rh antigens. Blood types are referred to as ABO and Rh.

ABO ANTIGENS

The ABO blood group consists of A and B antigens. An individual can receive from each parent an A antigen and a B antigen, or neither, called the O antigen. The A and B antigens are each dominant over the O antigen, but are codominant with each other. An individual who receives an A antigen from one parent and an A or an O from the other (AA or AO) will have type A blood. An individual who receives a B antigen from one parent and a B or an O from the other (BB or BO) will have type B blood. An individual who receives an A antigen from one parent and a B antigen from the other will have AB blood. Type O blood is possible only if an individual receives neither the A nor B antigen from either parent (OO).

THE RH ANTIGENS

On the red blood cell is also a complex group of antigens called the Rh antigens. If a particular type of this antigen is present on the red blood cells, an individual is considered to be Rh positive. If this antigen is not present, an individual is considered Rh negative. Each individual receives one Rh gene from each parent. The Rh-positive gene dominates, such that an individual with one Rh-positive gene and one Rh-negative gene is Rh positive. Rh antigens, when mismatched between mother and fetus, can be responsible for a severe reaction in the fetus. This reaction is characterized by red blood cell lysis and anemia (hemolytic disease of the newborn and erythroblastosis fetalis), which occurs when an Rh-negative mother (Rh negative, Rh negative) produces antibodies against the red cells of an Rh-positive fetus. Antibodies may cross the placenta and cause destruction of fetal red blood cells before or during birth.

IMMUNE REACTIONS AGAINST MISMATCHED BLOOD

An individual with type A blood given type B blood may develop a severe immune reaction against the B blood, a transfusion reaction. In a transfusion reaction, lysis and agglutination of donated red blood cells occur. Inflammation, blood clotting, and death may result. A similar reaction would occur if an individual with type B blood were to receive a donation of type A blood. An individual with Rh-negative blood who receives an Rh-positive blood transfusion may have an immunologic reaction, although typically the response is less intense.

Individuals with type A or type B blood can safely receive type O blood because type O blood will not stimulate an antibody reaction. Individuals with O-negative blood are called universal donors because they can supply blood to anyone. Individuals with AB-positive blood are considered universal recipients because they will not react against any type blood. O-negative is the blood of choice for an emergency trauma patient who has not been crossmatched (blood type determined).

Immunity

Immunity is the state in which one is protected from disease development. Immunity may be innate, passive, or acquired after exposure to a microorganism or toxin.

INNATE IMMUNITY

Innate immunity refers to species immunity. Humans are innately immune to many diseases that strike cattle, dogs, horses, and other animals. Innate immunity does not occur in response to a microorganism challenge; it is present before exposure to a microorganism occurs. Innate immunity probably occurs because human cells do not contain the appropriate "lock-and-key" receptors for certain microorganisms, and so cannot be infected by them. Innate immunity also includes protection provided by the skin and nonspecific mediators of inflammation.

PASSIVE IMMUNITY

Passive immunity refers to immunity provided to an individual by transfer of antibodies from someone else or by deliverance of a prepared antitoxin. Antitoxins are antibodies produced specifically against a certain bacterial toxin (i.e., diphtheria antitoxin). An example of passive immunity is when antibodies produced in one individual against the Hepatitis B virus are harvested and given to another individual who has been exposed to the virus, but whose cells have not yet been infected by it. Clinically, the transferred antibodies are referred to as Hepatitis B immunoglobulin. Likewise, an individual bitten by a rattlesnake may be given antivenom. The antivenom consists of antibodies produced by a person who was bitten by a rattlesnake and survived the bite. The hope in this situation is that the passively provided antibodies will take out of circulation the poisonous venom before the person is killed or seriously affected. Passive immunity also occurs when maternal IgG antibodies cross the placenta and when IgA and other antibodies are provided to the infant in breast milk.

Passive immunity works by providing a person with preformed, specific antibodies when that person is incapable of forming antibodies (a fetus or infant), or when there is insufficient time for antibodies to be produced before infection or death occurs. Passive immunity is temporary and does not provide a memory response.

ACTIVE IMMUNITY

Active immunity is the cellular and humoral immune response developed by an individual who has been significantly exposed to a microorganism or toxin. Exposure may occur in a disease process or as a result of an immunization. Active immunity is characterized by memory in the B and T cells and the production of specific antibodies and T cells.

An antibody titer (level) may be measured in a serum sample to document the development of immunity to a microorganism or toxin. A positive titer (except in an infant) implies active immunity.

IMMUNE STATUS OF THE FETUS AND NEWBORN

Cell-mediated (T-cell) immunity begins in utero. A primary humoral immune response (IgM) to various microorganisms can be stimulated in the fetus in the last trimester of gestation. Other immune responses to an antigen (IgG and IgA), neutrophil and macrophage phagocytosis, and the production of inflammatory mediators are not significantly present until 6 to 8 months after birth. This makes the fetus and newborn vulnerable to infection and disease. In utero, maternal IgG antibodies are actively transported across the cells of the placenta and can be detected in the newborn for at least 6 months after birth. These antibodies offer the fetus and infant passive immunity against various microorganisms. IgA and other immunoglobulins may pass to the newborn through breast milk.

A time of particular vulnerability for a newborn is at approximately 5 to 6 months after birth when maternal IgG levels are being cleared, yet the infant's own immune system is not yet working at its peak. This is especially true if the infant is not breastfeeding.

Pediatric Consideration

Before maternal antibodies are cleared from the infant's bloodstream, it is impossible to tell whether an infant showing IgG antibodies against a specific microorganism is reflecting maternal infection or whether the infant him or herself is actively infected by the microorganism. Maternal antibodies begin to decrease after 6 months; therefore, the infant's antibody titer (level) after 6 months should be measured to identify true infection versus passive immunity. This is important to keep in mind when identifying which infants of mothers infected with HIV are infected and which only carry maternal antibodies to the virus. Infants who are infected with the virus may benefit from drug therapies that would be unnecessary and possibly dangerous to noninfected infants. Recent attempts to measure IgA antibodies against HIV in non-breastfeeding infants born to women who are HIV-positive may allow earlier diagnosis of infant HIV status. This is possible because the presence of anti-HIV IgA in a non-breastfeeding infant would indicate active immunity because IgA does not cross the placenta.

The Inflammatory Response

The inflammatory response occurs after tissue injury or infection. Inflammation may precede an immune response or be initiated by one. There are two stages in an acute inflammatory reaction: vascular and cellular.

VASCULAR STAGE OF INFLAMMATION

The vascular stage of inflammation begins almost immediately after an injury or in response to infection or toxin exposure. Arterioles at or near the site briefly constrict and then undergo a prolonged vasodilation (relaxation). This occurs primarily as a result of mast cell degranulation with the release of chemical mediators (see later). Dilation of the arterioles causes increased fluid pressure in the downstream capillaries. At the same time, histamine and other chemicals cause the endothelial cells of the surrounding capillaries—normally tightly spaced—to pull apart, increasing the permeability of the capillary. Increased permeability combined with increased blood flow leads to increased movement of a plasma filtrate into the interstitial space. The result is swelling and edema of the interstitial space and increased viscosity of the blood left behind in the capillary. Occasionally red blood cells may also move into the area surrounding injured cells.

CELLULAR STAGE OF INFLAMMATION

The cellular stage of inflammation begins with the movement of white cells in the blood to the area of injury or infection. These cells and platelets are drawn to the area by chemicals released from mast cells, by complement activation, and by cytokine production that occurs after antibody-antigen binding. Attraction of white blood cells to an area of injury is called chemotaxis. Once at the site of injury, the various stimulants cause the capillary endothelial cells and the white blood cells, especially neutrophils and later monocytes, to express complementary adhesion molecules. The endothelial cells become sticky for the white blood cells, causing the white blood cells to move to the periphery of the capillary, in a process called margination. This leads to the emigration of the white blood cells through the capillaries to surround and phagocytize the damaged cells. Platelets entering the area stimulate clotting to isolate the infection and control bleeding. Cells brought to the site will eventually be responsible for healing the injured area.

THE MAST CELL

Inflammation begins with the rupture of specialized tissue cells, called mast cells. Mast cells are bags of granules found throughout the loose connective tissue surrounding the blood vessels. Mast cells burst open and release their intracellular contents during tissue injury, exposure to toxins, activation of the proteins of the complement cascade, and antibody-antigen binding. This bursting open of the mast cell is called mast cell degranulation. Histamine and other substances are released by mast cell degranulation and contribute to vasodilation, increased capillary permeability, and drawing white blood cells and platelets to the area.

CHEMICAL MEDIATORS OF INFLAMMATION

Histamine is the main chemical mediator of inflammation and is released by basophils, platelets, and mast cells. Histamine is in part responsible for both steps of the vascular response to inflammation: relaxation of blood vessels leading to increased blood flow and increased capillary permeability. Histamine is also active in nonvascular tissues. In the respiratory passages histamine causes constriction of bronchiolar smooth muscles. In the gut, histamine stimulates acid secretion. Histamine also causes itching. Histamine acts by binding to H_1 receptors in the respiratory passages and the vascular system, and to H_2 receptors in the gut. Binding to the H_1 receptors causes a decrease in further release of histamine from the mast cells, an example of a negative feedback response.

Neutrophil and **eosinophil chemotaxic** factors are chemicals released from white blood cells (neutrophils or eosinophils) that draw other cells to the area.

Prostaglandins especially of the E series, are produced from arachidonic acid found in the cell membrane. There are several different types of prostaglandins. Those of the E series are especially important in inflammation. These prostaglandins (PGE and PGE_2) increase blood flow and increase capillary permeability. They also potentiate the effects of histamine, cause fever in response to infection, and stimulate pain receptors. Prostaglandin synthesis is blocked by nonsteroidal anti-inflammatory drugs such as aspirin and ibuprofin.

Leukotrienes increase vascular permeability and affect the adhesion of white blood cells to the capillary during injury or infection. They also act as chemoattractant chemicals. One type of leukotriene, slow-reacting substance of anaphylaxis, plays an important role in the bronchiolar constriction of asthma, and in allergic reactions.

Cytokines are a family of peptides produced by a variety of immune and inflammatory cells, including macrophages, monocytes, neutrophils, and lymphocytes. They are also produced by noninflammatory cells including fibroblasts and endothelial cells. Cytokines are often referred to by specific names related to their function or numbered following the general term "interleukin." Cytokines function as local hormones that affect the host defense response to injury or infection. Each cytokine may have multiple effects on a variety of interrelated processes. In general, cytokines serve as communication links between different arms of the immune and inflammatory systems.

There are general categories of cytokines. Inflammatory cytokines (e.g., interleukin-1, interleukin-6, tumor necrosis factor, interferon-gamma) promote the inflammatory responses of fever and malaise, and stimulate T-cell activity. These inflammatory cytokines are released from macrophages and monocytes (interleukin-1, tumor necrosis factor) or activated T cells (interleukin-6, tumor necrosis factor, interferon) and are essential for activating B cells to become plasma cells and secrete antibody. Interleukin-2 is also secreted by activated T-helper cells. Interleukin-2 and tumor necrosis factor stimulate cytotoxic T cells to attack and kill cancer cells or cells infected with a virus. They also alert macrophages to increase phagocytosis. A variety of other cytokines are important for stimulating the bone marrow to increase white and red blood cell production (hematopoietic colony-stimulating factors). These cytokines cause the increase in white blood cells that typically accompanies infection. Noninflammatory cytokines (e.g., interleukin-10) decrease the activation of B cells.

Interferons are a type of cytokine specific for preventing intracellular infection by viruses or parasitic organisms. They are produced by T cells (interferon-gamma) or other white blood cells (interferon-alpha) or fibroblasts (interferon-beta) and function to alert neighboring cells to secrete chemicals that will prevent their becoming infected. The interferons have been used clinically to stimulate the immune system of patients with cancer and other diseases.

Chemokines are a type of cytokine that act as chemotactic agents to regulate leukocyte movement. Chemokines may act to attract all types of white blood cells, or may be specific for certain white blood cells. Chemokines interact with target white cells by binding to receptors on the cell membrane. Chemokines work by a variety of mechanisms, one of which is to cause the cell to express adhesion molecules complementary to those expressed by capillary endothelial cells. This makes the white blood cells sticky for the capillary, resulting in migration and emigration of the cells.

Complement System

The complement system consists of 20 or more plasma proteins that are activated one by one in a domino fashion when the first protein (C_1, the classical pathway) or the third protein (C_3, the alternative pathway) is activated. The C_1 protein is activated when the Fc portion of an IgG or IgM antibody is turned on after antigen binding to the Fab portion. The C_3 protein is usually activated by pieces of bacterial or fungal cell wall released during phagocytosis. Activation of complement is an effective mechanism for destroying extracellular microbes.

The first five complement proteins (C_1–C_5) stimulate mast cell degranulation, white blood cell chemotaxis, and opsonization of bacteria. Activation of complement proteins 6 through 10 (C_6–C_{10}) cause bacterial cell lysis by making the cell wall leaky to water.

Coagulation Pathway

The coagulation pathway involves another series of at least 13 proteins that activate in a step-by-step cascade. The coagulation cascade functions like the platelets (but more powerfully) to stop bleeding. The result of the coagulation cascade is the formation of an insoluble clot and a meshwork of fibers that entrap microorganisms and prevent the spread of infection.

The coagulation cascade can be stimulated by many substances present with inflammation or injury. The intrinsic pathway is activated when one of the plasma proteins, factor XII (the Hageman factor) comes into contact with an injured blood vessel. The extrinsic pathway is stimulated when a different plasma protein, factor VII, comes into contact with a substance called tissue thromboplastin, which is released by injured cells. Both pathways result in the formation of a fibrin clot. The coagulation pathway requires calcium ion for most steps. Coagulation is kept in check by a series of natural anticoagulants that act with naturally occurring heparin (from platelets) to stop the coagulation cascade and prevent uncontrolled thrombus formation.

PATHOPHYSIOLOGIC CONCEPTS

Local Signs of Inflammation

Local characteristics of inflammation include the following.

- Rubor, the redness that accompanies inflammation. Rubor results from increased blood flow to the inflamed area.
- Calor, the heat that accompanies inflammation. Heat results from increased blood flow.
- Turgor, the swelling of an inflamed tissue. Turgor results from increased capillary permeability, which allows plasma proteins and exudate to enter the interstitial space.
- Dolor, the pain of inflammation. Pain results from stretching of nerves caused by swelling and the stimulation of nerve endings by mediators of inflammation.

Fever

Fever is the elevation of the temperature set-point in the hypothalamus. With an increase in set-point, the hypothalamus sends out signals to increase body temperature. The body responds by shivering and increasing the basal metabolic rate.

Fever occurs in response to production of certain cytokines, including interleukin-1, interleukin-6, and tumor necrosis factor. These cytokines are considered to be endogenous pyrogens (heat producers). The pyrogenic cytokines are released by several different cells, including monocytes, macrophages, T-helper cells, and fibroblasts, in response to tissue infection or injury. The endogenous pyrogens appear to cause fever by producing a prostaglandin, probably PGE, that raises the hypothalamic thermoregulatory set-point. When the source of the pyrogen is removed (i.e., after a successful response of the immune system against a microorganism), its level decreases, which returns the set-point to normal. For a short time, body temperature will lag behind the return of the set-point and the hypothalamus will perceive the body temperature as too high. In response, the hypothalamus will stimulate responses such as sweating to cool the body. Aspirin and other nonsteroidal anti-inflammatory drugs inhibit fever by blocking prostaglandin synthesis.

Although the occurrence of endogenous pyrogens has been recognized for more than 20 years, it is still unknown how the interleukins transmit the message of infection from the periphery to the central nervous system. One hypothesis under investigation, is that interleukin-1 stimulates firing of the vagus nerve, which then transmits the information to the central nervous system, somehow causing the production there of PGE, which raises the set-point. An alternative hypothesis is that the interleukins may themselves cross the blood brain barrier, and directly stimulate hypothalamic PGE production.

Fever has been shown to occur in every observed animal, suggesting an evolutionary role in species survival. Research suggests that fever helps an organism fight off infection and thus is beneficial to the host. However, high fevers may damage cells, especially those of the central nervous system.

Leukocytosis

Leukocytosis is an increase in circulating white blood cells (leukocytes). An increase in neutrophils is responsible for the initial leukocytosis that accompanies an infection or inflammation. With infection, the number of immature cells (myeloid cells) increase in the blood as the mature neutrophils and other mature granulocytes are used up. This shift toward immature cells is called a **left shift.** With resolution of inflammation or infection, a right shift occurs as mature cells are released from the marrow and again dominate in the circulation.

Chronic Inflammation

Chronic inflammation is an inflammatory reaction lasting longer than 2 weeks. Chronic inflammation may follow acute inflammation, for example, an unresolved infection or a poorly healed wound. Chronic inflammation may also occur without a preceding acute inflammation, for example, if the body encounters a microorganism it cannot kill, it encloses the microorganism within a wall to isolate it. Examples of microorganisms that may lead to chronic inflammation include the mycobacteria responsible for tuberculosis and leprosy. These bacteria survive in macrophages, which group together to form a protective capsule of cells called a granuloma.

Hypersensitivity Reactions

Hypersensitivity reactions are abnormal immune and inflammatory responses. There are four types of hypersensitivity reactions.

TYPE I HYPERSENSITIVITY REACTIONS

These are allergic reactions mediated by the IgE antibody. In type I reactions, an antigen to which the individual is sensitive is bound to an IgE antibody that is bound to a mast cell or basophil. The IgE-antigen complex causes mast cell degranulation and the release of histamine and other mediators of inflammation. These mediators, as well as activated complement and eosinophil chemotaxic factor, cause peripheral vasodilation, increased capillary permeability, and local swelling and edema. Symptoms are specific according to where the allergic response is happening. Binding of the antigen in the nasal passages causes allergic rhinitis with nasal congestion and inflammation of the tissues, whereas binding of an antigen in the gut may cause diarrhea or vomiting.

A severe type I hypersensitivity reaction is an **anaphylactic reaction.** Anaphylaxis involves a rapid IgE-mast cell response after exposure to an antigen to which the individual is highly sensitive. Histamine-induced dilation of the entire systemic vasculature can occur, leading to collapse of the blood pressure. A severe decrease in systemic blood pressure during an anaphylactic reaction is called anaphylactic shock. Because histamine is a potent constrictor of bronchiolar smooth muscle, anaphylaxis involves closure of the respiratory passages. Anaphylaxis in response to some drugs such as penicillin, or in response to a bee sting, may be fatal in highly sensitized individuals, as a result of circulatory collapse or respiratory failure. Symptoms of an anaphylactic reaction include itching, abdominal cramps, flushing of the skin, gastrointestinal (GI) upset, and breathing difficulties.

TYPE II HYPERSENSITIVITY REACTIONS

Type II hypersensitivity reactions occur when IgG or IgM antibodies attack tissue antigens. Type II reactions result from a loss of self-tolerance and are considered autoimmune reactions. The target cell is usually destroyed.

In a type II reaction, antibody-antigen binding causes complement activation, mast cell degranulation, interstitial edema, tissue destruction, and cell lysis. Type II reactions lead to macrophage phagocytosis of the host cells. Examples of type II autoimmune diseases include Grave's disease, involving antibodies produced against the thyroid gland; autoimmune hemolytic anemia, involving antibodies produced against red blood cells; transfusion reactions, involving antibodies produced against donor blood cells; and autoimmune thrombocytopenic purpura, involving antibodies produced against platelets. Systemic lupus erythematous (SLE) also has aspects of type II reactions (described later).

TYPE III HYPERSENSITIVITY REACTIONS

Type III hypersensitivity reactions occur when circulating antibody-antigen complexes precipitate out in a blood vessel or in downstream tissue. Antibodies are not directed against those particular tissue sites, but are trapped in their capillary meshwork. In some cases, foreign antigens may adhere to tissues, causing formation of antibody-antigen complexes at those sites.

Type III reactions activate complement and mast cell degranulation, causing damage to the tissue or capillaries where they occur. Neutrophils are drawn to the area and begin to phagocytize the injured cells, causing release of cellular enzymes and the accumulation of cell debris. This continues the inflammation cycle.

Examples of type III hypersensitivity reactions include serum sickness, where antibodies form against foreign blood, often in response to intravenous drug use. The antibody-antigen complexes deposit in the vascular system, joints, and kidneys. With glomerulonephritis, antibody-antigen complexes form in response to an infection, often by streptococcal bacteria, and deposit in the glomerular capillaries of the kidneys. With systemic lupus erythematosus, antibody-antigen complexes form against collagen and cellular DNA and deposit in multiple sites throughout the body.

TYPE IV HYPERSENSITIVITY REACTIONS

In these T-cell-mediated reactions, cytotoxic (CD8+) or helper (CD4+) T cells are activated by an antigen, leading to destruction of the cells involved. Cell-mediated reactions are delayed, taking 24 to 72 hours to develop. They are characterized by the production of inflammatory cytokines that stimulate B-cell activation, activation of macrophage phagocytosis, and the stimulation of the coagulation cascade.

Examples of conditions caused by type IV reactions include autoimmune thyroiditis (Hashimoto's disease), in which T cells are produced against thyroid tissue, graft and tumor rejection, and delayed allergic reactions, such as poison ivy. The tuberculin skin test indicates the presence of cell-mediated immunity against the tuberculin bacillus.

Immune and Inflammatory Deficiencies

Immunodeficiency may result from impaired function of any or all white blood cells. Complement or coagulation proteins may also be deficient. Immune and inflammatory deficiencies may be congenital (present at birth) or acquired after illness, infection, or prolonged stress. Immune and inflammatory deficiencies inhibit the body's ability to respond to infection or injury. They may be temporary or permanent.

CONGENITAL IMMUNODEFICIENCY

Congenital immunodeficiency occurs as a result of a genetic defect. Congenital immunodeficiency may involve one type of T or B cell, all the T cells (DiGeorge syndrome), or all the B cells (Bruton's agammaglobulinemia). Most commonly, one immunoglobulin (usually IgA or IgG) is missing. Individuals with selective immunoglobulin deficiency may have an increased susceptibility to certain infections, or may be asymptomatic. Severe cases of IgG deficiency may be treated with replacement injections. Typically, selective IgA deficiency is not treated because patients may develop IgG antibodies to administered IgA, which may cause anaphylaxis. With total B-cell deficiency, the missing immunoglobulins can be provided to the individual by intravenous administration. Infants with primary T-cell deficiency have severely impaired ability to fight infection because T cells are required not only for cellular immunity but humoral immune responses as well. If the pluripotential bone marrow stem cells are dysfunctional, T and B cells and all other white blood cells may be deficient. This condition is called severe combined immunodeficiency syndrome (SCIDS). SCIDS used to be fatal in early childhood, but new treatments appear promising.

Congenital immunodeficiency may also occur if an individual is born without certain MHC proteins. Without these proteins, dysfunctional self-antigen presentation to the T cells occurs, leading to a failure of T-cell immune function. This condition usually causes death in early childhood.

ACQUIRED IMMUNODEFICIENCY

Acquired immunodeficiency is reduced functioning of the immune system developing after birth. Acquired immunodeficiency may arise in response to infection, malnutrition, chronic stress, or pregnancy. Systemic illnesses such as diabetes, renal failure, and cirrhosis of the liver can cause immunodeficiency. Individuals receiving corticosteroids to prevent transplant rejection or to reduce chronic inflammation are immunosuppressed, as are those receiving chemotherapeutic drugs and radiation therapy. Surgery and anesthesia may also depress the immune system.

Acquired immunodeficiencies can be of B- or T-cell function, or both. Because B cells require T-helper cell stimulation to successfully fight infection, T-cell deficiencies also cause dysfunction of the humoral immune system.

Geriatric Consideration

The elderly are often immunodeficient, in part because of the progressive decrease in function of the thymus as one ages, but also because of poor blood flow many elderly experience as a result of atherosclerosis. Other systemic diseases such as diabetes mellitus, which increases in incidence with age, contribute to a depressed immune response. Poor nutrition, caused by poverty, isolation, or bad dentition, contributes to poor immune function in the elderly.

CONSEQUENCES OF IMMUNODEFICIENCY

Immunodeficient individuals repeatedly develop frequent severe and unusual infections and are often unable to fight them. Individuals with T-cell deficiencies frequently develop viral and yeast infections; individuals with B-cell deficiencies are especially susceptible to infections by bacteria that normally require opsonization. The HIV virus destroys the T-helper (CD4+) cells and infects other white blood cells.

CONDITIONS OF DISEASE OR INJURY

Most diseases associated with alterations in immune function are presented elsewhere in this book. Only allergy, systemic lupus erythematosus (SLE), and HIV/AIDS are discussed in this chapter.

Allergy

An allergy is an overstimulation of inflammatory reactions that occurs in response to a specific environmental antigen. An antigen that causes an allergy is called an allergen. Allergic reactions may be antibody mediated or T-cell mediated. Type I hypersensitivity reactions are an example of antibody-mediated allergies, whereas Type IV hypersensitivity reactions comprise the T lymphocyte-mediated allergy.

An individual with a Type I hypersensitivity allergic response has developed sensitized IgE antibodies to an allergen. When the allergen is encountered by the antibody, the antibody overresponds, causing excessive mast cell degranulation and release of histamine and other inflammatory mediators. Type IV hypersensitivity reactions occur after transdermal (across the skin) transport of an allergen that is presented to T cells sensitized to that allergen. Manifestations of an allergic response depend on where the allergen is encountered: in food, in inhaled particles, or through the skin. The timing of an allergic reaction varies depending on if the response is type I (immediate) or type IV (delayed). A type I reaction involving the skin is called atopic dermatitis; a type IV reaction is called allergic contact dermatitis. The skin response to poison ivy in susceptible individuals is a type of **allergic contact dermatitis.**

CAUSE OF ALLERGIES

The cause of allergies is unclear although there appears to be a genetic predisposition. A predisposition may involve excessive IgE binding, easily provoked mast cell degranulation, or excessive T-helper cell response. Overexposure to certain allergens at any time, including gestation, may cause an allergic response.

Pediatric Consideration

Infants and children exposed to cigarette smoke are at greater risk of developing asthma and other respiratory allergies.

CLINICAL MANIFESTATIONS

- Localized swelling, itching, and redness of the skin, with skin exposure to an allergen. Type IV reactions are often characterized by blistering and crusting over of the affected area.

- Diarrhea and abdominal cramps, with exposure to a gastrointestinal allergen.
- Allergic rhinitis, characterized by itchy eyes and runny nose, with exposure to a respiratory allergen. Swelling and congestion occur. Breathing difficulties may occur because of histamine-mediated constriction of the bronchiolar smooth muscle of the airways.

DIAGNOSTIC TOOLS

- Skin tests help in diagnosing an allergy. A small amount of the suspected allergen is injected under the skin. Individuals allergic to that allergen will respond with marked erythema, swelling, and itching at the injection site.
- Serum immunoglobulin analysis may indicate increased basophil and eosinophil count.

COMPLICATIONS

- A severe allergic reaction may result in anaphylaxis, which is characterized by a decrease in blood pressure and closure of the airways. Itching, cramping, and diarrhea may occur. Without intervention, severe reactions can lead to cardiovascular shock, hypoxia, and death.
- Allergic contact dermatitis (i.e., with a poison ivy reaction) may lead to secondary infection from excessive scratching.

TREATMENT

- Antihistamines and drugs that block mast cell degranulation may reduce the allergy symptoms.
- Corticosteriods, inhaled or administered nasally, or taken systemically, act as anti-inflammatory agents and can reduce the symptoms of an allergy. Ihnaled or intranasal therapy needs to be used for extended periods of time before becoming effective. Inhaled corticosteroids exert their effects only on the respiratory passages and may have few systemic effects.
- Inhaled mast cell stabilizers reduce mast cell degranulation and may reduce type I allergic symptoms.
- Desensitization therapy, involving repeated injections of small amounts of an allergen to which an individual is sensitive, may cause the individual to build IgG antibodies against the allergen. These antibodies can act as blocking antibodies. When the individual is again exposed to the allergen, the blocking antibodies may bind to the allergen before the IgE antibodies. Because IgG binding does not cause excessive mast cell degranulation, allergic symptoms are reduced.

Systemic Lupus Erythematosus

Systemic lupus erythematosus (SLE) is a chronic autoimmune disease in which antibodies against several different self-antigens are produced. The antibodies are usually IgG or IgM and may be produced against DNA and RNA, proteins of the coagulation cascade, skin, red blood cells, white blood cells, and platelets. Antibody-antigen complexes can precipitate in the capillary networks, causing type III hypersensitivity reactions. Chronic inflammation can follow.

CAUSES OF SLE

The cause of SLE is unknown, although it often occurs in individuals with a genetic tendency for autoimmune disease. Evidence to support a genetic role is the high concurrence among identical twins, and an increased incidence in blacks compared to whites. It is suggested that the tendency to develop SLE may be related to alterations of specific MHC genes, and how self-antigens are expressed and recognized. Women are more likely to develop SLE than men, suggesting a role for the sex hormones. SLE can be brought on by stress, often related to pregnancy or childbearing. In some individuals, excessive exposure to ultraviolet radiation may initiate the disease. Typically affected are young women during their childbearing years. The disease may remain mild for years, or may progress and result in death.

CLINICAL MANIFESTATIONS

- Polyarthralgia (joint pain) and arthritis (inflammation of the joint).
- Fever from chronic inflammation.
- Facial rash, in a malar (butterfly) pattern across the nose and cheeks. The word lupus means wolf and refers to the wolflike appearance of the mask.
- Fingertip lesions and bluing caused by poor blood flow and chronic hypoxia.
- Sclerosis (tightening or hardening) of the skin of the fingers.
- Sores on the oral or pharyngeal mucous membranes.
- Scaling lesions on the head, neck, and back.
- Eye and feet edema may signify renal involvement and hypertension.
- Anemia, chronic fatigue, frequent infections, and bleeding are common because of the attack against the red and white blood cells and the platelets.

DIAGNOSTIC TOOLS

- Antinuclear antibodies are present in at least 95% of individuals with SLE, but may occur in those without the disease.
- Antibodies against double-stranded DNA are diagnostic for SLE.
- Protein in the urine signals renal damage.
- Antineuronal antibodies may be present.

COMPLICATIONS

- Renal failure is the most common cause of death in individuals with SLE. Renal failure may develop as a result of the deposit of antibody-antigen complexes in the glomeruli with resultant complement activation leading to cellular injury, an example of a type III hypersensitivity reaction.
- Pericarditis (inflammation of the pericardial sac surrounding the heart) may develop.
- Inflammation of the pleural membrane surrounding the lungs can restrict respirations. Bronchitis is common.
- Vasculitis of all peripheral and cerebral vessels may occur.
- Central nervous system complications include stroke and seizure. Alterations in personality, including psychosis and depression, may develop. Personality changes may be related to drug therapy or the disease.

TREATMENT

- Anti-inflammatory drugs including aspirin or other nonsteroidal anti-inflammatory agents are used to treat fever and arthritis. Systemic corticosteriods are used to treat or prevent renal and central nervous system pathology.
- Skin lesions are treated with antimalarial drugs.

Acquired Immunodeficiency Syndrome

Acquired immunodeficiency syndrome (AIDS) is a viral disease that causes collapse of the immune system. Until recently, once diagnosed with AIDS, an individual had a high probability of dying within 5 years. However, recent advances in treatment of patients with AIDS has made long-term survival a possibility. Since AIDS was first described in the late 1970s, much has been learned not only about this specific virus, but how all viruses work and about the important roles of all white blood cells in host defense. From the immeasurable sorrow and loss that has trailed this virus, knowledge that will provide hope and cure for diseases of all types has come.

AIDS is caused by infection with the human immunodeficiency virus (HIV). There are at least two known HIV viruses, HIV-1 and HIV-2. HIV-1 is common in the United States, whereas HIV-2 is found primarily in West Africa. HIV-1 was first identified in the early 1980s. It is a retrovirus, meaning it consists of a single strand of viral RNA that enters the host cell nucleus and is transcribed into the host DNA. Transcription of the virus into host DNA occurs by the actions of a specific enzyme called reverse transcriptase that the virus carries into the cell. Once a part of the host DNA, the virus replicates and mutates over the course of many years, slowly but steadily killing off cells of the immune system.

CELL INFECTION AND DEATH

HIV only infects cells that carry certain surface proteins, one of which is called the CD4 protein. The part of the virus that fits lock and key with the CD4 protein is known as the group 120 antigen. Cells that carry the CD4 protein, and so can be infected by HIV, include macrophages and T-helper (CD4+) cells. Most of the macrophages and CD4+ cells concentrate in the lymph nodes, spleen, and bone marrow, acting as a huge reservoir of virus-containing cells that continually pass the virus on to noninfected cells traveling through those sites. Because of the high density of infected cells lurking in secondary lymph organs, the number of circulating cells infected by the virus grossly underestimates the true number of infected cells, which means that even if the virus is undetectable in the blood, it may still exist in noncirculating cells.

In recent years it has become clear that to infect a T cell or macrophage, binding of the virus to the CD4 protein is not enough; the virus also has to bind a second surface receptor before it can enter the host cell. The second receptor is another protein found on the surface of macrophages, called the CCR5 receptor, or a protein found on the surface of T-helper cells, called a CXCR4 receptor. These receptors normally function as receptors for specific chemokines that are involved in the inflammatory response. A key point to understand is that naturally occurring HIV readily binds CCR5 receptors and so quickly infects macrophages, but ineffectively binds CXCR4 receptors. **This means that at first the virus infects primarily macrophages**. Once inside, HIV does not destroy the macrophage, but lives inside the cell for approximately a decade, replicating constantly, and mutating at random. Eventually a mutated strain develops that is equally capable of binding the CXCR4 receptor, and so the virus can infect T-helper cells as well as macrophages. This shift soon becomes deadly because HIV kills the helper cells it infects. Death of the T-helper cells leads to a decrease in circulating CD4+ cells to fewer than 200/mL of blood (normal levels are approximately 1,000/mL) and the development of opportunistic infections and other AIDS-defining illnesses.

HIV destroys the T-helper cells when it takes over the cell's genetic machinery and begins to reproduce. As the virus reproduces, it destroys the host cell membrane, perhaps by interfering with the cell's ability to protect itself from free radicals or by producing a superantigen that destroys the cell. Once HIV reproduces and kills a CD4+ cell, many more viruses are released into the circulation. These HIV go on to infect other cells. Contributing to the death of the CD4+ cells is the immune response the host killer cells mount, in an attempt to eliminate the virus and all infected cells. As the number of CD4+ cells decreases, the cell-mediated immune system becomes progressively weaker. B-cell and macrophage function is compromised by the loss of the T-helper cells. Loss of immune function allows microorganisms that would normally be kept in check to proliferate wildly, leading to disease and death from a variety of infections. Without immune surveillance, cancers develop, contributing to the high death rates seen in individuals infected with HIV.

THE COURSE OF HIV INFECTION

An individual infected with HIV may remain symptomless for 10 or more years during the time the infection is mostly restricted to the macrophages. Once the virus infects the CD4+ cells and symptoms of infection occur, the disease progresses rapidly, usually over the course of 2 to 5 years. An individual is diagnosed as having AIDS when the CD4+ count decreases to fewer than 200 cells/mL, or when an opportunistic infection, cancer, or AIDS dementia develops.

It should be emphasized that HIV infection is not AIDS, and some individuals infected by the virus have survived more than 12 years with no signs of AIDS developing. However, infection with the virus means the individual is contagious to others, whether symptoms of AIDS are present.

AIDS-RESISTANT GENES

Reports of HIV resistance have been described in the literature for many years. Approximately 10% to 20% of individuals repeatedly exposed to HIV will not become infected with the virus, and some people who become infected experience atypically long spans of time without symptoms. Recently it has been shown that some of the resistance to HIV results from a mutation in the gene coding for the CCR5 receptor. Specifically, it has been demonstrated that approximately 10% to 14% of the white population carries one mutant CCR5 gene, and approximately 1% of whites carry two mutant genes (one from each parent). If an individual is homozygous for a mutation in the CCR5 gene, he or she is usually incapable of becoming infected with HIV. If an individual is heterozygous for the mutant gene, he or she may become infected but will show a delay in the onset of overt AIDS by at least 2 to 3 years. Rates of resistance in populations other than whites are lower; only 3% of African Americans carry a single mutated gene offering resistance, and virtually zero Native Americans, native Africans, or East Asian people carry even one copy of the mutant gene.

Because of the presence of the mutant gene in Caucasians compared to other races, it has been hypothesized that the mutation in the CCR5 gene developed relatively recently in evolutionary terms; after the major races split from each other. It has been suggested that a mutation in the CCR5 gene survived in the white population because it conferred some sort of protection against a deadly disease experienced mostly by this group; this disease has been suggested to be the bubonic plague that ravaged Central Europe approximately 700 years ago. Research is underway to explore this hypothesis and to determine whether the

CCR5 protein can be disabled in those with two good copies, thereby offering AIDS-resistance to the rest of the population.

The astute reader will notice that it was mentioned earlier that an individual carrying two mutant copies of the CCR5 gene is "usually incapable of becoming infected with HIV." This caveat exists because even if an individual does not have the CCR5 protein, that individual could still become infected with HIV if exposed to already mutated HIV. This occurs most frequently if an individual is infected with the virus from someone in the late stages of infection; if this happens, the virus can go straight for the T cells without needing to infect the macrophages first.

PASSAGE OF HIV

HIV is passed between individuals during the exchange of body fluids, including blood, semen, vaginal fluid, and breast milk. Urine and gastrointestinal contents are not believed to be a source of contagion unless they visibly contain blood. Tears, saliva, and sweat may contain the virus, but in quantities thought to be too low to cause infection.

INDIVIDUALS AT RISK OF DEVELOPING HIV

Whether an individual exposed to HIV will become infected depends on several factors, including the individual's immune, nutritional, and general health status and the amount of virus to which the individual is exposed. The age and sex of an individual also influences risk.

Individuals at high risk for becoming infected with HIV include those who exchange blood with infected persons. This means anyone exposed to infected blood in a transfusion or through contaminated needles. A contaminated needle-stick exposure may occur accidentally in the health care setting or through the sharing of needles during drug use. The risk of becoming infected after an accidental needle-stick injury with a contaminated syringe is low (0.32%). The risk of becoming infected after a single exposure to contaminated injection-drug equipment is higher (0.67%). Although the risk of becoming infected from a transfusion with infected blood is very high (almost 100%), the blood supply in industrialized countries is routinely tested for the presence of antibodies to HIV. Contaminated blood is discarded. However, certain times after infection with the virus, antibodies may not appear in infected blood, making a contaminated transfusion possible. These times include the period after infection before antibody response has developed, and at the end stages of AIDS when an individual's immune system may be so depressed that antibody levels are negligible.

Other individuals at risk of becoming infected with HIV are those exposed to semen or vaginal fluid during sexual intercourse with an infected individual. In the United States, but not in other areas of the world, the incidence of infection in male homosexuals is greater than in heterosexuals, which may be related to the breakdown and bleeding of rectal cells that occurs during anal intercourse. The probability of HIV transmission after unprotected receptive anal intercourse is estimated to be 0.8% to 3.2%. Heterosexual transmission of the virus also occurs. This is true in all parts of the world, but is especially common in certain African countries and in countries where prostitution is common and acceptable. In general, heterosexual transmission more easily occurs from male to female; the probability of becoming infected from a single encounter with an infected partner is approximately 0.09% for a woman and 0.03% for a man.

The likelihood of becoming infected with the virus during heterosexual or homosexual intercourse depends on many factors. Exposure to HIV from a partner experiencing a primary infection (e.g., before an antibody response has developed) appears to increase the risk of infection compared to exposure from a partner who has had the infection for a longer period and has already produced antibodies. Similarly, a partner nearing the end of an infection has a higher titer of virus than at other times, and may show virtually no remaining immune resistance. The presence of a sexually transmitted disease in either partner also increases the risk of sexual transmission because of the occurrence of open wounds with some sexually transmitted diseases and the increased number of white blood cells in an area of infection. In women, cervical ectopy, a change in the structure of the cervix that causes it to be more fragile and likely to bleed, increases the likelihood of infection from a given exposure. Cervical ectopy is more common in teenagers, pregnant women, and women taking oral contraceptives, placing women from any of these categories at increased risk. Sex during menstruation may increase the risk of transmission from the male to the female, and the female to the male. And finally, the incidence of HIV in uncircumcised men is eight times as high as in men who are circumcised. This may be related to the co-occurrence of sexually transmitted diseases in uncircumcised men, or to the abundance of immune cells in the foreskin. There is also a greater risk of infection in sex partners of uncircumcised men. This finding may explain why some African countries show especially high rates of heterosexual transmission: these same countries also have been reported to show a cultural preference against circumcision.

SPREAD TO WOMEN AND CHILDREN

In the United States, HIV infection is increasing among women, usually after sexual intercourse with infected intravenous drug users or bisexual men. Women are more susceptible than men to infection during heterosexual intercourse because of the normal microscopic vaginal tears and bleeds that occur with intercourse. In addition, infected semen remains in the woman's vagina longer than the amount of time the penis is exposed to vaginal secretions.

A woman infected with HIV may pass the infection on to her infant across the placenta, usually during the third trimester, or after exposure of the infant to contaminated blood and amniotic fluid during the birth process. An infant born to an infected mother has approximately a 25% chance of becoming infected with the virus. The use of anti-HIV drugs administered to an infected mother during pregnancy and to an infant of an infected mother soon after birth, can significantly reduce the rate of infant infection. Some health workers and HIV advocates propose that because of this documented protection to the infant, all pregnant women should be tested for HIV infection as soon as pregnancy is confirmed. A woman may also acquire the virus after giving birth and pass it to her infant during breastfeeding.

Pediatric Consideration

In the United States, AIDS is the sixth leading cause of death in 15 to 24 year olds; it is the second leading cause of death among individuals 25 to 34 years of age. Because the median time for development of AIDS after HIV infection is 11 years, many of those dying of AIDS in their 20s and 30s were infected as teens. HIV infection in teens is related to a high level of unprotected intercourse, as evidenced by reports from The Centers for Disease Control and Prevention (CDC) that more than half of adolescents in the United States have had unprotected sexual intercourse by the age of 19. Educating teens about the risks of HIV infection and techniques to prevent infection is critical.

CLINICAL MANIFESTATIONS

- Flu-like symptoms, including a low-grade fever, aches, and chills, may develop a few weeks to a few months after infection. These symptoms correspond to the initial production of antibody to the virus. Symptoms resolve after the initial immune response reduces the number of virus particles, although the virus survives in other infected cells.
- During the latent period, an individual infected with HIV may be symptomless, or in some cases may experience persistent lymphadenopathy (swollen lymph nodes).
- Two to ten years after HIV infection, most individuals begin to experience opportunistic infections. These illnesses indicate the onset of AIDS and include vaginal and oral yeast infections, and various viral infections such as varicella zoster (chickenpox and shingles), cytomegalovirus, or persistent herpes simplex. Women may develop chronic yeast infections or pelvic inflammatory disease.
- Once AIDS is established, respiratory infections, often with the opportunistic organism Pneumocystis carinii, become frequent. Multiple-drug–resistant tuberculosis may develop because a patient with AIDS is unable to mount an effective immune response to fight the bacterium, even with the help of antibiotics. Patients

with AIDS who develop tuberculosis typically experience a rapidly worsening course of the disease, leading to death within a few months. The disease frequently spreads to extrapulmonary sites including the brain or bone.

- Central nervous system manifestations include headaches, motor defects, seizures, personality changes, and dementia. Patients may become blind and eventually comatose. Many of these symptoms result from opportunistic viral and bacterial infections of the CNS, which cause inflammation of the brain. HIV may also directly injure brain cells.
- Diarrhea and wasting away of body fat are common in patients with AIDS. Diarrhea results from viral and protozoal infections. Oral and esophageal thrush (yeast) infections cause extreme pain when chewing and swallowing, and contribute to the loss of body fat and failure to thrive.
- Various cancers occur at an increased rate in patients with AIDS because of the lack of a cell-mediated immune response against neoplastic cells. Especially common in patients with AIDS is the otherwise unusual cancer, Kaposi's sarcoma. Kaposi's sarcoma is a cancer of the vascular system characterized by red skin lesions. Most individuals who develop Kaposi's sarcoma have been infected through homosexual intercourse. Recent evidence suggests that coinfection with a unique herpes virus, herpesvirus 8, may be required for the development of Kaposi's sarcoma. Herpesvirus 8 is uncommon in the general population, but common in the U.S. homosexual population.

DIAGNOSTIC TOOLS

- Immediately after infection, CD4+ cell counts may decrease, but soon return to normal as the initial immune response contains the infection.
- Antibodies against HIV usually appear 4 to 6 weeks after infection, but may take 6 months or longer in some cases. If a serum sample is identified as HIV positive (having a positive antibody titer), a Western blot test will be performed to confirm infection. Uninfected infants born to infected mothers may appear HIV positive for more than a year after birth because of the presence of maternal antibodies.
- CD4 cell counts eventually begin to decrease. When levels reach fewer than 200 to 300 cells/mL of blood, opportunistic infections develop. The progress of the disease and the success of various treatments can be followed by measuring a patient's CD4+ cells over time.
- Tests to measure the viral load present at any given time in the blood of an infected individual have been shown to be highly accurate in predicting the occurrence of symptoms, the prognosis,

and the general state of health of an individual. Those found to have high amounts of virus have an accelerated progression of the disease regardless of the number of CD4+ cells. The greater the number of virus particles present in an individual, the greater the likelihood of transmission of virus between individuals during sexual intercourse and between mother and infant.
- Tests to measure HIV RNA also are predictive of host status. HIV RNA levels often are followed to evaluate the success of AIDS treatment.

TREATMENT

At this time, there is no cure for AIDS, thus prevention of HIV infection is essential. Prevention means not coming into contact with any HIV-contaminated body fluid. Because it is usually impossible to know in advance whether body fluid is contaminated with HIV, one should assume contamination unless proven otherwise. To avoid exposure to HIV one should:

- Practice sexual abstinence or mutually monogamous sexual intercourse with a noninfected partner.
- Be tested for the virus at least 6 months after the last unprotected sexual intercourse because it may take at least 6 months after exposure to the virus to build antibodies. Oral sex may also pass the virus.
- Use a latex condom if sexual intercourse occurs with a person whose HIV status is unknown. Although latex condoms can significantly reduce the risk of HIV transmission, they are unlikely to provide 100% protection against viral transmission.
- Refrain from sharing needles with anyone for any reason.
- Prevent infection to a fetus or newborn. A woman should know her and her partner's HIV status before pregnancy. If a pregnant woman is positive for HIV, anti-HIV drugs or antibodies can be given to her during pregnancy and to the infant after birth. Treatment in utero may also be effective in preventing transmission of the virus to the fetus or newborn. An infected mother should not breastfeed her infant. Breast pumps should not be shared.
- Postexposure prophylactic treatment with a reverse transcriptase inhibitor (AZT) after accidental needle stick or sexual exposure decreases the odds of acquiring primary HIV infection.

If infection occurs, drug treatment regimens are available that can dramatically change the course of infection. If infected with HIV, treatment involves:

- Anti-HIV drug therapy, involving a combination of two nucleoside reverse transcriptase inhibitors and a protease inhibitor. The reverse transcriptase inhibitors, such as azidothymidine (AZT), block the enzyme reverse transcriptase and thus block the ability of HIV to incorporate into host DNA. The protease inhibitor blocks the transcription of HIV RNA into protein. These drugs do not cure AIDS, but may dramatically prolong survival time for some people and are effective in reducing the number of infections that individuals with AIDS develop. Some studies suggest that initiating therapy early may prevent CD4+ cell infection. Early studies suggest that triple combination therapy is safe and effective in treating infants born to mothers infected with HIV.

- Side effects of the anti-HIV drugs include nausea, headaches, and bone marrow suppression, leading to anemia and fatigue. Protease inhibitor therapy is associated with hyperlipidemia and insulin resistance. Adherence to the triple therapy is difficult and may be impossible for some patients. Drugs must be taken frequently, in precise order and at certain times of the day. The cost of long-term combination therapy is enormous; HIV disproportionately affects the poor and therapy may be impossible for some countries and for uninsured individuals.
- Education to avoid alcohol and illicit drugs. A healthy diet and stress-free lifestyle are important. Stress, poor nutrition, alcohol, and other drugs are known to impair immune functioning. Smoking should be avoided.
- Avoidance of other infections because they could lead to activation of T cells and may accelerate the replication of HIV. To prevent infection, available vaccines should be administered as long as live viruses vaccines are not used.
- Treatment for specific infections and cancers as they arise.

Selected Bibliography

Beck, G. & Habicht, G. S. (1996). Immunity and the invertebrates. *Scientific American* 275, 60–66.

Borkowsky, W., Kasinski, K., Cao, Y., et al. (1994). Correlation of perinatal transmission of human immunodeficiency virus type 1 with maternal viremia and lymphocyte phenotypes. *Journal of Pediatrics* 125, 345–351.

Caldwell, J. C. & Caldwell, P. (1996). The African AIDS epidemic. *Scientific American* 276, 62–68.

Centers for Disease Control. Selected behaviors that increase risk for HIV infection among high school students—US. (1992). *MMWR* 41, 231–240.

Engelhard, V. H. (1994). How cells process antigens. *Scientific American* 271, 54–61.

Epstein, F. H. (1998). Antibodies to DNA. *New England Journal of Medicine* 338, 1359–1367.

Gueldner, S. H., Poon, L. W., LaVia, M., Virella, G., Michel, Y., Bramlett, M. H., Noble, C. A., & Paulling, E. (1997). Long term exercise patterns and immune function in healthy older women: a report of preliminary findings. *Mechanisms of Ageing and Development* 93, 215–222.

Huston, D. P. (1997). The biology of the immune system. *Journal of the American Medical Association* 278, 1804–1814.

Janeway, C. A., Jr. (1993). How the immune system recognizes invaders. *Scientific American* 269, 72–79.

Lichtenstien, L. M. (1993). Allergy and the immune system. *Scientific American* 269, 116–125.

Luzuriaga, K., Bryson, Y., Krogstad, P., et al. (1997). Combination treatment with zidovudine, didanosine, and nevirapine in infants with human immunodeficiency virus type I infection. *New England Journal of Medicine* 336, 1343–1349.

Luzuriaga, K., Bryson, Y., Martin, J. N., Ganem, D. E., Osmond, D. H., Page-Shafer, K. A., Macrae, D., & Kedes, D. H. (1998). Sexual transmission and the natural history of human herpesvirus 8 infection. *New England Journal of Medicine* 338, 948–954.

Nowak, N. A. & McMichael, A. J. (1995). How HIV defeats the immune system. *Scientific American* 273, 58–65.

O'Brien, S. J. & Dean, M. (1997). In search of AIDS-resistance genes. *Scientific American* 277, 44–51.

Palellta, F. J., Delaney, K. M., Moorman, A. C., et al. (1998). Declining morbidity and mortality among patients with advanced human immunodeficiency virus infection. *New England Journal of Medicine* 338, 853–860.

Royce, R. A., Sena, A., Cates, W., & Cohen, M. S. (1997). Sexual transmission of HIV. *New England Journal of Medicine* 336, 1072–1078.

Samet, J. H., Winter, M. R., Grant, L., & Hingson, R. (1997). Factors associated with HIV testing among sexually active adolescents: a Massachusetts survey. *Pediatrics* 100, 371–377.

Schur, P. H. (1992). Third International Conference on Systemic Lupus Erythematosus. *Arthritis Rheumatology* 35, 1238–1240.

Shaver, T. S., Harley, J. B., & Moser, K. L. (1997). Heredity and systemic lupus erythematosis: dissecting a complex genetic disease. *Kansan Medicine* 97, 18–22.

Smart, B. A. & Ochs, H. D. (1997). The molecular basis and treatment of primary immunodeficiency disorders. *Current Opinion in Pediatrics* 9, 570–576.

Timonen, T. (1997). Natural killer cells: endothelial interactions, migration, and target cell recognition. *Journal of Leukocyte Biology* 62, 693–701.

Volberding, P. A. & Deeks, S. G. (1998). Antiretroviral therapy for HIV infection. *Journal of the American Medical Association* 279, 1343–1344.

Weissman, I. L. & Cooper, M. D. (1993). How the immune system develops. *Scientific American* 269, 64–71.

Wiznia, A. A., Lamabert, G., Dobrosyzcki, J., et al. (1994). Virologic, immunologic, and clinical evaluation of HIV antibody status of symptom-free children born to infected mothers. *Journal of Pediatrics* 125, 352–355.

4 SYSTEMIC FOUNDATIONS OF HEALTH AND DISEASE

Good health is relative. For some, good health means being able to run a marathon or not miss a day of school the entire year. For others, good health means making it through the winter without a severe asthmatic attack or returning to work after recovery from a myocardial infarct. For all of us, however, there are basic physiologic requirements that must be met for a foundation of good health to exist. What comprises the foundation of good health and examples of what happens when this foundation is weakened are the bases for discussion in this chapter.

● ● ●

PHYSIOLOGIC CONCEPTS

Being Healthy

Being healthy means different things to different people, and different things to the same person throughout a lifetime. What is considered healthy at one age, for example, the deep slumber of infancy, would be abnormal or unusual in an elderly person. Likewise, although the onset of menses in a 13-year-old is a sign of normal growth and development, it would be an indication of pathology in a young child or a postmenopausal woman. What is considered healthy also is relative between people at the same age; is a 58-year-old male with well-controlled hypertension more or less healthy than a 58-year-old with normal blood pressure who smokes a pack and a half of cigarettes a day? And finally, what does it mean when our health status suddenly changes? For example, given that most cancers take 15 years or so to reach the stage where they can be clinically diagnosed, does it mean that a 48-year-old attorney who is diagnosed with breast cancer following a routine mammogram has been unhealthy for the last decade, even though during that time she would have described herself as in the best of health? What if she had skipped this year's mammogram; would she have continued to be in the best of health for one more year?

In addition to the dilemma of defining health is the very real fact that in our country and in our world, health is not equally distributed. Studies repeatedly have shown that low income and poor health are closely related. The effects of poverty on health may be seen acutely; for example, a woman living in poverty may not seek help for a nagging respiratory tract infection until it is full-blown pneumonia for which she needs to be hospitalized. Likewise, otitis media, a condition usually treated by antibiotics, is more likely to result in inpatient care in those without insurance and in those without access to medical care compared to those with insurance and access to medical care. The effects of poverty may also result in chronically worsened health. For example, persons who are uninsured or underinsured may not be able to purchase antihypertensive medications for daily use, or they may, to save money, take medication for diabetes every other day instead of daily, to increase the length of time they are medicated. Other examples of poor health that are linked to poverty include mothers diluting formula for infants to save money and those with AIDS who do not qualify for health insurance compared to those who can afford the new expensive therapies.

In addition to poverty, race also impacts health. An example of this is the decrease in birth weight of infants born to African- American women compared to white American women. Other conditions of poor health, such as hypertension and certain types of cancer, are increased or more aggressive in African-Americans. Reasons for this are multifactorial, but include reduced access to primary care and prevention, reduced access to screening examinations, and issues related directly to poverty. Genetics plays a role as well.

Another discrepancy in health care includes the inequalities between the sexes. There is an increased risk of unrecognized heart disease in women compared to men and a reduced likelihood that a woman with end-stage renal disease will receive a kidney transplant compared to a man. In addition, women are more likely than men to have their symptoms described as psychiatric in nature.

As the above paragraphs suggest, what it means to be healthy, and why some individuals have a better chance of being healthy than others, are ethical questions and considerations that cannot be easily reconciled. What we can do, however, is identify signs and standards of good health and recognize certain patterns that indicate when the foundations of good health have been shaken. Throughout life, normal growth and development, the maintenance of healthy sleep patterns, and the ability to fight off infection are some easily identified characteristics of a good health foundation. In addition, good health includes good mental health, which depends on feelings of self-worth, security, and love. Individuals without the foundations for good mental health may develop depression and behavioral disorders as well as physical ailments.

Growth and Development

Starting with embryogenesis, growth and development follow an accepted pattern that continues after birth and throughout the lifetime. Growth and development involves physical, cognitive, and emotional progression through well-identified stages. Our bodies go through the physical stages of infancy, "toddlerhood," early childhood, middle childhood, early adolescence, late adolescence, young adulthood, middle adulthood, and older adulthood. Cognitive and behavioral developmental patterns advance and mirror physical growth and development in healthy individuals. This preordained pattern of growth and development is determined by the genetic blueprint of an individual but can be modified by environmental factors including nutrition, infectious agents, and physical trauma. Indications that an individual is progressing along accepted norms of physical, cognitive, and behavioral development include expected increases in height and weight, the attainment of cognitive skills, and the reaching of developmental milestones.

HEIGHT AND WEIGHT

Height and weight are measured at birth and throughout a lifetime. Indeed, even prenatal measurements of fetal length can be used to indicate normal development. Physical growth typically follows an expected curve, based on previous height and weight measurements and family patterns. In the United States, height and weight are measured and graphed in children from birth to age 18 years at each well-child visit; a resulting growth chart (Figure 4.1) is kept in a child's permanent medical file. Head circumference also is measured from birth to the age of 2 years; this information is used to evaluate normal growth of the bones of the skull and to identify inappropriate closure or expansion. When an infant or child deviates from his or her growth curve significantly (usually defined as a change greater than two standard deviations on the growth curve), it may indicate a nutritional deficiency, an organic disease, or possibly a situation of neglect or abuse. A significant deviation in an infant or child's growth curve must be evaluated by a health care provider. Infants and children who do not receive regular well-child visits may lose or gain weight or height inappropriately without detection or follow-up.

In adulthood, height is less frequently tracked, at least until used as an indicator of osteoporosis in the elderly. Weight, however, is commonly measured at each visit to a health provider and by many adults at home. In fact, knowing that their weight will be measured and recorded has been identified as one reason that some people do not choose to schedule annual physical examinations.

Weight is usually evaluated in terms of height. For example, a standard recommendation for a woman is that for every inch over 5 feet she should add 5 pounds to 100 to determine her ideal weight (for example, a woman 5 feet 2 inches should ideally weigh 110 by this calculation). Another means of evaluating physical growth and development in adults is to determine an individual's **body-mass index**. The body-mass index is a ratio of a person's weight (in grams) to height (in meters). The equation for body-mass index is as follows:

$$\text{body weight (grams)}^2/\text{body height (meters)}^2$$

In pounds and inches: 1) multiply weight in pounds by 703; 2) multiply height in inches by height in inches; and 3) divide the answer in step

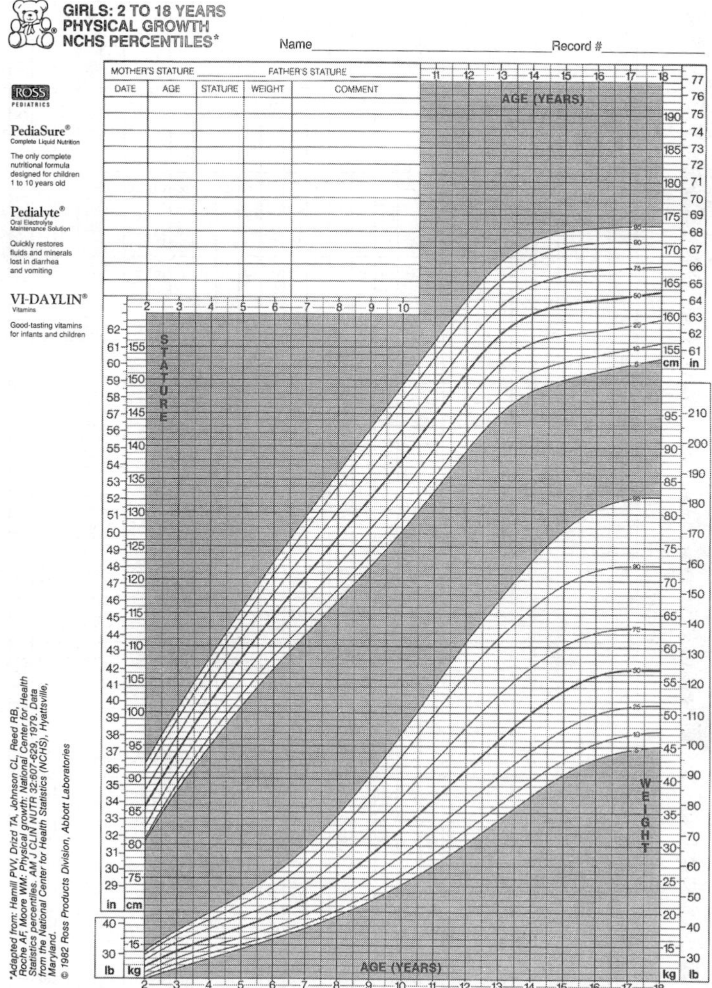

Figure 4-1. A growth curve for a female, from 2 to 18 years of age.

1 by the answer in step 2. Table 4.1 shows **body-mass** index values based on pounds and inches.

It is believed that in most cases, the body-mass index provides a better indication of the overall fat proportion of a person than does simply measuring body weight. Adults with a body-mass index of 20 to 24 are considered in a normal range; a **body-mass** index of 25 or above is considered overweight (a reduction from the previous limit of 27). Those with an index of 30 or more are classified as obese. In adults, as **body-mass** index rises above 25, the risk of high blood

Table 4-1. Body Mass Index

	HEIGHT (in)																											
	49	50	51	52	53	54	55	56	57	58	59	60	61	62	63	64	65	66	67	68	69	70	71	72	73	74	75	76
WEIGHT (lbs)																												
45	13	13	12	12	11	11	10	10	10	9	9	9	8															
50	15	14	13	13	12	12	12	11	11	10	10	10	9	9	9	9	8											
55	16	15	15	14	14	13	13	12	12	12	11	11	10	10	10	9	9	9										
60	18	17	16	16	15	15	14	13	13	13	12	12	11	11	11	10	10	10	9	9								
65	19	18	17	17	16	16	15	15	14	14	13	13	12	12	12	11	11	10	10	10	10							
70	21	20	19	18	17	17	16	16	15	15	14	14	13	13	12	12	12	11	11	11	10	10						
75	22	21	20	20	19	18	17	17	16	16	15	15	14	14	13	13	12	12	12	11	11	11	10					
80	24	22	21	21	20	19	19	18	17	17	16	16	15	15	14	14	13	13	13	12	12	11	11	11				
85	25	24	23	22	21	21	20	19	18	18	17	17	16	16	15	15	14	14	13	13	13	12	12	12	11			
90	27	25	24	23	22	22	21	20	19	19	18	18	17	17	16	15	15	14	14	14	13	13	13	12	12	12		
95	28	27	25	25	24	23	22	21	20	20	19	19	18	17	17	16	16	15	15	14	14	14	13	13	13	12	12	
100	29	28	27	26	25	24	23	22	22	21	20	20	19	18	18	17	17	16	16	15	15	14	14	14	13	13	13	12
105	31	30	28	27	26	25	24	24	23	22	21	21	20	19	19	18	17	17	16	16	16	15	15	14	14	13	13	13
110	32	31	30	29	27	27	25	25	24	23	22	22	21	20	19	19	18	18	17	17	16	16	15	15	15	14	14	13
115	34	32	31	30	29	28	27	26	25	24	23	23	22	21	20	20	19	18	18	17	17	16	16	16	15	15	14	14
120	35	34	32	31	30	29	28	27	26	25	24	24	23	22	21	20	20	19	19	18	18	17	17	16	16	15	15	15
125	37	35	34	33	31	30	29	28	27	26	25	25	24	23	22	21	21	20	20	19	19	18	17	17	17	16	16	15
130	38	37	35	34	32	31	30	29	28	27	26	26	25	24	23	22	22	21	20	20	19	19	18	18	17	17	16	16
135	40	38	36	35	34	33	31	30	29	28	27	27	25	25	24	23	22	22	21	20	20	19	19	18	18	17	17	16
140	41	39	38	36	35	34	32	31	30	29	28	27	26	26	25	24	23	22	22	21	21	20	20	19	19	18	18	17
145	43	41	39	38	36	35	34	33	31	30	29	28	27	27	26	25	24	23	23	22	21	21	20	20	19	19	18	18
150	44	42	40	39	37	36	35	34	32	31	30	29	28	28	27	26	25	24	24	23	22	21	21	20	20	19	19	18
155	46	44	42	40	39	37	36	35	33	33	31	30	29	29	27	26	26	25	24	23	23	22	22	21	21	20	19	19
160	47	45	43	42	40	39	37	36	35	34	32	31	30	29	28	27	27	26	25	24	24	23	22	22	21	21	20	19
170	50	48	46	44	42	41	39	38	37	36	34	33	32	31	30	29	28	27	27	26	25	24	24	23	23	22	21	21
175		49	47	46	44	42	40	39	38	37	35	34	33	32	31	30	29	28	27	27	26	25	24	24	23	22	22	21

pressure and elevated LDL cholesterol levels increase while HDL cholesterol levels decreases. The result is that coronary artery disease, stroke, hypertension, type II diabetes, gallbladder disease, osteoarthritis, and certain cancers—including cancer of the breast and endometrium—increase with a high body-mass index. It should be pointed out that the use of this index has primarily been studied in adults, and that studies are needed to validate and refine its use in children. It should also be mentioned that a very low body-mass index may indicate an eating disorder or a chronic illness. In addition, some individuals may show a high body-mass index because they have a more muscular physique, not because they are obese. Finally, the body-mass index cannot be evaluated in a vacuum; family history, past medical history, and high-risk behaviors such as smoking and alcohol consumption must also be considered.

COGNITIVE DEVELOPMENT

Just as physical development, cognitive development progresses along a relatively predictable path, especially during infancy and childhood. There are many different models used to predict normal cognitive development, one of which is Piaget's Model (Table 4.2). This model is frequently used to identify expected cognitive milestones. Cognitive development is assessed both formally and informally at each well-child medical visit. Cognitive development is especially evaluated by attainment of language skills and the ability to follow directions; often, parents are the first to express concerns regarding the development of these skills. In school-aged children, inability to attain a level of cognitive development within the range of others of the same age is often noticed by teachers. Physical causes of cognitive deficiency, such as hearing or vision defects, must be evaluated in children suspected of delayed attainment of cognitive skills.

Table 4-2. Piaget's Stages of Cognitive Development

PERIOD	AGE	CHARACTERISTICS
Sensorimotor	Birth to 24 months	Interprets and uses environment through senses.
Preoperational	2 to 7 years	Internalizes environment, rules and relationships. Is egocentric (self-centered in thought).
Concrete operations	7 to 11 years and older	Beginning of rational thought. Understands relationships and observable world.
Formal operations	12 years and older	Adult thinking. Considers multiple variables at once.

EMOTIONAL DEVELOPMENT

Emotional development also continues throughout a lifetime. Some emotions appear to be instinctive, for example, happiness, fear, and anger. Other emotions develop with experience, and are considered higher level, for example, hope, jealousy, and despair. Maslow's hierarchy of needs (Table 4.3) suggests that a lifetime of experiences sets the stage for emotional growth; only if the basic human needs of food and shelter have been met can one move to higher level needs such as the need for love and belonging or self-actualization. Erickson's model of emotional development suggests similarly that from infancy onward, the attainment of emotional milestones progresses in domino fashion beginning with the trust of infancy and ending with the ego integrity that comes with the successful completion of age-related tasks throughout the lifespan (Table 4.4). In this hierarchy, it is suggested that individuals who are not provided with the support at each stage to progress emotionally will stagnate and never reach full emotional satisfaction. Erickson's model has been questioned recently as being culture-specific and sex-specific; for example, autonomy is not necessarily seen as an important step to the highest level of self-fulfillment in some cultures.

Pediatric Consideration

The screening examinations used to test visual acuity in preschool-aged children offer an excellent opportunity to evaluate a child's age-

Table 4-3. Maslow's Hierarchy of Needs

Table 4-3. Maslow's Hierarchy of Needs
SELF-ACTUALIZATION To look for meaning of life
AESTHETIC Desire for beauty in art, music, and literature
SELF-ACTUALIZATION Acceptance of self and others
ESTEEM Self-respect, respect for others
LOVE AND BELONGING Affection, love, acceptance
SAFETY NEEDS Stability, sense of security
PHYSIOLOGIC NEEDS Basic human needs for food and shelter

Table 4-4. Erickson's Theory of Personality Development

STAGE OF DEVELOPMENT	DEVELOPMENTAL TASK
Infancy	**Trust vs. Mistrust**
Toddler	Autonomy vs. Shame and Doubt
Preschool	Initiate vs. Guilt
School Age	Industry vs. Inferiority
Adolescence	Identity Formation vs. Identity Confusion
Young Adult	Intimacy vs. Isolation
Middle Age	Generativity vs. Stagnation and Self-Absorption
Old Age	Ego Integrity vs. Self-Despair

appropriate physical, cognitive, and emotional development. In order to complete the vision examination, a child must not only visually focus on the chart, but also must be able and *willing* to follow complex directions, and be able and willing to pay attention for an extended period of time.

Sleep Patterns

Sleep is a necessary human condition. Sleep functions in a restorative fashion. Although the exact mechanism by which sleep allows the brain to restore itself is unknown, it is known that if a person's sleep patterns are repeatedly interrupted, health and mental functioning can become severely disturbed. Sleep naturally occurs in a diurnal pattern stimulated by the release of the hormone melatonin in early evening.

Sleep is divided into two phases: rapid eye movement (REM) sleep and non-REM sleep. Non-REM sleep is further divided into four stages, which are differentiated from each other and REM sleep by measurement of brain wave activity. With the onset of sleep, an individual begins moving through stages 1 to 4 of non-REM sleep. REM sleep usually occurs after 1 to 2 hours of non-REM sleep; however, it may start sooner if a person has been deprived of REM sleep. REM sleep lasts for approximately 90 minutes. Non-REM and REM sleep alternate throughout the night. When the sleep cycle is interrupted, a person must start over at the first stage of non-REM sleep. If this pattern continues, REM sleep may be lost. Most people require at least 7 to 8 hours of sleep a night in order to have true sleep balance. Less than that quantity, or poor-quality sleep (i.e., frequent interruptions in the cycle), can result in sleep deprivation, hallucinations, and even death. Individuals doing shift work, either long-term or short-term, must adjust the diurnal pattern of their sleep to sleep during the day. The neurologic pathways of sleep are described in Chapter 7.

Defense Against Infection

Our ability to fight infection depends on an adequate immune system, an adequate hematologic system, good nutrition, good blood flow to sites of infection and injury, and rest. Although healthy individuals occasionally do develop infections, a cornerstone of good health is the ability to respond to and defeat most infectious organisms. In some cases, an overresponsive immune system may result in a hypersensitivity reaction (allergy or autoimmune disease). The immune system is discussed in Chapter 3.

Tests of Health Status

DENVER II DEVELOPMENTAL SCREENING TEST

The Denver II Developmental Screening Test is a tool that uses a series of parental answers and direct observations to evaluate physical (fine motor and gross motor) and cognitive development in infants and children from birth to 6 years of age. For each question concerning a specific ability of the child and for each specific task observed by the clinician, a recording is made on a graph as to whether the child performed (passed) or did not perform the task. Performance for each task is related to expectations based on the child's age. Inability to perform an identified age-appropriate task raises a warning of developmental delay.

SLEEP OR NUTRITION DIARY

Individuals being evaluated for a sleep disorder are often asked to keep a diary of the hours spent in bed asleep. Likewise, individuals being evaluated for undernutrition or overnutrition are frequently asked to keep a food diary of all meals eaten. The length of time this information is recorded in these diaries varies, but ideally at least 2 weeks of records should be attained.

ELECTROENCEPHALOGRAMS

Specific tests to evaluate brain waves, including the electroencephalogram (EEG), may be used in patients with sleep disorders. Patterns of electrical currents are observed throughout the sequence of normal sleep. Disruptions or deficiencies in expected EEG patterns may indicate a sleep disorder.

● PATHOPHYSIOLOGIC CONCEPTS

Obesity

Obesity is defined as a weight-to-height ratio 120% or more above ideal and a triceps skin fold greater than the 85th percentile. Using the body-mass index, obesity is defined as an index of 30 or greater. Obesity is considered a risk factor for heart disease, certain cancers, type II diabetes mellitus, and musculoskeletal complaints. Obesity occurs when there is an imbalance in caloric intake versus output. There are a variety of genetic, social, and psychological variables that interact to cause obesity.

Anorexia

Anorexia is defined as a lack of desire for food. Anorexia may be due to physical conditions, for example, chemotherapy treatments or hepatitis, or may be emotionally induced. Anorexia nervosa is a condition where food is refused in a desire to be extremely thin. There is not a true lack of desire for food in anorexia nervosa.

Failure to Thrive

Failure to thrive is a condition primarily seen in childhood in which an infant or child does not progress along an expected growth curve, or falls two or more standard deviations from his or her previous level of growth. Failure to thrive may occur with a chronic illness, for example, cystic fibrosis, or may result from emotional or physical neglect or abuse. The concept of an individual experiencing failure to thrive can also be expanded to include adults who lose a significant amount of weight because of illness or neglect. This may be especially common in the elderly.

Insomnia

Insomnia is the inability to fall asleep or stay asleep for a specified length of time, usually considered at least 6 hours. Insomnia may result from physical or mental causes; it may be temporary or chronic.

Fatigue

The term "fatigue" can be used at the cellular level to describe a muscle fiber that is unable to contract in response to neural stimulation or the condition any cell might experience if its energy production is halted as a result of a lack of oxygen. Clinically, the term "fatigue" is used to describe a state of extreme tiredness during which an individual may have difficulty concentrating and staying awake. This definition emphasizes the subjective nature of fatigue. Fatigue may result from sleep deprivation, stress, or poor nutrition. During an acute infection, cytokines released by white blood cells may cause fatigue as may certain drug therapies, chronic illnesses, and severe anemia. Fatigue is also common during pregnancy.

Immunodeficiency

Immunodeficiency refers to a reduction in the number or functioning of the T lymphocytes, B lymphocytes, or both. Some or all of the different types of T lymphocytes and B lymphocytes may be affected. Causes and consequences of immunodeficiency are discussed in Chapter 3.

CONDITIONS OF DISEASE OR INJURY

Eating Disorder

The term "eating disorder" is used to describe one of two types of abnormal eating conditions: anorexia nervosa and bulimia. Both of these conditions are most commonly seen in young women and have a variety of physical and emotional causes and implications. They may also occur in some young men, especially male athletes who must achieve weight limits such as wrestlers or those who have suffered sexual abuse. The incidence of eating disorders has increased approximately 2 to 5 times in the United States in the last 30 years. Eating disorders are a problem of Western or Western-style nations; developing and underdeveloped nations very rarely report problems with anorexia nervosa or bulimia. The diagnostic criteria for anorexia nervosa and bulimia are established in the *Diagnostic and Statistical Manual of Mental Disorders, 4th edition* (DSM-IV).

ANOREXIA NERVOSA

Anorexia nervosa is a condition whereby an individual, usually a preteen, teen, or young adult woman, eats extremely sparingly out of a morbid fear of becoming fat. Anorexia nervosa likely has a number of different factors contributing to its cause, including pressures put on girls in our society to be unrealistically thin; parental and self-induced pressures for perfection in school, athletics, or behavior; and a biological vulnerability or predisposition. Family dynamics may be dysfunctional. The female to male ratio is 10 to 1, with bimodal age peaks at 14 and 18 years of age. Anorexia nervosa results in *or is caused by* an imbalance in the hypothalamic–pituitary–gonadal or adrenal axes. Anorexia nervosa may include restricting food, purging, or intense caloric expenditures (i.e., repeated daily bouts of extreme exercise) or combinations of all three methods of weight loss. The prevalence of anorexia in the United States is estimated to be approximately 0.48% in women 15 to 19 years of age.

Bulimia is characterized by the eating of a very large amount of food during a short period of time, after which the individual uses self-induced vomiting or laxatives, enemas, or diuretics to prevent weight gain. This type of bulimia is referred to as the "purging type." Excessive exercise may also be used following a binge of eating to prevent weight gain; this is referred to as the "nonpurging" type of bulimia. Patients with bulimia often feel out of control over their eating. Feelings of low self-esteem, depression, and self-destructive behavior have been described in association with bulimia. Bulimia has been suggested to have a prevalence of 1 to 5% in adolescent females in the United States; much higher rates, from 10 to 50% of older adolescents, admit to having had some experience with binging or purging.

CLINICAL MANIFESTATIONS

- The diagnostic criteria for anorexia nervosa include:
    1. A refusal to maintain a minimal normal body weight, leading to a weight less than 85% of that expected for height and age.
    2. An intense fear of gaining weight even though the person is obviously underweight.
    3. A disturbance in the perception of body weight, size, or shape.
    4. Secondary amenorrhea for three consecutive menstrual cycles in girls who have experienced menses. Amenorrhea may occur before significant weight loss develops, suggesting that hypothalamic dysfunction may precede physical signs of the disorder.
- Some girls, especially younger teens, may not meet all criteria for anorexia nervosa, for example, they may not say they are too fat, but feel their extreme thinness is normal. These girls, too, should be observed and treated because irreversible effects on growth and development may occur even without frank anorexia nervosa.
- The diagnostic criteria for bulimia include the following:
    1. Recurrent episodes of binge eating followed by an inappropriate compensatory behavior (purging or intense exercise), occurring on average at least twice a week for 3 months.
    2. Feelings of lack of control over eating and an overconcern with weight and body shape.
- Most patients with bulimia are not underweight, but are usually of normal or slightly higher-than-normal weight.

DIAGNOSTIC TOOLS

- It is important to screen all preteens, teens, and young adults for an eating disorder at each well-child examination or annual physical examination. All patients should be asked questions concerning dietary intake, eating habits and rituals, weight history, and body image. Information on a history of binging or purging should be gathered, and exercise habits should be evaluated.
- A good history and physical examination will usually allow diagnosis of an eating disorder. A complete physical examination includes documentation of vital signs and weight while the patient is wearing only a dressing gown.
- Observance of systemic signs of an eating disorder, including destruction of teeth enamel from vomiting, and thin, fragile hair and

nails in those suffering from anorexia, may indicate the disorder. Patients with anorexia nervosa may have a fine layer of hair covering their body and an intolerance to the cold.

COMPLICATIONS

- There is a 4% mortality rate associated with anorexia nervosa, owing to a variety of causes, including electrolyte disturbance and arrhythmia, heart failure, and suicide. Bradycardia, hypotension, and a decrease in fat and lean muscle mass occur. A decrease in cardiac muscle mass contributes to the cardiac pathology.
- Patients with an eating disorder may develop chronic constipation related to low bulk intake and laxative overuse. Tooth enamel may be destroyed from repeated vomiting.
- Patients with bulimia may have significant disturbances in electrolytes leading to hypokalemic, hypochloremic metabolic alkalosis. They may become dehydrated. They may also develop aspiration pneumonia from inhaling vomitus.
- There is some evidence of cerebral cortex atrophy and ventricular dilatation with anorexia nervosa. Attention, concentration, and learning may be impaired.
- Hormonal abnormalities including amenorrhea, growth retardation, and delayed sexual maturation may occur in anorexia nervosa. The amenorrhea may lead to early osteoporosis.

TREATMENT

- The first step in treatment is medical stabilization. Some patients will need to be hospitalized, including those 75% or less than ideal weight, and those with arrhythmias, severe dehydration and electrolyte disturbance, or uncontrollable binging and purging. Patients who have unsuccessfully undergone outpatient treatment, or those who are in acute food refusal, may also need to be hospitalized.
- Before any psychosocial therapy is initiated in patients requiring hospitalization, some nutritional rehabilitation must occur. This is important because some of the psychologic disorders associated with anorexia nervosa, such as depression and food obsession, may be starvation-induced and relieved by weight gain.
- After the patient has regained a certain predetermined amount of weight, psychologic counseling, using a variety of methods including behavioral modification, usually is begun. Treatment must be interdisciplinary and should include the family as much as possible. The interdisciplinary approach is important for outpatient and inpatient treatment.
- It is important to emphasize to patients that the goal of treatment is not to make them fat, but rather to return them to physical and emotional health.

Sleep Disorders

Sleep disorders include difficulties falling asleep and staying asleep and abnormalities in the progression through the stages of sleep. Excessive somnolence, meaning excessive daytime sleep, also is considered a sleep disorder, and is frequently related to poor-quality sleep at night. Individuals who experience frequent changes in their sleep–wake schedules, for example, individuals who fly between significantly different time zones or individuals who are shift workers, also experience a type of sleep disorder. For these workers, as well as for truckers who frequently skimp on sleep, and medical interns and residents who may be sleep-deprived, decreased concentration and vigilance may occur, resulting in increasing risks of accidents and poor judgments.

INSOMNIA

Insomnia refers to the inability to fall asleep or stay asleep. Insomnia may result from a variety of causes, including the use of stimulant drugs such as caffeine, amphetamines, bronchodilating agents, or steroids. Exercise or alcohol use prior to bedtime or poor bedtime sleep habits, for example, working in bed or watching television in bed, may also contribute to insomnia. Insomnia may be related to periods of personal stress or anxiety, or it may be a symptom of depression. Chronic pain also may interfere with a person's ability to fall asleep or stay asleep. In addition, chronic pain and depression may affect an individual's progression through the stages of sleep, shortening certain stages of restorative sleep, resulting in a poorer quality of sleep. Insomnia may be short-term or chronic, and periods of insomnia may come and go.

Geriatric Consideration

Changes in the sleep pattern and sleep cycle are common in the elderly. Although the cause of this shift is unclear, it may be related to changes in other hypothalamic set-points, for example, temperature regulation, which occur as one ages. Many elderly individuals are bothered by the changes in sleep they experience and may use over-the-counter sleep-aid medications. Practitioners should ask elderly clients about sleep problems or changes and be aware of the use of any drug that might interact with other prescribed medications.

Pediatric Consideration

Children frequently experience sleep disorders, including night terrors, enuresis (bed-wetting), and somnambulism (sleepwalking). Most conditions are benign and the child will outgrow them in time. Emotional support and protection against injury are important considerations. Physical causes of the disorder should be ruled out.

CLINICAL MANIFESTATIONS

- Fatigue is the most common symptom in patients with insomnia. The fatigue may interfere with an individual's ability to work or perform family functions.
- Patients may appear subdued, with darkened circles under their eyes.

DIAGNOSTIC TOOLS

- Asking a patient to fill out a sleep diary for at least 2 weeks, including time spent in bed, times awakened during the night, and time of arising in the morning, may allow an objective appraisal of sleep pattern. Included in the diary should also be exercise times, and the number of caffeine-containing beverages and alcoholic beverages ingested and at what time of day. All over-the-counter and prescription medications taken should be reported.
- Patients may be asked to rate their level of fatigue using a simple Likert scale.
- Patients should also be questioned about unusual stresses or worries, and they should be assessed for depression.
- Some sleep disorders may be diagnosed using EEG screening.

COMPLICATIONS

- Chronic sleep deprivation may result in serious psychological problems. Even less serious bouts of insomnia may be cause of great concern for an individual and result in anxiety as well as decreased productivity.
- Individuals doing shift work or those who work despite fatigue may have an increased risk of accidents.

TREATMENT

- Maintaining a sleep diary is important to establish usual routine.
- Initiating good sleep habits is essential for patients with insomnia. Good sleep habits include the following: using the bedroom only for sleeping and having sexual relations, not exercising after approximately 6:00 p.m., and limiting or eliminating all exposure to caffeine-containing drugs or beverages. In addition, medications that act as stimulants should be evaluated regarding their timing of administration. When a person does wake in the night or cannot fall asleep, it is recommended that he or she gets out of bed after approximately 15 minutes. This helps prevent the bedroom from becoming a place of great anxiety. Once arisen, the person is instructed to do something relaxing for a short period of time, for example, having a glass of milk or cup of herbal tea or reading a slow book, before going back to bed. Watching television and reading an exciting novel are discouraged. This cycle is to be re-

peated as necessary through the night. In addition, time to bed and time up in the morning should be standardized, regardless of the amount of sleep obtained, and daytime napping should be avoided.

- For shift workers, appropriately timed exposure to bright light may improve functioning.
- Melatonin therapy has been reported to improve patients' sleep quantity and quality in some studies. Melatonin appears to restore circadian sleep rhythm; thus, it may be suggested for shift workers or individuals traveling to a significantly different time zone. Optimal dosing and scheduling regimens for melatonin have not been clearly identified at this time, nor have all implications and risks related to its use been determined.
- Patients who suffer from depression may be placed on appropriate antidepressive medications.
- Patients who suffer from pain that interferes with sleep may also benefit from low doses of antidepressants. Pain management may require additional medications as well.

Chronic Fatigue Syndrome

The term chronic fatigue syndrome (CFS) has been adopted to identify a severely debilitating chronic condition of at least 6 months' duration, consisting of a low-grade fever, myalgia (muscle/body aches), and other "flu-like" symptoms, and that does not have a clearly defined cause. A fundamental characteristic of CFS is the abrupt development of the illness, usually following a viral illness in a person who previously had been functioning at a high level and feeling healthy. Many patients with CFS can pinpoint the day their illness began.

Laboratory studies of patients with CFS show a variety of immunologic changes including alterations in the numbers and activities of certain B and T cells, as well as deficiencies in natural killer (NK) cell function. Likewise, endocrine function appears to be affected with reduced levels of cortisol as a result of elevated levels of pituitary adrenocorticotropin hormone (ACTH), suggesting a hypothalamic–pituitary–adrenal feedback abnormality. Menstrual cycle abnormalities have also been reported as has dysregulation of sex hormone production. Women are more likely to be affected with CFS than are men.

The cause of CFS is unknown, but the best hypotheses suggest that it begins with the exposure of a susceptible host to an infectious agent, such as the Epstein-Barr virus or the cytomegalovirus, or perhaps a fungal infection with *Candida*. Although the person may effectively fight off the infection, an imbalance in immune and endocrine function remains. It is suggested that individuals might be predisposed, or susceptible, to the development of CFS because of certain physical, psychological, or personality traits present at the time of infection. For example, individuals experiencing a particularly high level of stress at the time of infection appear to be at higher risk of developing the disorder. In addition, the presence of depression and anxiety consistently overlap with the diagnosis of CFS, with depression often preceding development of the syndrome. It needs to be emphasized, however, that even though CFS is associated with depression and stress, and includes in its symptomology somatic complaints such as headaches and difficulty with concentration, it is not a psychiatric disorder. This understanding is emphasized when one considers the presence of nonsomatic symptoms, including pharyngitis, palpable or tender cervical or axillary nodes, and fever, which also make up the diagnosis.

CLINICAL MANIFESTATIONS

- Patients must have both of the following major criteria for CFS:
  - Persistent or relapsing fatigue for at least 6 months that does not resolve with bed rest.
  - Fatigue severe enough to reduce daily activity by at least 50%.
- Patients must also have six of the following minor criteria, the first three of which must be included and documented by a physician:
  - Mild fever (must be documented by physician).
  - Sore throat (must be documented by physician).
  - Anterior or posterior cervical node or axillary node enlargement or pain on palpitation (must be documented by physician).
  - Generalized muscle weakness.
  - Myalgia.
  - Prolonged fatigue following previously tolerable exercise.
  - Headaches.
  - Migratory, noninflammatory arthralgia (joint pain and swelling).
  - Sudden onset of the symptoms.
  - Neurologic symptoms related to loss of concentration, confusion, or depression.
  - Sleep disturbance.

DIAGNOSTIC TOOLS

- The diagnosis of CFS involves documenting the physical findings identified above as well as the subjective report of fatigue and an inability to function at previous levels. Other organic causes of fatigue should be ruled out using physical examination, radiographs when appropriate, and laboratory testing.
- Blood tests and laboratory analysis should include the following:
  - A complete blood count (CBC) with differential, and measurement of electrolytes, glucose, calcium, and phosphorous.
  - Renal and liver profiles.
  - Thyroid function tests.
  - Urinalysis.
  - Stool guaiac analysis.
  - Tests to screen for the presence of systemic autoimmune rheu-

matic diseases including systemic lupus erythematous may be performed.

COMPLICATIONS

- Family stress, loss of job and income, and severe depression may result.

TREATMENT

- Treatment of CFS needs to be holistic, in that there is no known "cure" for the syndrome, but emotional support and education on nutrition and exercise may improve quality of life for patients with CFS.
- Patients should be encouraged to eat healthy foods, with emphasis on low-fat, high-complex carbohydrates. Alcohol should be avoided.
- A program of limited exercise may improve functioning, beginning with just a few minutes a day of walking or other low-level exercise and slowly increasing in duration and intensity over several weeks.
- Nonsteroidal anti-inflammatory agents or acetaminophen may be used to treat the fever and muscle aches. Antidepressants may be used as part of a comprehensive plan to relieve depression.
- Family and individual counseling may improve outlook and reduce family tensions.

Developmental Delay

A developmental delay refers to the failure to attain one or more physical, cognitive, or emotional milestones for a given age. Examples of physical delays include an inability to walk well by 16 months of age, inability to hop in place or ride a tricycle by 36 to 48 months, or inability to begin menstruating by 16 years of age. Examples of cognitive delays include inability to use words by 18 months, inability to use two-word sentences by 24 months, or an inability to be understood by strangers 50% of the time by 36 months. Older children may show cognitive delays in reading or math, as evidenced by inability to progress in school or in tests to evaluate intellectual functioning. Emotional delay may be apparent in children who do not cry during separation from a primary caregiver at 9 months, are unable to play cooperatively in small groups during the preschool years, or are not interested in other people beginning in infancy. Severe, pervasive developmental disorders, for example, autism or mental retardation, may show a combination of delays.

Developmental delays may occur for no known reason or may result from genetic errors, infection, injury, or exposure to toxins prenatally or after birth. Nutritional deficits and emotional or physical neglect may cause delays as well. Sometimes, parents do not know what to expect of their infant or child; thus, they may not offer opportunities for the child to develop normally. For example, children to whom parents seldom talk may show a language delay, and 6-month-old infants who are never placed down on the floor may be slow to crawl or sit up.

CLINICAL MANIFESTATIONS

Developmental delays may be subtle or frank. Developmental delays should be viewed as a symptom, not a diagnosis. Clinical manifestations will depend on the particular skill or physical milestone being evaluated. Concerns about a developmental delay may be first related by a parent, a teacher, the child him or herself if older, or may be recognized during a visit to a health care provider.

DIAGNOSTIC TOOLS

- Diagnosis depends on knowing what physical, cognitive, and emotional milestones are expected for each age. A variety of tests are available to evaluate milestones, including the Denver II, the Stanford-Binet intelligence test, and several others, many of which are identified in the article by Rosenbaum and in various pediatric texts (see the bibliography section).

COMPLICATIONS

- Emotional or social isolation and low self-esteem may accompany developmental delays.

TREATMENT

- The most important step in treatment is identification of the disorder. This occurs by observing and listening to children and caregivers at each well-child visit or other scheduled appointment.
- Many developmental disorders may be relieved by education, for example, explaining to parents ways to stimulate a child, and anticipatory guidance about what to expect next.
- An early childhood evaluation team should evaluate children suspected of a significant developmental delay. It is essential that a child with a significant delay receive help early on in order to minimize negative long-term physical, psychological, and social outcomes.

Selected Bibliography

Beck-Little, R. & Weinrich, S. P. (1998). Assessment and management of sleep disorders in the elderly. *Journal of Gerontological Nursing* 24, 21–29.

Berlin, L. J., Brooks-Gunn, J., McCarton, C., & McCormick, M. C. (1998). The effectiveness of early intervention: examining risk factors and pathways to enhanced development. *Preventative Medicine* 27, 238–245.

Braver, E. R. & Pantula, J. F. (1997). The sleep of long-haul truck drivers. *New England Journal of Medicine* 338, 755–761.

Colson, E. R. & Dworkin, P. H. (1997). Toddler development. *Pediatrics in Review* 18, 255–259.

David, R. J. & Collins, J. W. (1997). Differing birth weight among infants of U.S. born blacks, African-born blacks, and U.S. born whites. *New England Journal of Medicine* 337, 1209–1214.

Erickson, E. (1963). *Childhood and society (2nd ed.)*. New York: W.W. Norton.

Flax, J. F. & Rapin, I. (1998). Evaluating children with delayed speech and language. *Contemporary Pediatrics* 15, 164–172.

Foster, H. W. (1997). The enigma of low birth weight and race. *New England Journal of Medicine* 337, 1232–1233.

Fukus, K., Straus, S. E., Hickie, I., et al. (1994). The chronic fatigue syndrome: a comprehensive approach to its definition and study. *Annals of Internal Medicine* 121, 953–959.

Houde, S. C. & Kampfe-Leacher, R. (1997). Chronic fatigue syndrome: an update for clinicians in primary care. *The Nurse Practitioner* 22, 35–36, 39–40.

Komaroff, A. L. & Buchwald, D. S. (1998). Chronic fatigue syndrome: an update. *Annual Review of Medicine* 49, 1–13.

Levine, R. L. (1995). Eating disorders in adolescents: a comprehensive update. *International Pediatrics* 10, 327–335.

Haas, J. (1998). The cost of being a woman. *New England Journal of Medicine* 338, 1694–1695.

Maslow, A. (1968). *Towards a psychology of being (2nd ed.)*. New York: D. Van Nostrand.

Mustard, C. A., Kaufert, P., Kozyrskyj, A., & Mayer, T. (1998). Sex differences in the use of health care services. *New England Journal of Medicine* 338, 1678–1683.

Newacheck, P. W., Stoddard, J. J., Hughes, D. C., & Pearl, M. (1998). Health insurance and access to primary care for children. *New England Journal of* Medicine 338, 513–519.

Piaget, J. (1963). *The origins of intelligence in children*. New York: W.W. Norton.

Rosenbaum, P. (1998). Screening tests and standardized assessments used to identify and characterize developmental delays. *Seminars in Pediatric Neurology* 5, 27–32.

Sedgwick, P. M. (1998). Disorders of the sleep–wake cycle in adults. *Postgraduate Medical Journal* 74, 134–138.

Sturner, R. A. & Howard, B. J. (1997). Preschool development 1: communicative and motor aspects. *Pediatrics in Review* 18, 291–301.

Sturner, R.A., Funk, S. G., & Green, J. A. (1994). Simultaneous technique for acuity and readiness testing (START): further concurrent validation of an aid for developmental surveillance. *Pediatrics* 93, 82–88.

VanRuth, O. (1998). Sleep and circadian disturbance in shift work: strategies for their management. *Hormone Research* 49, 158–162.

Zhdanova, I. V., Lynch, H. J., & Wurtman, R. J. (1997). Melatonin: a sleep-promoting hormone. *Sleep* 20, 899–907.

5 CANCER

Cellular reproduction is normally a tightly controlled process. Certain stimuli and growth factors, both physiologic and pathologic, can influence a cell's rate of reproduction. Uncontrolled cellular proliferation that knows no limits and serves no purpose, is called cancer or neoplasia.

• • •

PHYSIOLOGIC CONCEPTS

Cellular Reproduction

Although all cells reproduce during embryogenesis, only some cells continue to do so after the first few months after birth. Cells that reproduce, such as liver, skin, and gastrointestinal cells, copy their DNA exactly and then split into two new daughter cells. The process by which cells reproduce is called the **cell cycle**, described fully in Chapter 2. Cells that do not reproduce after birth, such as skeletal muscle cells, do not go through this cycle. Advancement through the cell cycle is tightly controlled and can be stopped or started depending on the conditions of the cell and the signals it receives.

Rates of Cellular Reproduction

Cells that reproduce do so at an inherent rate. This rate may be increased or decreased. Cells that reproduce slowly, or not at all, spend most of their time in the G1 or G0 stages of interphase. Cells that divide continually spend less time in these stages, and move frequently through the cell cycle.

Control of Cellular Reproduction

Cell cycling is controlled by the contributions of a variety of genes that respond to cues on cell crowding, tissue injury, and growth needs. In general, cells go through the cell cycle when stimulated to do so by hormones and growth factors secreted by distant cells, by locally produced growth factors, and by chemical cues released from neighboring cells including cytokines produced by immune and inflammatory cells. These external cues act by binding to specific receptors on the plasma membrane of the target cell. Once bound, the receptor complex activates a second messenger system, which delivers the growth signal to the nucleus. When the signal reaches the nucleus, certain proteins there, called **transcription factors**, turn on or off specific genes that in turn produce proteins that control cell proliferation. Activated genes also produce proteins that feed back on each of the steps of signaling and messenger stimulation to amplify or minimize the effects of the initial stimulus.

In the following discussion, the external cues controlling cell growth are described, followed by an example of an important second messenger system. Finally, a discussion of the two broad categories of genes whose end products ultimately control the cell cycle are presented. These categories of genes are the tumor suppressor genes and the proto-oncogenes.

HORMONES AND GROWTH FACTORS THAT CONTROL CELLULAR REPRODUCTION

Various hormones and growth factors may stimulate cells to increase or decrease their rate of reproduction. Epidermal growth factor, fibroblast growth factor, erythropoietin (which stimulates red blood cell proliferation), and insulin-like growth factors (which stimulate fat and connective tissue cell proliferation) can turn cellular reproduction on or off. Platelet-derived growth factor stimulates production of connective tissue cells. Some of these substances inhibit growth of other cells while stimulating cell division and growth in target cells. Some cancer cells overproduce membrane receptors that respond to stimulatory signals, or underproduce receptors for hormones that put the brakes on cell division. Cancer cells may also start producing their own growth factors that may stimulate neighboring cells, or, more importantly, may turn back and drive the cancer cell's own proliferation.

CHEMICALS THAT CONTROL CELLULAR REPRODUCTION

Various chemicals may stimulate cells to increase or decrease their rate of reproduction. These chemicals may be released by injured or infected neighboring cells or by immune and inflammatory cells drawn to an area after tissue injury. Many interleukins, released by cells of the immune system, stimulate cellular proliferation and differentiation. Cells possess receptors on their plasma membranes for immune and inflammatory mediators. Binding by some of these substances causes cells to produce more receptors for other immune proteins, thereby amplifying the initial response.

PHYSICAL CUES THAT CONTROL CELLULAR REPRODUCTION

Neighboring cells appear to communicate with each other about tissue crowding and tissue type by releasing locally active chemicals, and by passing ions and other small molecules through channels called gap junctions. Normal cells respond to physical and chemical cues put out by a large number of similar cells by slowing or stopping their rate of reproduction. This allows cellular growth and proliferation to be controlled based on tissue space requirements. These methods of communication allow cells to recognize other cells of the same type (i.e., kidney cells recognize other kidney cells).

CYTOPLASMIC MESSENGER CASCADE

The cytoplasmic signal cascade begins after a protein hormone, growth factor, or other chemical binds to a cell membrane receptor and turns on a specific second messenger system. Activated second messenger proteins relay the growth-controlling signal to the nuclear transcription proteins. An example of an important cytoplasmic messenger is the *ras* protein. The normal *ras* protein transmits stimulatory signals from bound growth factor receptors on a cell's membrane to other proteins down the line that ultimately turn on cell cycling. Many cancer cells show a mutation in the gene that produces the *ras* protein, such that it is always produced, even when growth factor receptors are not stimulated. This results in runaway cellular proliferation. Hyperactive *ras* proteins are found in approximately a fourth of all human tumors.

Tumor Suppressor Genes

Several different genes control cell cycling by coding for proteins that inhibit or stimulate cellular proliferation. Tumor suppressor genes (and proto-oncogenes) are vitally important in all normally functioning cells. As described later, cancer results from accumulated mutations in these genes.

Tumor suppressor genes are genes found in all cells that when activated, inhibit or slow the growth and reproduction of the cell. Some tumor suppressor genes act by producing proteins that slow down or stop the second messenger brigade, including proteins that interfere with the functioning of the stimulatory *ras* protein. Other tumor suppressor genes code for proteins that make up surface receptors that bind growth-*inhibiting* hormones or factors. And finally, some tumor suppressor genes have been identified that produce proteins that code for important brakes that act directly on cells about to commit to going through the cell cycle. These genes include the RB gene and the p53 gene.

THE RB GENE

The RB gene codes for the pRB protein—the master brake of the cell cycle. Without this protein, the cell cycle is constantly in the "on" mode, and cellular reproduction can occur nonstop. Mutations in this gene have been identified in a variety of human cancers including bone, bladder, small cell lung, and breast cancer, and the cancer after which the gene was named, retroblastoma.

THE P53 GENE

The p53 gene codes for the p53 protein that normally monitors the health of the cell and the integrity of cellular DNA. The p53 protein can act as a powerful brake to halt cell division before it is too late if errors in DNA transcription are present or cellular conditions are not right. The p53 protein can cause the cell to pause in the cycle indefinitely until the DNA error is corrected, or to commit cellular suicide (apoptosis). By controlling cellular replication, the p53 gene ensures that a genetic error is not passed on and only healthy cells reproduce. Mutations in the p53 gene are shown to occur in at least half of all types of human tumors.

Proto-Oncogenes

Proto-oncogenes are genes found in all cells that stimulate cellular growth and proliferation. These genes may stimulate cell cycling at all levels including: 1) producing proteins that make up membrane receptors for growth-*stimulating* hormones and chemicals, 2) increasing the production of second messenger proteins, including the *ras* protein, that transfer growth signals to the nucleus, and 3) producing transcription factors that turn on vital genes that force cell growth forward (i.e., the family of *myc* genes).

THE myc GENES

The *myc* genes are a type of proto-oncogenes that code for transcription factor proteins that drive cellular reproduction. *Myc* genes are normally activated only in response to growth factors acting on the cell surface. In many types of cancer, the *myc* gene is turned on constantly, even in the absence of growth factors. Cellular proliferation can occur without control when this gene is damaged.

When normal proto-oncogenes become overactive and cause uncontrolled cell division, they are called **oncogenes**, or cancer-causing genes.

Cellular Differentiation

Normal cells differentiate during development. Differentiation means that a given cell becomes specialized in structure and function, and aggregates with similar differentiated cells. For example, some embryonic cells are destined to become cells of the retina, whereas others are destined to become cells of the skin or heart. The more specialized a cell—that is, the more highly differentiated—the less frequently that cell goes through the cell cycle to reproduce and divide. Neural cells, which do not reproduce, are highly differentiated cells. Cells that seldom or never go through the cell cycle are unlikely to become cancerous.

MECHANISMS OF DIFFERENTIATION

Differentiation appears to occur from selective suppression of certain genes in some cells, whereas in other cells those same genes are active. Differentiation of each cell and tissue appears to affect differentiation of neighboring cells and tissues. Cells release specific growth factors that initiate or guide differentiation of neighboring cells.

Cell Recognition and Adhesion to Like Cells

Normal cells adhere to others of the same type and thus group together. Although the mechanism by which cells recognize each other is not well understood, it appears to involve chemical cues secreted only by certain cells and recognized only by similar cells. Surface proteins present on one cell type that match up with proteins on similar cell, also appear to assist in cells recognizing similar cells. These surface proteins are described as adhesion molecules, and appear to hold the cells together, in the manner of velcro. That cells recognize their own type is easily demonstrated by placing cells of many different types together in a petri dish; after a certain period, the cells will have moved into clusters with only same-type cells in each cluster.

Other adhesion molecules exist between cells and the underlying tissue matrix. These connections serve to anchor cells to one location. When normal cells become unattached from each other, or experience a loosening of their attachment to underlying tissue, they respond by initiating apoptosis (suicide), which prohibits cells from floating free of their tissue of origin.

The Cell Clock

Normal human cells reproduce a predictable number of times, after which they stop and become senescent. This implies that there is some counting system that cells possess that tells cells when to stop dividing. This is important because if cells divided indefinitely we would have many more cells than is compatible with life. The mechanism by which cells tick off their own divisions involves a telomere-based counting system.

Telomeres are described in Chapter 2. Telomeres are the end pieces of chromosomes that shorten with each division. When the telomere piece is of sufficiently short length (indicating that it has divided a certain number of times) the cell stops dividing. It is pertinent to note that putting the brake on cell division in response to telomere shortening requires that the cell has functioning RB and p53 proteins. Occasionally, a cell continues to divide after the telomere reaches its threshold length; usually these cells soon self-destruct as their chromosomes begin to chaotically fuse and randomly break.

Cell crowding also results in signals being released among neighboring cells that inhibit the further replication of cells. This is called contact inhibition.

PATHOPHYSIOLOGIC CONCEPTS

Uncontrolled Cellular Reproduction

Cancer cells do not respond to the normal cues controlling cellular reproduction. Instead they go through the cell cycle more often than normal, resulting in an overabundance of abnormal cells. Cancer cells spend little time in the gap stages of interphase and are frequently found in the M (mitosis) and S (DNA copying) stages.

Uncontrolled cellular reproduction occurs when cells become independent of normal growth control signals. This characteristic of cancer cells is called **autonomy**. Autonomy results when cells do not respond to the cues controlling contact inhibition, for example, growth inhibitors released by neighboring cells or inhibitory growth factors and hormones traveling in the circulation. Cancer cells may disregard these signals by not producing membrane receptors that bind the inhibitory growth signals, or by not activating appropriate second messengers that transmit inhibitory information to the nucleus. Cancer cells may also produce their own growth factors, which make them independent of any outside control. When placed in an in vitro experimental setting, cancer cells aggressively grow on top of each other and produce layers of disorderly cells, ignoring not only chemical signals but the tendency to respect neighboring borders. Autonomy is demonstrated in the tendency of cancer cells to detach from neighboring cells and spread to distant body sites. It has been suggested that the adhesion molecules that exist between cells of the same type and between normal cells and the extracellular matrix no longer exist for cancer cells. Cancer cell autonomy may result from the inactivation of tumor suppressor genes or the change from proto-oncogenes to oncogenes.

Anaplasia

Anaplasia refers to regression of a differentiated cell to a less differentiated stage. Cancer cells demonstrate various degrees of anaplasia. By undergoing anaplasia, a cancer cell loses its ability to perform previous functions and bears little resemblance to its tissue of origin. Highly anaplastic cells may appear embryonic and begin to express functions of a different cellular type. Some cancer cells may become ectopic sites of hormone production. For instance, antidiuretic hormone (ADH) or adrenocorticotrophic hormone (ACTH), hormones that are normally synthesized by cells of the hypothalamus and anterior pituitary, respectively, may be secreted by ectopic sites of hormone production. Lung cancers frequently become ectopic sites of hormone production.

Because the immune system poorly responds to embryonic antigens, the presence of highly anaplastic cells may interfere with the host's immune response to the tumor and usually indicates a particularly aggressive cancer.

Loss of the Cell Clock

Most cancer cells secrete an enzyme, telomerase, that functions to replace the telomere ends of chromosomes that shorten with each cell division. This leads to a destruction of the cell counting system and immortality of the cell. Not only does this allow a cancer cell to repeatedly divide, increasing its number, but it also gives the cancer cell time to accumulate more mutations, some of which may improve the cell's ability to evade the immune system or produce newer, more potent growth-stimulatory factors.

Nuclear and Cytoplasmic Derangement

Cancer cells often demonstrate multiple derangements of the nucleus, cytoplasmic organelles, and cytoskeleton. The nucleus is frequently enlarged and misshapen, with obvious chromosomal breaks, deletions, additions, and translocations. The rate of mitosis is usually increased.

In the cytoplasm, intracellular structures show disorganization and changes in size and shape. Changes in the microtubules that support the cell and are necessary for the control of virtually all intracellular functions are especially significant. The mitochondria become disorganized and misshapen.

Tumor Cell Markers

Some cancer cells release tumor cell markers, which are specific substances secreted by a tumor into the blood, urine, or spinal fluid of an individual with a particular cancer. Tumor cell markers may be specific antigens present on the cancer cells. Some tumor antigens are similar to fetal antigens and are called oncofetal antigens ("onco" referring to cancer). Because fetal antigens often do not provoke an immune response, they may mask the tumor against the host's immune system.

CLINICAL IMPLICATIONS OF TUMOR CELL MARKERS

Tumor cell markers are clinically important because they offer a means of identifying certain cancers and their progression can be studied before, during, and after treatment. For instance, if a specific tumor cell marker is identified in a patient, it suggests that cancer may exist in the person, and further diagnostic evaluation is necessary. Furthermore, in patients with a known malignancy, if after radiation or chemotherapy the tumor cell marker is nondetectable, it suggests that the cancer is in remission for that individual.

Examples of tumor cell markers include:

- Alpha-fetoprotein for liver and yolksac (ovarian and testicular) cancers.
- Carcinoembryonic antigen for colorectal cancer.
- Human chorionic gonadotropin for many tumors, including choriocarcinoma (usually cancer of the uterus).
- Acid phosphatase and prostate-specific antigen (PSA) for prostate cancer.
- Monoclonal immunoglobulin (one subtype of antibody) for multiple melanoma.

- CA-125 as a marker for ovarian cancer.

Although the presence of tumor cell markers may indicate the presence or recurrence of cancer, sole reliance on the presence or absence of cell markers is cautioned against. PSA is detectable in all adult men; only elevations above a certain age-dependent threshold are suggestive of disease. Likewise, pregnant women have increased human chorionic gonadotropin and CA-125 may be increased in women for reasons other than ovarian cancer. And finally, failure to detect a tumor cell marker does not mean that an individual is cancer-free.

Tumor Growth Rate

Each tumor grows at a certain rate dependent on characteristics of the host and the tumor itself.

CHARACTERISTICS OF THE HOST THAT AFFECT TUMOR GROWTH RATE

Important characteristics that affect a tumor's growth rate include age, sex, and overall health and nutritional status of the host. The status of the host's immune system is also important. An individual who is immunosuppressed may be unable to recognize a tumor as foreign, or may be unable to respond to a tumor that he or she recognizes. Certain hormonal states (i.e., pregnancy) may stimulate certain tumor growth rates.

CHARACTERISTICS OF THE TUMOR THAT AFFECT ITS GROWTH RATE

Important characteristics of the tumor that affect its growth rate include location in the body and blood supply. The degree of cellular anaplasia and the presence or absence of tumor growth factors are also important. Many tumors depend on circulating or self-produced growth factors to stimulate their growth. Therefore, tumors that grow most rapidly often stud their surface membranes with receptors for these factors. In addition, some tumor cells secrete chemicals that make the local environment more favorable to their growth. An example is tumor secretion of tumor angiogenesis factor.

Tumor Angiogenesis Factors

Tumor angiogenesis factors are substances secreted by tumor cells that stimulate the development of new blood vessel formation. To grow, all cells require an adequate blood supply to deliver oxygen and nutrients and to remove waste products. Once a group of cancer cells has grown to a certain size (approximately 1 to 2 mm in diameter), it will outgrow its original blood vessel supply and must stimulate the development of new blood vessels to grow further.

Recent experiments have demonstrated the feasibility of measuring tumor angiogenesis factors in the blood or urine, which may allow for early diagnosis of some cancers. Equally exciting are new treatments for cancer that involve blocking the production of tumor angiogenesis factors. Early experiments in mice demonstrate that without angiogenesis, tumors soon shrink and sometimes disappear. Therapeutic interventions to block tumor angiogenesis factors in humans with cancer are being studied.

Descriptions of Tumor Growth and Spread

Tumors may grow only locally, or may spread to distant sites in the process called metastasis. It is the metastasis of tumors that may ultimately lead to death of the individual. Growth and spread of a tumor is often described clinically. Some of the different terms used are presented, followed by a description of local growth and metastasis. Tumor treatment often depends on the grade and stage of the cancer.

- Grading: an assessment of the tumor based on the degree of anaplasia it demonstrates. For example, poorly differentiated cells (highly anaplastic) are assigned a high grade.
- Staging: a clinical decision concerning the size of a tumor, the degree of local invasion it has produced, and the degree to which it has spread to distant sites in a given individual.
- Doubling time: an estimate of the mean amount of time required for the division of the tumor cells. Tumor cells that rapidly divide have a short doubling time.

Local Growth of a Tumor

The term cancer refers to the crab-like projections put out by a growing tumor into the local tissue. Tumors spread locally when these crab-like projections injure and kill neighboring cells. Growing tumors injure and kill neighboring cells by compressing the cells and blocking off their blood supply. Tumor cells also appear to release chemicals or enzymes that destroy the integrity of a neighboring cell's membrane, causing the cell to lyse and die. When neighboring cells die, the tumor can easily grow to occupy that space. As described earlier, to grow beyond a certain size, tumors must stimulate the development of their own blood supply to meet their high metabolic demands.

Metastasis

Metastasis is the movement of cancer cells from one part of the body to another. Metastasis usually occurs through the spread of cancer cells from the original (primary) site in the blood or lymph to a new, secondary site. The term malignancy refers to the potential of a tumor to metastasize.

THE PROCESS OF METASTASIS

Steps involved in the metastasis of a primary tumor to a distant site include detachment, invasion, dissemination, and seeding.

Detachment

To metastasize, cancer cells must first detach from their primary cluster. Recall that normal cells are linked to neighboring cells and underlying matrix tissue, and thus detach with difficulty. In addition, if a normal cell senses that it has become detached from its neighbors, it undergoes apoptosis. Cancer cells, in contrast, lose adhesion with like cells and the extracellular matrix, allowing for relatively easy detachment. Likewise, a cancer cell may produce chemicals that mimic those secreted by neighboring cells, thereby fooling its internal checkpoints into thinking that it is still attached to other cells, and thus avoiding apoptosis. As cancer cells detach they begin to invade surrounding membrane barriers and enter the circulation.

Invasion

To spread to distant sites, detached tumor cells must gain entrance to a blood or lymph vessel. To do so, the tumor cells must: 1) cross the basement membrane (a thin layer of tissue) separating its tissue of origin from the rest of the body and 2) cross the basement membrane of a local blood or lymph vessel. To break down basement membrane walls and gain access to the circulation, tumor cells secrete specific enzymes that attack the integrity of the tissue. One such enzyme secreted preferentially by cancer cells to break down walls of a capillary is collagenase type IV. Collagenase type IV is effective in the spread of cancer cells because the new blood vessels formed in response to tumor angiogenesis factor are relatively thin and easily breached.

Dissemination and Seeding

Movement of tumor cells in the blood or lymph is called dissemination. Eventually—and especially if traveling in clumps—some tumor cells will get caught in a capillary or lymph network downstream from the primary site. Although many cells may die, a few tumor cells at this new site may survive and begin to seed the area. The more cells that detach from the primary tumor, the more likely that at least one will survive the journey and start a new tumor growth elsewhere.

When the secondary site has reached a critical size, the tumor cells will again begin to produce tumor angiogenesis factor and new blood vessel formation will be initiated to support growth of this secondary site. The processes of tumor detachment, invasion, dissemination, and seeding are shown in Figure 5-1.

PROGRESS OF A METASTASIZING TUMOR

Because cancer cells tend to be large, most lodge in the nearest lymph or capillary bed downstream from the primary tumor site. Because of this, the lungs, which receive systemic venous blood directly from most organs, are the most common sites of metastasis. Venous blood from the gastrointestinal (GI) tract and pancreas travels first to the liver through the hepatic portal blood flow system, causing the liver to be the most common site of cancers from these organs. Metastasis is evaluated by observing for secondary sites in the lymph nodes nearest, and then progressively further from, a primary tumor site. If exploration of the nodes closest to the primary site is negative for tumor cells, it is likely that more distant nodes will not have been seeded. Exceptions to this rule are tumor cells that show a striking

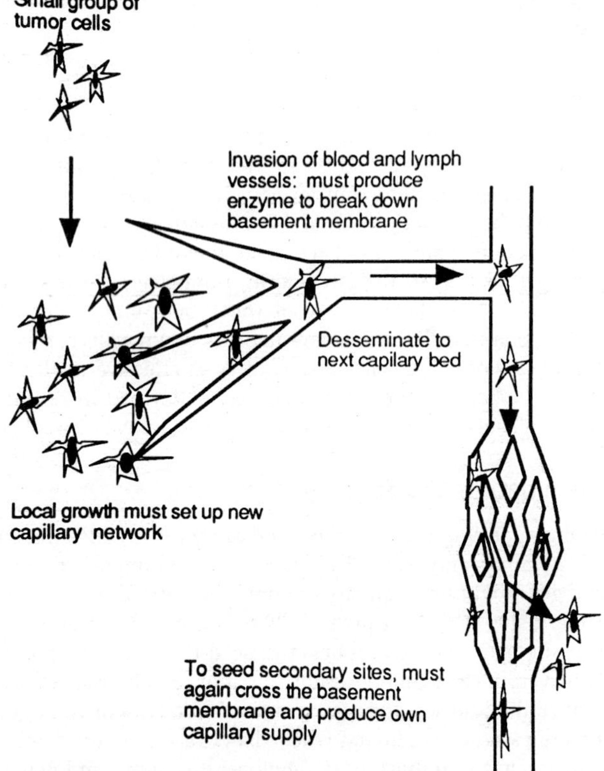

Figure 5-1. Tumor detachment, invasion, and dissemination.

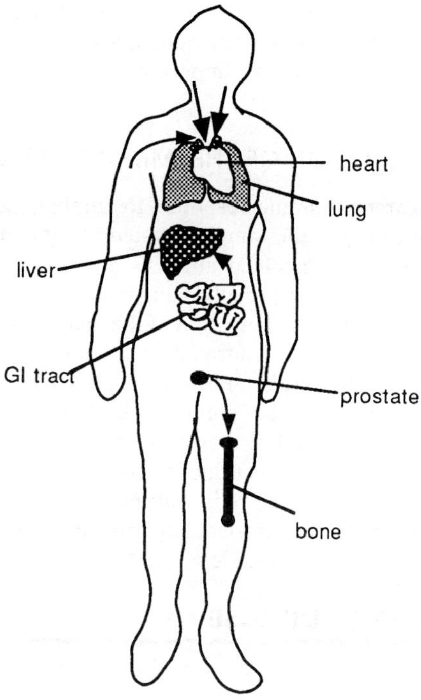

Figure 5-2. Spread of tumor cells from a primary site to a secondary site. Note: most tumors spread through blood or lymph to the lungs; GI tumors spread in portal flow to the liver; prostate tumors frequently spread to the bone.

preference to colonize certain tissues not necessarily downstream. The classic example of this is the tendency of prostate cancer to metastasize to bone. It has been suggested that in these cases, complementary adhesion molecules draw the tumor cells to the distant tissue. And finally, rough handling of a tumor during evaluation or surgery may cause cancer cells to break off from the primary site, thus increasing the likelihood of metastasis. Figure 5-2 identifies the typical metastasis pattern of tumors from various locations.

The Immune System and Cancer

The presence in the blood of antibodies, T cells, and natural killer (NK) cells produced against specific tumor antigens has been confirmed in individuals with cancer. In addition, individuals who are immunocompromised, including those with AIDS or those taking immunosuppressant drugs, have an increased chance of developing cancer. Potent anticancer cytokines, including tumor necrosis factor (TNF), have been identified that assist the immune system in identifying and destroying cancer cells. All of these findings demonstrate clearly that the immune and inflammatory systems have important roles in fighting and preventing cancer.

CANCER CELL EVASION OF THE IMMUNE RESPONSE

Despite an apparent immune response to tumors, cancer cells are frequently able to evade the immune system. Highly anaplastic cells that primarily express oncofetal antigens are most likely to evade immune detection and are especially malignant. Other cancer cells may demonstrate changes in the expression of the major histocompatibility antigens (MHC antigens) that normally stimulate a cell-mediated immune response, which may also allow cancer cells to evade the immune system. Cancer cells may also survive a host immune response by producing blocking antibodies that capture all host antibodies built against the tumor, allowing the tumor to continue to grow. These and other means by which tumor cells may escape immune recognition or destruction are being investigated. Experiments to boost the immune response to a tumor are also under way.

CONDITIONS OF DISEASE

Cancer

A cancer is a growth of abnormal cells that tend to invade neighboring tissue and spread to distant body sites. The term "cancer" refers to more than 100 forms of the disease, each with unique features and many features in common. Processes in common includes those related to how a cell loses control over its growth, how a cancer spreads, and how it evades detection. Unique features include how a tumor arises, where and how fast it spreads, and how it destroys its host.

There are several categories of cancer, and several theories as to how cancer develops. In this section, the categories of cancer are reviewed, followed by the theory of carcinogenesis.

CATEGORIES OF CANCER

Tumors are identified based on the tissue from which they develop. The suffix "oma" is usually added to the tissue term to identify it as a cancer. Several general categories of cancer are presented. Individual cancers are discussed in chapters pertaining to specific organs or systems.

Carcinoma is a cancer of the epithelial tissue, including cells of the skin, testis, ovary, mucus-secreting glands, melanin-secreting cells, breast, cervix, colon, rectum, stomach, pancreas, and esophagus.

Lymphoma is a cancer of the lymphatic tissue including the lymph capillaries, lacteals, spleen, various lymph nodes, and lymph vessels. The thymus and bone marrow may also be affected. Specific lymphomas include Hodgkin's disease (cancer of the lymph nodes and spleen) and malignant lymphoma.

Sarcoma is a cancer of the connective tissue, including cells found in the muscle and bone.

Glioma is a cancer of the glial (support) cells of the central nervous system.

Carcinoma in situ is a term used to describe abnormal epithelial cells that are as yet confined to a certain area and thus considered preinvasive lesions.

THE THEORY OF CARCINOGENESIS

Most evidence suggests that cancer development is a multistep occurrence that usually requires decades to develop. The first step in carcinogenesis is thought to be a mutation in the DNA of an individual cell during DNA transcription (copying). Although mistakes in DNA copying are not unusual, most mistakes are identified by "proofreading" enzymes that travel down the DNA strands to check for transcription errors, signaling the cell cycle to stop for repair when necessary. If a mistake cannot be repaired, the cell normally will be instructed to self-destruct. The theory of carcinogenesis suggests that in certain individuals an error may not be noticed, the cell cycle may not stop in time for repair, or a defective cell may not self-destruct. If any of these occur, the genetic mistake becomes a permanent mutation and will be passed to all daughter cells. This step is irreversible and is often called cellular "initiation." If the mutation has some significance related to cell proliferation, it may eventually cause the cell to develop uncontrollable growth and become cancerous (see Fig. 5-3).

For a cancer to develop from this irreversible event, years of interactions with the cell by various other factors must also occur, causing many more genetic errors, all of which must add up to produce cancer. These additive effects are often called "promoting events." Factors that promote the acceleration of the cell cycle through stimulation of oncogenic genes, and most importantly, those that break down the functioning of tumor suppressor genes are the most likely to result in a mutated cell becoming carcinogenic. This theory of carcinogenesis allows for the acceptance of many causes of DNA mutation, many different interacting variables, and roles for hereditary and environment in cancer development.

EFFECT OF FREQUENT CELL CYCLING ON TRANSCRIPTION ERRORS

The more times DNA is transcribed and a cell splits, the greater the chances of an error being made, a mistake being overlooked, and a mutation being passed on. Under some circumstances, these mutations

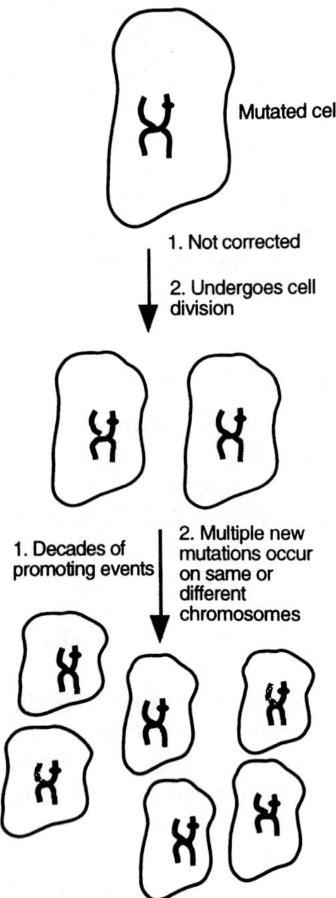

Figure 5-3. An uncorrected mutation passes to new daughter cells. If promoting events and new mutations occur, the cell may be released from normal growth controls and wildly proliferate.

may result in cancer. Cells that divide frequently are at greatest risk of becoming cancerous.

MONOCLONAL TUMOR DEVELOPMENT

When a tumor develops, it appears to do so from a single cell gone awry. This results in a monoclonal tumor from one ancestral cell. This theory is consistent with there being one mutated cell that eventually develops into a cancer.

CAUSES OF DNA TRANSCRIPTION ERRORS

Although some mistakes in DNA transcription occur randomly, certain physical agents, chemicals, and microorganisms are known to cause mutations. Such agents include ionizing radiation, ultraviolet radiation, components of cigarette smoke, aromatic hydrocarbons, certain dyes, nitrosamines (present in preserved meats), aflatoxin (present on moldy peanuts), and asbestos. Some of these physical agents appear to damage the DNA directly by breaking DNA base pair bonds, or indirectly by producing free radicals or other intermediates that react with and damage the DNA. Even aging itself may increase the risk of cancer through increased production of free radicals.

Certain viruses have been identified that can cause DNA mutations. These viruses may damage the DNA directly by causing a transcription error, or may insert into the host DNA and turn on cellular proliferation. Cancers known to be caused by a virus include Burkitt's lymphoma, caused by the Epstein-Barr virus, cervical cancer, caused by certain strains of the human papilloma virus, and liver cancer, caused by the Hepatitis B virus. Kaposi's sarcoma also may be caused by a virus and occurs especially in those suffering from AIDS.

In addition to directly altering the DNA and causing cancer, viruses and other microorganisms may irritate the cell and cause chronic inflammation. Inflammation may stimulate the cell to enter the cell cycle more frequently, thus increasing the likelihood that a DNA transcription error will occur.

Helicobacter pylori is a bacteria that appears to be responsible for causing some cases of stomach cancer. It is thought that it causes chronic gastric injury and inflammation, which leads to an increased rate of cell cycling.

EFFECT OF ANY MUTATING AGENT

Any physical, chemical, or viral agent may cause mistakes in DNA replication or destroy proofreading enzymes. The worst-case scenario is that a mutating agent may disrupt a proto-oncogene transforming it into an oncogene, or inactivate a tumor suppressor gene that produces the checkpoint proteins that normally control cell division. If one of these checkpoints is eliminated or rendered dysfunctional, cell proliferation may occur without control or without concern for DNA errors. Recall from the discussion earlier, a large proportion of human cancers result from mistakes in the p53, *ras*, or *myc* family of genes. Recall also, that there are two copies of each gene. It is hypothesized that cancer results from "two hits": damage to one gene must be followed by subsequent damage to the other. This requires more than one genetic error to occur in a cell over many years. Even then, cancer will not develop unless promoting effects have turned the mutation deadly.

PROMOTION

A mutated cell is not a cancerous cell; many years of promoting events must occur before that cell becomes cancerous. It is suggested that various promoting agents may act to cause a mutated cell to become cancerous by accelerating the proliferation of the cell. Promoters may stimulate cellular proliferation by stimulating oncogenes or inhibiting tumor suppressor function. The effects of a promoter on a mutated cell may be reversible if exposure to the promoter is stopped.

Examples of Promoting Agents

Examples of promoters include endogenous (produced in the body) hormones such as estrogen, certain food additives such as nitrates and salt, and drugs, especially, cigarette smoke and alcohol, which seem to have a synergistic effect. Some substances (tobacco) may act as an initiator of a mutation and a promoter of cell proliferation.

RISK FACTORS

Although some mistakes in DNA replication throughout a lifetime are inevitable, certain conditions or behaviors can increase or decrease the likelihood of a mutation arising and being stimulated to become cancerous.

Risk factors for cancer include exposure to any physical, chemical, or viral substance that is known to be mutagenic, and prolonged exposure to any promoter. Mutagens may be inhaled, eaten, or may act on the skin, such as ultraviolet radiation.

BEHAVIORAL RISK FACTORS

Certain behaviors increase the likelihood that an individual will be frequently exposed to cancer-causing agents. Behavioral risk factors include cigarette smoking and diets rich in animal fat and preserved meats. It has been estimated that at least a third of all cancers in the United States can be attributed to cigarette smoking, and a third to diet. Obesity may be an independent risk factor for cancer because of the increased accumulation of fat-soluble toxins and potentially carcinogenic hormones in fatty tissue. Even a low level of alcohol consumption is linked to an increase in breast cancer, as is a sedentary lifestyle. Next to smoking and diet, other environmental factors, including exposure to asbestos, radon, and coal tar account for a small percentage each of cancer cases. Even radiation exposure from sunlight, the primary cause of skin cancers, accounts for less than 2% of all cancers in the United States.

Other behavioral risk factors include those associated with sexual behavior. The number of sexual partners and an early onset of sexual activity increase the risk of becoming infected with the human papilloma virus associated with genital neoplasms and the AIDS virus associated with Kaposi's sarcoma. Some evidence suggests that infection with the sexually transmitted virus herpes simplex 2 may also increase cervical cancer risk. Hepatitis B virus can be passed sexually and increases the risk of liver cancer.

HORMONAL RISK FACTORS

Estrogen may act as a promoter for certain cancers, such as breast and endometrial cancer. Because estrogen levels are high in menstruating women, the risk for developing breast cancer is increased in women who started menstruating early and reached menopause late. Delayed childbearing or choosing not to bear children increases the risk of breast cancer. This appears to be related to many years of uninterrupted exposure to estrogen. Estrogen replacement therapy in postmenopausal women may be associated with a slight increase in the risk of breast cancer. However, estrogen replacement has been reported to decrease the risk of colon cancer.

INHERITED RISK FACTORS

A family history of cancer, especially clustered as one type, is a risk factor for developing cancer. Genetic tendencies for carcinogenesis may involve fragile tumor suppressor genes, susceptibility to certain mutagens or promoters, faulty proofreading enzymes, or a poorly functioning immune system. Inherited defects in the p53 gene and the RB gene have been documented to be associated with a high risk of cancer. Certain cancers have a higher tendency to run in families than others. For example, although most cases of colon cancer arise spontaneously, some families carry mutations that increase the risk of this disease. Likewise, although most cases of breast cancer arise without any clear genetic link, heritable breast cancer accounts for approximately 5% to 19% of all breast cancers. There have been two genes identified that increase a woman's chance of developing of breast cancer; BRCA1 and BRCA2. These genes are in the category of tumor suppressor genes, although their exact function in controlling normal cell proliferation is unknown. Mistakes in one or both of these genes are present in increased frequency in women with breast cancer compared to women without breast cancer, and may account for approximately half of the heritable cases of breast cancer. Having a mutation in either of these genes cannot predict the development of disease: it appears that a woman carrying a mutation in the BRCA1 gene has a 56% chance of developing breast cancer before the age of 70 and a 16.5% chance of developing ovarian cancer. Like other cancers with a genetic predisposition, familial cases of breast cancer tend to occur at a younger age.

Pediatric cancers likely have a genetic component. In children, the development of cancer is accelerated from several decades to only one or two. It has been suggested that this acceleration may occur if a child inherits in the germ line (egg or sperm) one defective gene controlling a tumor suppressor or proto-oncogene product or develops such a mutation early in embryogenesis. Later, a second gene error would cause early cancer growth. Similarly, inheriting defective genes for proofreading enzymes would also increase the risk of early cancer development.

It is likely that each of us has a certain genetic tendency toward developing cancer, which results in a small percentage of individuals developing cancer without known exposure to mutagens or promoters, whereas others with long-term exposures will remain cancer-free. In general, our genetic tendency toward cancer is overshadowed by risk factors we encounter in our environment and, most importantly, by risks we choose to accept in our lifestyles and behaviors.

FACTORS THAT ARE PROTECTIVE AGAINST CANCER DEVELOPMENT

Some studies suggest that women who breastfeed for at least 6 consecutive months have a reduced risk of developing breast cancer. In addition, women who have had multiple pregnancies have a reduced risk of breast cancer. These findings may relate to the decreased number of periods experienced by these women. Progesterone appears to be protective against breast cancer by inhibiting the stimulatory effects of estrogen. Progesterone is high during pregnancy, which may explain why women who have had many pregnancies have a reduced risk of breast cancer.

There is also a reduced risk of breast cancer in women who exercise even moderately. This finding may be related to reduction in estrogen levels or to a decrease in fat consumption and obesity.

Dietary factors are important in reducing cancer risk. Studies have shown that diets rich in substances known to scavenge or remove dangerous free radicals, called free-radical scavengers or antioxidants, can reduce the risk of certain cancers. These substances include vitamins A, E, and C, all of which are prevalent in colorful vegetables and fruits, and folic acid present in similar foods.

CLINICAL MANIFESTATIONS

Cancers may be diagnosed in routine examinations before any clinical manifestations appear. When clinical manifestations develop, they are usually specific to the tumor and its site. Some general clinical manifestations that most patients with cancer demonstrate include the following.

- Cachexia is a term used to describe the general wasting of fat and protein seen in many patients with cancer. Weight loss accompanies cachexia and is common in patients with cancer, many times being the presenting complaint. There appears to be a variety of causes of cachexia, including loss of appetite, poor digestion, and the increased metabolic rate of the cancer cells as they continue to go through the cell cycle and reproduce excessively. Cancer cells have high energy demands and steal nutrients needed by other cells for survival. Metabolism of food stuffs may be altered, especially if the cancer involves the liver. Cachexia also appears to be caused, at least in part, by the presence of certain cytokines produced by the immune system to fight the cancer, including tumor necrosis factor.

- Anemia occurs for many different reasons and in many different types of cancers. Most individuals with metastatic cancer eventually develop anemia. It occurs early in those with cancer of the blood-forming cells of the bone marrow. This is true whether the cancer specifically affects the red or white blood cells (leukemia). Cancers that result in chronic bleeding, such as colorectal or uterine cancer, cause anemia. Platelet abnormalities are common, contributing to blood loss. Some forms of chemotherapy and radiation may depress the bone marrow, causing anemia even in patients without previous bleeding or bone marrow disease.
- Fatigue frequently occurs as a result of poor nutrition, protein malnutrition, and poor oxygenation of tissues resulting from anemia. Certain cytokines produced to support the immune response against cancer also are known to cause fatigue. Growing tumors collapse the blood supply to healthy cells while stimulating their own blood supply. They take over the nutrient and oxygen supply of normal cells causing widespread fatigue.

DIAGNOSTIC TOOLS

- Diagnosis of cancer involves reviewing the patient's clinical presentation, gaining information on personal habits such as smoking, and investigating the patient's genetic background for cancer.
- Screening tests, such as Pap smears to detect cervical cancer, mammograms to detect breast cancer, and digital examinations of the prostate coupled with a blood assay for prostate-specific antigen to detect prostate cancer, can help to identify cancer early in its development.
- Advanced methods to diagnose and localize cancer include radiographs, CAT scans, and magnetic resonance imaging (MRI). Special bone scans may also be used.
- Diagnosis is confirmed by obtaining a tissue biopsy, which is submitted to various histologic (cell) studies.

COMPLICATIONS

- Infections are common in those with advanced cancers. Infections develop as a result of protein malnutrition, other dietary deficiencies, and the immune suppression (especially bone marrow suppression) that often follows conventional therapies. Hormones released in response to the long-term stress of cancer can also cause immune suppression. For example, adrenocorticotrophic hormone (ACTH) released from the anterior pituitary can cause immune suppression by stimulating cortisol release from the adrenal cortex gland. Surgery is another cause of frequent infection in patients with cancer. All of these factors make infection a major cause of disability and death in those with cancer.

- Pain may occur as a result of the invading tumor pressing on nerves or blood vessels in the area. Compression of the blood vessels can lead to tissue hypoxia, lactic acid accumulation, or cell death. Pain also occurs because the cancer cells release lytic enzymes that directly injure cells. Pain occurs as part of the immune and inflammatory reactions to the developing cancer. Fear and anxiety can worsen the pain for many patients with cancer. Most patients with advanced cancer experience pain. It is important for health care professionals to provide all treatment possible to reduce pain severity and frequency.

  Pain caused by compression of nerves and blood vessels occurs especially in tissues that exist in space-limiting compartments, such as in the bone or brain. For example, headaches are a common manifestation of advanced brain cancer and bone pain is common with childhood hematologic cancers and bone cancer at any age. GI pain occurs when the smooth muscle of the gut is stretched.

TREATMENT

Several treatments for cancer are available, as outlined below and shown in Table 5-1.

- Surgery has long been a treatment for cancer, with the first documented account of breast removal for cancer in 200 AD. Surgery has the best chance of curing a cancer if used on solid well-circumscribed tumors. Tumors that have metastasized may be treated with surgery to give the patient relief from pain of the pressure of the growing tumor on surrounding nerves. Surgery is also used to "debulk" the tumor, which reduces tumor burden and improves the response to chemotherapy or radiotherapy.
- Radiation therapy uses ionizing radiation to kill tumor cells. Radiation works on the principle that cells most susceptible to the damaging effects of radiation are those in the S or M stages of the cell cycle. Tumor cells are most likely to be found in those stages. Unfortunately, many normal cells are also in those stages of the cell cycle at any given time, and may be killed by the therapy. Until recently, it was thought that radiation killed cells through direct damage to the DNA. However, better understanding of tumor suppressor genes has revised the consensus on how radiation kills cells. It appears that radiation kills cells by altering the DNA enough that brakes on the cell cycle, especially put on by the p53 protein and the ras protein, are activated, leading to cell suicide. Unfortunately, many times cancer cells have inactivated normal braking genes, and therefore do not undergo apoptosis when DNA damage is present. This limits the usefulness of radiation therapy. Another

Table 5-1. Cancer Therapy, Actions, and Effects

CANCER THERAPY	MODE OF ACTION	ADVERSE EFFECTS
Surgery	Reduce size to alleviate pain; prevent metastasis if used early; diagnosis	Pain; deformity
Radiation	Damage dividing cells; stimulate apoptosis; halt cell cycle	Injures and leads to death of normal cells; bone marrow depression; skin desquamation
Chemotherapy	Multiple actions on cells to stop progression through cell cycle; may involve combination therapy and may selectively or nonselectively act	Injures and kills normal cells; anorexia; nausea; bone marrow depression
Immunotherapy/ Biotherapy	Activate host immune system to better recognize and destroy tumor cells; specifically blocks enzymes and growth factors required for metastasis; allows evaluation of treatment	Flu-like symptoms

limitation is the scarring of normal tissue that can occur, leading to fibrosis and reduced organ function. For some cancers radiation may be used alone for curative purposes, for example, in Hodgkin's disease. Often, radiation is used in addition to surgery or to shrink the tumor, reducing tumor load.

- Chemotherapy uses chemotherapeutic drugs of several different classes to destroy cells in the S, M, or initial G stages of the cell cycle. Tumors grow rapidly and therefore have the most number of replicating and dividing cells and so are most susceptible to chemotherapy. However, healthy cells are also susceptible to the damaging effects of chemotherapy. Chemotherapy is frequently used in addition to surgery or radiation therapy, but may be used alone. It also may be used for palliative purposes. Chemotherapy usually causes bone marrow suppression, which in turn causes fatigue, anemia, bleeding tendencies, and an increased risk of infection. One emerging type of adjuvant chemotherapy involves using reproductive hormone antagonists to fight reproductive cancers. The best example of this type of drug is tamoxifen, an antiestrogenic agent. Tamoxifen is used clinically to fight estrogen-dependent breast cancers. In addition, it has recently been reported to prevent the development of cancer in women at high risk of the disease. Tamoxifen and similar drugs, collectively known as selective estrogen receptor modulators, have been shown to exert estrogenic effects on some tissues, for example uterine endometrial tissue, bone, and the cardiovascular system, but antiestrogenic effects on the breast. This observation may allow different drugs to be tailored to the specific needs of each woman. Clinical trials to evaluate the use of tamoxifen to prevent the development of breast cancer are continuing.

- Immunotherapy is a newly developing form of cancer treatment that takes advantage of the two cardinal features of the immune system: specificity and memory. Immunotherapy may be used to identify a tumor and allow any sites of hidden metastasis to be discerned. Immunotherapy may stimulate the host's own immune system to respond more aggressively to a tumor, or tumor cells may be attacked by antibodies developed in the laboratory. Each of these options is described.
- Fluorescently labeled antibodies: To identify a tumor, antibodies can be produced in a culture against tumor-specific antigens taken from a patient. The antibodies can then be labeled with a fluorescent isotope and injected into the patient before, or at different times during, treatment. If the antibodies come on their specific type of tumor cells, the antibodies will bind to the tumor cells and the resulting fluorescence can be detected, located, and measured. This use of immunofluorescent antibodies allows clinicians to identify recurrent or metastasized tumors.
- Immune stimulants: Boosting the host's natural immune response to tumor cells involves activating B and T cells to "wake up and notice" the presence of a growing tumor. This approach has been used in skin tumors by injecting them with antigens capable of stimulating the immune system. Natural immune stimulants such as interferon or some interleukins administered to patients with certain cancers also appear to boost a cell-mediated response to these tumors.
- Attacking antibodies: Antibodies produced against specific tumor antigens are being used to attack and destroy tumor cells. For example, clinical trials involving the intravenous administration of monoclonal antibodies against malignant B cells in patients with lymphoma were begun in 1993. Preliminary evidence suggests that this technique may offer a viable means of destroying a cancer. Various other attacking antibodies also are available for use in cancer therapy.
- Therapies based on the unique molecular biology of tumor cells compared to noncancer cells are being developed. These treatments take advantage of the recent discoveries of how cancers grow to invade local tissues and metastasize into the blood or lymph. Examples of biologic therapies being developed against tumors include drugs that specifically block tumor angiogenesis

factors and enzymes such as collagenase type IV. Tumors make their own growth factors and stud their cell membranes with receptors for these factors and other substances that stimulate their growth. Drugs to block the production of tumor growth factors and the receptors for growth factors are also being investigated.

- Gene therapy is being developed to fight cancer. In gene therapy, pieces of DNA containing special messages are delivered to cancer cells with the hope that the cancer cell will take up the DNA and begin expressing the message for which the DNA codes. Although gene therapy is far from being available clinically, early studies have provided exciting leads. The most tantalizing development to date has been the recent attempts to incorporate genes that inhibit angiogenesis into mice suffering from various tumors. Other ideas include infecting cancer cells with genes that code for the production of toxic chemicals that destroy the cell when produced. Another idea involves providing cancer cells instructions to produce a therapeutic protein that would correct a faulty tumor suppressor gene or compensate for a variety of genetic errors. Other pieces of DNA may cause the cancer cell to produce a surface receptor that would bind a specific chemotherapeutic drug. And finally, the idea that it may be possible to vaccinate against a certain cancer uses the idea of gene therapy. In this scenario, a cancer cell may be tagged with certain genes that make it more visible to the immune system. This could improve the host immune response and lead to destruction of all cells carrying that tag. At this time the best candidate would be to tag the cancer cells with genes that express certain cytokines, which when produced, alert the immune system to the cancer. This approach combines immunotherapy with gene therapy.

CANCER PREVENTION

Cancer prevention is the ultimate goal. Although cancer will occur in some people no matter what their lifestyle or personal behaviors, certain types of lifestyles and behaviors increase cancer risk, whereas others reduce the risk of developing cancer. Cancer prevention includes the following.

Avoidance of cigarette smoking is the number one behavior that can have a positive influence on avoiding cancer, both for the individual who smokes and for family members and coworkers exposed to secondhand smoke. Children appear to be at increased risk of developing cancer after exposure to secondhand smoke even in utero. Chewable tobacco products also are associated with an increased risk of oral cancer and should be avoided. Chewing tobacco is a major health concern in adolescent medicine.

A diet rich in fruits and vegetables and low in animal fat has been associated with a reduction in cancer for many population groups.

Avoidance of sexually transmitted diseases reduces the risks of developing some types of cancer, such as cervical and liver cancer.

CANCER DETECTION

Early detection of cancer, while not a preventive measure, can serve to contain or destroy a cancer before it has metastasized throughout the body. Early detection depends on identifying risk factors for a specific patient, and using appropriate physical examination techniques. Early cancer detection tests include self breast examination and mammography, prostate examination, self testicular examination, and a thorough skin examination. Some screening tests, such as Pap smears, tests for intestinal polyps, and tests for occult rectal bleeding, may allow for intervention even before dysplastic cells (cells showing early signs of changes in cell organization) become cancerous.

Selected Bibliography

Bertwistle, D. & Ashworth, A. (1998). Functions of the BRCA1 and BRCA2 genes. *Current Opinion in Genetics and Development* 8, 14–20.

Blaese, R. M. (1997). Gene therapy for cancer. *Scientific American* 276, 111–115.

Braun, M. M., Caporaso, N. E., Page, W. F., & Hoover, R. N. (1994). Genetic component of lung cancer: cohort study of twins. *Lancet* 344, 440–443.

Brown, L. M. (1992). Smoking and the risks of leukemia. *American Journal of Epidemiology* 135, 763–768.

Cao, Y., O'Reilly, M. S., Marshall, B., Flynn, E., Ji, R. W., & Folkman, J. (1998). Expression of angiostatin cDNA in a murine fibrosarcoma suppresses primary tumor growth and produces long-term dormacy of metastasis. *Journal of Clinical Investigation* 101, 1055–1063.

Catalona, W. J., Smith, D. S., & Ornstein, D. K. (1997). Prostate cancer detection in men with serum PSA concentrations of 2.6 to 4.0 ng/ml and benign prostate examination: enhancement of specificity with free PSA measurements. *Journal of the American Medical Association* 277, 1452–1455.

Cavenee, W. K. & White, R. L. (1995). The genetic basis of cancer. *Scientific American* 272, 72–79.

Ellen, J. M., Moscicki, A. B., & Shafer, M. A. (1994). Genital herpes simplex virus and human papillomavirus infection. *Advanced Pediatric Infectious Disease* 9, 97–124.

Goolsby, M. J. (1998). Screening, diagnosis, and management of prostate cancer: improving primary care outcomes. *The Nurse Practitioner* 23, 11–41.

Grodstein, F., Stampfer, M. J., Colditz, G. A., Willett, W. C., Manson, J. E., & Josse, M. (1997). Postmenopausal hormone therapy and mortality. *New England Journal of Medicine* 336, 1769–1775.

Greider, C. W. (1998). Telomerase activity, cell prolifertion, and cancer. *Proceedings of the National Academy of Sciences, USA* 95, 90–92.

Halliwell, B. (1994). Free radicals, antioxidants, and human disease: curiosity, cause, or consequence? *Lancet* 344, 721–724.

Hellman, S. & Vokes, E. E. (1996). Advancing current treatments for cancer. *Scientific American* 275, 118–123.

Jain, M., Miller, A. B., & To., T. (1994). Premorbid diet and the prognoses of women with breast cancer. *Journal of the National Cancer Institute* 86, 1390–1397.

Kaminski, M., Zasadny, K. R., et al. (1993). Radioimmunotherapy of a Bcell lymphoma with [^{131}I] anti-B1 antibody. *New England Journal of Medicine* 329, 459–465.

Kjaer, S. K., Van den Brule, A. J., & Bock, J. E. (1996). Human papillomavirus—the most significant risk determinant of cervical intraepithelial neoplasia. *International Journal of Cancer* 65, 601–606.

Newcomb, P. A. & Storer, B. E. (1995). Postmenopausal hormone use and risk of large-bowel cancer. *Journal of the National Cancer Institute* 87, 1067–1070.

Nightengale, T. E. & Grube, J. (1994). Helicobacter and human cancer. *Journal of the National Cancer Institute* 86, 1505–1509.

Old, L. J. (1996). Immunotherapy for cancer. *Scientific American* 275, 136–143.

O'Reilly, M. S., Boehm, T., Shing, Y., et al. (1997). Endostatin: an endogenous inhibitor of angiogenesis and tumor growth. *Cell* 88, 277–285.

Ruoslahti, E. (1996). How cancer spreads. *Scientific American* 275, 72–77.

Schultz, M. Z., Ward, B., & Reiss, M. (1996). Breast diseases. In: Noble, J. (ed.). *Textbook of Primary Care Medicine (2nd ed.)*. St. Louis: Mosby.

Stewart, B. W. (1994). Mechanisms of apoptosis: integration of genetic, biochemical, and cellular indicators. *Journal of the National Cancer Institute* 86, 1286–1295.

Thune, I., Brenn, T., Lund, E., & Guard, M. (1997). Physical activity and the risk of breast cancer. *New England Journal of Medicine* 336, 1269–1275.

Trichopoulos, D., Li, F. P., & Hunter, D. J. (1996). What causes cancer? *Scientific American* 275, 80–87.

Weinberg, R. A. (1996). How cancer arises. *Scientific American* 275, 62–70.

Yeung, W., Pang, Y. K., Tsang, Y. S., Wong, S. W., & Leung, J. S. (1994). Short-duration in vitro interleukin-2-activated mononuclear cells for advanced cancer. *Cancer* 71, 3633–3639.

THE HEMATOLOGIC SYSTEM

The hematologic system includes all the blood cells, the bone marrow in which the cells mature, and the lymphoid tissue where the cells are stored when not in circulation. The hematologic system is designed to carry oxygen and nutrients, transport hormones, remove waste products, and deliver cells to prevent infection, stop bleeding, and promote healing. The hematologic system allows the body to feed and heal itself and to communicate between sites.

● ● ●

PHYSIOLOGIC CONCEPTS

Composition of the Blood

The blood is made up of approximately 45% formed elements and 55% plasma. The formed elements are the red blood cells (erythrocytes), the white blood cells (leukocytes), and the platelets (thrombocytes). The red blood cells account for 99% of the formed elements; the white blood cells and platelets the other 1%. The plasma is 90% water, with the other 10% made up of plasma proteins, electrolytes, dissolved gases, and various waste products of metabolism, nutrients, vitamins, and cholesterol. The plasma proteins include albumin, the globulins, and fibrinogen. **Albumin** is the most abundant of the plasma proteins and helps maintain the plasma osmotic pressure and blood volume. The **globulins** bind insoluble hormones and other plasma constituents in the plasma, and make them soluble. This allows these important substances to be transported in the blood from their site of production to their site of action. Examples of substances carried bound to plasma proteins include thyroid hormone, iron, phospholipids, bilirubin, steroid hormones, and cholesterol. Other globulin proteins, the immunoglobulins, are the antibodies that travel in the blood to fight infection. **Fibrinogen** is an important element in blood clotting.

Hematopoiesis

Red blood cells, white blood cells, and platelets are formed in the liver and spleen in the fetus, and in the bone marrow after birth. The process of blood cell formation is called **hematopoiesis.**

Hematopoiesis begins in the bone marrow with pluripotential stem cells (meaning "many possible"). Stem cells are the source of all blood cells. These cells continually self-renew and differentiate throughout a lifetime: their supply is endless and they are often described as immortal. After several stages of differentiation, a stem cell becomes committed to forming just one type of blood cell. This cell, called a "progenitor cell," remains in the marrow, and when instructed by specific growth factors, differentiates into a red blood cell, a white blood cell, or a platelet. The development of the blood cells from original pluripotential stem cells to differentiated cells is shown in Figure 6-1.

CONTROL OF PROGENITOR CELL DIFFERENTIATION

Progenitor cells are stimulated to proliferate and differentiate by a variety of hormones and locally produced agents that collectively are called **hematopoietic growth factors.** Each progenitor cell responds only to some of these growth factors, but many growth factors may be acting nonspecifically on several progenitor cells. Many hematopoietic growth factors are cytokines. Cytokines are released from immune and inflammatory cells and communicate to the progenitor cells the need for more cells to fight infection or help the body heal. Hematopoietic growth factors specific for the line of cells they stimulate are called **colony-stimulating factors.** For example, granulocyte colony-stimulating factor stimulates the production of white blood cells known as granulocytes (see later), whereas monocyte-macrophage colony-stimulating factor increases the proliferation of monocytes and macrophages. An example of an important colony-stimulating growth factor for red blood cells is the hormone **erythropoietin** produced by the kidney in response to low oxygen concentration in the blood. Other nonspecific cytokines may act on cells less differentiated than the progenitor cells, stimulating the production of a variety of blood cells.

The Red Blood Cell

The red blood cell (erythrocyte) contains no nucleus, mitochondria, or ribosomes. It cannot reproduce or undergo oxidative phosphorylation or protein synthesis. The red blood cell contains the protein hemoglobin that carries oxygen picked up in the lungs to all cells of the body. Hemoglobin takes up most of the red blood cell's intracellular space. Red blood cells are produced in the bone marrow in response to hemopoietic growth factors, especially erythropoietin, and require iron, folic acid, and vitamin B_{12} for their synthesis. As a red blood cell nears maturity, it is released from the bone marrow, completes its maturation in the bloodstream, and lives out its approximately 120-day life span. It then disintegrates and dies. Dying red blood cells are replaced with new ones released from the bone marrow. If red blood cell death is excessive, a larger than normal number of immature red blood cells, called *reticulocytes,* will be released from the bone marrow; elevated levels of circulating reticulocytes is suggestive of certain types of anemia.

CHARACTERISTICS OF RED BLOOD CELLS

Red blood cells are small, biconcave (two-sided) disks shaped like donuts without the hole. Their high surface area allows for rapid

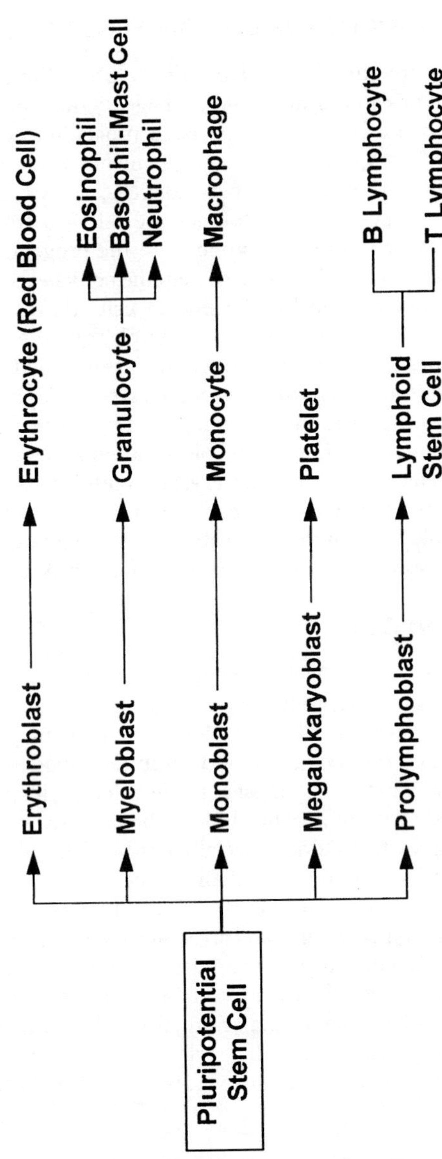

Figure 6-1. Examples of common anemias, their causes, and laboratory diagnosis.

diffusion of oxygen and carbon dioxide, while their small size (7 μm in diameter) and relative flexibility allows them to squeeze through even the smallest of capillary beds without damage. In a blood sample, the percentage of the blood that is taken up by red blood cells is called the **hematocrit**, which usually ranges from approximately 36% to 52% depending on age and sex. The concentration of hemoglobin in a blood sample (grams per 100 mL) usually is approximately a third the hematocrit. Red blood cells are described clinically by their size and by the amount of hemoglobin present in the cell. In the terminology, "cytic" refers to size, and "chromic" refers to the concentration of hemoglobin in the cell.

- Normocytic: cells of normal size.
- Normochromic: cells with normal amounts of hemoglobin
- Microcytic: cells too small in size
- Macrocytic: cells too large in size
- Hypochromic: cells with too little hemoglobin
- Hyperchromic: cells with too dense hemoglobin

RED BLOOD CELL ANTIGENS

The red blood cell has a variety of specific antigens present on its cell membrane that are not found on other cells. The most important of these antigens are known as A and B, and Rh.

ABO Antigens

An individual carries two alleles (genes) each coding for the A or B antigen, or neither antigen, which is designated O. One allele is received from each parent. The A and B antigens are codominant. Individuals with both the A and B antigen (AB) will have AB blood. Those with two A antigens (AA), or one A and one O (AO), will have A blood. Those with two B antigens (BB), or one B and one O (BO), will have B blood. Individuals with neither antigen (OO) will have O blood.

Individuals who have AB blood will accept A, B, or O blood. However, an immune response will develop if an individual without an A or B antigen is exposed to that antigen in a blood transfusion.

Rh Antigens

Rh antigens are the other main antigen group on the red blood cell and are also passed as genes from each parent. The main Rh antigen is called the Rh factor. An individual who carries the Rh antigen is considered Rh positive (Rh^+). An individual who lacks the Rh antigen is considered Rh negative (Rh). The Rh-positive gene is dominant; therefore, an individual must have two negative Rh factors to be Rh negative. Individuals who are Rh positive will accept Rh negative blood, but those who do not have the Rh antigen will develop an immune response if exposed to Rh-positive blood.

UNIVERSAL BLOOD RECIPIENTS AND DONORS

Universal blood recipients are those with AB-positive blood because their immune system will recognize as self the A or B antigen and the Rh-positive antigen. Therefore, they will accept blood with any ABO and Rh profile. Universal blood donors are those with O-negative blood. Although their immune systems will attack blood containing the A or B antigen, and the Rh factor, their blood can be given for transfusion to any recipient in an emergency. Other weaker antigens on red blood cells exist, however, and may provoke an immune reaction in a recipient.

HEMOGLOBIN

Hemoglobin consists of an iron-containing substance called heme and the protein globulin. There are approximately 300 hemoglobin molecules in each red blood cell.

Each hemoglobin molecule contains four binding sites for oxygen. Oxygen bound to hemoglobin is called oxyhemoglobin. Hemoglobin in the red blood cell may be partially or completely bound with oxygen on all four sites. Fully saturated hemoglobin is completely bound with oxygen, while partially saturated or deoxygenated hemoglobin is less than 100% saturated. Systemic arterial blood from the lungs is fully saturated with oxygen. Because hemoglobin releases oxygen to the cells, the hemoglobin saturation in venous blood is approximately 60%. The final job of the hemoglobin is to pick up carbon dioxide and hydrogen ions and carry them to the lungs where they are exhaled to the air.

There are at least 100 types of abnormal hemoglobin molecules that have been recognized in humans, resulting from a variety of different mutations. Most of these cause the hemoglobin molecule to carry oxygen more poorly than the normal molecule.

BREAKDOWN OF THE RED BLOOD CELL

When the red blood cell begins to disintegrate at the end of its lifetime, it releases hemoglobin into the circulation. Hemoglobin is broken down in the liver and spleen. The globulin molecule is converted into amino acids that are used again by the body. The iron is stored in the liver and spleen until it is reused. The rest of the molecule is converted to bilirubin, which is excreted in the stool as bile or in the urine. Normally, the rate of red cell breakdown is equal to the rate of synthesis. In certain conditions, synthesis or breakdown may outpace the other.

White Blood Cells

White blood cells are formed in the bone marrow from committed progenitor cells. On further differentiation, the progenitor cells become non–granular-appearing T and B lymphocytes, monocytes, and macrophages, or granular-appearing neutrophils, basophils, and eosinophils. The job of the white blood cells is to recognize and fight microorganisms in immune reactions, and to assist in the inflammation and healing processes. The platelets, which are not cells but fragments of bone marrow cells, are essential in the control of bleeding. In addition, they often function with the white blood cells in the inflammatory and healing processes.

TYPES OF WHITE BLOOD CELLS

B lymphocytes develop in the bone marrow and then circulate in the blood until they encounter the antigen to which they are programmed to respond. At this point, B lymphocytes mature further, become plasma cells, and begin secreting antibody, as described later.

T lymphocytes leave the bone marrow and develop during migration through the thymus. After leaving the thymus, they circulate in the blood or reside in lymphatic tissue until they encounter an antigen to which they are programmed to respond. Once stimulated by antigen, they produce chemicals to destroy the microorganism and alert other white blood cells that an infection is occurring, as described later.

Monocytes are formed in the bone marrow and enter the bloodstream in an immature form. At the site of injury or infection, the monocytes leave the blood and mature into macrophages in the tissues.

Macrophages may remain stored in the tissues, or may be used in an inflammatory reaction as soon as they mature.

Neutrophils, basophils, and eosinophils are granular-appearing white blood cells that assist in the inflammatory response. Macrophages, neutrophils, and eosinophils function as phagocytes—cells that destroy and digest microorganisms and accumulated cell debris. Although the exact function of the basophils is unclear, they appear to act like circulating mast cells (Chapter 3) that release vasoactive peptides that stimulate the inflammatory response.

The Spleen

The spleen is a small organ located in the upper left abdominal cavity. It is considered a secondary lymphoid organ, as opposed to the bone marrow and thymus. Like all lymphoid organs it is involved in the formation and storage of the blood.

The spleen is the site of hematopoiesis in the fetus. After birth, the spleen contains tissue macrophages and aggregates of lymphocytes. The spleen is well supplied with blood vessels that branch off from the splenic artery itself, a branch of the abdominal aorta. The intricate vasculature of the spleen circulates blood containing microorganisms, dead cells, and other debris past the macrophages and lymphocytes where they can be acted on or destroyed. After flowing through the splenic capillary networks, the blood vessels rejoin into venules and blood is delivered to the liver through the hepatic portal blood flow system.

FUNCTIONS OF THE SPLEEN

As blood passes through the spleen, residing macrophages act as phagocytes to clear the blood of cell debris (including lysed red blood cells) and to digest microorganisms. The macrophages present pieces of digested microorganisms to nearby B and T cells, initiating an immune response. Individuals who have lost their spleen (usually after trauma) are at a disadvantage in fighting certain infections compared to those with a functioning spleen. Other individuals may have their spleens removed surgically when platelet count is low and cannot be corrected. These individuals would also be at a disadvantage in fighting infection.

The spleen also serves as a reservoir for blood, capable of holding a few hundred milliliters in the adult. With a decrease in blood pressure, the spleen can expel this blood into the venous circulation to help return pressure. It also serves as a storage site for iron released during the catabolism of hemoglobin. Iron is stored in splenic macrophages until required for production of new red blood cells. Iron deficiency may occur without the spleen. The spleen also stores senescent red blood cells.

Lymph Nodes

Lymph nodes are small capsules of lymphoid tissue interspersed throughout the lymphatic system, near the lymphatic veins. Lymph flowing in the lymphatic vessels is filtered through many nodes.

Lymph nodes contain many lymphocytes, monocytes, and macrophages. These cells proliferate in the nodes and some are released into the circulation during infection or inflammation. Residing white blood cells entrap and phagocytize microorganisms that are delivered by the lymph flow, cleansing the lymph before it is returned to the general circulation. The lymph node closest to an infection is exposed to the highest number of microorganisms, which causes the macrophages and lymphocytes to proliferate and the node to enlarge. An active node may become tender as it fights to contain infection.

Hemostasis

The human body experiences frequent small capillary tears and occasional large blood vessel cuts. While unable to control large vessel bleeding without external support, the body is able to stop small vessel bleeding. Control of bleeding occurs by two steps—the formation of a platelet plug followed by the formation of a blood clot. These processes are interdependent, and occur one after the other in rapid succession. The control of bleeding is called hemostasis.

ROLE OF THE PLATELETS IN HEMOSTASIS

Platelets play an important role in both steps of hemostasis. Platelets normally circulate throughout the bloodstream without sticking to vascular endothelial cells. However, within seconds after damage to a blood vessel, platelets are drawn to the area in response to exposed collagen on the subendothelial layers of the damaged blood vessel. Platelets attach to proteins (called von Willebrand factors) expressed on the damaged surface of a blood vessel and release several vasoactive chemicals, including serotonin and adenosine diphosphate (ADP). Serotonin causes vasoconstriction, helping to reduce blood flow to the area and limit bleeding. Serotonin and other chemicals, including ADP, also cause the platelets to change shape and become sticky, beginning the formation of what is called a "platelet plug" inside the damaged blood vessel. Other platelets are drawn to the area and further build up the plug. **Thromboxane** A_2 is produced by the platelets and contributes to the attraction of more platelets to the area. **Fibrinogen**, a circulating plasma protein, connects between exposed sites on the platelets, serving like a bridge to add stability to the plug. The platelet plug effectively seals the damaged area. Deficiencies in any of the involved factors will result in excessive bleeding of even small capillary tears.

LIMITS ON PLATELET FUNCTION

Unimpeded platelet aggregation could cause a prolonged decrease in blood flow to the tissue or result in a plug becoming so enlarged that it may break off from the original site and travel downstream as an embolus, blocking downstream flow. To prevent either of these occurrences from happening, neighboring *undamaged* endothelial cells release other substances that limit the extent of platelet aggregation. The main substances released by neighboring endothelial cells to limit platelet aggregation are prostaglandin I_2, also called **prostacyclin**, and **nitric oxide**, an important vasodilator and an inhibitor of platelet aggregation.

Ultimately, the balance between pro-clotting and anti-clotting factors serve to keep the platelets active at the site of injury while preventing excessive platelet aggregation and spread of the platelet plug to uninjured vascular tissue. Platelet aggregation and the production of the platelet plug are shown in Figure 6-2.

BLOOD CLOT

The platelet plug becomes a true clot as it enlarges and traps circulating red cells and macrophages. The entire clot is stabilized and strengthened by a network of fibrin strands, produced from the fibronogen bridges mentioned earlier. The production of stabilized fibrin is the final step in the other essential component of homeostasis, the coagulation cascade.

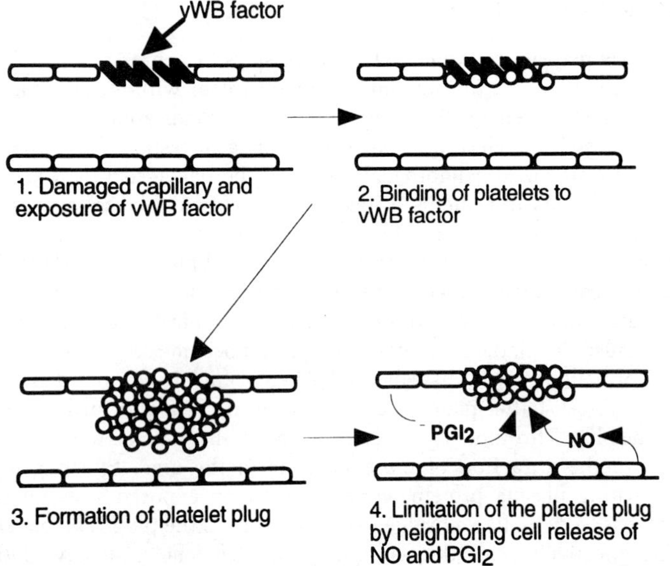

Figure 6-2. Steps involved in the formation of the platelet plug. The role of von Willibrand Factor (vWB), platelets, and prostaglandin I2 (PGI2) and nitric oxide (NO) released from neighboring endothelical cell is emphasized.

COAGULATION REACTIONS

Coagulation reactions involve a series of coagulation factors or proteins activated in domino fashion, leading to the coagulation (clotting) of the blood. There are a total of 13 proteins involved in the coagulation pathways, some activated in what is called the *intrinsic pathway* and some in the *extrinsic pathway*. Under most physiologic conditions, coagulation occurs first through the extrinsic pathway: activation of the extrinsic pathway then turns on the more powerful intrinsic pathway. Both pathways ultimately merge and function by activating one protein, factor X; the merging of the intrinsic and extrinsic pathways at factor X is called the final common pathway. Factor X is responsible for converting the plasma protein prothrombin to **thrombin.** Thrombin is the key catalyst that drives the conversion of fibrinogen to fibrin and causes coagulation. Thrombin also acts in a positive feedback manner to stimulate the proteins involved in its own production, furthering the coagulation cascade. Both pathways are shown in Figure 6-3.

The intrinsic pathway begins with the activation of the circulating coagulation factor, factor XII, also called the Hageman factor. Factor XII is activated when it comes into contact with damaged vascular tissue. Ultimately, activation of factor XII leads to the conversion of

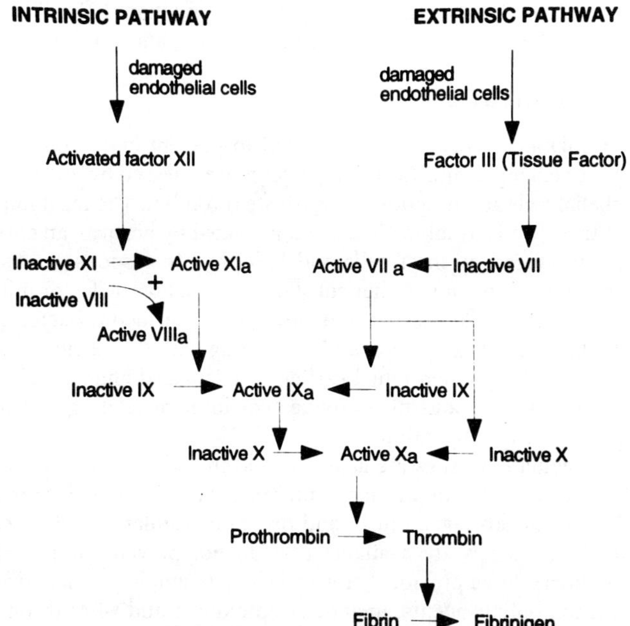

Figure 6-3. Simplified diagram of the intrinsic and extrinsic pathways of coagulation. Factor VII is highlighted to identify its pivotal role as a coenzyme in the intrinsic pathway. Letter "a" designates an activated factor.

prothrombin to thrombin. Factors XI and IX are important intermediate steps in the cascade, and factors V and VIII are important cofactors. Lack of any of these factors could interfere with coagulation.

The extrinsic pathway, the usual way of stimulating coagulation, begins with the release into the circulation of factor III, also called tissue factor or thromboplastin, from damaged vascular endothelial cells. When tissue factor encounters in the plasma another circulating coagulation factor, factor VII (also called serum prothrombin conversion factor), the extrinsic cascade is stimulated, again resulting in the production of factor X. The extrinsic pathway also can turn on the intrinsic pathway through activation of factor IX.

The blood does not continually and excessively clot even though factors XII and VII are always present in the circulation because healthy endothelial cells are smooth and intact. Therefore, they do not directly activate factor XII or produce tissue factor and activate factor VII. Healthy vascular endothelium repels coagulation factors and platelets. It is only when the endothelium is damaged by trauma, infection, forces of chronic hypertension, or accumulation of fat and cholesterol (Chapter 11) that a clot begins to develop.

Because several coagulation factors are produced in the liver in reactions involving vitamin K, liver disease or vitamin K deficiency can impair the production of coagulation factors and cause bleeding.

ANTICOAGULANTS

Anticoagulants are present in the blood to prevent clots from developing. For example, antithrombin proteins are released by undamaged endothelial cells and function to inactivate thrombin. The most important of these, antithrombin III, is itself activated by heparin, an anticoagulant produced by mast cells and basophils in response to tissue injury and inflammation. Other substances, called tissue factor inhibitors, circulate in the plasma and bind to tissue factor (factor III), directly blocking its activation and interfering with the extrinsic pathway. And finally, as mentioned earlier, nondamaged endothelial cells secrete prostacyclin and nitric oxide that limit platelet aggregation, and thus reduce coagulation.

Anticoagulation drugs are available and include the prostaglandin inhibitor aspirin, that in low doses inhibits the production of thromboxane A_2 but not prostaglandin I_2, and oral anticoagulants such as coumadin. Other drugs are available that do not prevent clotting, but serve to break down previously formed clots. Examples of these drugs, called thrombolytic agents, include streptokinase and t-PA; thrombolytic agents play an important role in the early treatment of myocardial infarct and thrombotic stroke.

Laboratory Tests of the Blood

THE COMPLETE BLOOD COUNT WITH DIFFERENTIAL AND PLATELET COUNT

The blood is frequently tested for the adequacy of cell number and function. The most common test is the complete blood count (CBC), which provides information on the number and concentration of red blood cells, white blood cells, and platelets present in a venous blood sample. The CBC with differential is age dependent and to a lesser extent, sex dependent. Exercise, reproductive status, and many drugs may cause test deviations. The CBC with differential is used as part of well physical examinations, to screen for specific conditions, and to determine preoperative health. The CBC is also used to evaluate treatment success.

Blood tests to evaluate red cell size (mean corpuscular volume [MCV]) and hemoglobin concentration (mean corpuscular hemoglobin concentration [MCHC]) give important information when evaluating patients with anemia. Other common blood tests include blood typing of ABO and Rh antigens and tests to identify the presence of microorganisms and antibody titers. The sedimentation rate (SED rate) is a test that evaluates the settling of red blood cells. The SED rate is often increased nonspecifically with inflammatory disease.

THE CBC WITH DIFFERENTIAL AND PLATELET COUNT (ADULT)

- Red blood cell count: 4.0 to 5.5 million/mL of blood
- White blood cell count: 5,000 to 10,000/mL of blood
- Platelet count: 150,000 to 400,000/mL of blood
- Hematocrit (% of red blood cells): 45% to 52% for males; 36% to 48% for females
- Hemoglobin: 14.0 to 17.5 grams/100 mL for males; 12.0 to 16.0 grams/100 mL for females
- Neutrophils: 50% to 62%
- Eosinophils: 0% to 3%
- Basophils: 0% to 1%
- Lymphocytes: 25% to 40%
- Monocytes: 3% to 7%

TESTS OF RED BLOOD CELL SIZE AND HEMOGLOBIN (ADULT)

- MCV: 76 to 96 fL/red cells
- MCHC: 30 to 35 pg/cell

SEDIMENTATION RATE

- SED Rate: 0 to 20 mm/hour

BLEEDING TIME

Bleeding time refers to the length of time bleeding occurs after a standardized puncture wound to the skin. Bleeding time is measured in minutes and indicates the functioning status of the platelets, specifically the effectiveness of the platelet plug. Bleeding time should not exceed 15 minutes (normal: 2.0 to 9.5 minutes) for a forearm stick.

PARTIAL THROMBOPLASTIN TIME/PROTHROMBIN TIME

Partial thromboplastin time (PTT) and prothrombin time (PT) detect deficiencies in the activity of various clotting factors. Both tests evaluate clotting in a venous blood sample.

PTT especially demonstrates the effectiveness of the intrinsic pathway of coagulation and should not exceed 90 seconds (normal: 30 to 45 seconds). This test is important in determining the effectiveness and safety of heparin therapy.

PT demonstrates the effectiveness of the vitamin K-dependent coagulation factors, especially the extrinsic and common pathways of coagulation. PT should not exceed 40 seconds, or 2 to 2.5 times a control level (normal: 10 to 14 seconds). PT is used to determine the effectiveness of warfarin (Coumadin) therapy.

Pediatric Consideration

Newborn values of red blood cells, white blood cells, hemoglobin, and hematocrit are elevated compared to older infants, children, and some adults. High values begin to decrease within 2 weeks of birth, reaching a plateau after approximately 6 months. Levels reach adult values at approximately 18 years of age. Bleeding time, especially PT is prolonged in infants because of a natural deficiency in vitamin K. At birth, infants in the United States are given injections of vitamin K to reduce the risk of bleeding.

PATHOPHYSIOLOGIC CONCEPTS

Anemia

Anemia is a decrease in the quantity of circulating red blood cells, an abnormality in the hemoglobin content of red blood cells, or both. Anemia can be caused by a disorder in red blood cell production or an elevated loss of red blood cells through chronic bleeding, sudden hemorrhage, or excessive lysis (destruction). All anemias result in decreased values for hematocrit and hemoglobin but may vary in values of MCV and MCHC. The symptoms associated with anemia depend on its duration, its severity, and the host's age and prior health status. All symptoms ultimately relate to a reduction in the delivery of oxygen to host cells and organs, thereby interfering with function and compromising health.

ANEMIA CAUSED BY A DISORDER IN RED CELL PRODUCTION

Anemias that result from a disorder in red cell production occur if there is inadequate or inaccessible iron, or a lack of folic acid, vitamin B_{12}, or globulin. Red blood cell production may also be insufficient if there is bone marrow disease, as would occur in leukemia or after radiation exposure. A deficiency in erythropoietin, as would occur in renal failure, would also lead to a decrease in red cell production. Disorders in production may result in a red cell that is too small (microcytic) or too large (macrocytic), and hemoglobin content that is abnormally low (hypochromic).

ANEMIA CAUSED BY SUDDEN OR CHRONIC HEMORRHAGE OR LYSIS

Anemias caused by sudden hemorrhage, a slow chronic hemorrhage, or lysis result in a decrease in the total number of circulating red cells. This type of anemia may be associated with an increased percentage of circulating immature red cells (reticulocytes). Normal red blood cells live approximately 120 days. Red cell destruction or loss occurring before 100 days is abnormal.

Common anemias, their causes, and laboratory profiles are shown in Table 6-1, and some are discussed more fully in the final section of this chapter.

Polycythemia

Polycythemia is an increase in the number of red blood cells. Primary polycythemia (polycythemia vera) is characterized by an increase in platelets and granulocytes as well as red blood cells, and is believed to be the result of a precursor cell abnormality.

Polycythemia may occur secondarily to chronic hypoxia. Chronic hypoxia causes an increased release of the renal hormone erythropoietin, which stimulates the production of red blood cells. Individuals who live at high altitude or suffer from chronic lung disease frequently experience secondary polycythemia. Athletes who "blood dope," meaning accept self-transfusions of previously collected packed red cells, demonstrate polycythemia. And finally, polycythemia may be relative, rather than absolute: for instance during dehydration. In this condition, a decrease in plasma volume is reflected as an increase in the concentration of red cells. Polycythemia from any cause is associated with an increased risk of thrombus formation and an increase in the workload of the heart.

Table 6-1. Common Anemias

COMMON TYPE OF ANEMIA	CAUSES	LABORATORY FINDINGS
Normocyticnor-mochromic	Acute hemorrhage Sickle cell anemia Malaria Aplastic anemia Thalassemia Anemia of chronic disease	↓ Hct ↓ Hemoglobin no change MCV no change MCHC normal iron normal ferritin
Microcytic hypo-chromic	Iron-deficiency slow chronic hemorrhage anemia of pregnancy	↓ Hct ↓ Hemoglobin ↓ Iron status (except sid-eroblastic) ↓ ferritin ↓ or no change MCV ↓ or no change MCHC
Megaloblastic anemia	Folic acid deficiency Vitamin B deficiency	↓ Hct ↓ Hemoglobin ↑ MCV normal MCHC

LEUKOPENIA

Leukopenia is a decrease in white blood cell number. Leukopenia may be caused by a variety of conditions, including prolonged stress, viral infection, bone marrow disease or destruction, radiation, or chemotherapy. Severe systemic disease such as lupus erythematosus, thyroid disease, and Cushing's syndrome may cause a decrease in white blood cells. All or one type of white cell may be affected. Leukopenia may predispose the individual to infection.

Leukocytosis

Leukocytosis is an increase in the number of circulating white blood cells. Leukocytosis is a normal response to infection or inflammation. It can be seen after emotional disturbance, after anesthesia or exercise, and during pregnancy. Abnormal leukocytosis is observed in certain malignancies and bone marrow disorders. Usually, only one type of white blood cell is affected. For example, allergic responses and asthma are specifically associated with increased numbers of eosinophils. Leukemia is characterized by an abnormally high level of one type of white cell, with deficiencies in the others.

Shift to the Left

Shift to the left is a term used to describe an increased proportion of immature leukocytes (usually neutrophils) seen in the blood of an individual fighting an infection. In a shift to the left, neutrophils will be released from the bone marrow before their final maturation, when the demand for white blood cells is excessive. In a shift to the left, the immature neurtrophils are frequently referred to as "bands" or "stabs." As the infection or inflammation begins to recede, the release of immature neutrophils stops and the blood is said to show a return shift to the right, as mature neutrophils again dominate a blood smear. The returning mature neutrophils are frequently referred to as "segmented" neutrophils.

Thrombocytopenia

Thrombocytopenia is a decrease in the number of circulating platelets. It is associated with increased risk of severe bleeding, even with small injuries or small spontaneous bleeds. Thrombocytopenia is characterized by small spots of subcutaneous bleeding, called *petechiae* or larger areas of subcutaneous bleeding, called *purpura*. Ecchymosis (bruising) may also be present.

Primary thrombocytopenia, also referred to as immune thrombocytopenia purpura, may occur idiopathically (for unknown reasons) or as a result of an autoimmune disorder characterized by antibodies built against the platelets. Secondary causes of thrombocytopenia include bone marrow damaging chemotherapeutic drugs and radiation, and certain viral infections including HIV. Thrombocytopenia also develops in the serious condition, disseminated intravascular coagulation (DIC), in which, after periods of extensive clotting, platelets begin to be consumed, leading to extensive bleeding and high mortality.

Thrombocythemia

Thrombocythemia is an increase in the number of circulating platelets. Thrombocythemia is associated with increased risk of thrombosis (clotting) in the vasculature. Depending on the site of clot formation or trapping, stroke, myocardial infarct, or respiratory distress may develop.

Primary thrombocythemia may occur with malignancy, polycythemia vera, and other diseases of the bone marrow. Secondary causes of thrombocythemia include acute infection, exercise, stress, and ovulation. Secondary thrombocythemia caused by these conditions is usually short-lived. However, prolonged secondary thrombocythemia may occur after removal of the spleen because this organ normally stores some platelets until they are needed in the circulation. Inflammatory diseases such as rheumatoid arthritis may also be associated with prolonged thrombocythemia.

Lymphadenopathy

Lymphadenopathy, or lymphoid hyperplasia, is the enlargement of the lymph nodes in response to a proliferation of B or T lymphocytes. Lymphadenopathy typically occurs after infection by a microorganism.

Regional lymphadenopathy indicates a localized infection. Generalized lymphadenopathy usually indicates a systemic infection such as AIDS, or an autoimmune disorder such as rheumatoid arthritis or systemic lupus erythematosus.

Splenomegaly

Splenomegaly is enlargement of the spleen. It is usually a result of the proliferation in the spleen of lymphocytes caused by an infection elsewhere in the body. Splenomegaly caused by macrophage proliferation occurs if there are excessive numbers of dead cells (especially red blood cells) needing to be cleared from the circulation.

Splenomegaly may also occur as a result of engorgement of the spleen with blood. This is usually a complication of portal hypertension. Splenic tumors or cysts may also cause splenomegaly. Splenomegaly in response to an infection is usually associated with lymphadenopathy; other causes of splenomegaly are not.

CONDITIONS OF DISEASE OR INJURY

Aplastic Anemia

Aplastic anemia is a normocytic, normochromic anemia caused by dysfunction of the bone marrow such that dying blood cells are not replaced. Aplastic anemia is usually associated with a deficiency in red blood cells, white blood cells, and platelets, although rarely it may affect only the red cells.

There are many causes of aplastic anemia, including cancers of the bone marrow, autoimmune destruction of bone marrow, vitamin deficiency, ingestion of many different drugs or chemicals, and high-dose radiation or chemotherapy. Aplastic anemia may also develop after various viral infections, including mononucleosis, hepatitis, and AIDS. Frequently the cause is unknown.

CLINICAL MANIFESTATIONS

- **Classic systemic signs of anemia** are common to all the anemias described in this chapter and include:
  - Increased heart rate as the body attempts to deliver more oxygen to the tissues.
  - Increased respiratory rate as the body attempts to provide more oxygen to the blood.
  - Dizziness caused by a decreased brain blood flow.
  - Fatigue caused by decreased oxygenation of various organs including cardiac and skeletal muscles.
  - Skin pallor caused by decreased oxygenation.
  - Nausea caused by decreased gastrointestinal and central nervous system blood flow.
  - Decreased hair and skin quality.
- In aplastic anemia if platelets and white blood cells are involved, additional symptoms include:
  - Bleeding from the gums and teeth, easy bruising including petechia and purpura.
  - Recurrent infection.
  - Poor healing skin and mucosal sores.

DIAGNOSTIC TOOLS

- CBC with differential and platelet count, MCV, and MCHC will diagnose anemia.
- Bone marrow biopsy will determine involved cells.

COMPLICATIONS

- Heart failure and death as a result of cardiac overload can occur with severe anemia.
- Death from infection and hemorrhage if white blood cells or platelets are involved.

TREATMENT

- Treat underlying disorder if known or remove causative agent.
- Transfusions to reduce symptomatology.

- Bone marrow transplant.
- Immunosuppression if an autoimmune disease is involved.
- Drugs to stimulate bone marrow function may be effective.

Hemolytic Anemia

Hemolytic anemia is a decrease in red blood cell number caused by excessive destruction of red cells. Remaining red cells are normocytic and normochromic. Red blood cell production in the bone marrow will increase to replace destroyed cells and the advancement into the blood of immature red cells, the reticulocytes, will be accelerated.

Hemolytic anemia can occur from many different causes, including a genetic defect in the red blood cell that accelerates its destruction, or the idiopathic development of autoimmune destruction of the cells. A severe burn, infection, incompatible blood exposure, or exposure to certain drugs or toxins may also cause hemolytic anemia. Depending on the cause, hemolytic anemia may occur once or repeatedly. Specific causes of hemolytic anemia that are discussed in detail include sickle cell anemia, malaria, hemolytic disease of the newborn, and transfusion reaction.

SICKLE CELL ANEMIA

Sickle cell anemia is an autosomal recessive disorder caused by inheritance of two copies of a defective hemoglobin gene, one from each parent. The defective hemoglobin, called hemoglobin S (HbS), becomes rigid and elongated and forms a sickle shape when exposed to low oxygen. The sickled red blood cell loses its ability to move easily through narrow vascular spaces and becomes trapped in the microvasculature. This causes a blockage in blood flow to downstream tissues, leading to painful tissue ischemia. Although sickling is reversible if oxygen saturation of the hemoglobin returns, the sickled cells are especially fragile and many are destroyed in the microvasculature, leading to anemia. Destroyed cells are filtered and removed from the circulation in the spleen, which places an extra demand on splenic function. Scarring and sometimes infarction (cell death) of various organs, especially the spleen and bone, may occur. Multiorgan dysfunction is common after many years.

Stimuli for sickling include hypoxia, anxiety, fever, and exposure to the cold. Because the spleen is an important immune organ, infections, especially of bacterial origin, are common and frequently stimulate a sickle cell crisis.

At birth, signs of sickle cell disease may not be apparent because all infants have a high level of a different type of hemoglobin, fetal hemoglobin. Fetal hemoglobin does not sickle, but only lasts until approximately 4 months after birth. It is at this time that signs of disease become apparent. These signs include the classic symptoms of anemia and signs related to the painful occlusions characteristic of the disorder.

Individuals with sickle cell disease carry two defective genes and thus have only hemoglobin S. Individuals who are heterozygous for the sickle cell gene (carry one defective gene) are said to carry the sickle cell trait. Heterozygotes usually express hemoglobin S in approximately 30 to 40% of their red cells, with normal hemoglobin carried in the rest of the red cells. These individuals are typically asymptomatic unless exposed to low oxygen levels, especially while exercising.

In the United States, sickle cell anemia primarily affects African Americans—up to approximately 10% of that population carry the trait and approximately one child in every 375 black live births has the disease. Sickle cell trait has been shown to offer protection against the destruction of the red blood cell after an infection with the microorganism responsible for malaria. It is thought that this protection allowed the sickle cell gene to survive during evolution in areas with endemic (widespread) malaria, such as equatorial Africa. Figure 6-4 shows a chi square diagram of the genetic inheritance of sickle cell anemia.

CLINICAL MANIFESTATIONS

- Systemic signs of anemia are present.
- Intense pain caused by vascular occlusion in a sickling episode.
- Serious bacterial infections caused by inadequate splenic filtering of microorganisms.
- Splenomegaly as the spleen removes the dead cells, sometimes leading to an acute crisis.

DIAGNOSTIC TOOLS

- Newborn screening for hemoglobinopathies are used to identify high-risk individuals. Hemoglobin electrophoresis is used to identify the presence of sickle cell hemoglobin and confirm the disease.
- Serial blood tests demonstrate decreased hematocrit, hemoglobin, and red cell count.

	Hb	**HbS**
Hb	HbHb	Hb**HbS**
HbS	HbHbS	**HbSHbS**

Figure 6-4. A chi square diagram showing the transmission of the sickle cell hemoglobin (HbS).

- Prenatal testing identifies the presence of the homozygote state in the fetus.

COMPLICATIONS

- Vaso-occlusive events leading to tissue infarct may cause intense pain and disability.
- A sudden trapping of blood in the spleen, called splenic sequestration, leading to hypovolemia, shock, and possibly death. Cause of splenic sequestration is unknown, but may occur with fever and pain. Frequently the spleen will be removed after an occurrence. Loss of the spleen compromises the individual's subsequent responses to infection.
- Stroke leading to weakness, seizures, or inability to speak may occur from occlusion of the cerebral vessels.
- Aplastic crisis, during which the bone marrow temporarily stops erythropoiesis, may occur.
- Avascular necrosis of the long bones of the leg or arm may occur from occlusion. Hip replacement is a common sequela of severe disability.
- Priapism, prolonged and painful erection, may occur with vaso-occlusion of the vessels of the penis, which may lead to impotence in some circumstances.

TREATMENT

- Newborn screening for sickle cell has dramatically improved the prognosis of infants with the disease. All identified infants are provided prophylactic antibiotics (penicillin or erythromycin) to prevent infections, from birth until at least 5 years of age.
- If at any time a fever or other sign of infection develops, the child should be evaluated immediately and parenteral antibiotics should be provided. Most children with a fever should be admitted to the hospital.
- Ibuprofin or acetaminophen should be administered to relieve minor pain, and more potent pain medication should be provided if needed.
- All childhood immunizations should be administered on schedule with the addition of the pneumococcal vaccine in the first 2 years of life and a booster dose at 5 years of age. This will reduce the main cause of mortality in children with sickle cell disease—infection leading to sepsis.
- Increased hydration by at least 1.5 to 2 times normal requirements may reduce the severity of a vaso-occlusive event.
- Avoidance of low oxygen situations or oxygen-demanding activities.
- Therapeutic drugs, including hydroxyurea, are available for patients' use.
- Red blood cell transfusions are frequently required but should be

limited when possible to reduce the risk of transmission of infectious agents.

- Bone marrow transplant with an HLA-matched donor may eliminate the production of sickled cells, but will not improve already damaged organs, and requires the subsequent lifelong use of immunosuppresants to block rejection.
- Genetic counseling for families allows for future informed childbearing decisions.

MALARIA

Malaria is a cause of hemolytic anemia related to an infection of the red blood cells by a protozoan of the genus Plasmodium that is transmitted to humans in the saliva of a mosquito. Malaria is endemic in tropical and subtropical environments of the world. It is an acute disease that can become chronic with repeated episodes of debilitation. Infants and children are frequently affected.

The Plasmodium microorganism first infects the cells of the liver and then passes into the erythrocytes. Infection causes massive hemolysis of the red blood cells. At this point more parasites are released into the circulation and subsequent cycles of infection occur. Red cell hemolysis leads to acute and chronic anemia. Cycles of infection typically occur approximately 72 hours apart. The host response to infection includes activation of the immune system, including production of various cytokines designed to increase the immune response. These cytokines, including tumor necrosis factor and interleukins 1 and 6, are key in fighting against the parasite, but also are responsible for most of the clinical manifestations of the disease, especially fever and myalgia (muscle aches). Individuals usually recover, but may relapse.

CLINICAL MANIFESTATIONS

- Systemic signs of anemia are present.
- Cyclic (usually every 72 hours) fever spikes.
- Chills and sweating with the fever.
- Headache.
- Myalgia.
- Hepatomegaly and splenomegaly.
- Jaundice may occur from excessive red blood cell lysis and release of bilirubin.

DIAGNOSTIC TOOLS

- Blood analysis will demonstrate the occurrence of anemia and the presence of red blood cell parasites.

COMPLICATIONS

- With severe disease, hypoglycemia, respiratory distress, shock, and coma may develop.

- Some strains of the parasite are becoming resistant to traditional drug therapy.

TREATMENT

- Prophylactic therapy against malaria is advised for travelers to endemic areas.
- Prevention in endemic areas involves elimination of standing sources of water and the use of insecticides, mosquito nets, and repellents.
- Antimalarial drugs are available to treat the disease if contracted, although resistance to all available drugs, including the chloroquine-related drugs is high.
- Blood transfusions are occasionally performed; however, transmission of HIV has resulted in endemic areas.
- Vaccines against malaria are being developed, including DNA vaccines that may stimulate the immune response to infection. Some vaccines in use do not prevent infection by the parasite, but may reduce the severity of the disease.

HEMOLYTIC DISEASE OF THE NEWBORN

Hemolytic disease of the fetus and newborn is a normocytic, normochromic anemia seen in an Rh-positive fetus or infant born to an Rh-negative mother who has previously been exposed to Rh-positive blood, and has developed antibodies to the Rh antigen. The development of antibodies usually occurs only after multiple maternal exposures to the antigen, during previous pregnancies, abortions, or miscarriages, or during amniocentesis. The maternal antibodies, usually IgG, are transferred to the fetus through the placenta, and attack fetal red blood cells, leading to excessive red cell lysis and anemia. If the condition is mild, the maternal circulation effectively eliminates for the fetus the waste products of hemoglobin metabolism, including bilirubin, and the fetus suffers few ill effects in utero. Occasionally, maternal destruction of the fetal cells may be excessive, leading to a severe anemia and *hydrops fetalis*, a fatal condition characterized by massive edema and heart failure.

After delivery in the less affected infant, clinical signs of anemia may occur. More significant in the neonatal period is the development of severe jaundice, as the breakdown products of hemoglobin are ineffectively cleared by the infant's immature liver. A dramatic elevation in bilirubin can lead to a significant neurologic disorder, called **kernicterus**, as the unconjugated bilirubin precipitates out in the infant's brainstem, causing brain damage.

Hemolytic disease of the newborn in response to Rh incompatibility is uncommon and has become rarer with fewer pregnancies experienced by each woman and important prophylactic interventions (see later). As a result of these factors, the incidence of hemolytic disease of the newborn has dropped by at least 80% in the last few decades. More common than Rh incompatibility is ABO incompatibility. In this condition maternal antibodies are produced as a result of ABO incompatibility, even during a first pregnancy. The presence of antibodies against the A or B antigens seldom leads to full-blown newborn hemolytic disease. Hemolytic disease of the newborn is described further in Chapter 17.

CLINICAL MANIFESTATIONS

- Mild hemolytic disease may be relatively asymptomatic with slight hepatomegaly and minimally elevated bilirubin.
- Moderate and severe disease manifest with pronounced signs of anemia.
- Hyperbilirubinemia, resulting from excessive red cell lysis, may occur, leading to jaundice.

COMPLICATIONS

- Kernicterus.
- Severe anemia may cause heart failure.
- *Hydrops fetalis*. Affected fetuses often abort spontaneously at approximately 17 weeks' gestation.
- In one study, 10% of school-aged children who had received in utero transfusions for severe Rh incompatibility, showed neurologic abnormalities, most likely related to asphyxia and anemia at birth.

TREATMENT

- Prevention of Rh-induced hemolytic disease begins with the prenatal visit and documention of a woman's Rh-negative status and the presence or absence of Rh antibodies. Women who are confirmed Rh negative and who do not show Rh-positive antibodies, are administered an anti-Rh antibody preparation called RhoGAM at 28 weeks' gestation, or at the time of a miscarriage, abortion, or amniocentesis. If after birth, the infant is deemed to be Rh positive and the woman is still Rh negative, she is again given RhoGAM within 72 hours. The RhoGAM injection provides passive immunity to the woman such that she does not develop her own antibodies against the Rh factor. A woman who is found to be Rh positive at any time is not given RhoGAM, but she and her fetus are observed closely during pregnancy and after delivery.
- If a woman becomes Rh positive during pregnancy, the fetus is observed by serial amniocentesis to determine bilirubin level. Mildly affected fetuses are delivered at term; moderately affected fetuses may be delivered before term; severely affected fetuses may receive an intrauterine transfusion and be delivered before term.
- In the newborn with hemolytic disease, exchange blood transfusions

may be required. Transfusion is with Rh-positive blood not containing Rh antibody. Treatment should begin within 24 hours of birth and be repeated until twice the blood volume of the infant has been exchanged.
- In mild cases, phototherapy to reduce the levels of unconjugated bilirubin may be sufficient.

Transfusion Reaction

A transfusion reaction is an immune-mediated destruction of incompatible red blood cells received in a blood transfusion. Transfusion reactions against donated white blood cells occur more frequently, but are typically mild. Although host and donor blood antigens are always identified (typed) for ABO and Rh compatibility before a transfusion is given, an error in red blood cell typing or a mix-up in the blood supplies may occur. Transfusion reactions may also develop as a result of an immune reaction to bacteria transferred in contaminated blood products.

CLINICAL MANIFESTATIONS

- Immediate, life-threatening reactions occur with ABO incompatibility. Manifestations include:
  - Immediate flushing of the face.
  - A feeling of warmth in the vein receiving the blood.
  - Fever and chills.
  - Chest, flank, or low back pain.
  - Abdominal pain with nausea and vomiting.
  - Decreased blood pressure with increased heart rate.
  - Dyspnea (a sensation of breathing difficulty).
- Transfusion reactions against white blood cells are milder and usually include fever and occasionally chills.

COMPLICATIONS

- Renal failure may result from red blood cell casts and hemoglobin obstruction of the nephrons.

TREATMENT

- The transfusion must be stopped immediately.
- Fluids may be given to reduce the risk of renal damage.
- Anaphylactic responses are treated by anti-inflammatory drugs including antihistamines and steroids.
- Leukocyte-cleansed blood is available, which will eliminate reactions to white blood cells.

Posthemorrhagic Anemia

Posthemorrhagic anemia is a normocytic, normochromic anemia that results from sudden loss of blood in an otherwise healthy individual. The hemorrhage may be obvious or hidden.

Blood pressure decreases with sudden hemorrhage. Reflex responses to decreased blood pressure and tissue hypoxia include increased activation of the sympathetic nervous system. This results in increased vascular resistance, heart rate, and stroke volume, all of which serve to return blood pressure toward normal. Respiratory rate increases to improve oxygenation. Renal responses to decreased blood pressure include decreased urine output and increased release of the hormone renin. Salt and water reabsorption in the kidney increase, serving to return blood pressure toward normal. Renal secretion of erythropoietin is stimulated, leading to increased red cell production.

CLINICAL MANIFESTATIONS

- Increased heart rate and respiratory rate, with a decrease in blood pressure. Consciousness may be impaired.
- The cause of the hemorrhage will present with individual clinical manifestations.

DIAGNOSITIC TOOLS

- Reduction in red cell count, hematocrit, and hemoglobin on the CBC as interstitial fluid moves into the vascular compartment in an attempt to increase blood volume.

COMPLICATIONS

- Hypovolemic shock with the possibility of renal failure, respiratory failure, or death.

TREATMENT

- Restore blood volume with intravenous infusion of plasma or type-matched whole blood (or O negative). Saline or albumin may also be infused.

Pernicious Anemia

Pernicious anemia is a megablastic anemia characterized by abnormally large red blood cells (MCV > 100) with immature ("blastic") nuclei. Pernicious anemia is caused by a deficiency in vitamin B_{12}. Vitamin B_{12} is essential for DNA synthesis in red blood cells and for neuronal functioning. Vitamin B_{12} is provided in the diet and is absorbed across the stomach into the blood. A gastric hormone, *intrinsic factor,* is essential for absorption of vitamin B_{12}. Intrinsic factor is secreted by the parietal cells of the gastric mucosa. Most causes of pernicious anemia result from intrinsic factor deficiency, but dietary deficiency of vitamin B_{12} may occur. Usually, B_{12} deficiency is a slowly developing disorder, and frequently goes unnoticed until symptoms are severe. Typically, patients affected are elderly; it is rare for an individual younger than 30 to suffer pernicious anemia unless it is present at or soon after birth.

Intrinsic factor deficiency may occur congenitally or may develop after atrophy or destruction of the gastric mucosa as a result of chronic gastric inflammation or an autoimmune disease. There appears to be a genetic susceptibility to autoimmune causes. Surgical removal of all or part of the stomach will also result in intrinsic factor deficiency.

CLINICAL MANIFESTATIONS

- Systemic signs of anemia are present.
- Dementia related to neurologic deterioration.
- Ataxia (poor muscle coordination) and sensory loss resulting from myelin degeneration.

DIAGNOSTIC TOOLS

- Blood analysis will demonstrate anemia characterized by macrocytic cells with normal hemoglobin (elevated MCV, normal MCHC).
- A decrease in serum B_{12} will confirm the disease.

COMPLICATIONS

- Severe anemia may cause heart failure, especially in the elderly.

TREATMENT

- Lifelong intramuscular injections of vitamin B_{12}.

Geriatric Consideration

The elderly are most prone to suffer from a dietary deficiency of vitamin B_{12}, as a result of poor diet. Any elderly person demonstrating fatigue, rapid heart rate, and mental and physical sluggishness should be evaluated for vitamin B_{12} deficiency.

Folate-Deficiency Anemia

Folate (folic acid) deficiency anemia is a megablastic anemia characterized by large red cells with immature nuclei. Folic acid deficiency is caused by a lack of the vitamin folate. Folate is essential for red blood cell production and maturation. It is also important for DNA and RNA synthesis and for the function of several DNA proofreading enzymes (Chapter 2). Folic acid is provided in the diet, but deficiency is relatively common, especially in young women, anyone malnourished, and in those abusing alcohol. Folic acid absorption occurs across the small intestine and does not require intrinsic factor. Because of widespread folic acid deficiency and its recognized importance in maintaining health, folic acid supplementation of cereals and other grains is soon to be initiated in the United States. Folic acid supplementation is especially important for pregnant women, as described later.

CLINICAL MANIFESTATIONS

- Systemic signs of anemia are present.

DIAGNOSTIC TOOLS

- Blood analysis will demonstrate anemia characterized by macrocytic cells with normal hemoglobin (elevated MCV, normal MCHC). Typically, the MCV will be elevated less than in pernicious anemia, and there will be no vitamin B deficiency.

COMPLICATIONS

- Maternal deficiencies in folic acid are associated with an increased risk of fetal malformations, especially neural tube defects. Adult deficiency may be associated with an increased risk of cardiovascular disease.

TREATMENT

- Administration of oral folate. Women intending to become pregnant should begin vitamin supplementation at least 3 months before conception. It is important not to confuse folate-deficiency anemia with pernicious anemia because treatment with folic acid is contraindicated in pernicious anemia.
- Blood transfusions may be required in severe cases.

Iron-Deficiency Anemia

Iron-deficiency anemia is a microcytic-hypochromic anemia that results from a diet deficient in iron, or the slow, chronic loss of blood. Iron is an essential component of the hemoglobin that makes up a large part of the red blood cell. Iron deficiency is a problem in toddlers and children with increased growth demands. Pregnant women are frequently iron-deficient because of the iron demands of the growing fetus. Menstruating women tend to be iron deficient because of iron loss each month and an iron-deficient diet. Menstruating women who exercise are at increased risk because exercise increases metabolic demands of muscle cells. In men, iron deficiency usually occurs with an ulcer or liver disease characterized by bleeding. Iron deficiency develops slowly. Decreased red blood cell numbers prompt the bone marrow to increase the release of abnormally small, hemoglobin-deficient red cells.

CLINICAL MANIFESTATIONS

- Systemic signs of anemia are present once hemoglobin decreases to less than 12 g/100 mL in an adult. Individuals usually do not seek treatment for symptoms until hemoglobin decreases to 8 g/100 mL or below.
- In addition to the previously described systemic signs of anemia, pale palms, conjunctivae, and earlobes may also be present.

DIAGNOSTIC TOOLS

- Blood analysis demonstrates anemia characterized by microcytic-hypochromic cells and decreased serum iron. Iron-binding capacity in the blood is high because proteins that bind iron are in less demand.
- Stool test for occult blood may be positive, suggesting a GI bleed or carcinoma.

COMPLICATIONS

- A hemoglobin value of less than 5 g/100 mL can lead to heart failure and death.

TREATMENT

- An iron-rich diet containing red meat and dark green vegetables, such as spinach.
- Oral iron supplementation.
- Treat the cause of abnormal bleeding if known.

Sideroblastic Anemia

Sideroblastic anemia is a microcytic-hypochromic anemia characterized by the presence of abnormal red cells (sideroblasts) in the circulation and the bone marrow. Sideroblasts carry iron in the mitochondria rather than in the hemoglobin molecules, and thus are unable to transport oxygen to the tissues. There is no iron deficiency.

Poor transport of oxygen causes hypoxia. This is sensed by erythropoietin-secreting kidney cells. Erythropoietin stimulates new red cell production in the bone marrow, which causes the marrow to become congested and increases the production of sideroblasts, worsening the anemia.

Primary sideroblastic anemia can occur as a result of a rare genetic defect on the X chromosome (primarily seen in males) or may occur spontaneously, especially in the elderly. Secondary causes of sideroblastic anemia include certain drugs (i.e., some chemotherapeutic agents) and lead ingestion.

CLINICAL MANIFESTATIONS

- Systemic signs of anemia are present.
- Iron accumulation results in hepatomegaly and splenomegaly.

DIAGNOSTIC TOOLS

- Blood analysis demonstrates anemia characterized by microcytic hypochromic cells, with elevated plasma iron and normal iron-binding capacity.
- A bone marrow examination demonstrates the presence of iron accumulations, sideroblasts, and phagocytic macrophages.

COMPLICATIONS

- Some cases progress to myelodysplastic syndrome and acute myeloblastic leukemia.

TREATMENT

- The cause of the disease, if related to a drug, is removed.
- The drug pyridoxine may successfully treat the disease, especially in persons with no evidence of neutropenia or thrombocytopenia. Iron is not given.

Acute Infectious Mononucleosis

Mononucleosis is an acute infection of the B lymphocytes, usually caused by the Epstein-Barr virus, or less frequently, by the cytomegalovirus. Most adults were exposed to these viruses in early childhood and at that time successfully fought off active infection to gain lifelong immunity. Usually, individuals who develop mononucleosis are children who do not fight off the infection, or teenagers and young adults who are exposed to the virus for the first time. Transmission of the virus occurs primarily through oral secretions and appears to require repeated exposures. In the teenage to young adult years, the immune system may be less active, or depressed by poor dietary and sleep habits, making those age groups especially susceptible to infection.

CLINICAL MANIFESTATIONS

- The classic triad of symptoms of mononucleosis include: severe sore throat, fever, and swelling of the cervical lymph nodes.
- Overwhelming or mild fatigue may be present.
- Swelling of all lymphoid tissues, including spleen, tonsils, and other neck nodes, may be present. The lymph nodes are usually tender.
- The liver may be enlarged and tender.

Geriatric Consideration

Although mononucleosis is usually seen in young adults or children, the elderly may contact the disease. When infected, the elderly may be difficult to diagnose because of the absence of the classic triad of symptoms. Jaundice may be present.

DIAGNOSTIC TOOLS

- The liver may be palpable and liver function tests are abnormal in 95% of cases. Jaundice is rare in young people.
- Laboratory findings demonstrate a brief leukopenia followed by proliferation first of the infected B cells, and then immunoactive T cells. Many white cells are atypical.
- Blood tests, especially the monospot agglutination test, demonstrate antibodies to the Epstein-Barr virus.

COMPLICATIONS

- Complications are rare, but may include hepatitis, meningitis, encephalitis, and Guillain-Barré syndrome. Rarely, Burkitt's lymphoma or B lymphoma may develop.

TREATMENT

- Mononucleosis is usually self-limiting. Treatment is supportive and encourages adequate rest and hydration.
- Avoidance of contact sports so not to injure or rupture the spleen is important.
- Ibuprofin and acetaminophen may be given. Aspirin is not recommended because of its association with Reye's syndrome.

Leukemia

Leukemia is a cancer of one class of white blood cells in the bone marrow, which results in the proliferation of that cell type to the exclusion of other types.

Leukemia appears to be a clonal disorder, meaning one abnormal cancerous cell proliferates without control, producing an abnormal group of daughter cells. These cells prevent other blood cells in the bone marrow from developing normally, causing them to accumulate in the marrow. Because of these factors, leukemia is called an accumulation and a clonal disorder. Eventually, leukemic cells take over the bone marrow. This reduces blood levels of all nonleukemic cells, causing the many generalized symptoms of leukemia.

TYPES OF LEUKEMIA

Leukemia is described as acute or chronic, depending on the suddenness of appearance and how well differentiated the cancerous cells are. The cells of acute leukemia are poorly differentiated, whereas those of chronic leukemia are usually well differentiated.

Leukemia is also described based on the proliferating cell type. For instance, acute lymphoblastic leukemia, the most common childhood leukemia, describes a cancer of a primitive lymphocyte cell line. Granulocytic leukemias refer to leukemias of the eosinophils, neutrophils, or basophilis. Leukemia in adults is usually chronic lymphocytic or acute myeloblastic. Long-term survival rates for leukemia depend on the involved cell type, but range to more than 75% for childhood acute lymphocytic leukemia, which is a remarkable statistic for what was once a nearly always fatal disease.

RISK FACTORS FOR DEVELOPING LEUKEMIA

Risk factors for leukemia include a genetic predisposition coupled with a known or unknown initiator (mutating) event. Siblings of children with leukemia are 2 to 4 times more likely to develop the disease than other children. Certain abnormal chromosomes are seen in a high percentage of patients with leukemia. Likewise, individuals with certain chromosomal abnormalities, including Down syndrome, have an increased risk of developing leukemia. Exposure to radiation, some drugs that depress the bone marrow, and various chemotherapeutic agents have been suggested to increase the risk of leukemia. Environmental agents such as pesticides and certain viral infections also have been implicated.

Previous illness with a variety of diseases associated with hematopoiesis (blood cell production) have been shown to increase the risk of leukemia. These diseases include Hodgkin's disease, multiple myeloma, polycythemia vera, sideroblastic anemia, and myelodysplastic syndromes. Chronic leukemia may sometimes transform into acute leukemia.

CLINICAL MANIFESTATIONS

Acute leukemia has marked clinical manifestations. Chronic leukemia progresses slowly and may have few symptoms until advanced.

- Pallor and fatigue from anemia.
- Frequent infections caused by a decrease in white blood cells.
- Bleeding and bruising caused by thrombocytopenia and coagulation disorders.
- Bone pain caused by accumulation of cells in the marrow, which leads to increased pressure and cell death. Unlike growing pains, bone pain related to leukemia is usually progressive.
- Weight loss caused by poor appetite and increased caloric consumption by neoplastic cells
- Lymphadenopathy, splenomegaly, and hepatomegaly caused by leukemic cell infiltration of these lymphoid organs may develop.
- Central nervous system symptoms may occur.

DIAGNOSTIC TOOLS

- Laboratory findings include alteration in specific blood cell counts, with overall elevation or deficiency in white blood cell count variable, depending on the type of cell affected.

- Bone marrow tests demonstrate clonal proliferation and blood cell accumulation.
- Cerebral spinal fluid is examined to rule out central nervous system involvement.

COMPLICATIONS

- Children who survive leukemia have an increased risk of developing a new malignancy years later when compared to children who have never had leukemia, most likely related to the aggressiveness of chemotherapeutic regimens.
- Treatment regimes, including bone marrow transplant, are associated with temporary bone marrow depression, and increase the risk of developing a severe infection that could lead to death.

TREATMENT

- Multiple drug chemotherapy.
- Antibiotics to prevent infection.
- Transfusions of red blood cells and platelets to reverse anemia and prevent bleeding.
- Bone marrow transplant may successfully treat the disease. Blood products and broad spectrum antibiotics are provided during bone marrow transplant procedures to fight and prevent infection.
- Immunotherapy, including interferons and other cytokines, are used to improve outcome.
- Therapy may be more conservative for chronic leukemia.
- The treatments described earlier may contribute to the symptoms by causing further bone marrow depression, nausea, and vomiting. Nausea and vomiting may be controlled or reduced by pharmacologic and behavioral intervention.
- Even with successful treatment and remission, leukemic cells may still persist, suggesting residual disease. Implications for prognosis and cure are unclear.

Pediatric Consideration

Some evidence suggests the risk of developing childhood leukemia increases if the child's mother or father smokes, before or after the child's birth. Other reports suggest that childhood leukemia may be caused by a leukemia-causing virus. Both of these factors are under study.

Hodgkin's Disease

Hodgkin's disease is a cancer of the lymphoid tissue, usually of the lymph nodes and spleen. It is one of the most common cancers in young adults, especially young males. There is a second peak in incidence in the 6th decade of life. There are four major classifications of Hodgkin's disease, based on the cells involved and whether the neoplasms are nodular in form. Staging of Hodgkin's disease is important because it guides treatment and strongly influences outcome. Early stages of Hodgkin's, stages I and II, are usually curable. Cure rates for stages III and IV tend to be 75% and 60%, respectively.

Hodgkin's disease is a clonal disorder, arising from one abnormal cell. The abnormal cell population appears to be derived from a B cell or, less frequently, a T cell or monocyte. Neoplastic cells of Hodgkin's are called Reed-Sternberg cells. These cells intersperse among normal lymph tissue present in the lymph organs.

The cause of Hodgkin's disease is unknown. However, individuals with the disease and in remission from it demonstrate reduced T-cell-mediated immunity. In addition, sporadic case clusters suggest that a virus, perhaps one of the herpes strains, especially the Epstein-Barr virus, may be involved. There is likely a genetic tendency to develop the disease.

Geriatric Consideration

Elderly patients with Hodgkin's disease have a poorer response to therapy compared to young patients. This is largely because of the increased morbidity associated with aggressive chemotherapy. A more advanced stage of disease at the time of diagnosis also may be involved. Concurrent disease in the elderly (lung, cardiac, and renal) may affect the response to chemotherapy and radiation.

CLINICAL MANIFESTATIONS

- Painless enlargement of lymph nodes, especially in the neck and under the arms.
- Evening fevers and night sweats may occur.
- Weight loss accompanies advanced stages of the disease.

DIAGNOSTIC TOOLS

- Lymph node biopsy can diagnose Hodgkin's disease.

COMPLICATIONS

- Secondary malignancies and cardiotoxicity may develop after aggressive treatment.

TREATMENT

- Multidrug chemotherapy.
- Radiation therapy.
- Bone marrow transplant.

Non-Hodgkin's Lymphoma

Non-Hodgkin's lymphomas are cancers of the lymph tissue that are not Hodgkin's disease. Non-Hodgkin's lymphoma usually occurs in older adults and is typically discovered at a more advanced stage than Hodgkin's disease. Non-Hodgkin's lymphoma is not confined to a single group of lymph nodes as in Hodgkin's disease, but rather is diffusely spread throughout the lymphoid organs, including the lymph nodes, liver, spleen, and occasionally the bone marrow. Disease may also be found in the sinuses. Like Hodgkin's disease, non-Hodgkin's disease is classified under several divisions, primarily related to whether the neoplastic tissue is nodular or diffuse.

Non-Hodgkin's disease appears to develop from a malignancy of the B cells primarily, but T cells and macrophages may also be the original site of the cancer. Causes of non-Hodgkin's lymphoma are unclear, but a viral infection, including HIV infection, appears to be responsible for at least some cases. Overall, non-Hodgkin's lymphoma has a poorer prognosis than Hodgkin's disease, but there are multiple types of this disease—some aggressive and others less so; therefore, prognosis varies greatly.

CLINICAL MANIFESTATIONS

- Painless enlargement of lymph nodes.
- Splenomegaly.
- GI complications may occur.
- Fever.
- Fatigue.
- Weight loss.
- Back and neck pain with hyperreflexia.

DIAGNOSTIC TOOLS

- Lymph node biopsy can diagnose non-Hodgkin's lymphoma.

TREATMENT

- Aggressive chemotherapy is used for advanced disease. Diffuse disease usually requires more aggressive therapy.
- Conservative chemotherapy may be used for slow-growing lymphomas and for palliative treatment.
- Radiotherapy is also used, as is surgery to remove large tumors.
- Bone marrow transplant may be performed.

Multiple Myeloma

Multiple myeloma is a clonal disorder characterized by proliferation of one type of B lymphocyte, and plasma cells derived from that lymphocyte. These cells disperse throughout the circulation and deposit primarily in the bone, causing bone breakdown, inflammation, and pain. Antibodies produced by the plasma cells are usually clonal IgG or IgA. Monoclonal fragments of these antibodies may be found in the urine of patients with the disease. These fragments are called Bence Jones proteins. The cause of multiple myeloma is unknown, but risk factors are believed to include occupational exposures to certain materials and gases, ionizing radiation, and possibly multiple drug allergies. Survival rate is low, although some patients may live a long time with this disease.

CLINICAL MANIFESTATIONS

- Bone pain and fracture may occur if bones are involved.
- Weight loss and fatigue may occur.
- Neurologic dysfunction resulting from high blood calcium levels is seen with bone breakdown.
- Recurrent infections from reduced B-cell function are common.

DIAGNOSTIC TOOLS

- Bone biopsy and blood analysis confirms the disease. Urine may also be diagnostic with the presence of Bence Jones proteins.
- Hypercalcemia may be present when bones are involved.

COMPLICATIONS

- Renal failure may develop as a result of Bence Jones proteins depositing in the renal tubules.

TREATMENT

- Chemotherapy may prolong life.
- Radiation therapy is used to reduce the size of bone lesions and relieve pain.
- Bone marrow transplant may be successful in some patients.

Hemophilia A

Hemophilia A, also called classic hemophilia, is an X-linked recessive disease resulting from an error in the gene coding for coagulation factor VIII. Classic hemophilia is the most common inherited coagulation disorder. It is seen in boys who inherit the defective gene on the X chromosome from their mother. The mother is usually heterozygous for the disorder and shows no symptoms. However, 25% of cases come from new X chromosome mutations. The defective gene may result from one of several different deletions or point mutations.

Without factor VIII, the intrinsic coagulation pathway is interrupted and extensive bleeding from small wounds or microvascular tears occurs. Bleeding is frequently into the joints and can cause significant pain and disability.

OTHER TYPES OF HEMOPHILIA

Other forms of hemophilia exist. These hemophilias result in the absence of different coagulation factors. Hemophilia B is an X-linked disorder caused by a lack of factor IX. Hemophilia C is an autosomal disorder caused by a lack of factor XI. Von Willebrand disease is an autosomal-dominant disease resulting from an abnormality of von Willebrand factor (vWF). This factor is released from endothelial cells and platelets and is essential for the formation of the platelet plug. With a reduction vWF factor, factor VIII levels are also reduced.

CLINICAL MANIFESTATIONS OF CLASSIC HEMOPHILIA

- Spontaneous or excessive bleeding after a minor wound.
- Joint swelling, pain, and degenerative changes.

DIAGNOSTIC TOOLS

- Laboratory studies show a normal bleeding time, but prolonged PTT. Measurement of factor VIII is reduced.
- Prenatal testing for the gene is possible.

COMPLICATIONS

- Intracranial hemorrhage may occur.
- Infection with HIV was common before artificial production of factor VIII.

TREATMENT

- Factor VIII replacement. Factor VIII may be from a frozen plasma concentrate donated from the father of the boy with hemophilia or may be produced by monoclonal antibody techniques. Multiple donor plasma extracts of Factor VIII are no longer used because of the risk of transmission of viral infections such as HIV and hepatitis B and C.

Liver Disease and Vitamin K Deficiency

The liver is the site of synthesis for many coagulation factors, several of which are vitamin K dependent. Disease of the liver or inadequate plasma levels of vitamin K will interrupt the coagulation pathways. Vitamin K is a fat-soluble vitamin absorbed in the diet with bile. Because bile is produced in the liver, a healthy liver and a clear bile duct are required for successful coagulation. Vitamin K is synthesized by bacteria in the gut. Newborns are vitamin K deficient because of a lack of vitamin K, producing bacteria in the intestine and immature liver function.

CLINICAL MANIFESTATIONS

- Bleeding characterized by petechia (small hemorrhage spots on the skin) and purpura (purplish discoloration of the skin).

TREATMENT

- Vitamin K is administered intramuscularly to the neonate and orally in children or adults.

Disseminated Intravascular Coagulation

Disseminated intravascular coagulation (DIC) is a unique condition characterized by the formation of multiple blood clots throughout the microvasculature. Eventually, the components of the blood clotting cascade and the platelets are used up, and hemorrhages begin to occur at all bodily orifices, any site of injury or venous puncture, and throughout many organ systems.

DIC is never a primary condition. Instead, it occurs as a complication to major clinical incidents or trauma such as shock, widespread infection, a major burn, myocardial infarct, or obstetric complication. Hypoxemia and acidemia develop, which damage the endothelial cells of the vasculature. Multiple endothelial cell injuries initiate extensive activation of the platelets and the intrinsic coagulation pathway, leading to microthrombi throughout the vascular system. Tissue damage, occurring as the precipitating event or after hypoxia and acidemia, causes the production of thromboplastin, which activates the extrinsic coagulation pathway. Clotting is extensive, with fibrin strands firming and holding the emboli.

As the coagulation cascades proceed, fibrinolytic processes (breaking down of fibrin strands) are accelerated. These processes result in the release of anticoagulation enzymes into the circulation. Eventually, clotting factors and platelets are used up and hemorrhage and oozing of blood into mucous membranes occur. The loop is completed with bleeding and clotting occurring simultaneously.

CLINICAL MANIFESTATIONS

- Hemorrhage from puncture sites, wounds, and mucous membranes in a patient with shock, obstetric complications, sepsis (widespread infection), or cancer. If bleeding is under the skin, vascular lesions will be apparent.
- Altered consciousness indicates a cerebral thrombus.
- Abdominal distention indicates a GI bleed.
- Cyanosis and tachypnea (increased respiratory rate) caused by poor tissue perfusion and oxygenation are common. Mottling of the skin indicates tissue ischemia.
- Hematuria (blood in urine) caused by hemorrhage or oliguria (decreased urine output) caused by poor renal perfusion.

DIAGNOSTIC TOOLS

- Blood tests demonstrate accelerated clotting and decreased platelets.
- Fibrin degradation products are elevated. Platelets, and plasma fibrinogen levels are reduced.

COMPLICATIONS

- The many clots cause obstruction to blood flow in all organs of the body. Widespread organ failure may occur. Mortality is greater than 50%.

TREATMENT

Treatment is difficult because of the combination of hemorrhage and clotting. Prevention of DIC and early identification of the condition is essential. Treatment is geared toward:

- Removal of the precipitating event.
- Heparin therapy may be initiated if organ failure caused by hypoxia is imminent. Heparin is not suggested when DIC is caused by sepsis or if central nervous system bleeding occurs.
- Fluid replacement is important to maintain organ perfusion as high as possible.
- Plasma-containing factor VIII, red cells, and platelets may be administered.

Selected Bibliography

Babior, B. M. & Stassel, T. P. (1994). *Hematology: a pathophysiological approach (3rd ed)*. New York: Churchill Livingstone.

Barat, L. M. & Blikabd, P. B. (1997). Drug resistance among malaria and other parasites. *Infectious Disease Clinics of North America* 11, 969–987.

Bowman, J. (1997). The management of hemolytic disease in the fetus and newborn. *Seminars in Perinatology* 21, 39–44.

Brown, L. M. (1992). Smoking and the risks of leukemia. *American Journal of Epidemiology* 135, 763–768.

Daniels, J. L., Olshan, A. F., & Savitz, D. A. (1997). Pesticides and childhood cancers. *Environmental Health Perspectives* 105, 1068–1077.

Dich, J., Zahm, S. H., Hanberg, A., & Adami, H. O. (1997). Pesticides and cancer. *Cancer Causes and Control* 8, 420–443.

Friebert, S. E. & Shurin, S. B. (1998). ALL: Diagonsis and outlook. *Contemporary Pediatrics* 15, 118–136.

Guyton, A. C. & Hall, J. E. (1996). *Textbook of medical physiology (9th ed.)* Philadelphia: W.B. Saunders.

Hickey, S. M. & Strasburger, V. C. (1997). What every pediatrician should know about infectious mononucleosis in adolescents. *Pediatric Clinics of North America* 44, 1541–1556.

Hoffman, S. L., Doolan, D. L., Sedegah, M., et al. (1997). Toward clinical trials of DNA vaccines against malaria. *Immunology and Cell Biology* 75, 376–381.

Janssens, H. M., DeHaan, M. J., vanKamp, I. L., Brand, R., Kanhai, H. H., & Veen,

S. (1997). Outcome for children treated with fetal intravascular transfusions because of severe blood group antagonism. *Journal of Pediatrics* 131, 373–380.

Long, M. W. & Mann, K. G. (1993). Bone marrow as a source of osteoprogenitor cells. In: *The hematopoietic microenvironment,* Long, M. W. & Wicha, M. S. (eds.). Baltimore: The Johns Hopkins University Press.

Mani, S. & Duffy, T. P. (1995). Anemia of pregnancy. *Perinatal Hematology* 22, 593–607.

Oakley, G. P., Jr. (1993). Folic acid–preventable spina bifida and anencephaly. *Journal of the American Medical Association* 269, 1292–1293.

Petridou, E., Revinthi, K., Alexander, F. E., Haidas, S., Tzortzatou, F., & Trichopoulos, D. (1996). Space-time clustering of childhood leukaemia in Greece: evidence supporting a viral aetiology. *British Journal of Cancer* 73, 1278–1283.

Porth, C. M. (1998). *Pathophysiology concepts of altered health states (5th ed.)* Philadelphia: J.B. Lippincott.

Quaglino, D., DiLeonardon, G., Furia, N., Recchia, F., Pasquoloni, E., & Ciarrocchi, G. (1997). Therapeutic management of hematological malignancies in elderly patients. Biological and clinical considerations. Part II: Non-Hodgkins lymphomas and Hodgkin's disease. *Aging* 9, 310–319.

Richards, A. L. (1997). Tumour necrosis factor and associated cytokines in the host's response to malaria. *International Journal for Parasitology* 27, 1251–1263.

Roberts, W. M., Estrov, Z., Ouspenskaia, M. V., Johnston, D. A., McClain, K. L., & Zipf, T. F. (1997). Measurement of residual leukemia during remission in childhood acute lymphoblastic leukemia. *New England Journal of Medicine* 336, 317–323.

Schlehofer, B., Blettner, M., Geletneky, K., et al. (1996). Sero-epidemiological analysis of the risk of virus infections for childhood leukaemia. *International Journal of Cancer* 65, 584–590.

Schwartz, R. S. (1997). Hodgkin's disease—time for a change. *New England Journal of Medicine* 337, 495–496.

Skarin, A. T. & Dorfman, D. M. (1997). Non-Hodgkin's lymphoma: current classification and management. *Ca: A Cancer Journal for Clinicians* 47, 351–372.

Straus, D. J. (1997). HIV-associated lymphomas. *Current Opinion in Oncology* 9, 450–454.

Vander, A. J., Sherman, J., & Luciano, D. (1998). *Human physiology (7th ed.)* Boston: McGraw-Hill.

Werler, M. M. (1993). Periconceptual folic acid exposure and the risk of occurrent neural tube defects. *Journal of the American Medical Association* 269, 1257–1261.

Yuen, R. R. & Horning, S. J. (1995). Recent advances in Hodgkin's disease. *Current Opinion in Hematology* 2, 262–267.

Zharhary, D. (1994). Age-related decline in B and T cell immunity. In: *Handbook of B and T Lymphocytes,* Snow, E. C. (ed.). San Diego: Academic Press.

Zimmerman, S. A., Ware, R. E., & Kinney, T. R. (1997). Gaining ground in the fight against sickle cell disease. *Contemporary Pediatrics* 14, 154–177

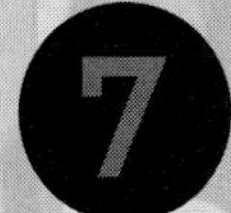

THE NERVOUS SYSTEM

The nervous system and the hormonal system are the means by which different parts of the body communicate. The nervous system can be separated into the central nervous system, consisting of the nerve pathways of the brain and spinal cord, and the peripheral nervous system, consisting of nerves that innervate the rest of the body. The coordination of our central and peripheral nervous systems allows us to move, talk, think, and respond.

● ● ●

PHYSIOLOGIC CONCEPTS

The Neuron

The neuron, also called a *nerve cell,* is the functional unit of the nervous system and is a highly specialized cell. Neural maturation occurs before or soon after birth, and once mature, the neuron does not undergo cellular reproduction and cannot be replaced. Each neuron functions to receive incoming stimuli from, and to send outgoing stimuli to, other nerves or muscles. Neurons pass and receive signals through changes in the flow of electrically charged ions back and forth across their cell membranes.

PARTS OF THE NEURON

Most neurons have four parts: the dendrite, an afferent end that receives incoming signals; the cell body, a central area containing the nucleus; the axon, a long extension on which the signal passes; and the axon terminals, which branch off the axon and deliver the signal to other cells. A typical neuron is shown in Figure 7-1.

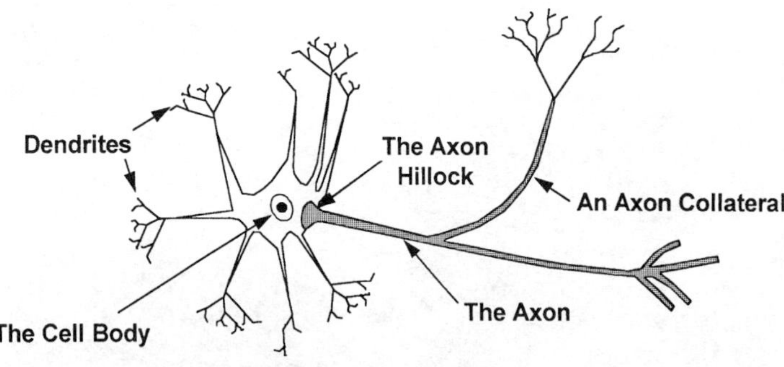

Figure 7-1. The neuron.

Dendrites

A dendrite is a neural extension from the cell body. The dendrite is the part of the neuron that receives stimulation from other nerves. Each neuron may have many dendritic branches. Excitation of a neuron typically begins at the dendrite. The dendrite passes its excitation on to the adjacent segment, the cell body.

Cell Body

The cell body contains the cell nucleus, the ribosomes, and all the genetic information necessary for making various cellular products including proteins, enzymes, and neurotransmitters. The cell body delivers these substances as needed to the rest of the neuron. Although neural excitation typically begins with excitation of the dendrites, a cell body sometimes may be stimulated directly by incoming stimuli from other neurons and by chemical and electrical stimuli. The cell body delivers the electrical signal to the next segment, the axon.

Axon

Projecting from the cell body is the axon, the beginning of which is called the *initial segment* or trigger zone. The axon is a long fiber on which passes the electrical signal initiated in the dendrites and cell body. The axon transmits the original signal to another neuron or to a muscle or gland. Branching off the main stem of the axon may be multiple collateral fibers. Collaterals convey information to many other interconnected nerve cells, increasing the influence of the neuron throughout the nervous system. Down the length of the axon, contractile proteins and microtubules transport substances produced in the cell body.

The axon is also called a *nerve fiber;* many nerve fibers (axons) traveling together in a bundle are called a *nerve.*

In some nerves, the axons are covered by an insulating, lipid sheath, called **myelin.** Myelin is produced when support cells wrap their plasma membranes around an axon. In the peripheral nervous system, the support cells are the *Schwann cells.* In the central nervous system myelin is produced by a specialized type of cell, the *oligodendroglia.* Myelin increases the velocity with which an electrical signal is transmitted down an axon, as described later.

Axon Terminals

At the end of the main axon stem and each collateral, the branching becomes extensive. These final divisions of the axon are called axon terminals. It is across axon terminals that the electrical signal is passed to the dendrites or the cell body of a second neuron. In the peripheral nervous system the signal may also pass to a muscle or glandular cell.

CATEGORIES OF NEURONS

Neurons that carry information from the periphery to the central nervous system are called sensory or **afferent neurons.** These neurons are the only type of nerve cell that do not have dendrites, but possess receptors on their distal ends that sense physical or chemical stimuli. Neurons that carry information out of the central nervous system to various target organs (a muscle cell, another nerve, or a gland) are called motor or **efferent neurons.** A third group of neurons, which make up most of the central nervous system neurons, pass messages between afferent and efferent neurons. These neurons are called **interneurons.** Almost 99% of all neurons in the body are interneurons, and all interneurons are in the central nervous system.

THE SYNAPSE

A synapse is the point of junction between two neurons. Neurons communicate with each other by releasing chemicals into the small cleft (synaptic cleft) separating one from the other. The chemical released from a particular neuron is called a neurotransmitter. Usually, a neurotransmitter is released from the axon terminal of one neuron, diffuses across the synaptic cleft, and binds to the dendrite or cell body of the other neuron. However, a synapse can occur between dendrites, between dendrites and a different cell body, or between an axon and an axon terminal. The cell that releases the neurotransmitter is called the **presynaptic neuron.** The neuron that completes the synapse is called the **postsynaptic neuron.** One postsynaptic neuron may receive input from thousands of presynaptic neurons. The postsynaptic neuron integrates and responds to the many signals influencing it. A synapse with two presynaptic neurons is shown diagrammatically in Figure 7-2.

NEUROTRANSMITTERS

Many neurotransmitters are used in the nervous system. Each neurotransmitter is synthesized in the cell body and transported down the axon to the axon terminal. Because neurotransmitters are released only from presynaptic neurons, synaptic transmission is always in one direction: from the presynaptic to the postsynaptic neuron. Neurotransmitters act rapidly to affect the postsynaptic neuron. To respond to a particular neurotransmitter, the postsynaptic cell must have specific receptors for it on its cell membrane.

Most neurons release just one neurotransmitter, although some neurons may also release a cotransmitter. Frequently, cotransmitters are a slightly different type of chemical than the neurotransmitter, called a **neuromodulator.** Neuromodulators typically take longer to act compared to a neurotransmitter, and may function to increase or decrease DNA transcription and protein synthesis. Neuromodulators

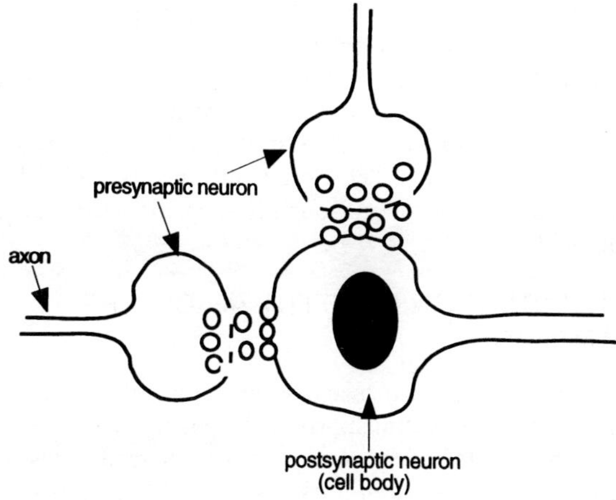

Figure 7-2. At a synapse, a presynaptic neuron releases chemicals that diffuse across the synaptic cleft and bind to a postsynaptic cell.

often affect the response of a postsynaptic cell to a neurotransmitter, and are associated with more long-term functions such as learning, mood, and development.

EXAMPLES OF NEUROTRANSMITTERS AND NEUROMODULATORS

Examples of neurotransmitters and neuromodulators include the following: monoamines—norepinephrine, serotonin, dopamine, and histamine; amino acids—gamma-aminobutyric acid (GABA), glycine, glutamate, and aspartate; acetylcholine; and the neuropeptides, including the endorphins, enkephalins substance P, vasoactive intestinal peptide (VIP), and adenosine triphosphate (ATP). Even some gases may serve as neurotransmitters, including nitric oxide and carbon dioxide. Gases do not bind postsynaptic receptors, but diffuse into the postsynaptic cell to exert an action.

A few neurotransmitters (i.e., acetylcholine and norepinephrine) can excite or inhibit a postsynaptic cell. However, a neurotransmitter usually has the same effect (excitatory or inhibitory) on all cells it binds. Examples of inhibitory neurotransmitters include GABA and nitric oxide. Dopamine is an example of an excitatory neurotransmitter. The neurotransmitters mentioned earlier may function in the central nervous system or the peripheral nervous system.

The Membrane Potential

The separation of electrical charge across any structure sets up an electrical potential. Nerve cells, like all cells, have a separation of electrical charges across their cell membrane such that the inside of the cell is negatively polarized (charged) compared to the outside. The separation of charge across a cell is called the membrane potential.

The membrane potential results from a balance between concentration and electrical gradients that exist across the cell membrane and drive the movement of ions. These gradients unequally distribute electrically charged ions inside and outside the cell, setting up a membrane potential.

THE CONCENTRATION GRADIENT ACROSS THE CELL MEMBRANE

A concentration gradient exists across all cell membranes because the sodium-potassium pump transports three positively charged sodium ions out of the cell for every two positively charged potassium ions it pumps in. The separation of ions is shown in Figure 7-3. This sets up a concentration gradient with potassium in higher concentration inside the cell than outside, while sodium is in higher concentration outside the cell than inside (Chapter 1). Because potassium and sodium can readily move across the membrane, both tend to diffuse down their concentration gradients—potassium diffusing out of the cell, and sodium diffusing into the cell. Potassium is more than 50 times more permeable across the membrane than sodium is. Therefore, more positive charge moves out of the cell than comes in, making the inside negative.

THE ELECTRICAL GRADIENT ACROSS THE CELL MEMBRANE

Opposing the concentration gradient is an electrical gradient set up by potassium and sodium diffusion, and by the accumulation of *negatively charged proteins inside* the cell. Because the inside of the cell is negative, potassium, sodium, and other positively charged ions are drawn inside

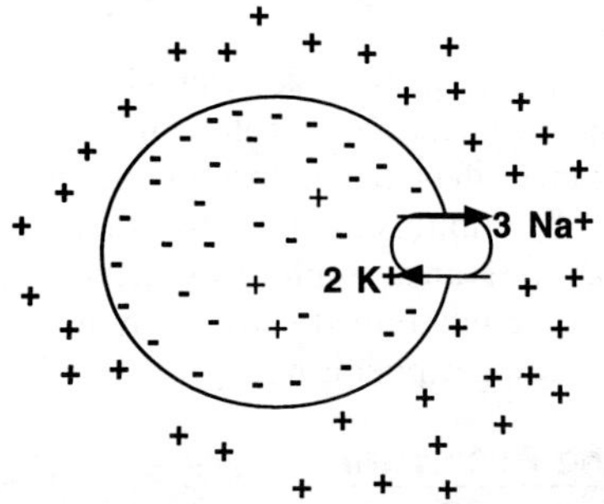

Figure 7-3. Excess positive charge on the outside of the membrane compared to the inside contributes to the membrane potential.

the cell; negatively charged ions such as chloride tend to leave the cell, which sets up an electrical gradient across each cell.

Net Result of Concentration and Electrical Gradients

The final balance reached between the electrical gradient and the concentration gradient across a resting cell is called the **resting membrane potential.** For any given cell the resting membrane potential may range from 5 to 100 millivolts (mV), with the inside negative relative to the outside.

Changes in the Membrane Potential of Nerve and Muscle Cells

Cell membranes of neurons and muscles are unique because their permeability to sodium, potassium, chloride, and sometimes calcium can be changed by electrical or chemical stimulation. This allows the membrane potential of neurons and muscle cells to vary from the resting potential.

For neurons at rest, the membrane potential is approximately −70 mV (inside negative). If the inside of the cell becomes less negative, the cell is said to have become **depolarized.** If the cell becomes more negative inside, the cell is said to become **hyperpolarized.** When the cell potential returns to its resting potential, it is said to be **repolarized.** Changes in the cell membrane potential of a nerve cell may cause a local change in electrical current, called a graded potential, or may cause a large, propagated change in electrical current, called an action potential. It is through graded potentials and action potentials that the nervous system sends and receives signals.

Graded Potentials

A graded potential is an electrical potential that can vary in amplitude and duration. There are many examples of graded potentials in neurophysiology, including the synaptic potential, the receptor potential, and the muscle end-plate potential (discussed in Chapter 11). Graded potentials are usually produced at a small site on the neuron (synapse, receptor, muscle end-plate) and die out as their charge spreads. Graded potentials are produced by chemical or electrical stimuli, and may be excitatory (depolarizing) or inhibitory (hyperpolarizing). If they are highly excitatory, they may cause an adjacent area of the neuron to fire an action potential.

SYNAPTIC POTENTIALS

When a neurotransmitter is released from the presynaptic and binds to the postsynaptic neuron, it will electrically excite (depolarize) or inhibit (hyperpolarize) the postsynaptic cell. If the transmitter depolarizes the postsynaptic cell, the synaptic signal is called an **excitatory**

presynaptic potential (EPSP). EPSPs occur if the transmitter opens channels that allow the passage of positive ions, such as sodium or potassium, into the postsynaptic cell. If binding of the neurotransmitter to the postsynaptic neuron hyperpolarizes the postsynaptic cell, the synaptic signal is called an **inhibitory postsynaptic potential** (IPSP). IPSPs occur if the transmitter opens channels that allow the passage of negative ions, usually chloride, inside the postsynaptic cell. Of the thousands of incoming signals on a postsynaptic neuron, some will be excitatory, others will be inhibitory. The electrical potential generated in the postsynaptic membrane varies in size, depending on the summation between the IPSPs and EPSPs it receives, and the amount of neurotransmitter released from each presynaptic cell.

If at the postsynaptic cell, the summation of all EPSPs and IPSPs results in significant excitation of the postsynaptic dendrite or cell body, the electrical excitation will be passed on to the postsynaptic cell. If the summation of EPSPs and IPSPs is inhibitory, it is unlikely that the postsynaptic cell will pass the electrical signal further.

Changes in Membrane Potential of a Muscle Cell

The resting membrane potential of a muscle cell is approximately −90 mV. Stimulation by a motor neuron always causes depolarization at the site where the motor neuron synapses on the muscle cell, called the motor end plate. This depolarization is called an end-plate potential (EPP). The EPP is also a graded potential and spreads locally through the muscle fiber and usually causes contraction of the muscle. One motor neuron typically innervates many muscle fibers. One motor neuron and the fibers it innervates is called a **motor unit.**

RECEPTOR POTENTIALS

A receptor potential is the electrical potential produced at the distal end of an afferent neuron after electrical or chemical stimulation.

Specialized cells in sensory organs produce receptor potentials that activate neurons in response to touch, sight, sound, smell, or taste.

A receptor potential is a graded potential; it varies in amplitude and duration and spreads through local current flow. When the receptor potential reaches the cell body, if it is large enough to cause the cell body to depolarize to threshold, the neuron will reach threshold and fire an action potential.

The Action Potential

An action potential is a rapid change in the membrane potential of a neuron or muscle cell. An action potential occurs when depolarization is great enough to cause voltage- sensitive sodium gates, present throughout the membrane, to burst open. Once the gates open, sodium ions rush inside the cell. The incoming rush of sodium ions causes the charge inside the cell to rapidly become more positive, reaching approximately +30 mV in a nerve cell. As the cell becomes more positive, the sodium gates begin to snap shut. At this time, the potassium gates, also affected by the change in membrane potential, open, allowing potassium ions to rush out of the cell, which causes the cell to again become negatively charged on the inside. In muscle cells, the action potential also opens calcium gates.

The action potential is an active, transient state of dramatic cell depolarization. Action potentials are different from graded potentials in that they do not vary in amplitude or duration. Instead, action potentials are considered "all or none": if the electrical or chemical stimulus, or the EPSPs, are great enough to open enough voltage-dependent sodium channels to sufficiently depolarize the membrane, the action potential will occur. If the stimulus is insufficient to cause a certain level of depolarization, the action potential will not occur. The level of depolarization great enough for a neuron to fire an action potential is called the **threshold** potential. In muscles, it takes one EPP to cause the muscle cell to reach threshold and contract.

SPREAD OF AN ACTION POTENTIAL

When a nerve fiber reaches threshold and fires an action potential, the action potential is propagated at exactly the same level, down the entire length of the axon, to the axon terminals. Propagation of the action potential occurs because neighboring sites on the axon are affected by the change in current generated by the original action potential. The change in current produced by an action potential *will* be great enough to cause depolarization at a neighboring site on the neuron, and the action potential *will* be repeated. As the action potential passes down the axon, the part of the axon that has just fired will be refractory for a period of time until the membrane potential returns to the resting level. Propagation of an action potential compared to the local spread of a graded potential is shown in Figure 7-4.

The speed at which an action potential passes along a nerve fiber depends on the diameter of the fiber and whether the fiber is covered by myelin. Because large fibers present less resistance to the flow of current than small fibers, large fibers transmit action potentials faster than small fibers. Fibers coated with myelin pass an action potential faster than uncoated fibers because the myelin acts like insulation to prevent the current from leaking out across the membrane. This allows the action potential to spread by jumps down the axon, in process called **saltatory conduction**, rather than step by step. As shown in Figure 7-5, areas where myelin is absent on the axon, called the nodes of Ranvier, contain a large density of sodium channels that open in response to the spread of current and quickly depolarize to threshold,

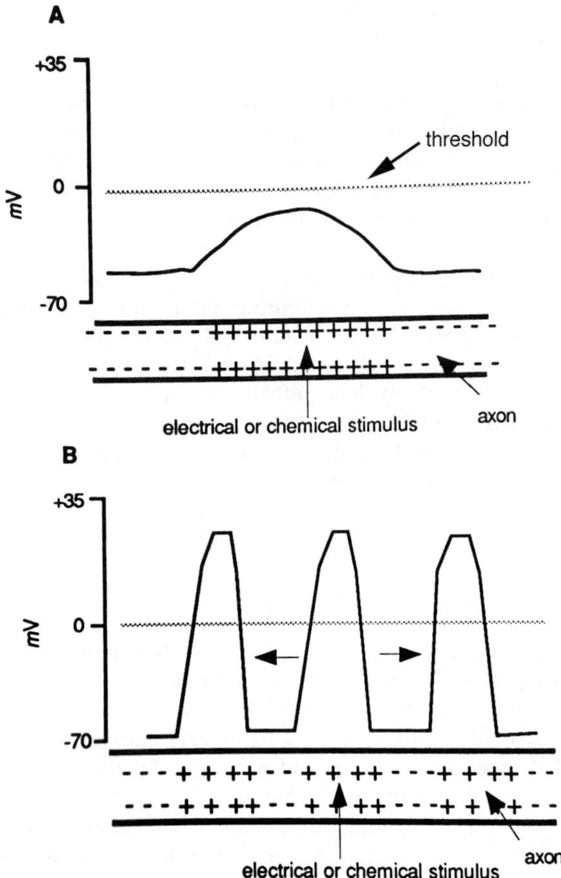

Figure 7-4. A graded potential (**A**) does not reach threshold and passes only a short distance on the membrane and dies out. An action potential (**B**) fires when depolarization reaches threshold and is repeated along the entire length of the axon. A neuron is capable of propagating an action potential in both directions, although in vivo an action potential starts at one end and travels unidirectional.

propagating the signal with great speed. Without myelin covering, the current must depolarize each adjacent area of the axon, a process that slows neural transmission considerably.

SYNAPTIC TRANSMISSION OF AN ACTION POTENTIAL

Once an action potential reaches the axon terminals, it causes the opening of sodium and calcium channels. When calcium ions enter the presynaptic terminal, packets of that nerve's neurotransmitters are released into the synaptic cleft. The more calcium that enters, the more neurotransmitter released. In response to the neurotransmitter, the postsynaptic neuron will become adequately depolarized and fire its own action potential, or the summation of incoming signals on the postsynaptic neuron will not be enough to cause depolarization to threshold, and the signal will not pass on to the next neuron in the chain.

The Central Nervous System

The brain is a large mass of neural tissue located in the cranium (skull). The brain includes nerve cells and nonneural support cells. The brain is where reflexes are integrated to maintain the internal environment. It is also the source of several hormones and the site of integration of all sensory information. The brain receives approximately 15% of the cardiac output. Brain cells require glucose for energy metabolism and production of ATP. Figure 7-6 shows the central nervous system divided into the forebrain, midbrain, hindbrain, and spinal cord. The midbrain and hindbrain make up the brainstem. The cerebellum is described separately.

THE FOREBRAIN

The forebrain includes the diencephalon located in the core of the brain, and the left and right cerebral hemispheres. The outer shell of the cerebral hemispheres is called the cerebral cortex. The cerebral hemispheres are connected together across a longitudinal fissure by

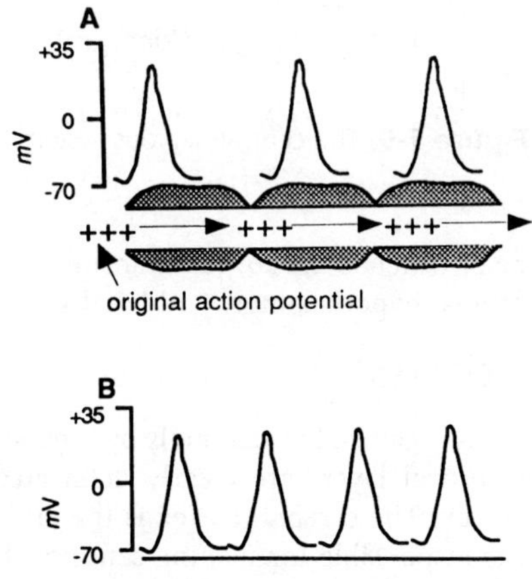

Figure 7-5. Propagation in myelinated fiber (**A**) compared to an unmyelinated fiber (**B**). Action potentials pass by rapid saltatory conduction in myelinated fibers.

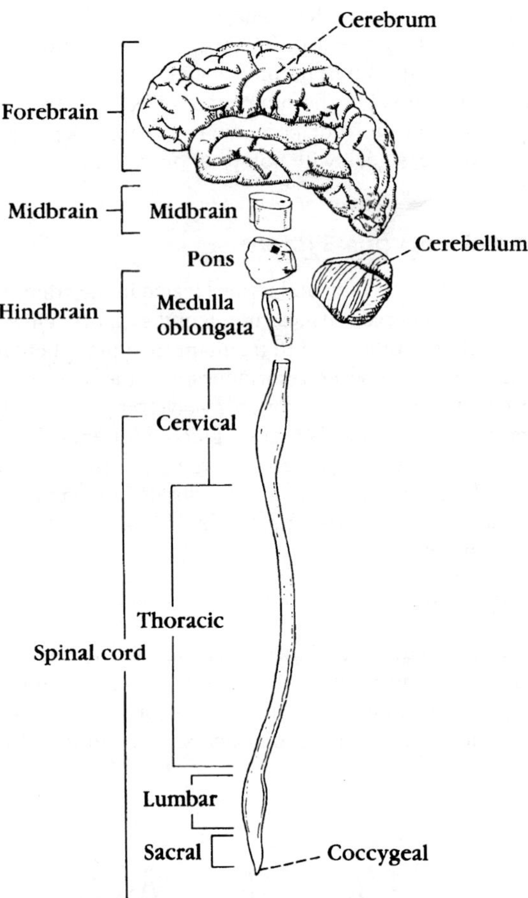

Figure 7-6. The central nervous system.

axon bundles, one of which is the corpus callosum. The diencephalon includes the thalamus, hypothalamus, and basal ganglia.

THE CEREBRAL CORTEX

The cerebral cortex is organized horizontally by function and vertically into layers. The vertical layers are clearly delineated and repeated throughout the cortex. The cerebral cortex is the most advanced part of the brain and is responsible for making sense of the environment and initiating thought and goal-oriented behavior. The cortex is called gray matter because of the preponderance of neural cell bodies as opposed to neuronal axons. Different sections of the cerebral cortex, called lobes, perform different functions. Some parts of the cerebral cortex function as primary sensory areas and directly receive incoming sensory stimuli. These areas are bordered by secondary sensory areas that help interpret sensory stimuli. Other association areas receive information from primary and secondary sensory areas, and from other sites in the cortical and subcortical brain. Association areas allow for complex movements, interpretation and production of language, and appropriate response to friends, enemies, and strangers. The lobes of the cortex are shown in Figure 7-7.

The Frontal Lobe

The frontal lobe includes the part of the cerebral cortex forward from the central sulcus (fissure or furrow) and above the lateral sulcus. It contains the motor and premotor areas. Broca's area is in the frontal lobe and controls the expression of speech. Many association areas in the frontal lobe receive information from throughout the brain and incorporate the information into thoughts, plans, and behavior. The frontal lobe is responsible for goal-oriented behavior, moral decision making, and complex thought. The frontal lobe modifies emotional surges produced in the limbic system and the vegetative reflexes of the brainstem.

Cell bodies in the primary motor area of the frontal lobe send axon projections to the spinal cord, most of which travel in pathways

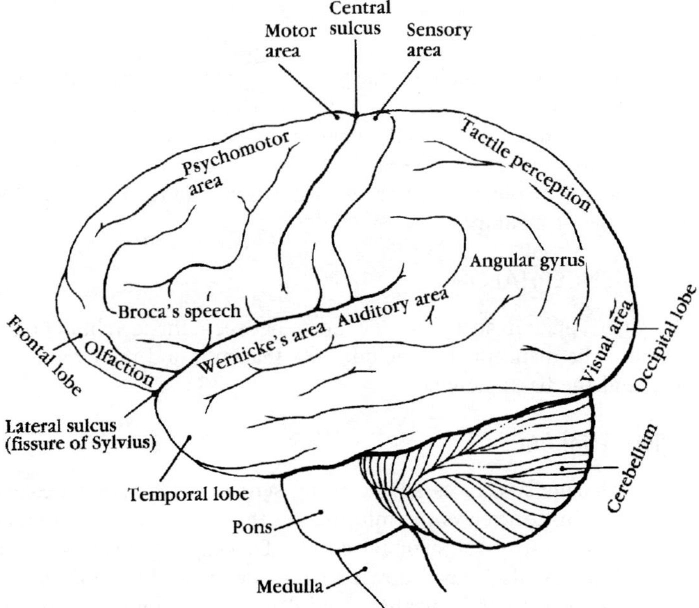

Figure 7-7. The brain.

belonging to what is described as the corticospinal tract. In the corticospinal tract, motor neurons cross sides; motor information from the left side of the cerebral cortex passes down the right side of the spinal cord and controls motor movements of the right side of the body, and vice versa. Other axons from the motor area travel in extrapyramidal pathways. These fibers control fine motor movement and run outside the corticospinal tract to the spinal cord.

The Parietal Lobe

The parietal lobe is the area of the cortex located behind the central sulcus, above the lateral fissure, and extending back to the parieto-occipital fissure. It is the primary sensory area of the brain for touch and hearing. Cells of the parietal lobe act as secondary association areas to interpret incoming stimuli. The parietal lobe passes sensory information to many other areas of the brain, including the neighboring motor and visual association areas.

The Occipital Lobe

The occipital lobe is the posterior lobe of the cerebral cortex. It lies posterior to the parietal lobe and above the parieto-occipital fissure, separating it from the cerebellum. This lobe is the primary visual association center of the cortex. It receives information that originated as signals in the retina of the eye.

The Temporal Lobe

The temporal lobe includes the part of the cerebral cortex extending down from the lateral fissure and posteriorly to the parieto-occipital fissure. The temporal lobe is the primary association area for auditory information and includes Wernicke's area where language is interpreted. It is also involved in interpretation of smell and is important for the storage of memory.

THE DIENCEPHALON

The diencephalon structures lie deep between the cerebral hemispheres. The diencephalon includes the thalamus and the hypothalamus, and the basal ganglia.

The Thalamus

The thalamus receives all incoming sensory information (except smell) and in turn relays the information through numerous afferent tracts to the rest of the cerebral cortex. Descending fibers from the cerebral cortex also travel down to the thalamus. Function of the cerebral cortex depends on thalamic relay. The thalamus is also part of the reticular activating system, an extensive group of neurons essential in arousal of the individual. The thalamus receives pain information and relays it to the cerebral cortex.

The Hypothalamus

The hypothalamus makes up the base of the diencephalon. It is an important endocrine and neural organ responsible for maintaining homeostasis—constancy of the internal environment. The hypothalamus integrates and directs information concerning temperature, hunger, autonomic nervous system activity, and emotional status. It also regulates several hormone levels, including the pituitary hormones (Chapter 8).

The Basal Ganglia

The basal ganglia are islands of gray matter lying deep in the diencephalon on either side of the thalamus and upper midbrain, which process and influence information in the extrapyramidal nerve tracts. The basal ganglia are important for controlling highly skilled movements that require patterns and quickness of response without intentional thought. The precision of a baseball player and the grace of a ballerina require significant basal ganglia control.

The basal ganglia are composed of several structures that can be anatomically or physiologically separated, including the caudate nucleus, the putamen, and the globus pallidus. The basal ganglia are intimately associated with the substantia nigra, and the subthalamic and red nuclei. Virtually all projections to and from the basal ganglia go through the thalamus. Lesions of the basal ganglia cause repetitive movements, grimaces, and tremors, as seen with Huntington's disease (chorea) and Parkinson's disease.

THE LIMBIC SYSTEM

The limbic system is a diffuse grouping of neurons from different areas of the brain. Neurons in the limbic system include fibers from all lobes of the forebrain and extensive connections from the hypothalamus and thalamus. Midbrain and hindbrain areas also send projections that contribute to the limbic system. The limbic system is the part of the brain associated with production of emotions. Learning and behavior are also influenced by limbic system structures.

THE BRAINSTEM

The brainstem, or stalk of the brain, is made of up of the pons, medulla oblongata, and mesencephalon (midbrain). In the brainstem are cells that control cardiovascular and respiratory system functions. Neurons pass through the brainstem and carry motor information up and down from the cerebral cortex, controlling equilibrium. Ten of the twelve cranial nerves that control motor and sensory function of the eyes, face, tongue, and neck leave from the brainstem. The secretory and motor functions of the gastrointestinal (GI) tract and the sensory functions of hearing and taste are also controlled by the cranial nerves.

RETICULAR FORMATION

Running through the brainstem is a network of many small, branched neurons, called the reticular formation. These neurons include ascending and descending tracts, some of which cluster to form centers that control swallowing, vomiting, and respiratory and cardiovascular reflexes. The reticular formation is also essential for wakefulness and is necessary to focus attention. Functioning of the reticular formation is essential for life.

Wakefulness

Various neurons in the reticular formation send information to higher brain areas to maintain wakefulness and arousal. These neurons and their projections are part of a functional rather than anatomic group of cells, called the **reticular activating system** (RAS). The RAS maintains wakefulness, attention, and concentration. The RAS is stimulated by all sensory stimulation, including painful stimuli.

Sleep

The process of sleep is also under the control of the reticular formation. Like wakefulness, sleep is an active process that occurs when certain centers in the brainstem send inhibitory signals to neurons throughout the RAS. These inhibitory signals appear to result from release of the neurotransmitter serotonin by the reticular formation cells. Serotonin inhibits RAS firing, temporarily ending conscious behavior. Serotonin levels in the brain eventually decrease, and the person wakes up. Sleep and wakefulness normally follow a cyclic pattern unless the pattern is blocked, changed, or interrupted.

THE CEREBELLUM

The cerebellum sits in the hindbrain posterior to the brainstem. The cerebellum helps maintain balance and is responsible for the smooth skeletal muscle responses that give grace and direction to voluntary movements. It controls fast, repetitive movements required for activities such as typing, piano playing, and bike riding.

The Spinal Canal

The spinal canal or vertebral column is a long, thin column extending from the base of the skull to the sacrum (tailbone). Running down the center of the spinal canal is the spinal cord. It is filled with cerebrospinal fluid (CSF) and surrounded by the bony vertebral column, which extends beyond the end of the spinal tract and offers protection to the delicate nerves inside. The spinal cord consists of interneurons whose axons travel up and down in organized tracts. Incoming to the ascending tracts are axon terminals that carry sensory information from peripheral afferent neurons. Many axon terminals synapse in the cord on an interneuron. If the summation of the various incoming IPSPs and EPSPs results in the interneuron reaching threshold, the interneuron will fire an action potential and pass the information further into the central nervous system. The sensory neuron may also stimulate a spinal reflex. This is accomplished by synapsing in the spinal canal directly on the dendrites or cell body of a motor neuron (monosynaptic reflex), or by synapsing on an interneuron that secondarily activates a motor neuron (polysynaptic reflex).

Descending interneurons that innervate dendrites and cell bodies of efferent nerves are also in the spinal cord. These efferent nerves leave the spine in tracts and innervate muscle or endocrine cells.

DORSAL AND VENTRAL ROOTS

Groups of afferent nerves entering at each level of the cord on the dorsal (toward the back) side are called dorsal roots. Efferent nerves leave each level of the cord in groups on the ventral (toward the front) side. These are called ventral roots. Dorsal and ventral roots at a given level of the spinal cord join together outside the cord to form 1 of 31 pairs of spinal nerves.

GRAY AND WHITE MATTER

The spinal cord can be separated into gray and white matter. Gray matter occupies the center of the tract and is filled with interneurons, cell bodies, dendrites of efferent neurons, axons of afferent neurons, and various support cells. The white matter, consisting mostly of myelinated ascending and descending tracts, surrounds the gray matter.

The Meninges

The meninges are thin, fluid-filled membranes surrounding the brain and spinal cord. There are three meninges: the dura mater ("thick mother") on the outside, the arachnoid ("spider-like") as a middle layer, and the pia mater ("little mother") lying immediately above the brain. Spaces between the layers are filled with CSF.

References to the meninges include the terms epidural (the space above the dura mater) and subdural (the space below the dura mater, but above the arachnoid). The epidural and subdural spaces contain many small blood vessels. Damage to these vessels leads to blood accumulating in the epidural or subdural spaces. Cerebral spinal fluid circulates in the subarachnoid space (beneath the arachnoid, above the pia mater).

Cerebrospinal Fluid and the Ventricles

Cerebrospinal fluid is a clear fluid surrounding the brain and spinal cord. The CSF circulates in the subarachnoid space, and offers the brain protection against physical jarring. There is some exchange of nutrients and waste products between the CSF and the neural tissue. Although CSF is formed from plasma that flows through the brain, its concentration of electrolytes and glucose differs from plasma.

FORMATION OF CEREBROSPINAL FLUID

Cerebrospinal fluid is formed as a result of filtration, diffusion, and active transport across special capillaries into the ventricles (cavities) of the brain, especially the lateral ventricle. The capillary network responsible for CSF formation is called the choroid plexus. Once in the ventricles, CSF flows toward the brainstem. Through small holes in the brainstem, CSF circulates to the surface of the brain and spinal cord. At the surface of the brain, CSF enters the venous system and returns to the heart. Thus, CSF is continually recirculated through and over the central nervous system. If the ventricle conduction pathways for CSF become blocked, fluid can accumulate, which results in a buildup of pressure inside or on the surface of the brain.

The Blood-Brain Barrier

The blood-brain barrier refers to the capability of the brain vascular system to manipulate the composition of cerebral interstitial fluid compared to interstitial fluid in the rest of the body. The blood-brain barrier results from tightly fused endothelial cells present in the brain capillaries, and from cells lining the ventricles that limit diffusion and filtration. Special transport functions regulate what fluid crosses out of the general circulation to bathe brain cells. The blood-brain barrier protects delicate brain cells from exposure to potentially harmful substances. Many drugs and chemicals cannot cross the blood-brain barrier.

Brain Blood Flow

The brain receives approximately 15% of the cardiac output. This high rate of blood flow is required to meet the brain's continually high demands for glucose and oxygen.

BRAIN METABOLISM

The brain is unique in that it normally uses only glucose as a source for oxidative phosphorylation and the production of adenosine triphosphate (ATP). Unlike other cells, brain cells do not store glucose as glycogen; therefore, the brain must continually receive oxygen and glucose through brain blood flow. Oxygen deprivation for as little as 5 minutes, or glucose deprivation for 15 minutes, can cause significant brain damage. Brain function depends so much on blood flow that it is possible to identify which parts of the brain are performing different tasks by measuring brain blood flow during specific brain activities.

Studies have shown that in performing a burst of mental work, the brain initially produces ATP by anaerobic glycolysis, rather than oxidative phosphorylation. Anaerobic glycolysis depends on glucose but does not require oxygen. The brain does this even if oxygen is readily available. The result is a rapid utilization and depletion of glucose, with a corresponding increase in oxygen levels. Within a short period, the brain begins oxidative phosphorylation.

Intracranial Pressure

The pressure inside the cranium is called intracranial pressure (ICP). ICP is determined by the volume of blood in the brain, the volume of CSF, and the volume of brain tissue. Normally, ICP ranges from 5 to 15 millimeters of mercury (mmHg).

The Peripheral Nervous System

The peripheral nervous system consists of nerves traveling between the brain or spinal cord and the rest of the body. There are 12 nerve pairs traveling to and from the brain and 31 pairs from the spinal cord. The peripheral nervous system can be separated into afferent and efferent divisions. Afferent and efferent fibers travel together in opposite directions, in all spinal nerves and most cranial nerves. Some cranial nerves carry only afferent information. Afferent neurons convey information to the central nervous system from all sensory organs, pressure and volume receptors, temperature receptors, stretch receptors, and pain receptors. Efferent neurons deliver neural stimulation to muscles and glands. Efferent neurons belong to the autonomic or somatic nervous system.

THE AUTONOMIC NERVOUS SYSTEM

Autonomic nerve fibers leave the spinal cord and innervate smooth and cardiac muscle and the endocrine and exocrine glands. Autonomic nerves fibers are considered involuntary because there is little conscious control over their function. The two divisions of the autonomic nervous system, the sympathetic and parasympathetic divisions, are shown in Figure 7-8. Sympathetic and parasympathetic nerves innervate many of the same organs but typically cause opposite responses. The cell bodies of these neurons lie in the brain or spinal cord. In both divisions of the autonomic system, two nerve fibers participate in the efferent pathway.

THE SYMPATHETIC NERVOUS SYSTEM

The first fibers of the sympathetic nerves, called the *preganglionic fibers,* leave from the thoracic or lumbar regions of the spine. Soon

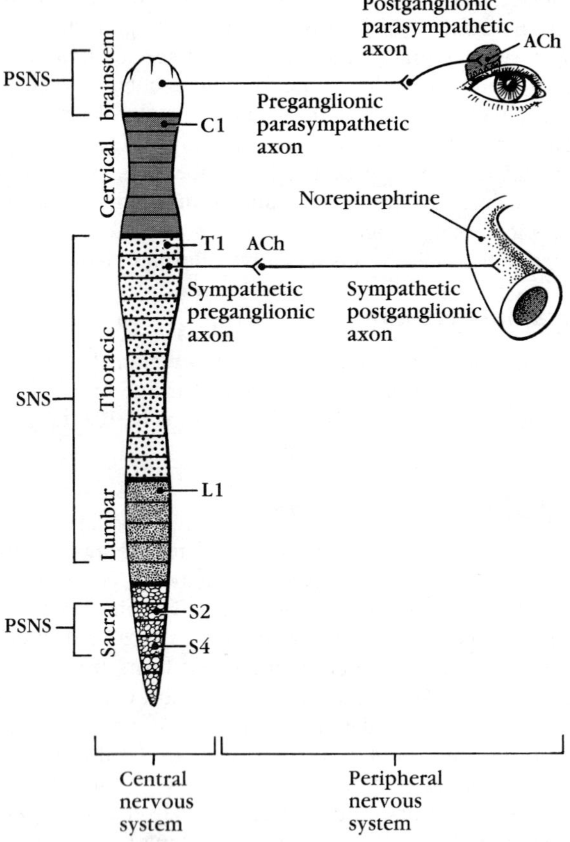

Figure 7-8. Sympathetic and parasympathetic system.

after leaving the spine, a preganglionic fiber joins other preganglionic fibers to form an autonomic ganglia. At this point, the preganglionic fiber synapses on the second nerve fiber of the system, the postganglionic fiber, and releases acetylcholine, which causes the *postganglionic fiber* to fire an action potential. From the autonomic ganglia, the postganglionic fiber travels to its target organ, the muscle or gland. The sympathetic postganglionic fiber usually releases the neurotransmitter norepinephrine. Target organ receptors for norepinephrine are called **adrenergic receptors.**

THE PARASYMPATHETIC NERVOUS SYSTEM

The fibers of the parasympathetic nervous system leave the brain in the cranial nerves or leave the spinal cord from the sacral area. The preganglionic fiber of the parasympathetic system is typically long and travels to an autonomic ganglia located near the target organ. Preganglionic parasympathetic nerves release acetylcholine that then stimulates the postganglionic fiber. The parasympathetic postganglionic fiber then travels a short distance to its target tissue, a muscle or a gland. This nerve also releases acetylcholine. Preganglionic acetylcholine receptors for sympathetic and parasympathetic fibers are called **nicotinic receptors.** Postganglionic acetylcholine receptors are called **muscarinic receptors.** These names relate to the receptor being stimulated by nicotine or muscarine (a mushroom poison).

Functions of the Sympathetic and Parasympathetic Nerves

The sympathetic nervous system innervates the heart, causing an increase in heart rate and strength of contraction. Sympathetic nerves innervate all large and small arteries and veins, causing constriction of all vessels except the arterioles supplying skeletal muscle. Sympathetic nerves innervate the smooth muscle of the gut, causing decreased motility, and the smooth muscle of the respiratory tract, causing bronchial relaxation and decreased bronchial secretions. Sympathetic stimulation affects the liver, stimulates secretions of the sweat glands, and is responsible for ejaculation during male orgasm.

Parasympathetic fibers innervate the heart, slowing the heart rate, and innervate the gut, causing increased motility. Parasympathetic nerves innervate bronchial smooth muscle, causing airway constriction, and innervate the genitourinary tract, causing erection in the male.

THE SOMATIC NERVOUS SYSTEM

Somatic nerves of the peripheral nervous system consist of efferent motor neurons that leave the brain or spinal cord and synapse directly on skeletal muscle cells. Motor neurons are large myelinated nerves that release acetylcholine at the neuromuscular junction. Acetylcholine binds to receptors on a specialized area of the muscle cell called the end plate. Binding of acetylcholine causes the muscle cell to reach threshold, resulting in an action potential and the opening of calcium channels (gates) in the membrane. This leads to an increase in intracellular calcium and contraction of the skeletal muscle fiber. There are no inhibitory motor neurons.

Support Cells

Cells in the central and peripheral nervous systems function to support nerve cells by providing nutrients, forming an insulated coating called myelin, and clearing away cell debris from the neuronal area. In the central nervous system, these cells are called neuroglia and are more numerous than nerve cells. Examples of neuroglia include astrocytes, which provide nutrients and act as contact points for blood vessels, the oligodendroglia cells, which make myelin, and microglia that support immune function in the central nervous system. In the peripheral nervous system, the Schwann cells provide a source of nutrients for the neurons and produce myelin.

How the Brain Works

Advances in technology, especially positron emission tomography (PET) and magnetic resonance imaging (MRI), have offered insights into how the brain functions to allow us to think, remember, interpret stimuli, and understand and use language.

It appears that the mind breaks down complex functions into discreet components of a specific job, and delegates these components to specific neuronal networks. The outcomes from the different networks are then reassembled in a pattern that allows the brain to perform the activity or to give meaning to a stimulus.

COMMUNICATION PATHWAYS

Perhaps best studied are the many steps involved in participating in a conversation. To begin with, spoken sounds are carried from auditory receptors in the ears through the thalamus, to the primary auditory area of the cortex, while at the same time, nonverbal visual clues are sent from the retina through the thalamus, to the primary visual area. From the auditory cortex, signals travel to an area in the left temporal lobe, called Wernicke's area, where meaning is assigned to the words; and to associative areas where the impact of the words is perceived by the listener. To respond verbally, an area of the frontal lobe, called Broca's area, is activated, and an appropriate response is formulated. The reply is then spoken by activating the primary motor area of the brain, and passing the motor signals through the thalamus and down the spinal cord, resulting in activation of motor neurons to the face and throat.

The processing of various tasks by the brain is adaptable; as one becomes proficient at a task, the patterns of processing can change, become faster, and often more efficient. One can learn to speak "before thinking" and listen without paying attention.

MEMORY

Memory is the internal recording of a prior event. The formation of memory is a multistep process that involves: 1) focusing attention on a selected event, name, or number, to the exclusion of background events, 2) rehearsing the information, and 3) consolidating the information into chemical storage in the brain.

Focusing attention on one event or piece of information allows that information to enter short-term memory storage. This is an active state wherein the new event is compared with previous experiences. Short-term memory is considered to be the working memory; it is of limited capacity and if the information is not continually **rehearsed**

or attended to, it will be lost when a new input arrives to distract attention. However, if the information is rehearsed, it will stay in short-term storage until it can be **consolidated** into long-term memory storage. Long-term memory is theoretically unlimited and permanent. Long-term memory depends on several excitatory neurotransmitters, including acetylcholine, dopamine, norepinephrine, and glutamate, and on hormones released with stressful events, including adrenocorticotropic hormone (ACTH), vasopressin, and epinephrine. Inhibitory transmitters, including GABA, can reduce the likelihood of consolidating memory from short-term storage to long-term.

When a short-term memory is consolidated into a long-term memory, it is done so by breaking the information to be remembered into separate units that are then processed in specific areas of the brain. For example, a visual experience is broken down into discreet attributes of color, shape, and size, and these attributes are stored separately. There are also two general types of long-term memory. **Declarative** memory is conscious memory for facts and events. This type of memory requires a well-functioning medial temporal lobe and structures in the diencephalon. A declarative memory is stored in the cerebral cortex. **Nondeclarative** memory is involved with skill learning, repetition, and classical conditioning. Nondeclarative memory involves unconscious recollection and requires an intact cerebral cortex, basal ganglia, and cerebellum. With most types of dementia, declarative memory is lost before nondeclarative memory. Strokes (brain attacks) may interfere with nondeclarative and declarative memory.

● PATHOPHYSIOLOGIC CONCEPTS

Alterations in Consciousness

Consciousness is the full awareness of self, location, and time in any environment. To be fully conscious, an intact reticular activating system is required, as is the functioning of higher brain centers in the cerebral cortex. Connections through the thalamus must also be intact.

Alterations in consciousness typically begin with disruption in diencephalon functioning, characterized by dullness, confusion, lethargy, and finally stupor as the person becomes difficult to arouse. Continued decreases in consciousness appear with midbrain dysfunction and are characterized by deepening of the stupor state. Finally, dysfunction of the medulla and pons may occur, resulting in coma. This progressive decrease in consciousness is described as rostral-caudal progression.

Alterations in Pupil Responses

The ability of our eyes to dilate or constrict, rapidly and equally, depends on an intact brainstem. Likewise, cerebral hypoxia and many drugs change pupil size and reactivity. Therefore, pupil size and reactivity offer valuable information concerning brain integrity and function.

Important pupil changes seen with brain damage are pinpoint pupils seen with opiate (heroin) overdose and bilaterally fixed and dilated pupils usually seen with severe hypoxia. Fixed pupils are typically seen with barbiturate overdose. Brainstem injury presents with pupils fixed bilaterally in the midposition.

Alterations in Eye Movements

In a fully conscious person, the steady gaze of the eyes at rest results from an intact cerebral cortex exerting control over the brainstem. With brain injury and loss of cortical function, the eyes typically rove and move together toward or away from the side of the brain injured, depending on the type of injury. Loss of higher brain centers results in reflective eye movements, called doll's head movements. A doll's head movement is that which occurs when the eyes stare forward, always following the position of the head. Normally, when an individual's head is passively turned to one side, the eyes move to face the previous, forward direction.

With injury to the brainstem, loss of ocular movement occurs, and the eyes become fixed in a direct forward position. A skewed deviation, with one eye looking up and one down, suggests a compressive injury to the brainstem. Normal involuntary cyclic movements of the eyeball (nystagmus responses) in response to ice water delivered into the ear are lost with cortical and brainstem dysfunction.

Alterations in Breathing Pattern

BRAINSTEM DAMAGE

The respiratory center in the lower brainstem controls respiration based on hydrogen ion concentration in the surrounding CSF. Damage to the brainstem causes irregular and unpredictable patterns of breathing. Opiate overdose damages the respiratory center and results in a gradual decline in the breathing rate, until respiration ceases.

CEREBRAL DAMAGE

A higher brain center normally maintains the rhythmic, regular breathing patterns seen in healthy individuals. This control center is lost with cerebral damage, and the individual begins to breathe in a pattern dependent on brainstem carbon dioxide and the hydrogen ion it produces. This type of carbon dioxide-dependent breathing is called posthyperventilation apnea. In this pattern, respirations cease (apnea) until carbon dioxide builds up to a certain threshold, which causes the individual to hyperventilate (increase his or her respiratory rate) until carbon dioxide is removed. At this point respirations cease again.

Cheyne-Stokes respirations also involve breathing based on carbon dioxide levels. In this case the respiratory center is overresponsive to carbon dioxide, which results in a breathing pattern of smooth increases in rate and depth (crescendo breathing) that progresses until a certain carbon dioxide level is reached. The rate and depth of respirations then decrease smoothly until apnea occurs (decrescendo breathing). Cheyne-Stokes is like postventilation apnea, seen with damage to the cerebral hemispheres, and is often associated with metabolically induced coma.

Alterations in Motor Responses and Movement

Abnormal motor responses include inappropriate or absent movements in response to painful stimuli. Brainstem reflex such as sucking and grasping responses will occur if higher brain centers have been damaged. Flexion and rigidity of limbs also are motor responses indicative of brain damage. Muscle movements that indicate abnormal brain function include hyperkinesia (excessive muscle movements), hypokinesia (decreased muscle movements), paresis (muscle weakness), and paralysis (loss of motor function). Specific loss of cerebral cortex functioning, but no loss of brainstem function, results in a particular body posture called *flexor posturing*. Flexor posturing is characterized by flexion of the upper extremities at the elbows and external rotation and extension of the lower extremities. This posture may be unilateral or bilateral. *Extensor posturing* occurs with severe injury to higher brain centers and the brainstem and is characterized by rigid extension of the limbs and neck.

Dysphasia

Dysphasia is impairment of language comprehension or production. Aphasia is total loss of language comprehension or production. Dysphasia usually results from cerebral hypoxia, which is often associated with a stroke but can result from trauma or infection. Brain damage leading to dysphasia usually involves the left cerebral hemisphere.

BROCA'S DYSPHASIA

Broca's dysphasia results from damage to Broca's area in the frontal lobe. Persons with Broca's dysphasia will understand language, but their ability to meaningfully express words in speech or writing will be impaired. This is called expressive dysphasia.

WERNICKE'S DYSPHASIA

Wernicke's dysphasia results from damage to Wernicke's area in the left temporal lobe. With Wernicke's dysphasia, verbal expression of language is intact, but meaningful understanding of spoken or written words is impaired. This is called receptive dysphasia.

Agnosia

Agnosia is the failure to recognize an object because of the inability to make sense of incoming sensory stimuli. Agnosia may be visual, auditory, tactile, or related to taste or smell. Agnosia develops from damage to a particular primary or associative sensory area in the cerebral cortex.

Cerebral Death

Cerebral death refers to irreversible loss of functioning of the cerebral hemisphere, leading to a state in which a person is unresponsive to the external environment. This state is also referred to as a persistent vegetative state and can occur after several different types of brain injuries. Although consciousness is lost, brainstem and cerebellum function is intact; therefore, respiration, cardiovascular control, maintenance of body temperature, and certain brainstem reflexes such as yawning, grasping, and sucking will continue. Eyes may be open or shut, and a sleep–wake cycle will be followed, but there is no conscious perception of events or deliberate action.

A coma is somewhat similar, except there is no opening of the eyes, and no sleep–wake cycle. Coma and cerebral death have legal and ethical implications for the family and for society.

Brain Death

Brain death is irreversible loss of cerebral hemisphere, brainstem, and cerebellum function. Consciousness is lost, as is maintenance of respiration, cardiovascular, and temperature control function. There is no sleep–wake cycle. The electroencephalogram (EEG) is flat in an individual with brain death.

LEGAL IMPLICATIONS OF BRAIN DEATH

A patient cannot be legally discontinued from life support without prior living will instructions unless brain death is established. Organ donation is allowed only when brain death is established. Unfortunately, a donated organ is more likely to be healthy when taken from an individual before brain death.

Dementia

Dementia is a loss of intellectual functioning without a loss of arousal or vegetative functioning. Memory, general knowledge, abstract thought, judgment, and interpretation of written and oral communication may be affected. Dementia may be caused by infection, drugs, trauma, or tumors. Biochemical disturbances and metabolic imbalance may also cause dementia. Some dementia is reversible if the initiating insult can be relieved. Other types of dementia, such as that caused by Alzheimer's disease, are progressive and irreversible.

Increased Intracranial Pressure

Intracranial pressure may increase with increases in cranial blood, CSF, or tissue. A significant increase in intracranial pressure is called intracranial hypertension. Intracranial hypertension causes delicate neurons and capillaries in the brain to become compressed, leading to hypoxia, neuronal injury and death, and progressive deterioration of brain function. If intracranial pressure reaches systemic mean arterial pressure, blood flow to the brain will stop and the individual will die.

CAUSES OF INCREASED INTRACRANIAL PRESSURE

Shifts in intracranial pressure are common, and occur with stimuli such as straining at stool, coughing, and sneezing. More significant increases in intracranial pressure can occur with conditions that increase blood flow to the brain, or that block blood flow out of the brain. Anything that significantly increases CSF production or blocks CSF outflow can increase intracranial pressure. Any increase in tissue mass (i.e., that associated with a growing brain tumor) can increase intracranial pressure.

EDEMA AND SWELLING OF THE INTERSTITIAL SPACE

Important sources of increased intracranial pressure are any stimuli that lead to edema and swelling of the interstitial fluid compartment. Infection and inflammation are associated with interstitial swelling and edema as a result of the release of vasoactive mediators of inflammation that stimulate increased capillary blood flow and increased capillary permeability (Chapter 3). Bacterial toxins also cause significant cellular destruction and initiate capillary destruction, again causing interstitial swelling. Therefore, infection and inflammation significantly increase intracranial pressure.

Severe hypertension may increase intracranial pressure by causing filtration of plasma into the interstitial space, leading to edema and swelling. Severe trauma to the head, a burst aneurysm, or a hemorrhagic stroke cause bleeding in the brain, which increases intracranial pressure by acting as a source of expanding tissue (blood) and by causing swelling and edema.

THE STAGES OF INTRACRANIAL HYPERTENSION

As volume in the brain increases, the brain directs response mechanisms designed to minimize increases in pressure and reduce the extent of brain damage. The response of the brain to increased intracranial pressure is called compensation. However, if the volume in the brain continues to increase, compensation will eventually lose its effectiveness. The brain goes through four stages in response to increased intracranial pressure.

Stage 1

An increase in one of the three volumes in the brain (blood, CSF, or tissue) is normally compensated for by a decrease in one or both of the other volumes. If successful, compensation will allow intracranial pressure to remain near normal even with a significant increase in one of the brain volumes. If there is increased volume in one compartment, but near normal intracranial pressure because of compensation, the brain is said to be in stage 1 of intracranial hypertension. Usually, this stage involves decreased CSF production or increased CSF reabsorption, if possible, followed by venous constriction to increase blood flow out of the brain. Persons in stage 1 may demonstrate only subtle behavioral changes, primarily drowsiness and slight confusion.

Stage 2

If the volume continues to increase despite early compensatory mechanisms, intracranial pressure begins to increase significantly and the individual is said to be in stage 2. This stage would occur with the progression of a tumor or continual bleeding from a severed artery or vein. During stage 2, the brain responds by constricting cerebral arteries in an attempt to further reduce pressure by reducing blood volume. However, reduced blood flow causes development of cerebral hypoxia and hypercapnea (increased carbon dioxide levels) and deterioration of brain function. Obvious clinical signs include decreased level of consciousness, alterations in breathing pattern, and pupillary changes.

Stage 3

Brain hypoxia and deterioration of brain function cause the cerebral arteries to respond with reflex dilation and blood volume increases. Intracranial pressure increases further and worsens the situation. This is called decompensation. With the onset of decompensation, the individual is said to enter stage 3 of intracranial hypertension.

In stage 3, the volume-pressure curve develops so that small changes in intracranial volume produce large changes in pressure. Fast-rising pressure compresses the arterioles and capillaries, worsening the hypoxia and the hypercapnea, and damaging the neural cells. The result is pronounced decreased consciousness, altered respiratory pattern, and loss of pupillary reflexes. As the brain senses worsening hypoxia and hypercapnia, it responds with reflexes geared toward increasing systemic mean arterial pressure in an attempt to increase its own oxygenation. A dramatic increase in systemic blood pressure only serves to further increase intracranial pressure, accelerating the destruction of the brain cells. Cerebral blood flow slows, and consciousness and reflexes are usually lost.

Stage 4

As the swelling and pressure in one compartment of the brain become very high, herniation (bulging) into another compartment occurs. Herniation increases pressure in the other compartment and eventually the whole brain is involved. When intracranial pressure reaches mean systolic pressure, cerebral perfusion stops. The volume-pressure curve demonstrating the stages of increased intracranial pressure is shown in Figure 7-9.

TREATMENT OF INTRACRANIAL HYPERTENSION

Treatment of intracranial hypertension includes osmotic diuretics (mannitol) to reduce blood volume and steroids to decrease inflammation. It is essential that patients suspected of suffering from increased intracranial pressure have accurately measured cerebral perfusion pressure. Hyperventilation is contraindicated under most conditions because it worsens cerebral ischemia.

Tests of Neurologic Functioning

There are several methods to measure neuronal and brain electrical activity and to observe for malformations, injuries, or tumors. Some of these techniques are presented briefly.

ELECTROMYOGRAPHY

Electromyography (EMG) is a technique to measure peripheral nerve function by recording the electrical activity of a motor nerve-muscle cell unit. EMG is used to diagnose, describe, and monitor neuromuscular pathology in patients who are suspected of suffering a disorder in neural transmission or muscle cell function.

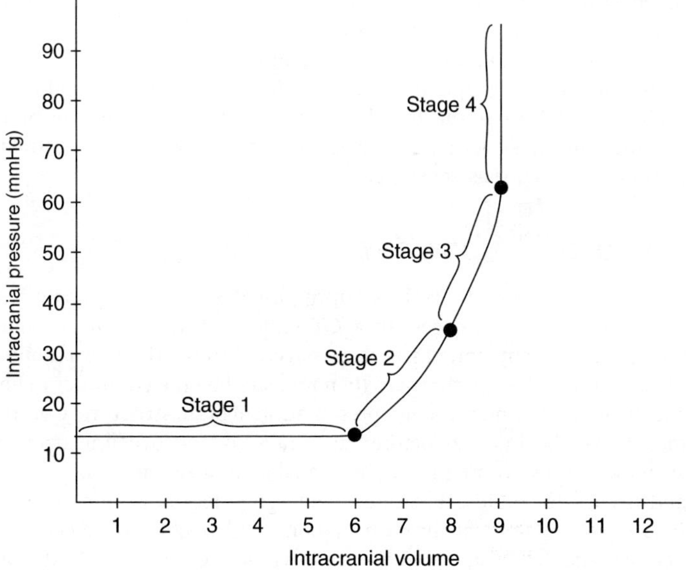

Figure 7-9. Intracranial volume versus pressure.

ELECTROENCEPHALOGRAPHY

Electroencephalography measures electrical activity occurring in the brain through electrodes placed on the scalp. This technique offers a fast, real-time picture of brain activity. EEG is capable of picking up unusual brain wave signals indicative of brain damage or seizure activity. It is limited by an inability to accurately identify which area of the brain is generating the electrical signal, especially when the areas of desired evaluation are located deep in the brain.

MAGNETIC RESONANCE IMAGING

Magnetic resonance imaging captures the physiologic changes happening in the brain before and while an individual performs a task. MRI relies on the principle that each atom in the body will act like a little compass needle and line up in a predictable direction when exposed to a magnetic field. Signals unique to each atom are emitted and images can be formed from this information using specific computer programs. Organs are reproduced in more anatomic detail than by radiograph alone.

Magnetic resonance imaging has made a dramatic impact on the study of brain function and pathophysiology. It allows an investigator to noninvasively study oxygen concentration in the brain as an individual performs a task. Because the brain quickly shifts to anaerobic glycolysis with an activity spurt, oxygen levels increase in venous blood leaving an area performing a task. By looking for areas with high oxygen levels, active areas of the brain can be identified and blood flow patterns can be identified. With MRI, tissue structure and integrity can be imaged clearly. Advantages of MRI include the absence of ionizing radiation and the high sensitivity the technique offers. It is the imaging technique of choice for most neurologic conditions. A limitation of MRI is the length of time required to scan the brain, although ultrafast MRI imaging is available. However, the ultrafast techniques are not as sensitive.

COMPUTED TOMOGRAPHY

Computed tomography (CT) scanning involves computer analysis of multiple radiologic images. In a CT scan, an x-ray beam is rotated around the patient, and passes successively through tissue from multiple directions. The pictures are then recreated by the computer to give a realistic three-dimensional representation of brain structure. Contrast media may be injected before the x-rays to improve fine detail of structures. CT scanning is readily available in most emergency rooms, and is used for rapid evaluation of emerging neurologic emergencies. It is excellent for visualization of bone and is able to detect acute hemorrhage. It is also the technique of choice compared to MRI when patients cannot undergo MRI because of the presence of foreign objects in the eye, pacemakers, or metal protheses. Limitations of a CT scan involve multiple x-ray exposure and less detailed pictures compared to MRI.

POSITRON EMISSION TOMOGRAPHY

Positron emission tomography involves intravenous injection or inhalation of a positron-emitting isotope, followed by sequential radiographs of the skull that monitor the decay of the isotope in tissues that take up the label. This procedure allows the investigator to study the distribution of a particular substance in the brain. It also allows the investigator to anatomically map the brain and determine blood flow patterns. Observing the flow of blood or the uptake of the isotope in different areas of the brain, as an individual performs a task, can identify which areas of the brain are most responsible for that task. Radiolabeled water is often injected when determining cerebral blood flow, radiolabeled fluorodeoxygelucose is used to measure cerebral glucose metablolism, and carbon-11 is used to identify biochemical changes in the brain indicative of multiple sclerosis and Parkinson's disease.

A technique similar to PET scanning, single-photon emission computed tomography (SPECT) also involves the injection of a radionuclide to provide information on metabolic processes and blood flow, but involves decay to only a single photon. SPECT is typically less expensive than PET but offers poorer resolution of structure and metabolic activity.

Typically, blood flow patterns are determined at rest and during a specific task. Limitations to PET and SPECT involve the invasive nature inherent in injecting a radionucleotide, although the ones chosen typically emit low levels of radiation and decay rapidly. Another limitation to these techniques is that neurons typically react faster than blood flow pattern can change, thus some brain activity will be missed.

ULTRASONOGRAPHY

Ultrasound techniques use reflected sound to measure blood flow velocity, which is important for assessment of cerebral blood flow when evaluating ischemic cerebrovascular disease. Ultrasound is used during surgical procedures on the brain to study in real time the development of vascular spasm or blockage. It is limited by the high degree of user proficiency required for its performance.

CONDITIONS OF DISEASE OR INJURY

Seizure Disorder

A seizure is the sudden, uncontrolled discharge of brain neurons, which produces changes in brain function. Seizures result when certain cerebral neurons exist in a hyperexcitable or easily depolarized state. These neurons appear to have a less negative than normal membrane potential at rest, or are missing important inhibitory connections. As a result, this group of neurons, called an epileptogenic focus, is always closer to the threshold potential required for firing an action potential. Neurons of the epileptogenic focus respond to levels of stimuli that do not produce disorderly discharge in other neurons.

Once an epileptogenic focus begins to fire action potentials, resulting current can spread to neighboring cells, causing them to discharge also. It may spread to both sides of the brain and throughout cortical, subcortical, and brainstem areas. If the seizure begins diffusely throughout the cerebral cortex and includes both sides of the cortex, it is called a generalized seizure, and consciousness is always lost. If the seizure arises from a discreet focus and is limited to one side of the brain, it is called a partial seizure, and consciousness is usually not lost. Partial seizures may progress and become generalized. The time of unconsciousness after any generalized seizure is called the postictal phase.

As a seizure continues, inhibitory neurons in the brain fire and cause the neuronal discharge to slow, then stop. If one seizure is followed by a second or third seizure before the individual regains consciousness, status epilepticus is said to occur.

SEIZURE SYNDROMES

Generalized seizures include *tonic-clonic* seizures characterized by sudden onset of rigid, intense contractions of arm and leg muscles (tonic seizure), followed by rhythmic contractions and relaxation of the muscles (clonic seizure). This is the most common type of generalized seizure and has been formally termed a grand mal seizure. Other generalized seizures may be purely *tonic*, purely *clonic,* or *atonic*. *Absence* seizures, frequently seen in children, are characterized by staring and sudden cessation of activity. Generalized seizures may occur idiopathically (for no known reason) or after brain trauma, infection, tumor, or bleeding.

Partial or focal seizures include *simple partial* seizures during which consciousness is not impaired and *complex partial* seizures in which consciousness is impaired. Partial seizures may occur idiopathically or after brain damage.

CONSEQUENCES OF A SEIZURE

During a seizure, cerebral oxygen demand increases more than 200%. If this oxygen demand cannot be met, brain hypoxia and brain damage may occur. Seizures that continue for extended periods, or the occurrence of status epilepticus, greatly increase the chance of brain damage.

Other consequences of a seizure, especially repeated seizures, include social isolation and reduced employment. Even the mildest forms of childhood epilepsy are associated with lifelong social effects, including a reduced likelihood of marriage, childbearing, and academic achievement, even with normal intellectual functioning.

CAUSES OF SEIZURE DISORDERS

Seizures can occur in anyone who experiences severe hypoxemia (decreased oxygen in the blood), hypoglycemia (decreased glucose in the blood), acidemia (increased acid in the blood), alkalemia (decreased acid in the blood), dehydration, water intoxication, or high fever. Drug withdrawal, drug abuse, and toxemia in pregnancy also may cause seizures. Some people seem to have a lower seizure threshold and are therefore more prone to seizures than others, suggesting a genetic tendency toward seizures. Seizures caused by metabolic disturbances are reversible if the initiating stimulus is removed. Syncope (fainting) is often misdiagnosed as a seizure because some muscle movements may be similar. Unconsciousness and muscle jerking related to fainting rarely last longer than 5 to 10 seconds, and is not associated with postictal symptoms such as fatigue.

EPILEPSY

Epilepsy refers to a seizure that occurs without a reversible, metabolic cause. Epilepsy may be a primary or secondary condition. Primary epilepsy develops spontaneously, usually in childhood, and has a genetic predisposition. Mapping of several genes associated with primary epilepsy is under way. Secondary epilepsy occurs as a result of hypoxemia, head injury, infection, stroke, or central nervous system tumor. Adult-onset epilepsy is usually caused by one of these incidents.

CLINICAL MANIFESTATIONS

- Partial seizures may be associated with:
  - facial movements or grimaces
  - jerking beginning in one part of the body, which may spread
  - sensory experiences of sights, smells, or sounds
  - tingling
  - an alteration in level of consciousness
- Generalized seizures may be associated with:
  - unconsciousness, usually accompanied by a fall, except with childhood absence seizures
  - uncontrolled jerking of arms and legs
  - a short period of apnea (breathing cessation)
  - salivation and frothing at the mouth
  - tongue biting
  - incontinence
  - a postictal stage of stupor or coma, followed by confusion, headache, and fatigue

- A prodroma may occur with any seizure type. A prodoma is a certain feeling or symptom that may precede a seizure by hours or days.
- An aura may occur with any seizure type. An aura is a certain sensory sensation that frequently or always immediately precedes a seizure.

DIAGNOSTIC TOOLS

- A detailed medical history is required for an accurate diagnosis of a seizure.
- Basic laboratory evaluation must be performed to rule out metabolic causes or drug-induced seizures.
- Lumbar puncture is performed to rule out meningitis or encephalitis if suspected.
- MRI is the imaging modality of choice to identify brain lesions such as tumor, abscess, or vascular malformation as the cause of the seizure.
- A CT scan may be used for patients with emerging neurologic symptoms who need immediate diagnostic information.
- An EEG may allow diagnosis of the type and location of the occurring seizure. Multiple EEG recordings increase the diagnostic potential.

COMPLICATIONS

- Hypoxic brain damage and mental retardation may follow repeated seizures.
- Depression and anxiety may develop. As described earlier, long-term social isolation may develop.

TREATMENT

- Identification of the type of seizure is essential for optimal treatment.
- Reverse the cause of the seizure disorder if possible.
- Medications are available that may decrease the number of seizures an individual experiences. The goal of seizure treatment is zero seizure occurrence with a minimum of treatment-induced side effects. The medication selected must be appropriate for the seizure type.
- Resective surgery to excise the epileptogenic focus is becoming more common and is indicated in patients in whom antiepileptic drugs do not completely control seizures. Surgery may also be used to remove connections between the cerebral hemispheres to limit seizure occurrence (called corpus callostomy).
- Vagus nerve stimulation involves an electrical device implanted in the infraclavicular area that provides a certain pattern of vagal stimulation to patients with seizures refractory to treatment. This

treatment is a relatively new, nonpharmacologic alternative to drug therapy. Vagal nerve stimulators have been shown to be effective in reducing the frequency of seizures in some patients.

- Counseling for the patient and family is advised.

Pediatric Consideration

Seizures in infants and young children brought on by a rapid increase in body temperature, known as febrile convulsions, are common. Children who have febrile seizures do not appear to experience any long-term intellectual, academic, or behavioral effects.

Head Injury

Head injuries may be open (penetrating through the dura mater) or closed (blunt trauma, without penetration through the dura). Open head injuries allow environmental pathogens direct access to the brain. Damage will occur in either type of injury if blood vessels, glial cells, and neurons are destroyed or torn. Brain damage may develop after severe injury if bleeding and inflammation cause increased intracranial pressure.

CAUSES OF HEAD INJURIES

Causes of head injuries include automobile accidents, fights, falls, and sporting injuries. Open head injuries are often caused by bullet or knife wounds.

Pediatric and Geriatric Consideration

Falls are a major cause of head injuries in children and the elderly. Falls may be related to poor vision, slippery rugs or tubs, and poor muscle strength in the elderly population. Head injuries in toddlers often are related to falls down the stairs or at playgrounds. An infant or young child who receives a head injury should be evaluated for nonaccidental head injury, often referred to as "shaken-baby syndrome." This type of injury occurs from violently shaking an infant or small child, and usually involves striking the head of the child against a hard surface. This type of injury is characterized by subdural or subarachnoid hemorrhage. An elderly person who receives a head injury may be the victim of elder abuse.

TYPES OF HEAD INJURIES

Several different types of head injuries are possible. Some involve an immediate loss of consciousness; others show delayed effects. Some head injuries result in obvious bleeding into the brain; others show no obvious signs of structural damage, but symptoms may develop.

Concussion

A concussion is a closed head injury usually characterized by loss of consciousness. Concussion results in a brief period of apnea. A concussion can be mild, moderate, or severe, depending on the length of time the person is unconscious. A longer period of unconsciousness is predictive of a worse outcome. However, even mild concussions may be associated with subtle behavioral or cognitive changes, even if no obvious brain pathology exists. The condition, called postconcussive syndrome, may last for more than a year.

Epidural Hematoma

An epidural hematoma is the accumulation of blood above the dura mater. An epidural hematoma occurs acutely and is usually caused by a life-threatening arterial bleed.

Subdural Hematoma

A subdural hematoma is the accumulation of blood under the dura mater, but above the arachnoid membrane. It is usually caused by a venous bleed, but occasionally a subdural arterial bleed may occur. A subdural hematoma may develop rapidly, called an acute subdural hematoma, or may result from a slow bleed, called a subacute subdural hematoma. The elderly or the chronic alcohol abuser may experience a slowly developing hematoma over a period of months after a mild head injury, and may not show any obvious symptoms from the hematoma until it is large. This is called a chronic subdural hematoma. A chronic subdural hematoma is possible because the elderly and the chronic alcohol abuser have reduced brain tissue, which allows the cranium to accommodate an expanding hematoma without a significant increase in pressure.

Subarachnoid Hemorrhage

A subarachnoid hemorrhage is the accumulation of blood under the arachnoid membrane, but above the pia mater. This space normally contains only CSF. A subarachnoid hemorrhage usually results from a burst intracranial aneurysm, severe hypertension, an arteriovenous malformation, or a head injury. Blood accumulating on top or under the meninges causes increased pressure on the underlying brain tissue.

CLINICAL MANIFESTATIONS

- With a concussion, consciousness is usually lost immediately and for variable amounts of time.
- Respiratory patterns may become progressively abnormal.
- Pupillary responses may be absent or progressively deteriorate.
- Headache may occur immediately or develop with increasing intracranial pressure.

- Vomiting may occur as a result of increased intracranial pressure.
- Behavioral, cognitive, and physical changes in speech and motor movements may occur immediately or develop slowly. Amnesia related to the event is common.

DIAGNOSTIC TOOLS

- A skull radiograph may locate fractures or a developing bleed or blood clot. A CT scan or an MRI may pinpoint the site and extent of injury. A CT scan is usually the diagnostic tool of choice in the emergency room, although results of CT may be misleadingly normal. An MRI is a more sensitive and accurate tool, capable of diagnosing diffuse axonal injury, but is costly and less accessible at most facilities.

COMPLICATIONS

- Bleeding inside the brain, called an **intracerebral hematoma,** may accompany a severe closed head injury, or more commonly, an open head injury. With bleeding in the brain, intracranial pressure increases, and neuronal and vascular cells are compressed. This is a type of secondary brain injury. With a hematoma, consciousness may be lost immediately, or may decrease later as the hematoma expands and the interstitial edema worsens.

TREATMENT

- Mild and moderate concussions are usually treated with observation and bed rest.
- Surgical ligation of a bleeding vessel and evacuation of a hematoma may be required.
- Surgical debridement (removal of foreign material and dead cells) may be required, especially for an open head injury.
- Decompression through drilling of holes, called Burr holes, into the brain may be required.
- Mechanical ventilation may be required.
- Antibiotics are required for open head injury to prevent infection.
- Methods to decrease intracranial pressure may include the administration of diuretics and anti-inflammatory drugs.

Spinal Injury

Spinal injury usually involves a fracture or other injury to the vertebral bones. The spinal cord, running through the vertebral column, may be sliced, pulled, twisted, or compressed. Damage to the vertebral column or cord may occur at any level. Damage to the cord may involve the entire cord or be restricted to one half. Damage to the spine may result in temporary dysfunction, or permanent damage if the cord is transected (cut).

CAUSES OF SPINAL INJURY

The most common causes of spinal injury are automobile accidents, motorcycle accidents, falls, sports injuries, and wounds from guns and knives.

RESULTS OF SPINAL INJURY

Microscopic Hemorrhages

Small hemorrhages develop with all vertebral or spinal cord injuries. These small bleeds, accompanied by inflammatory reactions that lead to swelling and edema, cause increased pressure in and surrounding the cord. Increased pressure compresses the nerves and decreases the vascular supply, which causes hypoxia and dramatically increases the extent of cord injury. Scar tissue can develop, causing the nerves in the area to become blocked or tangled irreversibly.

Loss of Sensation, Motor Control, and Reflexes

With severe spinal injury, sensation, motor control, and reflexes at and below the level of cord injury are lost. The loss of all reflexes is called **spinal shock.** Swelling and edema surrounding the cord may extend two vertebral segments above the site of injury. Therefore, sensory and motor loss and spinal shock may develop starting from two segments above the injury. Spinal shock typically goes away, but the permanent loss of sensation and motor control will continue if the cord has been transected or if severe swelling and hypoxia has occurred.

Spinal Shock

Spinal shock involves immediate loss of all reflexes from two segments above and below the site of cord injury. The lost reflexes include those controlling posture, bladder and bowel function, blood pressure, and maintenance of body temperature. Spinal shock appears to occur from sudden loss of all tonic discharge normally carried in neurons descending from the brain, which acts to maintain the function of the reflexes. Spinal shock typically lasts 7 to 21 days, but may last longer. As spinal shock regresses, hyperreflexia may occur, characterized by muscle spasticity and reflex bladder and bowel emptying.

Autonomic Hyperreflexia

Autonomic hyperreflexia is characterized by the reflex activation of sympathetic nerves, which leads to a dangerous increase in blood pressure. This condition can occur anytime after the cessation of spinal shock. Autonomic hyperreflexia occurs when a painful sensory stimulus is relayed to the spinal cord and initiates a spinal reflex involving the activation of the sympathetic nervous system. With sympathetic activation, constriction of the blood vessels occurs and systemic blood pressure increases.

In individuals with an intact cord, such an increase in blood pressure would immediately be sensed by baroreceptors that monitor blood pressure (Chapter 13). In response to normal baroreceptor activation, the cardiovascular center in the brain would increase parasympathetic stimulation to the heart, thereby slowing the heart rate. In addition, the sympathetic nervous response would be blocked and dilation of the blood vessels would occur. The parasympathetic and sympathetic changes would serve to rapidly return blood pressure toward normal. In an individual with a cord lesion, although parasympathetic activation will reach and slow heart rate and vasodilation above the site of injury will occur, descending nerves cannot pass through the cord lesion, thus sympathetic reflex vasoconstriction below that level will continue.

With an occurrence of autonomic hyperreflexia, blood pressure can increase more than 200 mmHg systolic, leading to stroke or myocardial infarct. Stimuli that typically cause autonomic hyperreflexia include a distended bladder or bowel, or the stimulation of surface pain receptors. Autonomic hyperreflexia is more likely to happen the higher the spinal cord lesion.

Paralysis

Paralysis is the loss of sensory and voluntary motor function. With spinal cord transection, paralysis is permanent. Paralysis of the upper and lower extremities occurs with transection of the cord at level C6 or higher and is called quadriplegia. Paralysis of the lower half of the body occurs with transection of the cord below C6 and is called paraplegia. If only one half of the cord is transected, hemiparalysis may occur. Permanent paralysis may occur even when the cord is not transected as a result of the destruction of the nerves that follows cord hemorrhage and swelling. In addition, demyelination of the axons in the cord can lead to "clinically complete" lesions, even though the spinal cord may not be transected. Demyelination of the axons most likely occurs as part of the inflammatory response to cord injury.

CLINICAL MANIFESTATIONS

- Loss of sensation, motor control, and reflexes below the level of injury, and up to two levels above, will occur. Body temperature will reflect ambient temperature, and blood pressure will be reduced.
- The pulse rate is often normal with low blood pressure.

DIAGNOSTIC TOOLS

- Physical examination coupled with CT and MRI will document vertebral and spinal injury and edema.

COMPLICATIONS

- If damage and swelling around the cord is in the cervical spine (down to approximately C5) respirations may cease because of compression of the phrenic nerve, which exits between C3 and C5 and controls the movement of the diaphragm.
- Autonomic hyperreflexia is characterized by high blood pressure with bradycardia (low heart rate), and sweating and flushing of the skin on the face and upper torso.
- In the past, individuals suffering from a C2 or higher transection invariably died as a result of respiratory arrest. Although this is still true for many, recent advances in treatment modalities and better emergency rescue service responses have resulted in the survival of many individuals with high cord transection.
- Virtually all systems of the body are affected to some degree by a severe spinal cord injury. Commonly, urinary tract and kidney infections, skin breakdown, and muscle atrophy occur. Depression, marital and family stress, loss of income, and large medical expenses are some of the psychosocial complications.

TREATMENT

- Immobilization to prevent cord severing or additional damage after any head or neck injury is essential, even if a cord injury is not obvious.
- Early surgical intervention to relieve pressure on the cord caused by broken vertebral or collapsed disks may reduce long-term disability.
- Immediate (within the first hour) large-dose administration of steroids has been shown to reduce cord swelling and inflammation and to limit the extent of permanent damage. Strategies to stimulate axon regeneration, or to return impulse conduction along preserved but demyelinated axons, will likely lead to improved outcomes of patients with spinal cord injuries.
- Surgical fixation of the vertebral column hastens and supports healing.
- Physical therapy, including speech therapy if the lesion interferes with speech and respiratory movements, is begun soon after the patient's condition stabilizes.
- Education on avoidance and recognition of autonomic hyperreflexia can reduce the risk of stroke or myocardial infarct.
- Treatment of autonomic hyperreflexia includes antihypertensive medications and the removal of the initiating stimulus.
- For patients with permanent damage, education and counseling about long-term expectations and complications of skin, reproductive, and urinary systems are essential. Including family members in education and counseling sessions is essential.

Cerebral Vascular Accident

A cerebral vascular accident (CVA), often called a stroke or a brain attack, is a brain injury related to an obstruction in brain blood flow. Especially at risk of suffering a CVA are the elderly with hypertension, diabetes, hypercholesterolemia, or heart disease. With a CVA, cerebral hypoxia leading to neuronal cell death and injury occurs. Brain damage after a CVA occurs as a result of swelling and edema, which follow 24 to 72 hours after neuronal cell death.

There are two general classifications of CVAs: ischemic and hemorrhagic. Ischemic CVAs develop from a prolonged blockage in arterial blood flow to a part of the brain. Arterial blockage may occur as a result of a thrombus (a blood clot in the cerebral artery) or an embolus (a blood clot that has traveled to the brain from elsewhere in the body). Hemorrhagic CVAs occur as a result of bleeding into the brain.

THROMBOTIC STROKE

A thrombotic stroke occurs from occlusion of blood flow, usually resulting from severe atherosclerosis. Frequently, an individual will experience one or more transient ischemic attacks (TIAs) before a true thrombotic stroke occurs. A TIA is a brief, reversible disruption in brain function resulting from cerebral hypoxia. It is likely that a TIA occurs when an atherosclerotic vessel undergoes a spasm, or when the oxygen demand of the brain increases and this demand cannot be met because of advanced atherosclerosis. By definition, a TIA lasts fewer than 24 hours. Frequent TIAs suggest a true thrombotic stroke is likely.

A thrombotic stroke typically develops over a period of 24 hours. During the period in which a stroke is progressing, the individual is said to be suffering from a stroke in evolution. At the end of that period the individual is said to have suffered a completed stroke.

EMBOLIC STROKE

An embolic stroke develops after arterial occlusion by an embolus formed outside the brain. Common sources of emboli leading to stroke include the heart after a myocardial infarct or atrial fibrillation, and emboli breaking off the common carotid arteries or the aorta.

HEMORRHAGIC STROKE

A hemorrhagic stroke occurs when a blood vessel in the brain is broken, leading to ischemia (reduced flow) and hypoxia downstream. Causes of hemorrhagic stroke include hypertension, a burst aneurysm, or an arteriovenous malformation (abnormal connection). Hemorrhage into the brain significantly increases intracranial pressure, worsening the resulting brain injury.

CLINICAL MANIFESTATIONS

- Symptoms of a TIA may include temporary numbness of the face or limbs, slurring of words, confusion, dizziness, and changes or blackouts in vision. If any of these occurs, an individual should immediately seek medical assistance.
- With a CVA, which area of the brain becomes ischemic determines the presenting clinical manifestations. Mentation, emotions, speech, vision, or movement can be affected. Many changes are irreversible, but some are reversible.
- A hemorrhagic stroke is frequently accompanied by a severe headache and loss of consciousness.

DIAGNOSTIC TOOLS

- Rapid diagnosis of a CVA is essential to minimize damage. A CT scan is the method of choice for assessment of an acute presentation of a CVA. CT is highly sensitive to hemorrhage, an important consideration because there are vital differences in the treatment of ischemic versus hemorrhagic strokes. CT scans are also readily accessible, even in small or rural hospitals.
- Most MRI devices, although even more sensitive than CT at identifying early brain damage from a CVA, are slower than CT, thus are used less often in this emergent situation. However, after the initial CT scan, MRI is frequently used to determine the exact location of damage and to monitor the lesion.

COMPLICATIONS

- An individual suffering a major CVA to the part of the brain controlling respiration or cardiovascular response may die. Hypoxic destruction of expressive or receptive areas of the brain may lead to communication difficulties. Hypoxia of motor areas in the brain may lead to paresis. Emotional changes may occur with damage to the cortex, including the limbic system.
- An intracerebral hematoma may result from a burst aneurysm or a hemorrhagic stroke, causing secondary brain injury as intracranial pressure increases.

TREATMENT

- In patients in whom the cause of the CVA can be clearly identified as ischemic in nature, thrombolytic agents, such as tissue plasminogen activator (TPA), can be administered. TPA should be given as early as possible to be most effective in preventing long-term damage (at least within the first 3 hours of the attack). However, it would be dangerous to treat a hemorrhagic stroke with a thrombolytic because this would increase bleeding and worsen outcome.

- A hemorrhagic stroke is treated with emphasis on stopping the bleeding and preventing another occurrence. Surgery may be required.
- All strokes are treated with bed rest and a reduction of external stimuli to reduce cerebral oxygen demands. Measures to reduce intracranial edema and pressure may be instituted.

Central Nervous System Infection

A central nervous system infection may involve the brain tissue (encephalitis), or the meninges (meningitis). With encephalitis and meningitis, inflammatory and immune responses cause increased swelling and edema in or around the brain, increasing intracranial pressure. Encephalitis is associated with death of the neurons caused by the infecting microorganism.

ENCEPHALITIS

Encephalitis is usually a viral infection of the brain. It is often carried by a mosquito vector or related to infection with herpes simplex 1 or cytomegalovirus. Nerve cell degeneration is widespread and edema and swelling are severe.

MENINGITIS

Meningitis is usually caused by bacteria, but fungi, viruses, or toxins are also causes. Meningitis frequently occurs from the spread of an infection elsewhere in the body, for example, the sinuses, ears, or upper respiratory tract. A posterior basilar skull fracture with a ruptured eardrum may also cause meningitis. With bacterial meningitis, released toxins destroy meningeal cells and stimulate immune and inflammatory reactions. Secondary encephalitis may occur.

Until recently, most cases of meningitis were in children younger than the age of 5, and most often the causative agent was *Haemophilus influenzae (H. influenzae)*. Since 1990, a vaccine against *H. influenza* has become available and is administered to most children in the United States and other countries as a series of three injections, beginning in the second month of life. As a result of this important intervention, the incidence of meningitis in children ages 1 month to 5 years has decreased 87%. Because of the dramatic decline in *H. influenzae*-type meningitis in this population, cases of bacterial meningitis overall in the United States have dropped 55%.

Meningitis occurs most commonly in adults ages 19 to 59. In this age group, the most common cause of bacterial meningitis is *Streptococcus pneumoniae (S. pneumoniae)*. The next greatest incidence is in children ages 2 to 18, and is most often caused by *Neisseria meningitidis*. In those older than 18, including those older than 65, S. pneumoniae is usually the causative agent. In the neonate, the cause is most often group B streptococcus; in infants aged 1 to 23 months the causes are nearly split between *S. pneumoniae* and *N. meningitidis*.

CLINICAL MANIFESTATIONS

- Symptoms of increased intracranial pressure may develop with meningitis and encephalitis, including headache, decreased consciousness, and vomiting. Papilledema (swelling of the area around the optic nerve) may occur in severe cases. Typically the symptoms are worse with encephalitis.
- Fever from infection is common in meningitis and encephalitis.
- Photophobia (painful response to light) from irritation of the cranial nerves frequently accompanies meningitis and encephalitis.
- Inability to flex the chin to the chest without pain (nuchal rigidity) occurs in meningitis and encephalitis as a result of irritation of the spinal nerves.
- Encephalitis typically presents with dramatic signs of delirium and a progressive decrease in consciousness. Seizures and abnormal movements may occur.

DIAGNOSTIC TOOLS

- In patients suspected of having an acute bacterial meningitis, and in whom there is no clinical contraindication, the CSF is collected through lumbar puncture, and examined for white blood cells and microorganism sensitivity. Elevated protein and reduced glucose in the CSF indicate meningitis. After collection of CSF, a broad spectrum antibiotic is administered. Culture results will determine subsequent antibiotic treatment.
- Rapid diagnosis of CNS infection is essential; this is especially true of meningitis. CT scan and MRI may be used to evaluate the degree of swelling and sites of necrosis. CT is very rapid and of most use in emergent situations.

COMPLICATIONS

- Individuals may suffer permanent disability, brain damage, or die from encephalitis or, less commonly, meningitis.
- Seizures may develop.

TREATMENT

- A broad spectrum antibiotic is administered after CSF collection and will be changed if necessary after culture results.
- An antiviral drug will be administered for encephalitis.
- Measures to reduce intracranial pressure will be initiated, especially for encephalitis.

- Some types of meningitis will require the patient to be isolated in the hospital.

Alzheimer's Disease

Alzheimer's disease is a progressive dementia characterized by the widespread death of brain neurons, especially in an area of the brain called the nucleus basalis. Nerves from here normally project throughout the cerebral hemispheres to areas of the brain responsible for memory and cognition. These nerves release acetylcholine, which has been shown to be essential in building short-term memory at the biochemical level. The enzyme responsible for the production of acetylcholine, choline acetyltransferase, is reduced up to 90% in the brains of individuals who have died of Alzheimer's disease compared to those who have died of other causes. Therefore, lack of acetylcholine can account for at least some of the forgetfulness and loss of cognitive function seen in individuals with Alzheimer's disease. Other neurotransmitters also appear to be absent in individuals with the disease, as does a reduced ability to focus attention on selected information, a requirement for the consolidation of memory.

Alzheimer's disease typically develops after the age of 65, causing senile dementia. However, it may occur earlier and result in presenile dementia. There appears to be a genetic tendency to develop the disease, especially early onset disease.

PATHOLOGY

The pronounced autopsy findings of patients with Alzheimer's disease are widespread development of neuronal tangles, the axons of which coalesce into plaques, called senile plaques. The senile plaques include remnants of the dying nerve terminals, aluminum deposits, and abnormal protein fragments. The protein fragments always include pieces of a protein known as the amyloid precursor protein (APP).

DEVELOPMENT THEORIES

One theory concerning the development of Alzheimer's disease suggests that abnormal processing of the APP allows pieces of the protein to stick out of nerve cell membranes, somehow initiating the tangles and killing the cells. Support for this theory comes from the finding that the gene coding for APP lies on chromosome 21, which when present in triplicate (rather than as a pair), causes Down syndrome. Virtually all individuals with Down syndrome who live into their 40s will develop Alzheimer's disease. However, at least two other chromosomes have also been linked to Alzheimer's disease in different groups of patients, suggesting that there may be more than one genetic cause of the disease.

A second theory as to the cause of Alzheimer's disease involves the discovery that the risk of developing the disease increases with inheritance of a certain gene coding for a specific type of cholesterol-shuttling protein, called apolipoprotein E (APO-E4). Inheritance of the gene for APO-E4, as opposed to one of the other varieties of this protein, APO-E2 or APO-E3, may somehow destabilize the nerve cell membrane, leading to tangling and neuronal cell death. Homozygotes for APO-E4 are at increased risk of developing the disease compared to heterozygotes.

CLINICAL MANIFESTATIONS

The diagnosis of Alzheimer's disease is usually a clinical one, based on history, physical, and biochemical and radiologic examinations. A clinical diagnosis of Alzheimer's is typically highly sensitive in diagnosing positive cases, but may misdiagnose falsely, especially in the very old. Clinical manifestations include:

- Insidious, slowly progressing forgetfulness, decreased judgment, behavioral and personality changes developing over a period of up to 10 years.
- Short-term memory loss and problems with math concepts are common.

DIAGNOSTIC TOOLS

- There is no definitive means of diagnosing Alzheimer's disease during an individual's lifetime, other than by eliminating metabolic or vascular causes of the mental deterioration. However, increasingly sensitive MRI, PET, and SPECT scans can provide clinical support for the diagnosis. Newer techniques are likely to become available for more accurate identification of neuronal tangles and senile plaques.
- Although Alzheimer's disease is the most common cause of dementia, approximately one-third of suspected cases are caused by reversible disorders, including metabolic imbalance, drug effects, CVA, vitamin deficiencies, and depression. These causes must be ruled out using CT or MRI, a complete blood count, and metabolic studies.

TREATMENT

- Patient and family education regarding memory aids, diet, and safety issues may slow the progression of symptoms.
- Medications (Cognex) for the slowing or reversal of early Alzheimer's symptoms are available and may delay the progression of symptoms in some patients. Long-term efficacy is undetermined.

Parkinson's Disease

Parkinson's disease is a progressive brain disorder characterized by the degeneration of dopamine-secreting neurons deep in the cerebral hemisphere in a part of the brain called the basal ganglia. Onset of the disease typically occurs in the sixth or seventh decade of life.

Dopamine acts as an inhibitory neurotransmitter in nerve projections that travel from the basal ganglia throughout the brain. In the basal ganglia, dopamine is normally in balance with the excitatory neurotransmitter acetylcholine. Without dopamine, neurons in the basal ganglia and projections to the cortex and thalamus are overstimulated by acetylcholine, resulting in excess muscle tone characterized by tremor and rigidity. A fixed facial tone projects a lack of emotional responsiveness, although there is often no emotional or cognitive deficit in patients with Parkinson's.

CAUSE

The cause of Parkinson's disease is unknown. There does not appear to be a genetic likelihood of developing the disease. Viruses and toxins have been implicated in some studies.

OTHER CONDITIONS WHOSE SYMPTOMS RESEMBLE PARKINSON'S

Symptoms of Parkinson's disease can develop in persons without Parkinson's disease who suffer from certain types of brain trauma, infection, or tumors. Likewise, individuals who suffer from schizophrenia and require therapy with certain psychotropic drugs such as the phenothiazines may develop symptoms of Parkinson's disease. Some symptoms of secondary Parkinson's can be relieved by treatment of the injury or infection, or removal of the tumor or drug, but others may remain.

CLINICAL MANIFESTATIONS

- A tremor at rest.
- Drooling and dysphagia (difficulty swallowing).
- A shuffling gait, muscle rigidity, and stiffness.
- Akinesia, which is described as a poverty of movement, including movements involved with facial expressions, and other voluntary movements, characterize the disease.
- Loss of postural reflexes leading to loss of equilibrium and a tendency to stoop cause the typical bent over posture seen in patients with Parkinson's.

DIAGNOSTIC TOOLS

- In patients with parkinson-like symptoms, diagnosis is often made based on history and physical. A positive response to levodopa is strongly indicative of Parkinson's.

COMPLICATIONS

- Many patients with Parkinson's develop dementia.

TREATMENT

- Dopaminergic (l-dopa) or anticholinergic drugs may be administered to reduce symptoms.
- Transplanting cells from the basal ganglia or adrenal medulla (where dopamine is also produced) of fetuses into the brains of patients with Parkinson's disease has been successful in some studies.

Huntington's Disease

Huntington's disease (chorea) is a rare, degenerative disease of the basal ganglia and cerebral cortex. It is passed genetically as an autosomal-dominant disorder, apparently caused by expansion of a repeating codon located on chromosome 4. Onset of the disease typically occurs in the fourth or fifth decade of life.

With degeneration of the basal ganglia and cerebral cortex, several different neurotransmitters are lost. Many complications of the disease result from the loss of the inhibitory neurotransmitter GABA. There also appear to be gross abnormalities in energy production by the neuronal cell mitochondria.

Characteristic movements seen in patients with Huntington's disease include extreme involuntary jerking, called chorea. These abnormal movements can occur all over the body and lead to physical exhaustion. Persons with Huntington's disease undergo progressive loss of mental functioning, leading to dementia. Death usually results within 10 years.

CLINICAL MANIFESTATIONS

- Choreic (jerking) movements.
- Personality changes, depression, and slowly progressing dementia.

DIAGNOSTIC TOOLS

- Identification of the gene responsible for Huntington's disease allows the diagnosis of the trait prenatally or before the onset of symptoms in an adult.
- Occasionally, MRI is used to image the brain. Atrophy is apparent in late disease. PET scan may be used to demonstrate hypometabolism of specific areas of the brain.

TREATMENT

- There is no treatment for Huntington's disease. Because genetic identification of symptomless individuals who will likely develop the disease is possible, counseling is essential for those who choose to know their status and those who do not so choose.

Multiple Sclerosis

Multiple sclerosis is an autoimmune disease characterized by antibodies produced against self-antigens that lead to the destruction of neurons in the central nervous system. The peripheral nervous system is unaffected. Until recently, it was thought that the immune attack was primarily against the myelin, which subsequently resulted in the slowing of neural transmission down the axon. Currently, it is thought that the immune attack may begin against the axon itself, causing severing of the axon and subsequent destruction of the myelin. In either case, the transmission of neural impulses in the brain and spinal cord is slowed, leading to dramatic alterations in movements, reflexes, and, in some cases, changes in mental status. Continued inflammatory responses contribute to the disease by producing swelling and edema, which further injure the neurons and cause the development of scar tissue plaques on the myelin.

CATEGORIES OF MULTIPLE SCLEROSIS

There are four categories of multiple sclerosis, called syndromes, based on the original nerve tracts affected. These syndromes are the coriticospinal syndrome, the brainstem syndrome, the cerebellar syndrome, and the cerebral syndrome. Initial symptoms usually fit into one of these syndromes. As the disease progresses, different tracts are affected and the symptoms become more widespread.

Besides separate neural tracts involved, multiple sclerosis can also take different forms based on the rate of progression of the disease. In the first type, **relapsing-remitting form**, the course of the disease is characterized by exacerbations of symptoms, followed by partial or full remission back to the preceding state. The second type, called **primary progressive form**, is characterized by a quick downhill course, without remission, from the beginning of the disease. The third type, **secondary progressive form**, begins as the relapsing-remitting type, and then changes to a fast progression without remission.

CAUSES OF MULTIPLE SCLEROSIS

The cause of multiple sclerosis is unknown, but there appears to be a genetic tendency toward developing this and other autoimmune diseases. Some evidence suggests that a childhood viral infection, perhaps measles or a type of herpes infection, may initiate the immune response. It has been suggested that a breakdown in the blood-brain barrier during the time of the viral infection may have allowed a B-cell lymphocyte, developed against the virus, to gain entrance to and colonize the brain. An IgG clone (IgG from one B-cell line) is often present in the CSF of an individual with multiple sclerosis. These clones increase in number with the many exacerbations of the disease.

In support of this theory are observations that viral infections and multiple sclerosis occur more frequently in individuals who live at northern latitudes. An individual's risk of developing multiple sclerosis appears to be related to the latitude in which the individual lived for approximately the first 15 years of life.

CLINICAL MANIFESTATIONS

- Episodes of motor, visual, or sensory disturbances that partially resolve and then recur.
- Bladder dysfunction may occur with some types of multiple sclerosis.
- Some individuals may develop cognitive or emotional disorders.
- Symptoms are frequently precipitated by stress. Stresses may include the birth of an infant, illness, fever, fatigue, or high temperatures.

DIAGNOSTIC TOOLS

- Clonal IgG bands in the CSF are found using electrophoresis techniques in approximately 90% of patients.
- Elevations in other types of CSF and plasma IgG are frequently present.
- MRI, and to a lesser degree CT scans, may allow for visualization of central nervous system plaques. MRI may identify disease activity even in the absence of acute clinical findings, and is capable of differentiating between old and new lesions.
- Techniques to measure muscle cell discharge will demonstrate delayed muscle excitation in some types of the disease.

COMPLICATIONS

- Severe neurologic deficits including loss of sight, increasing fatigue, and intellectual deterioration may develop over the course of the disease.
- Depression, loss of social support, family and spousal stress, and financial problems are common.

TREATMENT

- Aggressive immunosuppressant therapy at the start of the disease and with any exacerbation may limit the autoimmune destruction of the neuron or myelin.
- Antiviral drugs may slow the progress of the disease.
- Subcutaneous injections of the immune substance beta-interferon may reduce the number and severity of exacerbations in some patients with multiple sclerosis.
- Education on bladder training, sexual functioning, and avoidance of complications associated with reduced mobility may increase lifestyle satisfaction and overall health.

- Education regarding the need to avoid overfatigue and high temperatures may reduce symptoms.
- Innovative drug therapies are being tried that aim to foster antigenic self-tolerance by providing myelin protein for ingestion. These therapies are based on the hypothesis that an individual may tolerate (not attack in an immune response) a substance that enters the body through the GI tract.

Amyotrophic Lateral Sclerosis

Amyotrophic lateral sclerosis (ALS) is a degenerative disease of the upper and lower motor neurons resulting in near total paralysis. The loss of motor neurons does not include cranial nerves III, IV, and VI. Therefore, some facial movements, including blinking, are maintained. ALS is also known as Lou Gehrig's disease and usually occurs in the fourth or fifth decade of life. The disease is usually fatal within 5 years, although some individuals may live much longer. There is no known cause of ALS, although viral infection, metabolic disturbances, and trauma have been suggested. Degeneration of the motor neurons occurs without any obvious inflammation. Although the myelin is not a primary site of degeneration, loss of the nerve axon causes the subsequent loss of myelin, and scarring occurs.

CLINICAL MANIFESTATIONS

- Initial weakness develops in one muscle group, which progresses to weakness and paralysis in all skeletal muscles except the extraocular muscles.
- Intellectual and sensory functioning remain normal until death.

COMPLICATIONS

- ALS may be difficult to diagnose. Once confirmed, depression may occur. Immense family hardship develops as the disease, in most cases, quickly progresses.

DIAGNOSTIC TOOLS

- Muscle biopsy demonstrates lower neuron degeneration and confirms a strong clinical diagnosis.

TREATMENT

- Psychological support is essential for the individual and family, as is education on maintaining eye communication.

Myasthenia Gravis

Myasthenia gravis is a peripheral nervous system disorder characterized by autoantibody production against the receptors for acetylcholine present on the motor end-plate region of skeletal muscles. The IgG autoantibodies competitively bind to the acetylcholine receptors, prevent acetylcholine from binding to the receptors, and therefore prevent muscle contraction. Eventually, receptors at the neuromuscular junction are destroyed.

Myasthenia gravis may first cause weakness of the muscles controlling eye movements (ocular myasthenia gravis) or may affect the entire body (generalized myasthenia gravis). Progression of the disease is variable and may be slowly progressing, with or without remissions, or rapidly progressing, leading to death by respiratory paralysis and failure.

The cause of myasthenia gravis is unknown but appears to be associated with a familial tendency toward developing autoimmune disease. The thymus gland is frequently hyperplastic and appears to function as it did in early childhood, suggesting it may be initiating or perpetuating the immune response.

CLINICAL MANIFESTATIONS

- Weakness of the muscles of the eyes, causing pitosis (drooping of the eyelids).
- Weakness of face, neck, and throat muscles, causing difficulty eating and swallowing.
- Continued spread of muscle weakness. Initially there is easy fatigue with recovery of strength after rest. Eventually there is no recovery of strength after rest.

DIAGNOSTIC TOOLS

- Normally acetylcholine is broken down at the neuromuscular junction by the enzyme acetylcholinesterase. A clinical diagnosis of myasthenia gravis can be confirmed on the basis of the return of muscle strength after intravenous administration of a medication that prevents the activity of acetylcholinesterase, thereby prolonging the half-life of acetylcholine. This medication, edrophonium chloride (Tensilon), allows acetylcholine to have a better chance of binding its receptors, allowing voluntary muscle contraction. The effect of Tensilon lasts several minutes, after which muscle weakness reappears.
- Electromyography (EMG) measurements of skeletal muscle action potentials show reduced amplitude on motor neuron stimulation.

COMPLICATIONS

- Myasthenia crisis, characterized by severe worsening of skeletal muscle function culminating in **respiratory distress** and death as the diaphragm and intercostal muscles become paralyzed, may occur after a stressful experience such as an illness, emotional upset, surgery, or during pregnancy.

- Cholinergic crisis is a toxic response occasionally seen with the use of too much anticholinesterase drug. A hypercholinergic state can develop that is characterized by increased intestinal motility, pupillary constriction, and bradycardia. The individual may develop nausea, vomiting, sweating, and diarrhea. Respiratory distress may occur.

TREATMENT

- Frequent rest periods during the day conserve strength.
- Anticholinesterase medications are provided to prolong the half-life of acetylcholine at the neuromuscular junction. The medications must be taken on schedule each day to prevent muscle fatigue and collapse.
- Anti-inflammatory medications are used to limit the autoimmune attack.
- A myasthenia crisis may be treated with additional medication, and respiratory support if necessary.
- A cholinergic crisis is treated with atropine (acetylcholine blocker) and respiratory support, until symptoms resolve. Anticholinesterase therapy is withheld until toxic levels of the drug are reversed.
- Myasthenia crisis and cholinergic crisis present similarly, but are treated differently and to a degree, oppositely. Tensilon administration is used to differentiate the two disorders.
- Plasmapheresis (blood dialysis with the removal of IgG antibodies) and thymectomy (surgical removal of the thymus) are sometimes performed with variable long-term results.

Guillain-Barré Syndrome

Guillain-Barré syndrome is a peripheral nervous system disease characterized by the sudden onset of muscle paralysis or paresis. Guillain-Barré results from an autoimmune attack against the myelin surrounding the peripheral nerves. With destruction of the myelin, the axons can be damaged. Symptoms of Guillain-Barré disappear as the autoimmune attack ceases and the axons regenerate. If destruction of the cell body occurred during the attack, some degree of disability may remain. Although the cause of Guillain-Barré is unknown, the disease usually occurs 1 to 4 weeks after a viral infection or immunization.

The muscles of the lower extremities are usually affected first, with paralysis advancing up the body. Respiratory muscles may be affected, leading to respiratory collapse. Cardiovascular function may be impaired because of interruption of autonomic nerve function.

CLINICAL MANIFESTATIONS

- Ascending muscle weakness or paralysis.

DIAGNOSTIC TOOLS

- Nerve conduction tests will demonstrate neuronal dysfunction.
- Elevated protein in the CSF is common.

COMPLICATIONS

- Respiratory or cardiovascular collapse may cause death.

TREATMENT

- Ventilatory support may be required if the respiratory muscles are affected.
- Anti-inflammatory medications may limit the autoimmune attack.

Spina Bifida

Spina bifida is a congenital neural tube defect characterized by a failure of the vertebral arches to close. This results in a cyst-like protrusion of the meninges alone (meningocele) or of the meninges and the spinal cord (myelomeningocele) out of the vertebral column. In the case of a meningocele, neural tissue is unexposed, thus neural deficits are absent or minor. With a myelomeningocele, the spinal cord, in the cyst-like protrusion with its nerves, suffers injury, inflammation, and scarring. The result is some loss of neural function, often including paralysis. Another type of spina bifida is one in which minor irregularities in the vertebral arches exist that are not obvious at birth. This is called spina bifida occulta (hidden).

A meningocele can occur in any area of the spine; cranial or upper cervical meningoceles are frequently associated with hydrocephalus. A myelomeningocele typically occurs in the lumbar or lumbosacral areas.

CAUSES OF SPINA BIFIDA

Although the cause of spina bifida is unknown, a genetic predisposition may exist. Increased risk of the disorder occurs with maternal folic acid deficiency. Folic acid deficiency is common in women; therefore, it is strongly recommended that all women anticipating pregnancy begin taking folic acid vitamin supplements at least 3 months before conception.

CLINICAL MANIFESTATIONS

- Spina bifida occulta may be symptomless or associated with:
  - hair growth along the spine
  - midline dimple, usually in the lumbosacral area
  - gait or foot abnormalities
  - poor bladder control
- A meningocele may be symptomless or associated with:
  - a sac-like protrusion of meninges and CSF from the back

    - club foot
    - gait disturbance
    - bladder incontinence
- A myelomeningocele is associated with:
    - protrusion of meninges, CSF, and spinal cord
    - neurologic deficits at and below the site of exposure

DIAGNOSTIC TOOLS

- Elevated levels of a fetal protein, called alpha-fetoprotein, in maternal serum may indicate fetal spina bifida.
- Ultrasound may diagnose the condition in utero.

COMPLICATIONS

- Hydrocephalus may occur with a meningocele or myelomeningocele.

TREATMENT

- No treatment may be required for spina bifida occulta or meningocele.
- Surgical repair of the myelomeningocele, and sometimes the meningocele, is required.
- If surgical repair is performed, placement of a shunt to allow for CSF drainage is necessary to prevent hydrocephalus and a subsequent increase in intracranial pressure.
- Planned cesarean section before the initiation of labor can be important in reducing the neurologic damage seen in an infant with a spinal cord defect.

Hydrocephalus

Hydrocephalus ("water on the brain") is characterized by an accumulation of CSF anywhere in the ventricles of the brain. Hydrocephalus may result from overproduction of CSF, obstruction of the flow of CSF within the ventricular system, or a decrease in the absorption of CSF out of the ventricles. Hydrocephalus can be apparent with a sonogram before birth, or it may develop in adulthood. In adults, hydrocephalus may develop suddenly after a head injury or slowly in response to a growing tumor.

TYPES OF HYDROCEPHALUS

There are two types of hydrocephalus: noncommunicating and communicating.

Noncommunicating Hydrocephalus

Noncommunicating hydrocephalus occurs as a result of obstruction of CSF flow within the ventricular system. This type of hydrocephalus may occur with a tumor or as a result of a congenital irregularity in the ventricular pathways.

Communicating Hydrocephalus

Communicating hydrocephalus occurs as a result of a blockage in the absorption of CSF. Causes of this type of hydrocephalus include a buildup of tissue (usually a neoplasm) or blood in the subarachnoid space. Head injuries may cause communicating hydrocephalus.

EFFECT OF HYDROCEPHALUS

Intracranial pressure increases with hydrocephalus, which can directly injure underlying nervous tissue and compromise cerebral blood flow and the neuronal supply of oxygen and glucose. Compensation to increased ICP may occur with slowly developing hydrocephalus. With an acute brain injury, rapidly developing hydrocephalus dramatically increases intracranial pressure and compensation is usually ineffective.

CLINICAL MANIFESTATIONS

- Newborns with hydrocephalus may have an enlarged head and a high-pitched cry.
- Acutely developing hydrocephalus causes a rapid increase in intracranial pressure and may present with a severe headache, decreased consciousness, papilledema, and vomiting.
- Slowly progressing hydrocephalus may present with irritability and changes in cognition and behavior.

DIAGNOSTIC TOOLS

- Ultrasound may allow diagnosis in utero.
- After birth, diagnosis is made by clinical inspection, measurements of head circumference, and observation of cranial suture lines.

COMPLICATIONS

- Mental retardation may result.

TREATMENT

- Placement of a shunt to drain CSF in utero or after birth may be performed.
- Treatment of the underlying cause is required.

Cerebral Palsy

Cerebral palsy is brain damage that occurs in an infant before, during, or soon after birth. It results in some degree of motor dysfunction. Cerebral palsy is nonprogressive and is caused by cerebral hypoxia or increased intracranial pressure after physical trauma to the brain. Increased intracranial pressure may directly damage neuronal cells or may cause hypoxia by compressing the blood vessels. Frequently, hemorrhage is the cause of increased intracranial pressure.

CLINICAL MANIFESTATIONS

- Cerebral palsy may result in a motor deficiency in any or all limbs and usually involves muscle spasticity.
- Vision disturbances, mental impairment, and seizures may occur.

DIAGNOSTIC TOOLS

- Typically the infant is diagnosed based on clinical signs at birth or in early infancy.

COMPLICATIONS

- Developmental and social delay are common and may lead to family and marital stress.

TREATMENT

- Treatment depends on the extent of the physical impairment, mental status, and the occurrence of seizures. Surgery may be required to relieve contractions.
- All treatment regimens must include physical therapy.
- Counseling is important for the family and the child.

Selected Bibliography

Ashizawa, T., Wong, L. J. C., Richards, C. S., Caskey, C. T., & Jankovic, J. (1994). CAG repeat size and clinical presentation in Huntington's disease. *Neurology* 44, 1137–1143.

Boechxstaens, G. E. & Pelckmans, P. A (1997). Nitric oxide and the non-adrenergic noncholinergic neurotransmission. *Comparative Biochemistry and Physiology. Part A, Physiology* 118, 925–932.

Brenner, D. E., Kukull, W. A., Stergachis, A., et al. (1994). Postmenopausal estrogen replacement therapy and the risk of Alzheimer's disease. *American Journal of Epidemiology* 140, 262–267.

Bullock, B. L. & Rosendahl, P. P. (1996). *Pathophysiology. Adaptations and alterations in function (4th ed)*. Philadelphia: J.B. Lippincott.

Chase, T. N. (1998). The significance of continuous dopaminergic stimulation in the treatment of Parkinson's disease. *Drugs* 55 (Suppl), 1–9.

Delgado-Escueta, A.V., Serratosa, J. M., Liu, A., et al. (1994). Progress in mapping human epilepsy genes. *Epilepsia* 35 (Suppl), S29–S40.

Duhaime, A., Christian, C. W., Rorke, L. B., & Zimmerman, R. A. (1998). Nonaccidental head injury in infants—the shaken-baby syndrome. *New England Journal of Medicine* 338, 1822–1829.

Feldman, Z. & Reichenthal, E. (1994). Intracranial pressure monitoring. *Journal of Neurosurgery* 81, 329–330.

France, J. K. (1993). Huntington's disease: helping the patient retain function. *American Journal of Nursing* 93, 62–64.

Gabrieli, J. D. (1998). Cognitive neuroscience of human memory. *Annual Review of Psychology* 49, 87–115.

Gilman, S. (1998). Imaging the brain: first of two parts. *New England Journal of Medicine* 338, 812–820.

Gilman, S. (1998). Imaging the brain: second of two parts. *New England Journal of Medicine* 338, 889–896.

Gruen, P. & Liv, C. (1998). Current trends in the management of head injury. *Emergency Medicine Clinics of North America* 16, 63–83.

Guyton, A. C. & Hall, J. A. (1997). *Textbook of medical physiology (9th ed)*. Philadelphia: W.B. Saunders.

Jenkins, B. G., Koroshetz, W. J., Beal, M. F., & Rosen, B. R. (1993). Evidence for impairment of energy metabolism in vivo in Huntington's disease using localized 1H NMR spectroscopy. *Neurology* 43, 2689–2695.

Kampen, D. L. & Sherwin, B. B. (1994). Estrogen and verbal memory in healthy postmenopausal women. *Obstetrics and Gynecology* 83, 979–983.

Marks, W. J. & Garcia, P. A. (1998). Management of seizures and epilepsy. *American Family Physician* 57, 1589–1600.

Mayeux, R., Saunders, A. M., Shea, S., et al. (1998). Utility of the apolipoprotein E genotype in the diagnosis of Alzheimer's disease. *New England Journal of Medicine* 338, 506–511.

McLatchie, G. & Jennett, B. J. (1994). ABC of sports medicine. Head injury in sport. *British Medical Journal* 308, 1620–1624.

Paganini-Hill, A. & Henderson, V. W. (1994). Estrogen deficiency and risk of Alzheimer disease in women. *American Journal of Epidemiology* 140, 256–261.

Poirier, J., Davignon, J., Bouthillier, D., Kogan, S., Bertrand, P., & Gauthier, S. (1993). Apolipoprotein E polymorphism and Alzheimer's disease. *Lancet* 342, 697–699.

Raichle, M. E. (1994). Visualizing the mind. *Scientific American* 270, 58–65.

Rose, D. J. (1997). A multilevel approach to the study of motor control and learning. In: *Memory and learning*. Boston: Allyn & Bacon. pp. 189–213.

Schuchat, A., Robinson, K., Wenger, J. D., Harrison, L. H., Farley, M., Reingold, A. L., Lefkowitz, L., & Perkins, B. A. (1997). Bacterial meningitis in the United States in 1995. *New England Journal of Medicine* 337, 970–976.

Sillanpaa, M., Jalava, M., Kaleva, O., & Shinnar, S. (1998). Long-term prognosis of seizures with onset in children. *New England Journal of Medicine* 338, 1715–1722.

Scott, J. (1993). Apolipoprotein E and Alzheimer's disease. *Lancet* 342, 696–699.

Terry, R. D. (1994). Neuropathological changes in Alzheimer disease. *Progress in Brain Research* 101, 383–390.

Trapp, B. D., Peterson, J., Ransohoff, R. M., Rudick, R., Mork, S., & Bo, L. (1998). Axonal transection in the lesions of multiple sclerosis. *New England Journal of Medicine* 338, 278–285.

Vander, A. J., Sherman, J., & Luciano, D., (1998). *Human physiology (7th ed)*. Boston: McGraw-Hill.

Verity, C. M., Greenwood, R., & Golding, J. (1998). Long-term intellectual and behavioral outcomes of children with febrile seizures. *New England Journal of Medicine* 338, 1723–1728.

Waxman, S. G. (1998). Demyelinating diseases—new pathological insights, new therapeutic targets. *New England Journal of Medicine* 338, 323–325.

Werler, M. M., Shapiro, S., & Mitchell, A. A. (1993). Periconceptional folic acid exposure and risk of occurrent neural tube defects. *Journal of the American Medical Association* 269, 1257–1261.

Zeman, A. (1997). Persistent vegetative state. *Lancet* 350, 795–799.

8 THE ENDOCRINE SYSTEM

The endocrine system, like the nervous system, allows for communication between distant sites in the body. There are three components to the endocrine system: endocrine glands that secrete chemical messengers into the bloodstream; the chemical messengers, called hormones; and target cells or organs that respond to the hormones.

• • •

PHYSIOLOGIC CONCEPTS

Endocrine Glands

Endocrine glands are organs that synthesize, store, and secrete hormones into the bloodstream. There are many endocrine glands in the body, including the pancreas, thyroid, parathyroid, and some cells of the gut and kidney. The endocrine glands reviewed in this chapter are the hypothalamus, the anterior and posterior pituitary glands, and the endocrine glands that function as target organs for certain pituitary hormones.

THE HYPOTHALAMUS

The hypothalamus is a small area of the brain located in the section of the forebrain called the diencephalon. The hypothalamus is a neural and an endocrine organ. It is concerned with maintaining homeostasis, that is, keeping the body's internal environment constant. The hypothalamus is also essential in controlling behavior and allowing appropriate responses to multiple incoming stimuli. It continually receives information from the central and peripheral nervous systems concerning temperature, pain, pleasure, feeding, hunger, body mass, and metabolic status. It also receives input from most all other hormones of the body and receives neural extensions from most other areas of the brain.

The hypothalamus, in turn, responds to all the incoming stimuli by sending neural projections throughout the brain and by synthesizing and secreting its own hormones. Nerve cell bodies in the ventral hypothalamus synthesize several hormones and send them in axon projections to be released into the blood and delivered to the anterior pituitary gland. Other nerve cell bodies in the hypothalamus synthesize hormones that are sent down axon projections to the posterior pituitary where they are stored until released into the bloodstream. These two routes by which the hypothalamus controls hormone release by the anterior and posterior pituitary are shown in Figure 8-1.

THE ANTERIOR PITUITARY

The anterior pituitary, also called the adenohypophysis, is composed of nonneural tissue. It is anatomically separate from the hypothalamus,

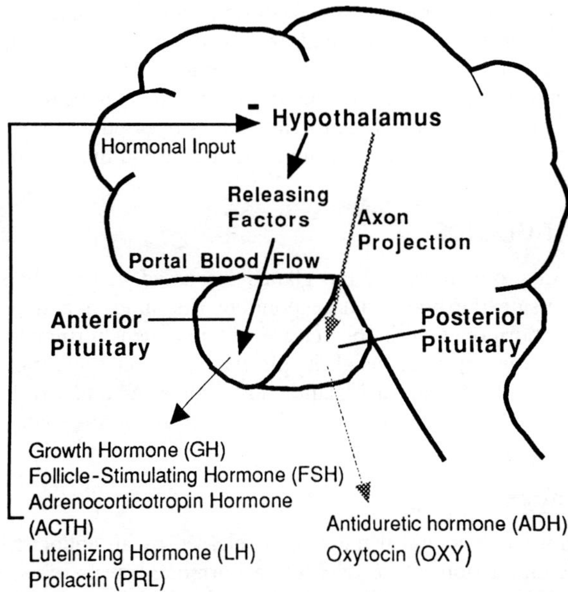

Figure 8-1. The hypothalamic-pituitary system. The hypothalamus is connected through the blood to the anterior pituitary while the posterior pituitary is a neural outgrowth.

but functionally connected to it through its blood supply. The anterior pituitary receives its blood through venous drainage from the hypothalamus. When blood flowing in a vein breaks into another capillary network instead of flowing back to the vena cava, the system is called a portal venous system. Thus, the hypothalamus and the anterior pituitary are connected by the **hypothalamic-anterior pituitary portal blood flow system**. Because this blood has already been used by the hypothalamus, it is poorly oxygenated but rich in hormonal messages put out by the hypothalamus into the median eminence (see later). The anterior pituitary is, therefore, a major target organ for hypothalamic hormones and responds to hypothalamic hormones with release of its own hormones.

THE POSTERIOR PITUITARY

The posterior pituitary, also called the neurophysis, is true neural tissue derived embryologically from the hypothalamus. There are three parts to the posterior pituitary: the median eminence (sometimes considered hypothalamic tissue) into which the hypothalamus secretes the anterior pituitary-releasing hormones; the infundibular stem connecting the hypothalamus with the posterior pituitary; and the infundibular process, which is the terminal end of the posterior pituitary.

Nerve cell bodies in the supraoptic and paraventricular nuclei of the hypothalamus synthesize two hormones: antidiuretic hormone and oxytocin. The hypothalamus sends these hormones in axon projections through the infundibular stem to the infundibular process. They are stored there until the hypothalamus stimulates them to be released into the general circulation. Thus, the hormones released by the posterior pituitary are hypothalamic in origin and depend on the hypothalamus for their release.

TARGET GLANDS

The third group of endocrine glands discussed in this chapter are those outside the brain that respond to the anterior and posterior pituitary hormones with the release of their own hormones. These glands are the target organs of the pituitary hormones and include the thyroid gland, the adrenal gland, and the testes and ovaries. The pancreas, which secretes insulin, is also an endocrine gland and is mentioned later.

Hormones

A hormone is a chemical messenger released by an endocrine gland into the circulation. Once released, a hormone travels in the bloodstream and affects only cells in the body that have receptors (binding sites) specific to it. Cells that respond to a particular hormone are called **target cells** for that hormone. Typically, a hormone is released in bursts from an endocrine gland in a pattern that often follows an inherent daily (diurnal) rhythm. The burst of hormone release can be increased or decreased above or below baseline level by various inputs to the gland. Inputs that affect hormone release involve: 1) stimulation by another hormone or neurotransmitter, or 2) stimulation by a decrease or increase in a certain ion or nutrient. Examples of hormones that cause an increase or decrease in another hormone's release include all the hypothalamic hormones affecting the anterior pituitary. Examples of neurotransmitters affecting a hormone's release include the release of insulin in response to epinephrine and norepinephrine stimulation. Ions that influence the release of a hormone include calcium ion's effect on parathyroid hormone, and sodium ion's effect on aldosterone. Nutrients that affect the release of hormones include amino acids that stimulate the release of insulin and growth hormone. Frequently, one endocrine gland is stimulated simultaneously by several different inputs.

There are three broad categories of hormones: peptide, steroid, and amino acid. Most hormones are peptide hormones and include all the hypothalamic hormones and pituitary hormones. The amino acid hormones are made from the amino acid tyrosine. The steroid hormones are made from cholesterol and are soluble across the cell membrane.

PEPTIDE HORMONES

Peptide hormones range in size from just a few amino acids to relatively large protein complexes. Peptide hormones circulate dissolved in the plasma to their target organs and exert their effects by binding to specific receptors present on the outside of target cell membranes. By binding to its receptor, a protein hormone changes the permeability of the cell to water, electrolytes, or organic molecules such as glucose, or causes the activation of intracellular messengers, which then causes enzyme activation or protein synthesis. Examples of intracellular messengers include the G proteins, which many protein hormones first activate during receptor binding, and the second messengers such as cyclic adenosine monophosphate (cyclic AMP) and calcium, which are subsequently activated by the G proteins. See Table 8-1 for a list of the peptide hormones.

STEROID HORMONES

Steroid hormones are cholesterol-based, lipid-soluble molecules produced by the adrenal cortex or the sex organs. Because they are lipid-soluble, they can cross the cell membrane and bind to receptors or carriers inside the cell. Once inside a cell, the steroid hormone travels to the cell nucleus where it influences the cell by affecting DNA replication, transcription of DNA into RNA, or translation of RNA into proteins. Steroid hormones are discussed in this chapter and in Chapter 21. See Table 8-2 for a list of steroid hormones.

AMINE HORMONES

The amine hormones are derivatives of the amino acid tyrosine and include thyroid hormone and the catecholamines (epinephrine, norepinephrine, and dopamine). Epinephrine, norepinephrine, and dopamine also act as neurotransmitters in the central and peripheral nervous systems. The catecholamine hormones travel dissolved in the blood to their target cell and bind to the plasma membrane at specific receptor sites. Binding of catecholamine activates the cyclic AMP second messenger system and alters enzyme activity or membrane permeability. Thyroid hormone travels in the blood mostly bound to carrier proteins with a smaller amount circulating free. Once at the target cell, free thyroid hormone crosses the cell membrane and binds to the nuclear DNA, directly affecting DNA transcription. Therefore, free hormone, although in lesser quantity, is the active hormone. Table 8-3 lists the amine hormones.

Feedback

In the endocrine system, feedback refers to the response of a target tissue after stimulation by a hormone, which influences the continued release of that hormone.

Each hormone is stimulated to be released by a specific signal. Once released, a hormone affects its target organ, causing a response that usually reduces further hormone release. This type of feedback, shown in Figure 8-2, is called negative feedback, and allows tight control over hormone levels. Positive feedback is uncommon and

Table 8-1. Protein Hormones

HYPOTHALAMIC-RELEASING AND -INHIBITING HORMONES AND FACTORS
Thyrotropin-releasing hormone (TRH)
Corticotropin-releasing hormone (CRH)
Growth hormone-releasing factor (GRF)
Somatostatin (growth hormone-inhibiting hormone)
Gonadotropin-releasing hormone (GnRH)
Prolactin-inhibiting factor (PIF)
Prolactin-releasing hormone (PRH)
Substance P

ANTERIOR PITUITARY PROTEIN HORMONES
Thyroid-stimulating hormone (TSH)
Adrenocorticotropic hormone (ACTH)
Growth hormone (GH)
Follicle-stimulating hormone (FSH)
Luteinizing hormone (LH)
Prolactin
Melanocyte-stimulating hormone

POSTERIOR PITUITARY HORMONES
Antidiuretic hormone (ADH)
Oxytocin

HORMONES OF DIGESTION AND METABOLISM (CHAPTERS 15, 16, AND 17)
Insulin
Glucagon
Calcitonin
Parathyroid hormone
Cholecystokinin
Gastrin
Secretin

HORMONE OF BLOOD PRESSURE AND ELECTROLYTE BALANCE (CHAPTERS 11 AND 13)
Angiotensin II

HORMONE FOR RED BLOOD CELL DEVELOPMENT (CHAPTER 5)
Erythropoietin

HORMONE TO MODULATE STRESS AND PAIN (CHAPTERS 7 AND 8)
Endorphin

Table 8-2. Steroid Hormones

Gonadal Hormones
Estrogens
Progesterone
Androgens (primarily testosterone)
HORMONES OF THE ADRENAL CORTEX
Aldosterone
Glucocorticoids (primarily cortisol)
Androgens (primarily testosterone)
Estrogens

Table 8-3. Amine Hormones

Thyroid hormones
Epineiphrine
Norepinephrine
Melatonin (from the anterior pituitary)

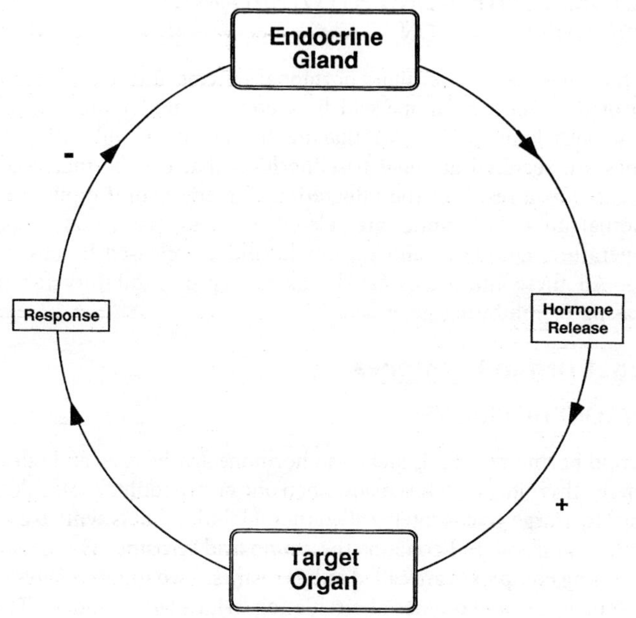

Figure 8-2. Feedback: general.

occurs when the response by a target tissue to hormonal stimulation increases the further release of that hormone.

Factors Controlling Hormone Secretion

FACTORS CONTROLLING ANTERIOR PITUITARY HORMONE SECRETION

The stimuli that control the secretion of the pituitary hormones (except melanocyte-stimulating hormone) are the hormones secreted by the hypothalamus that travel in the portal blood to the anterior pituitary. These hormones are hypothalamic-releasing or hypothalmic-inhibiting hormones depending on whether they increase or decrease the release of the pituitary hormone they control. When a hypothalamic-releasing hormone is secreted, its corresponding anterior pituitary hormone is released. When a hypothalamic-inhibiting hormone is secreted, synthesis and release of the anterior pituitary hormone over which it has control is inhibited. Once secreted, the pituitary hormones then act to stimulate another target organ or cell to perform a function or release a hormone of its own.

The pituitary hormone and the subsequent response to it by its target organ may feed back on the hypothalamus to decrease further release of the hypothalamic hormone. The target organ response may also inhibit further release of the pituitary hormone.

FACTORS CONTROLLING HYPOTHALAMIC HORMONE SECRETION

For the hypothalamic-pituitary hormonal systems, ultimate determination of whether a hormone will be secreted is under the control of the hypothalamus. The hypothalamic-releasing or -inhibiting hormones are secreted at some baseline level that can be increased or decreased as a result of the integration of many neural inputs to the hypothalamus. The inputs are related to stress, pain, body weight, temperature, emotions, and various hormones released by target organs. All these influences can be excitatory or inhibitory for each releasing or inhibiting hormone.

Target Organ Hormones

THYROID HORMONE

Thyroid hormone (TH) is an amino hormone synthesized and released from the thyroid gland. It is made when one or two iodine molecules are joined to a large glycoprotein called thyroglobulin that is synthesized in the thyroid gland and contains the amino acid tyrosine. These iodine-containing complexes are called iodotyrosines. Two iodotyrosines then combine to form two types of circulating TH, called T_3 and T_4. T_3 and T_4 differ in the total number of iodine molecules they contain (three for T_3 and four for T_4). Most (90%) of the TH released into the bloodstream is T_4, but T_3 is physiologically more potent. In passage through the liver and kidney, most T_4 is converted to T_3. T_3 and T_4 are carried to their target cells in the blood bound to a plasma protein, but enter the cell as free hormone. T_3 and T_4, collectively are referred to as TH.

Effects of Thyroid Hormone

Target cells for TH include almost all cells of the body. The primary effect of TH is to stimulate the metabolic rate of its target cells by increasing the metabolism of protein, fat, and carbohydrate. TH also appears to stimulate the rate of the sodium-potassium pump in its target cells. Both functions serve to increase utilization of energy by the cells, thereby increasing basic metabolic rate (BMR), burning calories, and increasing heat production by each cell.

Thyroid hormone also increases the sensitivity of target cells to catecholamines, thus increasing heart rate and causing heightened emotional responsiveness. TH increases the rate of depolarization of skeletal muscle, which increases the speed of skeletal muscle contractions, often leading to a fine tremor. TH is essential for normal growth and development of all cells of the body and is required for the function of growth hormone.

Factors Controlling Thyroid Hormone Secretion

The stimulus for the secretion of TH is thyroid-stimulating hormone (TSH) released into the bloodstream from the anterior pituitary. The stimulus for the release of TSH is thyroid-releasing hormone (TRH) secreted from the hypothalamus into the portal bloodstream. Thyroid hormone appears to act on the hypothalamus, to decrease the further release of TRH, and on the pituitary, to decrease the release of TSH. TSH may also act on the hypothalamus to decrease further release of TRH.

Factors Controlling Thyroid-Releasing Hormone Secretion

Stimuli responsible for increasing TRH secretion include exposure of the body to cold temperature, physical and perhaps psychologic stress, and low levels of TH. When the secretion of TRH is stimulated by cold temperature, the result is an increase in TH, which increases BMR, thereby increasing body heat and reducing the demand for a further increase in TRH (Fig. 8-3). This is an example of negative feedback.

GLUCOCORTICOIDS

Glucocorticoids are steroid hormones released from the cortex (outer layer) of the adrenal gland that affect many aspects of metabolism,

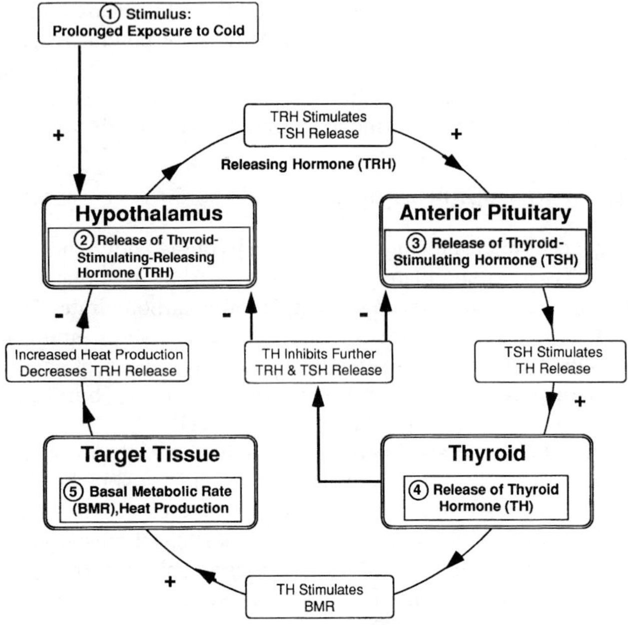

Figure 8-3. Feedback: thyroid hormone.

especially glucose metabolism. In humans the main glucocorticoid is cortisol. The glucocorticoids also affect many other systems of the body, including the cardiovascular and immune systems. Glucocorticoids are released in a diurnal (daily) manner, peaking at approximately 8 AM.

Effects of the Glucocorticoids

The glucocorticoids increase the level of blood glucose by stimulating gluconeogenesis (conversion in the liver of fats and proteins into glucose). Glucocorticoids also increase blood glucose levels by stimulating muscle, adipose (fat), and lymphatic tissues to use free fatty acids for energy instead of glucose. Likewise, the glucocorticoids stimulate protein breakdown and inhibit protein synthesis in all body cells. They also stimulate hunger, promote fat buildup in the trunk and facial regions, and inhibit growth by suppressing growth hormone and by antagonizing the effects of growth hormone on protein synthesis. The glucocorticoids increase the effect of growth hormone on adipose tissue and increase the effect of thyroid hormone on its target tissues. They also increase the effects of the catecholamines, causing increased heart rate and blood pressure. Many of these glucocorticoid effects are essential in times of trauma and stress. They allow one to survive blood loss, periods of hunger or starvation, or prolonged exposure to environmental extremes.

A nonmetabolic effect of cortisol that occurs with high circulating levels of hormone is the inhibition of immune and inflammatory functions. The glucocorticoids exert this effect by blocking almost every component of the immune and inflammatory responses, which include depressing cytotoxic T-cell function and suppressing the production, release, and activation of many chemical mediators of inflammation including interleukins, prostaglandins, and histamine. Levels of cortisol high enough to inhibit immune and inflammatory function may be reached with pharmacologic administration of cortisol for immunosuppression, with tumors of the adrenal gland or with long-term stress. In addition, cortisol, or a metabolite of cortisol, appears to have a strong effect on emotional stability and mood.

Factors Controlling Glucocorticoid Release

Glucocorticoids are released from the adrenal gland in response to circulating adrenocorticotropic hormone (ACTH) from the anterior pituitary. ACTH is released in response to corticotropin-releasing hormone (CRH) carried in the portal blood from the hypothalamus. CRH also stimulates the release of endorphins by the anterior pituitary and perhaps elsewhere. When released, glucocorticoids feed back on the hypothalamus and on the anterior pituitary to decrease further release of CRH and ACTH, respectively.

Factors Controlling Corticotropin-Releasing Hormone

Corticotropin-releasing hormone is released from the hypothalamus in a diurnal pattern that sets the subsequent release pattern of ACTH and cortisol. Stimuli for an increase in the release of CRH include stress, hypoglycemia (low blood glucose), and decreased circulating levels of glucocorticoids. The feedback cycle of CRH release in response to hypoglycemia is shown in Figure 8-4.

Other Effects of Adrenocorticotropin Hormone

Adrenal androgens are released in response to ACTH stimulation of the adrenal gland. Adrenal androgens are the primary source of androgens in women and children. ACTH is similar in structure to another anterior pituitary hormone, melanin-stimulating hormone (MSH), which causes the cells of the skin to produce the tanning substance melanin. Therefore, high levels of ACTH will have crossover effects on the skin and cause bronzing and can cause masculizing effects in women and children. A limited amount of ACTH appears to be essential for the synthesis of another adrenal cortical hormone, aldosterone. Without aldosterone, salt wasting and death occur.

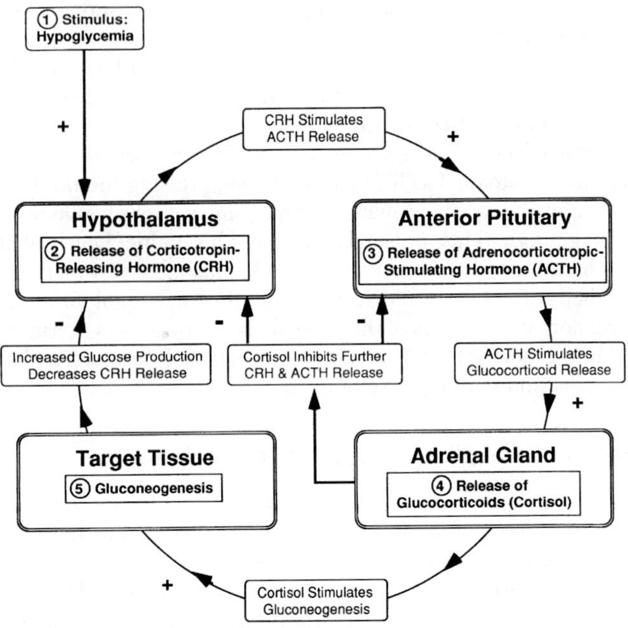

Figure 8-4. Feedback: glucocorticoids.

GROWTH HORMONE

Growth hormone (GH), also called somatotropin, is a protein hormone released in a diurnal pattern over 24 hours. Approximately 70% of daily secretion occurs in a burst 1 to 4 hours after the onset of sleep. Accelerated GH release occurs during puberty and pregnancy.

Effects of Growth Hormone

Growth hormone increases protein synthesis in all cells of the body, especially muscle cells. GH stimulates the growth of cartilage and stimulates activity of osteoblasts, the bone-producing cells of the body. GH is essential for longitudinal bone growth and for continual remodeling of bone that occurs throughout life. Effects of GH on bone and cartilage occur through intermediary peptides, called somatomedins or insulin-like growth factors (IGF), released from the liver in response to growth hormone. GH directly stimulates the growth of most all other organs of the body including the heart muscle, skin, and endocrine glands.

Growth hormone causes breakdown of fats and subsequent use of fatty acids for energy. Because fats are being used as an energy source, GH results in increased circulating blood glucose. GH also induces an insensitivity to insulin. With a decreased sensitivity to insulin, most cells will not transport glucose intracellularly, further increasing plasma glucose levels.

Factors Controlling Growth Hormone Release

Growth hormone is released from the anterior pituitary in response to a balance between two hypothalamic hormones; growth hormone-releasing hormone (GHRH) and growth hormone-inhibiting hormone, also called somatostatin. GH acts on the hypothalamus to decrease further release of GHRH.

Factors Controlling Growth Hormone-Releasing Hormone

Increased GHRH occurs in response to increased levels of circulating amino acids, hypoglycemia, fasting or starvation, physical and emotional stress, and decreased GH. Exercise stimulates the release of GHRH, directly or through the effects of hypoglycemia and physical stress. The reproductive hormones, estrogen and testosterone, appear to increase the secretion of GH, either by acting directly on the pituitary or through stimulation of GHRH. The feedback pattern of GHRH secretion in response to increased plasma amino acids is shown in Figure 8-5.

Factors Controlling Somatostatin Release

The hypothalamus releases an inhibitory hormone for GH, called somatostatin. Somatostatin is released in response to high blood glucose, free fatty acids, obesity, and cortisol. Emotional influences, including stress, stimulate somatostatin, most likely through increased cortisol, and reduce growth.

Pediatric Consideration

Children release more of their GH in the nocturnal burst than do adults. In children, GH is essential for the longitudinal bone growth that occurs throughout gestation, infancy, childhood, and puberty. Infants and children suffering emotional or physical neglect may develop failure to thrive syndrome, characterized by a decrease in longitudinal growth and weight gain. It has been suggested that a stress-induced increase in the release of somatostatin as a result of neglect may play a role in the syndrome of failure to thrive.

GONADOTROPINS

The gonadotropins include two anterior pituitary hormones: follicle-stimulating hormone (FSH) and luteinizing hormone (LH). Target tissues of FSH and LH are the ovary in women and the testis in men (Chapter 21).

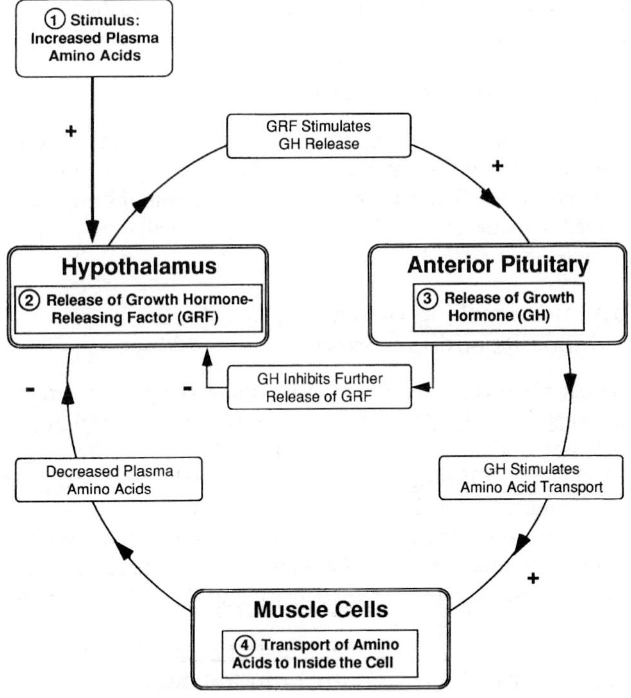

Figure 8-5. Feedback: growth hormone.

Effects of the Gonadotropins

In response to FSH and LH in women, the ovary secretes the steroid hormones estrogen and progesterone. Estrogen feeds back on the hypothalamus and anterior pituitary in a complicated manner, with a negative effect on increasing the release of FSH and a positive effect on the release of LH, ultimately resulting in ovulation (rupture) of an ovarian follicle. With ovulation, the egg, also called the ovum, is released (Chapter 21) and becomes available for fertilization by a sperm. Progesterone appears to feed back on the anterior pituitary to limit secretion of FSH and LH.

In men, FSH stimulates cells of the testes to initiate and support spermatogenesis (production of sperm). Cells of the testes predominantly affected by FSH in the male are Sertoli cells. Sertoli cells make up the inner lining of the seminiferous tubules, the site of spermatogenesis, and are important in providing nutrients to the developing sperm (Chapter 21). A hormone produced by Sertoli cells, inhibin, influences the production of testosterone by acting directly on the pituitary gland to decrease the release of FSH.

LH also is released from the anterior pituitary in men. LH causes interstitial cells of the testes to produce and secrete testosterone. Estrogen and testosterone are also synthesized by the adrenal gland, in men and women, in response to stimulation by ACTH.

Factors Controlling Gonadotropin Release

The gonadotropins are released from the pituitary in response to gonadotropin-releasing hormone (GnRH) from the hypothalamus. It appears that one hypothalamic hormone controls the release of both of the pituitary gonadotropins. GnRH is sometimes referred to as luteinizing hormone-releasing factor (LHRF). An increase in GnRH synthesis and release causes the onset of puberty.

Factors Controlling Gonadotropin-Releasing Hormone

Before puberty, the circulating level of GnRH is very low. With maturation of the hypothalamus and perhaps attainment of a certain body mass, GnRH increases and initiates puberty. When sexual maturation is established, the circulating level of GnRH is controlled in a negative feedback manner by estrogen and testosterone. Stress, starvation, and fear may affect the release of GnRH at any time, influencing the release of estrogen and progesterone in females and testosterone in males, and altering reproductive function.

ESTROGENS

Estrogens are steroid hormones that affect their target tissues by altering the rate of DNA replication, transcription, or RNA translation. Although the effects of estrogen are most apparent in females, males also produce and are affected by estrogens. There are three main types of estrogens in humans: estrone, estradiol, and estriol.

Effects of Estrogens

- Development in utero of female internal and external sex organs.
- Female distribution of body fat.
- Pigmentation of the nipples.
- Stimulation of breast development during pregnancy.
- Stimulation of growth of the endometrial lining of the uterus each month to prepare for implantation of the embryo.
- Maintenance of pregnancy.
- Stimulation of lactation.
- Stimulation of bone formation throughout life in males and females.
- Limiting bone resorption (breakdown) by direct action on bone or by limiting bone response to parathyroid hormone in males and females.
- Affecting liver protein production of lipoproteins (stimulates HDL, decreases LDL), coagulation factors, and carrier molecules for steroid hormones and thyroxine in males and females.

- Acting to reduce the risk of coronary artery disease, most likely as a result of increasing HDL, in males and females.
- Stimulating the kidneys to retain sodium in males and females.
- Influencing brain neural signaling in males and females, affecting behavior and mood.
- Estrogen excess in men can cause gynecomastia (breast enlargement).

Pediatric Consideration

Estrogen acts during puberty in a girl to cause the development of female secondary sex characteristics, including the development of breasts and axillary and pubic hair growth. Estrogen also acts along with growth hormone and the androgens to cause skeletal growth during puberty and causes the closure of the epiphysial bone plates to halt growth at the end of puberty in males and females. Estrogen can pathologically affect children, causing precocious (early) onset of menstruation in girls and breast development in girls and boys.

Geriatric Consideration

Menopause occurs in women when the aging ovaries no longer respond to the gonadotropins. Estrogen levels decrease, and LH, FSH, and GnRH levels increase because any negative feedback by estrogen has been removed. The lack of estrogen in postmenopausal women has many effects, including decreased bone density, increased risk of cardiovascular disease, and drying of the skin and vaginal membranes. Studies suggest that the decrease in estrogen increases the risk of the development of certain dementia, such as Alzheimer's disease.

PROGESTERONE

Progesterone, like estrogen, is a steroid hormone. In women, progesterone is synthesized by thecal cells of the developing follicle, and later the corpus luteum, in response to stimulation by LH and, to a lesser extent, FSH.

Effects of Progesterone

- Progesterone is released from an ovarian follicle after the follicle has ruptured during ovulation. It causes the endometrial lining of the uterus to become secretory in anticipation of fertilization of the ovum and embryo implantation in the uterus. The ruptured follicle becomes the corpus luteum, which continues progesterone secretion.
- If the ovum is fertilized and the embryo implants in the uterus, the corpus luteum and later the placenta maintain the pregnancy by secreting progesterone. If progesterone decreases, the pregnancy terminates. If pregnancy does not occur, the corpus luteum degener-

ates over the next 14 days, progesterone levels decline, and menstruation (sloughing off of the uterine lining) occurs.
- Progesterone works with estrogen and prolactin to stimulate breast development during puberty and pregnancy.
- Progesterone relaxes smooth muscles, including the uterus and the vascular smooth muscle of the arterioles.
- Progesterone appears to be protective against some sorts of cancer development.

TESTOSTERONE

Testosterone, also a steroid hormone, is the most abundant of the powerful androgen hormones. Testosterone synthesis occurs in specialized cells of the testes called Leydig cells, and in women, in the adrenal gland.

Effects of Testosterone

- Development in utero of male internal and external sex organs.
- Maintenance of sperm production throughout a man's lifetime.
- Male distribution of muscle.
- Stimulation of bone formation throughout life in males and females.
- Stimulation of red blood cell formation in males and females.
- Stimulation of anabolism (buildup) of proteins in males and females.
- Involved in brain neural signaling, affecting behavior and mood, in males and females.
- Testosterone excess in women can cause clitoral enlargement, voice deepening, and beard development.

Pediatric Consideration

Testosterone acts during puberty to cause the development of male secondary sex characteristics, including growth of the penis and scrotum, and the development of male axillary and pubic hair patterns. Testosterone is also important for skeletal growth during puberty, especially in males. Testosterone can pathologically affect children, causing precocious development of the penis and scrotum and voice deepening in boys, and clitoral enlargement in girls.

Geriatric Consideration

The testes continue to respond to the gonadotropins as a man ages, although at a reduced level. Testosterone synthesis and release by the testes continues, as does sperm production, throughout a man's lifetime, albeit at some declining rate. Testosterone levels adequate to maintain sperm production and muscle mass continue into a man's seventh decade, at least.

PROLACTIN

Prolactin is a protein hormone released from the anterior pituitary.

Effects of Prolactin

When a girl reaches puberty, prolactin acts in concert with estrogen, progesterone, and GH to promote breast tissue development. All of these hormone levels increase dramatically during pregnancy, resulting in further stimulation of breast development. With birth of the infant, prolactin acts on the breast to stimulate lactation (milk production), allowing the infant to breastfeed.

In nonpregnant women, high prolactin levels inhibit the release of two other anterior pituitary hormones: FSH and LH. Because FSH and LH are essential for ovulation and pregnancy, high prolactin levels in women who are breastfeeding full-time may offer some protection against another pregnancy occurring.

In addition to prolactin, the posterior hypothalamic hormone oxytocin is also required for successful breastfeeding. A role for prolactin in men has not been identified, although recent evidence suggests that in men and women, prolactin may have effects on the immune system, possibly by modulating the release of certain cytokines.

Factors Controlling Prolactin Release

The secretion of prolactin from the anterior pituitary is controlled by the release of a prolactin-inhibitory hormone (PIH) from the hypothalamus, recently identified as the catecholamine dopamine. A decrease in the release of dopamine stimulates prolactin release. There may also be a prolactin-stimulating hormone released from the hypothalamus, although it is yet to be identified.

Stimulation for increased prolactin release during pregnancy appears to be an estrogen-dependent decrease in the hypothalamic release of PIH. Stimulation for prolactin release after pregnancy is suckling of the nipple during breastfeeding by the infant. Stimulation of the nipple by suckling appears to cause increased prolactin by decreasing the hypothalamic release of PIH.

The major hypothalamic and anterior pituitary hormones and their target organ effects are listed in Figure 8-6.

ANTIDIURETIC HORMONE

Antidiuretic hormone (ADH) is a protein hormone made in the supraoptic nuclei of the hypothalamus and stored in and released from the posterior pituitary. It is also called vasopressin, which means "vascular tensor."

Effects of Antidiuretic Hormone

Antidiuretic hormone primarily causes cells of the renal collecting ducts to become more water permeable. This increases the reabsorption

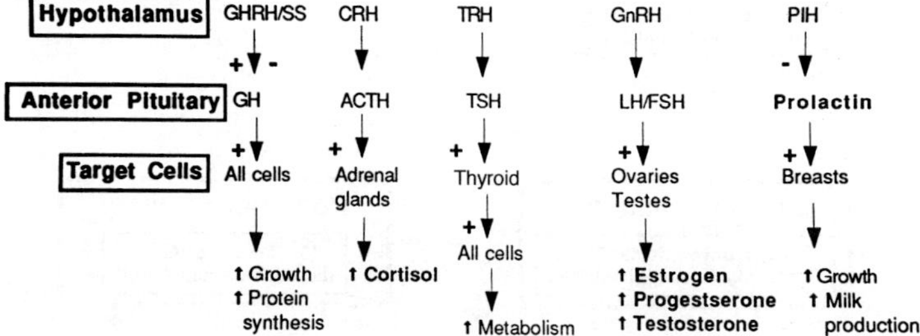

Figure 8-6. The major hypothalamic and anterior pituitary hormones. Note that decreased PIH increases prolactin release.

of water into the blood, decreasing urine diuresis (flow). This is the antidiuretic effect of ADH.

At very high levels, ADH causes vascular smooth muscle contraction, increasing total peripheral resistance and blood pressure (Chapter 15).

Factors Controlling Antidiuretic Hormone Release

The major stimulus for ADH release is increased plasma osmolality (increased solute concentration). Increased plasma osmolality is sensed by osmoreceptors in the hypothalamus. Normal plasma osmolality is approximately 280 mL mOsm/kg. ADH-induced antidiuresis returns a high plasma osmolality toward normal by diluting the plasma (increasing its water concentration) as shown in Figure 8-7.

Other stimuli for ADH release include decreased blood pressure (sensed by the carotid and aortic baroreceptors), stress, pain, and exercise. ADH secretion is inhibited by decreased plasma osmolality, increased blood pressure, and alcohol.

OXYTOCIN

Oxytocin is a protein hormone made in the paraventricular nuclei of the hypothalamus and stored in and released from the posterior pituitary.

Effects of Oxytocin

Oxytocin stimulates contraction of the smooth muscle lining the milk ducts of the breast, causing increased intramammary pressure and subsequent letdown of stored milk into the nipples.

Oxytocin also stimulates contraction of the uterine smooth muscle. Its exact role in initiating labor in a pregnant woman is unclear. However, it causes increased intensity of uterine contractions as labor progresses and delivery approaches. The drug Pitocin is a derivative of oxytocin and is used clinically to initiate and speed labor.

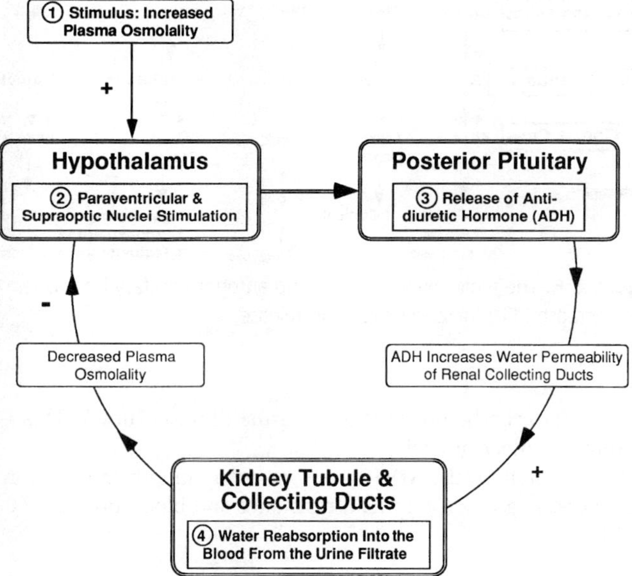

Figure 8-7. Feedback: Antidiuretic hormone.

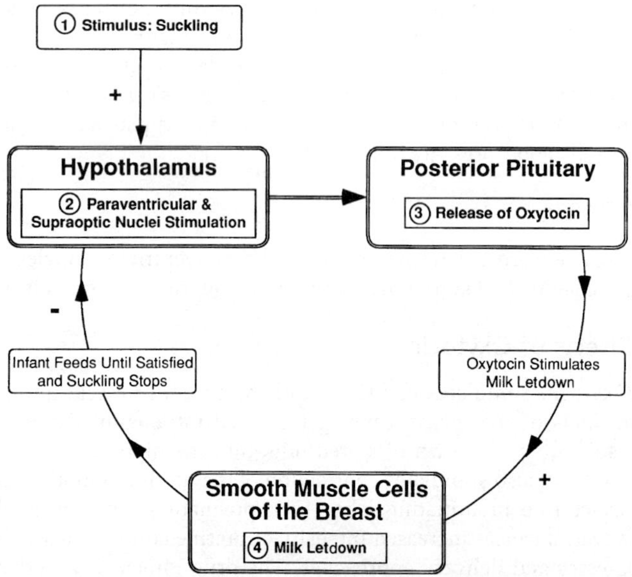

Figure 8-8. Feedback: oxytocin.

Factors Controlling Oxytocin Release

The primary stimulus for the release of oxytocin is suckling on the nipple of the breast in women. As shown in Figure 8-8, suckling leads to milk letdown, which allows the infant to feed. This reduces the drive for suckling and the stimulus for oxytocin release is decreased—a clear example of negative feedback. Stress or fear may inhibit synthesis of oxytocin.

PATHOPHYSIOLOGIC CONCEPTS

Hypopituitarism

Hypopituitarism refers to low secretion of any anterior pituitary hormone. Panhypopituitarism refers to low secretion of all anterior pituitary hormones.

CAUSES OF HYPOPITUITARISM

Hypopituitarism can result from malfunction of the pituitary gland or the hypothalamus. Causes include:

- Infection or inflammation.
- An autoimmune disease.
- A tumor (adenoma). Typically, a tumor of one type of hormone-producing cell expands to the point that it begins to interfere with the function of other hormone-producing cells, leading to reduced secretion of one or more other hormones.
- Feedback from a malfunctioning target organ, for example, decreased secretion of TSH from the pituitary would occur if a diseased thyroid gland were secreting excessively high levels of TH.
- Hypoxic necrosis (death caused by lack of oxygen) of the pituitary or hypothalamus resulting from decreased blood flow or decreased oxygenation. Hypoxia can destroy any or all of the hormone-producing cells. An example of this is Sheehan's syndrome, which develops after maternal hemorrhage during or after a woman gives birth.

Hyperpituitarism

Hyperpituitarism is the excess secretion of an anterior pituitary hormone. Hyperpituitarism typically involves just one of the pituitary hormones. The other pituitary hormones are often secreted in reduced levels.

CAUSES OF HYPERPITUITARISM

Hyperpituitarism can result from malfunction of the pituitary gland or the hypothalamus. Causes include:

- A primary adenoma of one type of hormone-producing cell, usually GH, ACTH, or the prolactin-producing cells.
- A lack of feedback from a target gland, for example, increased TSH may occur in response to decreased or absent secretion of TH by the thyroid gland.

CONDITIONS OF DISEASE OR INJURY

Hypothyroidism

Hypothyroidism results from decreased levels of circulating thyroid hormone. It is sometimes referred to as myxedema.

CAUSES OF HYPOTHYROIDISM WITH SPECIFIC HORMONAL PATTERNS

Hypothyroidism may result from malfunction of the thyroid gland, the pituitary, or the hypothalamus. If it results from thyroid gland malfunction, low TH levels are accompanied by high TSH and high TRH because of the lack of negative feedback on the pituitary and hypothalamus by TH.

If hypothyroidism results from pituitary malfunction, low levels of TH are caused by low TSH. TRH from the hypothalamus is high because there is no negative feedback on its release by TSH or TH. Hypothyroidism caused by hypothalamic malfunction would result in low TH, low TSH, and low TRH.

DISEASES OF HYPOTHYROIDISM

- Hashimoto's disease, also called autoimmune thyroiditis, results from autoantibody destruction of thyroid gland tissue. This results in decreased TH, with increased TSH and TRH levels caused by minimal negative feedback. The cause of autoimmune thyroiditis is unknown, but there appears to be a genetic tendency to develop the disease.
- Endemic goiter is hypothyroidism caused by a dietary deficiency of iodide. A goiter is an enlargement of the thyroid gland. Goiter occurs with a deficiency of iodide because the thyroid cells become overactive and hypertrophic (larger) in an attempt to sequester all possible iodide from the bloodstream. Low TH levels are accompanied by high TSH and TRH because negative feedback is minimal.
- Thyroid carcinoma may cause hypothyroidism or hyperthyroidism. Treatment of this rare cancer may include thyroidectomy, TSH suppression drugs, or radioactive iodine therapy to destroy thyroid tissue, and all of these treatments may result in hypothyroidism. Exposure to radiation, especially during childhood, is a cause of thyroid cancer. Iodine deficiency may also increase the risk of

developing thyroid cancer because it stimulates thyroid cell proliferation and hyperplasia.

CLINICAL MANIFESTATIONS

- Sluggishness, slow thinking, and clumsy, slow movements.
- Decreased heart rate, enlarged heart (myxedemic heart), and decreased cardiac output.
- Bogginess and edema of the skin, especially under the eyes and in the ankles.
- Intolerance to cold temperatures.
- Decreased metabolic rate, decreased caloric requirements, decreased appetite and nutrient absorption across the gut.
- Constipation.
- Change in reproductive function.
- Dry, flaky skin and brittle, thin body and head hair.

DIAGNOSTIC TOOLS

- A good history and physical examination will help diagnose hypothyroidism.
- Blood tests measuring levels of TH (both T_3 and T_4), TSH, and TRH will allow diagnosis of the condition and localization of the problem at the level of the central nervous system or the thyroid gland.

COMPLICATIONS

- Myxedema coma is a life-threatening situation characterized by exacerbation (worsening) of all symptoms of hypothyroidism including hypothermia without shivering, hypotension, hypoglycemia, hypoventilation, and a decrease in consciousness resulting in coma. Death can occur without TH replacement and stabilization of symptoms.

TREATMENT

- Treatment always includes replacement of thyroid hormone with synthetic thyroxine.
- For endemic goiter, iodide replacement may relieve symptoms.
- If the cause of hypothyroidism is related to a central nervous system tumor, it may be treated with chemotherapy, radiation, or surgery.

Pediatric Consideration

Infants born without a thyroid gland or with defects in TH synthesis will develop congenital hypothyroidism, a disease sometimes referred to as cretinism. Congenital hypothyroidism is characterized by low TH, with high TSH and TRF. TH is permissive (necessary for the functioning) of all cells of the body, including cells of the central nervous system (CNS). Development of the CNS occurs in utero and for approximately 1 year after birth. Because an infant with congenital hypothyroidism was exposed to maternal TH in utero, it will be born neurologically intact. If the condition is unrecognized after birth and TH is not replaced pharmacologically, further development of infant CNS will be compromised and severe mental retardation will result. Growth will be stunted and skeletal deformity will develop. Many states require measurement of infant TH levels at birth. With thyroxine-replacement therapy, CNS damage can be avoided.

Hypothyroidism at birth may also occur if maternal antithyroid antibodies attack the fetal thyroid during pregnancy. Likewise, if a pregnant woman is severely deprived of iodide, her infant may also have hypothyroidism after birth. Long-term neurologic prognosis for either of these conditions depends on the extent of thyroid deficit.

Geriatric Consideration

Myxedema coma is usually seen in elderly persons who are not being adequately treated for hypothyroidism. It may also occur after an acute illness in this population. Prolonged exposure of an elderly individual to cold weather may precipitate the disorder.

Hyperthyroidism

Hyperthyroidism is excessive levels of circulating TH.

CAUSES OF HYPERTHYROIDISM WITH SPECIFIC HORMONAL PATTERNS

Hyperthyroidism can result from dysfunction of the thyroid gland, the pituitary, or the hypothalamus. Increased TH caused by malfunction of the thyroid gland is accompanied by decreased TSH and TRF, as a result of the negative feedback on their release by TH.

Hyperthyroidism caused by malfunction of the pituitary results in high TH and high TSH. TRF would be low because of negative feedback from TH and TSH. Hyperthyroidism caused by malfunction of the hypothalamus would show high TH accompanied by excess TSH and TRH.

DISEASES OF HYPERTHYROIDISM

- Grave's disease, the most common cause of hyperthyroidism, is an autoimmune disorder usually characterized by production of autoantibodies that mimic the action of TSH on the thyroid gland. These IgG autoantibodies, termed thyroid-stimulating immunoglobulins, turn on the production of TH, but are not negatively inhibited by high TH. TSH and TRH levels are low because they respond to high TH. The cause of Grave's disease is unknown; however, there appears to be a genetic predisposition to autoimmune disease. Women in their 20s and 30s are most often diagnosed, although the disease may start during the teen years.

- Nodular goiter is an increase in the size of the thyroid gland caused by increased demand for thyroid hormone. Increased demand for thyroid hormone occurs during periods of growth or excess metabolic demand such as puberty or pregnancy. In this case, increased TH is caused by metabolically driven activation of the hypothalamus, and therefore is accompanied by increased TRH and TSH. When the demand for thyroid hormone is lessened, the thyroid gland usually returns to its previous size. Occasionally, irreversible changes may have occurred and the gland does not regress. The enlarged thyroid may continue to produce excess TH. If the individual remains hyperthyroid, the condition is referred to as a toxic nodular goiter. Pituitary adenomas of TSH-producing cells or hypothalamic diseases rarely occur.

CLINICAL MANIFESTATIONS

- Increased heart rate.
- Increased muscle tone, tremors, irritability, increased sensitivity to catecholamines.
- Increased basal metabolic rate, increased heat production, intolerance to heat, excess sweating.
- Weight loss, increased hunger.
- A "staring" appearance.
- Exophthalmus (bulging of the eyes) may develop.
- Increased number of bowel movements.
- Goiter (usually), which is an increase in the size of the thyroid gland.
- Changes in skin and hair condition may occur.
- Reproductive irregularities.

DIAGNOSTIC TOOLS

- A good history and physical examination will help diagnose hyperthyroidism.
- Blood tests measuring levels of TH (both $T_3$and T_4), TSH, and TRH will allow diagnosis of the condition and localization of the problem at the level of the CNS or the thyroid gland.
- Decreased serum lipids may accompany hyperthyroidism.
- Decreased sensitivity to insulin, which may result in hyperglycemia.

COMPLICATIONS

- Arrhythmias are common in patients with hyperthyroidism and are frequently the presenting symptom of the disorder. Any person complaining of arrhythmia should be evaluated for thyroid disorder.
- A life-threatening complication of hyperthyroidism is thyrotoxic crisis (thyroid storm), which may develop spontaneously in patients

with hyperthyroidism undergoing therapy, during surgery on the thyroid gland, or may occur in undiagnosed patients with hyperthyroidism. The result is a large burst of TH release that causes tachycardia, agitation, tremors, hyperthermia (up to 106°F), and, if untreated, death.

TREATMENT

Treatment depends on the site and cause of hyperthyroidism.

- If the problem is at the level of the thyroid gland, treatment usually involves antithyroid drugs that block TH production or beta-blocking drugs to decrease sympathetic hyperresponsiveness.
- Drugs that destroy thyroid tissue may also be used. For instance, radioactive iodine (I^{131}) administered in oral form is actively taken up by hyperactive thyroid cells. Once incorporated, I^{131} destroys the cells. This is a permanent treatment for hyperthyroidism and frequently results in the individual becoming hypothyroid and requiring lifelong TH replacement.
- Partial or total thyroidectomy may also be a treatment choice. Total thyroidectomy results in hypothyroidism, as often does partial thyroidectomy.

Adrenal Insufficiency

Adrenal insufficiency is a decrease in the circulating level of the glucocorticoids. The mineralocorticoid, aldosterone, may also be reduced.

CAUSES OF ADRENAL INSUFFICIENCY WITH SPECIFIC HORMONAL PATTERNS

Adrenal insufficiency may be caused by dysfunction of the adrenal gland called primary adrenal insufficiency, or by dysfunction of the pituitary or hypothalamus. Both of these latter conditions cause secondary adrenal insufficiency.

Primary adrenal insufficiency is characterized by low levels of glucocorticoids, especially cortisol, accompanied by high ACTH and high CRH because there will be no negative feedback on their release. Adrenal androgens and aldosterone levels may be normal, increased, or decreased depending on the cause of the glucocorticoid deficiency.

If the entire adrenal gland is destroyed or malfunctioning, adrenal androgens and aldosterone will be low. If only the glucocorticoid-secreting cells are malfunctioning, the high ACTH levels that accompany primary adrenal insufficiency will cause high levels of circulating adrenal androgens. Aldosterone secretion is primarily determined by the renin-angiotensin system, but may be slightly increased by elevated ACTH.

If the cause of adrenal insufficiency is secondary to a pituitary dysfunction, low glucocorticoids will be accompanied by low ACTH and high CRH. In this case, adrenal androgens will also be low. If there is zero ACTH, aldosterone levels will be reduced.

If adrenal insufficiency is caused by a hypothalamus malfunction, the glucocorticoids, ACTH, and CRH will be low.

DISEASES OF ADRENAL INSUFFICIENCY

- Primary adrenal insufficiency, called Addison's disease, occurs as a result of destruction of the adrenal cortex. The disease is usually autoimmune, and results from IgG antibodies directed against all or part of the adrenal gland. Addison's disease may also result from infectious causes, such as tuberculosis. Tuberculosis of the adrenal gland is a common cause of adrenal insufficiency in developing countries and does not typically resolve with treatment of the infection. Destructive adrenal gland tumors may also lead to adrenal insufficiency.
- Addison's disease is characterized by low glucocorticoid levels accompanied by high ACTH and high CRH. Total loss of the adrenal gland results in the loss of adrenal androgens and aldosterone. Aldosterone deficiency results in increased loss of sodium in the urine, leading to hyponatremia (decreased sodium concentration in the blood), dehydration, and hypotension (because water loss in the urine frequently accompanies the loss of sodium). Decreased potassium excretion in the urine will lead to hyperkalemia (increased potassium concentration in the blood).
- Secondary adrenal insufficiency can occur as a result of hypopituitarism or hypothalamic dysfunction. With secondary adrenal insufficiency, ACTH is not released, so the adrenals do not secrete glucocorticoids or androgens. Aldosterone synthesis may also be affected.
- Secondary adrenal insufficiency can occur if cortisol is used therapeutically for anti-inflammatory purposes. When taking pharmacologic levels of corticosteroids, the pituitary secretion of ACTH is inhibited in a negative feedback manner. If the prescribed medication is abruptly discontinued, the pituitary remains in a refractory period and does not secrete ACTH for an extended period of time. Even a few weeks of oral glucocorticoid therapy can result in the suppression of ACTH, and hence secondary adrenal insufficiency, for several months. Treatment of inflammatory illnesses for fewer than approximately 10 days will not result in pituitary suppression.

CLINICAL MANIFESTATIONS

- Depression because cortisol levels influence mood and emotions.
- Fatigue, related to hypoglycemia, and decreased gluconeogenesis.
- Anorexia, vomiting, diarrhea, nausea.
- Hyperpigmentation of the skin if ACTH levels are high (primary adrenal insufficiency) as a result of ACTH having melanin-stimulating hormone-like effects on the skin.

- Sparse body hair in women if the adrenal cells producing androgens are destroyed or if ACTH levels are very low.
- Inability to respond to stressful situations, perhaps leading to severe hypotension and shock.

DIAGNOSTIC TOOLS

- A good history and physical examination will help diagnose glucocorticoid deficiency.
- Blood tests measuring levels of CRH, ACTH, and different glucocorticoids will allow diagnosis of the condition and localization of the problem at the level of the CNS or adrenal gland.
- Hyponatremia, hyperkalemia, and hypotension may be present if the adrenal cells that produce aldosterone are destroyed or if ACTH levels are undetectable.

COMPLICATIONS

- Adrenal crisis may occur after physical or mental stress in an affected individual. This can be life-threatening and is characterized by volume depletion, hypotension, and vascular collapse.

TREATMENT

- Cortisol replacement is essential. If cells producing aldosterone are destroyed, aldosterone must be provided. Glucocorticoid administration may need to be increased during periods of stress, including infection, trauma, and surgery. Morbidity and mortality are high without treatment.
- If the cause of adrenal insufficiency is related to a pituitary tumor, it may be treated with chemotherapy, radiation, or surgery.

Glucocorticoid Excess

Glucocorticoid excess refers to any condition that results in very high levels of circulating glucocorticoids.

CAUSES OF GLUCOCORTICOID EXCESS WITH SPECIFIC HORMONAL PATTERNS

If the cause of glucocorticoid excess is primary adrenal gland hypersecretion, there is usually an adrenal tumor present. In this situation, low ACTH and low CRH levels will be seen as a result of negative feedback from high glucocorticoids. Adrenal androgen levels will be low because ACTH is low. Bronzing of the skin will not occur.

Most commonly, glucocorticoid excess is a secondary result of an adenoma of the pituitary cells producing ACTH. In this case, elevated ACTH will result in excess adrenal androgen production and excess glucocorticoids. Bronzing of the skin will occur because of crossover in effects of ACTH with melanin-stimulating hormone. CRH levels will be low as a result of negative feedback from ACTH and the glucocorticoids.

Excess ACTH may occur as a result of the production of ACTH by a nonpituitary tumor. This is referred to as an ectopic source of ACTH, meaning a source other than the normal one. Many tumors demonstrate ectopic production of ACTH, especially lung tumors. Excess adrenal androgens and bronzing of the skin will accompany high ACTH.

High levels of glucocorticoids may result from chronic administration of high-dose corticosteroids, especially cortisol, for treatment of inflammatory conditions. Disease states in which long-term administration of corticosteroids occur include asthma and several different autoimmune diseases.

DISEASES OF EXCESS GLUCOCORTICOIDS

- Cushing's syndrome refers to any condition of high glucocorticoids and includes glucocorticoid excess caused by therapeutic administration of corticosteroids.
- Cushing's disease refers to high glucocorticoids caused specifically by malfunction of the anterior pituitary resulting in excess ACTH.

CLINICAL MANIFESTATIONS

- Altered fat metabolism leading to fat pads on the back (subclavian "buffalo hump"), moon face, protruding abdomen with thin extremities, stretch marks on breasts, thighs, and abdominal surface.
- Muscle weakness from protein breakdown.
- Hypertension as a result of increased catecholamine responsiveness.
- Weight gain resulting from strong appetite stimulation. Because of effects on hepatic gluconeogenesis, a reversible form of diabetes mellitus may result.
- Inhibition of immune and inflammatory reactions, leading to poor wound healing.
- Extreme emotional swings (lability), sometimes causing psychosis and occasionally resulting in suicide.
- Masculinization of women and children as a result of adrenal androgen stimulation if ACTH levels are high.
- Bronzing of the skin if ACTH levels are high.

DIAGNOSTIC TOOLS

- A good history and physical examination will help diagnose glucocorticoid excess.
- Blood tests measuring levels of CRH, ACTH, and different glucocorticoids will allow diagnosis of the condition and localization of the problem at the level of the CNS or adrenal gland.
- Loss of normal diurnal (morning) pattern of cortisol release.

- Hyperglycemia.
- Hypernatremia and hypokalemia may be present because of aldosterone-like properties of the glucocorticoids. This can contribute to hypertension and cardiac and neural irregularities.

COMPLICATIONS

- There are many complications of excess glucocorticoid levels. Morbidity and mortality are high without treatment and approximately 50% of individuals die within 5 years. Causes of death include suicide, overwhelming infections, and coronary artery disease from severe hypertension.

TREATMENT

Correction of high glucocorticoid levels depends on the cause of the problem.

- Surgery for tumors of the adrenal, pituitary, or other tissue (i.e., the lung) is frequently performed.
- Radiation therapy if a tumor is present.
- Drugs that block steroid synthesis may be used if the tumor is inoperable.
- Discontinue corticosteroid therapy, by weaning down, if syndrome is caused by medication.

Congenital Adrenal Hyperplasia

Congenital adrenal hyperplasia is total or relative unresponsiveness of the adrenal glucocorticoid-producing cells to ACTH during gestation.

Congenital adrenal hyperplasia results in masculinization of the genitalia of a female fetus. Female masculinization occurs because the adrenal androgen-producing cells are still responsive to ACTH and ACTH levels are extremely high because there is little or no negative feedback on ACTH release.

CAUSES OF CONGENITAL ADRENAL HYPERPLASIA

Congenital adrenal hyperplasia occurs as a result of an autosomal-recessive genetic alteration whereby there is a deficiency in one or more of the five enzymes needed to produce cortisol. Mineralocorticoid production (aldosterone) may be affected by this enzyme deficiency. The most common enzyme deficiencies are of 21-hydroxylase or 11-β-hydroxylase. Enzyme deficiencies may be partial or total. Carriers of the disorder do not appear to be affected.

CLINICAL MANIFESTATIONS

- Masculinization of the female infant is apparent at birth and may include ambiguous genitalia with an enlarged clitoris, fused labia, and malformation of the urogenital area. The degree of abnormality is variable. Male fetuses are usually normal at birth or have slightly enlarged genitalia.

- If aldosterone production is blocked, salt wasting, dehydration, vomiting, hyperkalemia, and hypotension develop.
- In the rare case of enzyme 11-deoxycorticosterone deficiency, mineralocorticoid levels increase, resulting in salt retention, hypokalemia, and hypertension.

DIAGNOSTIC TOOLS

- Physical examination at or soon after birth will help diagnose the condition in females. Blood tests will demonstrate enzyme deficiency in either sex.

COMPLICATIONS

- Because cortisol is essential to surviving even relatively minor stresses, illnesses or surgeries in the newborn period may be fatal, if the diagnosis of congenital adrenal hyperplasia has not been made.

TREATMENT

- Cortisol, and possibly aldosterone, replacement therapy, will be required lifelong. Therapy must be monitored and adjusted appropriately for growth and in times of excess physical stress.
- Masculinized females may require reconstructive surgery. With successful treatment, sexual functioning and fertility will be unaffected.

Growth Hormone Deficiency

Growth hormone deficiency is the decrease in circulating levels of GH. Most cells of the body will be affected. GH deficiency is usually clinically recognized only in children.

CAUSES OF GROWTH HORMONE DEFICIENCY

Growth hormone deficiency is usually caused by a pituitary adenoma of another anterior pituitary hormone-producing cell type. It can also be a result of hypoxic necrosis (death caused by lack of oxygen) and inflammation of the pituitary. The cause of GH deficiency may also be at the hypothalamic level, and result from malnutrition, sleep deprivation, or stimulation of somatostatin released during periods of prolonged physical or emotional stress. For example, some studies suggest that growth potential may be reduced in adolescent female athletes as a result of intense physical exercise and reduced nutritional intake caused by dieting. Low estrogen levels are frequently seen in female athletes, which may also affect growth.

DISEASES OF GROWTH HORMONE DEFICIENCY

- Dwarfism.
- Reduction of growth potential.
- Alteration in metabolic functioning in adults.

CLINICAL MANIFESTATIONS

- In children, GH deficiency results in proportional short stature (below the third percentile for their age). Affected children have decreased muscle mass and increased subcutaneous fat stores. They are typically bright mentally.
- Short stature different from predicted based on familial patterns may be observed if a reduction in growth potential occurs.
- Delayed onset of puberty may accompany GH deficiency, especially if abnormalities in the gonadotropins occur concomitantly.
- Adult-onset GH deficiency may result in nonspecific changes in functioning, including alterations in physical and mental well-being.

DIAGNOSTIC TOOLS

- A good history and physical examination will help diagnose growth hormone deficiency.
- Blood tests measuring decreased levels of GH will support diagnosis of the condition.

TREATMENT

- Treatment of GH deficiency in children involves subcutaneous injections of recombinant GH multiple times per week during the pubertal years or earlier. GH deficiency in adults may also be treated with GH injections.

Pediatric Consideration

Reduced growth in children may occur as a result of a normal genetic predisposition (i.e., short parents) or may accompany certain genetic abnormalities such as Turner's syndrome. Illness, including renal disease, and autoimmune disease treated with chronic corticosteroids may also result in stature shorter than expected from parental heights. Asthma chronically treated with oral steroids has been reported to reduce final growth, as have medications used to treat attention-deficit disorder. The term "constitutional short stature" is used to describe children who are shorter than others their age, and those growing at a reduced velocity without a known cause. Under certain circumstances, GH treatment may be used in these children to increase final growth.

Growth Hormone Excess

Growth hormone excess is the increase in circulating levels of GH. Increased levels of GH result in increased somatomedin levels and increased growth of bone, cartilage, and other tissues. Direct effects of GH on the breakdown of carbohydrates and the increase in protein synthesis also occur.

CAUSES OF GROWTH HORMONE EXCESS

Growth hormone excess is usually caused by a GH-secreting tumor of the anterior pituitary.

DISEASES OF GH EXCESS

- Gigantism, a disease of excess longitudinal growth of the bones of the skeleton, is seen as a result of GH excess before puberty.
- Acromegaly, a disease of connective tissue proliferation, is seen in adults with GH excess. Because long bone growth has stopped in adults, GH excess cannot cause growth of the skeleton. Instead it is associated with growth of the cartilage of the hands and feet, nose, jaw, chin, and facial bones. Connective tissue proliferation of internal organs, including the heart, also occurs.

CLINICAL MANIFESTATIONS

- Tall stature, with gigantism.
- Thickening of the fingers, jaw, forehead, hands, and feet with acromegaly.
- Because GH excess is usually caused by an aggressively growing adenoma, other hormone-secreting cells of the anterior pituitary are frequently destroyed. Therefore, symptoms of GH excess often include those associated with deficiencies of other hormone systems. For example, if the growing tumor crowds out the gonadotropin-secreting cells of the anterior pituitary, decreased reproductive functioning may occur. If the tumor affects any other hormone-producing cells, manifestations particular to that missing hormone will prevail. Increased intracranial pressure can also occur with a growing tumor. Symptoms include headache, vomiting, and papilledema (swelling at the site where the optic nerve enters the eye chamber).

DIAGNOSTIC TOOLS

- A good history and physical examination will help diagnose growth hormone excess.
- Blood tests measuring increased levels of GH will support diagnosis of gigantism or acromegaly.
- Increased blood glucose levels may be present with either condition.

- The secretory pattern of GH release is no longer predictable and is unrelated to sleep with either condition.

COMPLICATIONS

- Complications of acromegaly include cardiac hypertrophy and hypertension. Diabetes mellitus can occur from the effect of GH on increasing blood glucose and decreasing cellular insulin sensitivity.

TREATMENT

- Treatment of GH excess is usually by surgical excision of the GH-secreting tumor.
- Radiation therapy may also be applied.
- Bromocriptine, a dopamine antagonist, may be effective in decreasing GH levels.

Pediatric Consideration

Elevated growth in children may occur as a result of a normal genetic predisposition (i.e., tall parents) or may accompany certain genetic abnormalities such as Marfan's syndrome and Klinefelter's syndrome. The term "constitutional tall stature" is used to describe children who are taller than others their age, and those growing at an accelerated velocity. Occasionally, treatment may involve the judicial administration of sex hormones (birth control pills in girls) to retard excess growth.

Gonadotropin Deficiency

Gonadotropin (GnRH) deficiency is the decrease in circulating levels of FSH and LH.

CAUSES OF GONADOTROPIN DEFICIENCY

Gonadotropin deficiency is usually caused by pressure exerted on the gonodotropin-producing cells by a pituitary tumor of another hormone-producing cell type. Oversecretion of the target gland hormones, estrogen, progesterone, or testosterone, can also act in a negative feedback manner to cause gonadotropin deficiency. Prolactin is known to inhibit pituitary secretion of the gonadotropins, and prolactin-secreting tumors can cause gonadotropin deficiency. Finally, the hypothalamus may decrease its secretion of gonadotropin-releasing hormones under periods of physical stress, obesity, starvation, or emotional trauma.

CLINICAL MANIFESTATIONS

- Amenorrhea (lack of menstrual periods), vaginal, uterine, and breast atrophy in women.
- Testicular atrophy and reduction in beard growth in men.

DIAGNOSTIC TOOLS

- Blood tests measuring the levels of estrogen, testosterone, and the gonadotropins will allow diagnosis of the condition and localization of the problem at the level of the CNS or the ovary or testicle.

TREATMENT

- Surgery if a tumor is present.
- Gonadotropin, estrogen, or testosterone replacement may be considered.
- Stress reduction, weight gain or loss.

Hypoprolactemia

Hypoprolactemia is a decrease in circulating levels of prolactin.

CAUSES OF HYPOPROLACTEMIA

Hypoprolactemia may occur as a result of hypothalamic dysfunction leading to increased release of prolactin-inhibiting hormone. It may also occur because of dysfunction of prolactin-secreting cells of the pituitary. Dysfunction of pituitary cells may be caused by increased pressure from a pituitary tumor of another cell type. More commonly, hypoprolactemia is diagnosed after an episode of pituitary ischemia and necrosis.

DISEASES OF HYPOPROLACTEMIA

- Sheehan's syndrome is a condition seen in women of hypopituitarism resulting from an intrapartum or postpartum hemorrhage (during or after delivery of an infant). With a significant loss of blood volume during the birth process, blood flow to the anterior pituitary may be reduced. Complicating the problem further is that during pregnancy the anterior pituitary grows and becomes very active metabolically. This is especially true for cells that produce prolactin, TSH, and GH. The result is a very high oxygen demand. In addition, anterior pituitary blood flow is venous blood coming from the hypothalamus through the hypothalamic-pituitary portal system, and is therefore relatively deoxygenated. Thus, the anterior pituitary is particularly susceptible to ischemic damage with a birth hemorrhage. Sheehan's syndrome may manifest after delivery of the infant when the woman experiences an inability to breastfeed. Other pituitary hormones may also be deficient.

CLINICAL MANIFESTATIONS

- Inability to breastfeed in women.
- In Sheehan's syndrome, other symptoms will depend on which hormone-producing cells were affected by the ischemia.

DIAGNOSTIC TOOLS

- Blood tests measuring decreased levels of prolactin will allow diagnosis of the condition.

TREATMENT

- Treatment is related to needs of the individual, and may involve hormone replacement therapy.

Hyperprolactemia

Hyperprolactemia is the increase in circulating levels of prolactin.

CAUSES OF HYPERPROLACTEMIA

Hyperprolactemia may be caused by a decrease in secretion of prolactin-inhibiting hormone by the hypothalamus, or as a result of a prolactin-secreting tumor of the pituitary. Certain phenothiazine drugs, used to treat psychosis, sometimes cause hyperprolactemia, probably by affecting the hypothalamus.

CLINICAL MANIFESTATIONS

- Infertility, hypogonadism, anovulation, and amenorrhea in women as a result of prolactin-mediated decreases in LH or FSH secretion by the pituitary. No clinical signs are apparent in men.

DIAGNOSTIC TOOLS

- Blood tests measuring the increased level of prolactin will allow diagnosis of the condition.

TREATMENT

- A prolactin-secreting tumor may be surgically resected.
- If the condition is drug related, further use of the drug should be evaluated if the patient is concerned about her reproductive status.

Syndrome of Inappropriate ADH

Syndrome of inappropriate ADH (SIADH) is characterized by increased release of ADH from the posterior pituitary in the absence of normal stimuli for ADH release. Increased ADH release usually occurs in response to increased plasma osmolality (a decrease in plasma water concentration) or, to a lesser extent, decreased blood pressure. With SIADH, *plasma osmolality is low in the face of high ADH*. Plasma osmolality continues to decrease because of ADH stimulating water reabsorption by the kidneys. Release of ADH continues without feedback control, in spite of low osmolality and increased blood volume.

CAUSES OF SIADH

Causes of SIADH include disease, injury, or tumors of the CNS, pain, stress, temperature extremes, and certain drugs. Surgery may result in a transient occurrence of SIADH. Tumors outside the CNS, especially bronchogenic carcinomas, frequently produce ADH ectopically.

CLINICAL MANIFESTATIONS

- Water retention and weight gain.
- Decreased urinary output.
- Nausea and vomiting worsening with the degree of water intoxication.

DIAGNOSTIC TOOLS

- Blood tests measuring increased level of ADH with decreased plasma osmolality and hyponatremia (decreased sodium concentration, mild: serum sodium decreased to 130 mEq/L; severe: serum sodium below 126 mEq/L) will allow diagnosis of the condition.

COMPLICATIONS

- Neurologic symptoms may range from headache and confusion to muscle twitching, seizures, coma, and death as a result of hyponatremia and water intoxication.

TREATMENT

- For mild cases, fluid restriction is adequate to control symptoms until the syndrome spontaneously regresses. If the condition is more severe, diuretics and drugs that block ADH action on the collecting tubules will be administered. A hypertonic solution of sodium chloride may occasionally be used to increase plasma sodium concentration.
- If ADH is coming from ectopic tumor production, treatment will be aimed at eliminating the tumor.

Diabetes Insipidus

Diabetes insipidus is a disease of decreased ADH production, secretion, or function. The term diabetes insipidus refers to the quantity and quality of the urine—copious amounts of dull, or tasteless, urine. Without ADH, the renal-collecting tubules cannot reabsorb water and cannot concentrate the urine.

CAUSES OF DIABETES INSIPIDUS

Diabetes insipidus may result from a partial or total lack of ADH production by the hypothalamus, or decreased release of ADH from the posterior pituitary. These deficits may result from a tumor or head injury. Diabetes insipidus may also result from the kidney not responding to circulating ADH because of a receptor or second messenger deficit. This type of diabetes insipidus is called nephrogenic, that is, originating in the kidney. Causes of nephrogenic diabetes insipidus include a genetic, X-linked recessive trait, kidney disease, hypokalemia, or hypercalcemia.

CLINICAL MANIFESTATIONS

- Large volumes of dilute urine.
- Polydipsia (excessive thirst).

DIAGNOSTIC TOOLS

- Blood tests measuring decreased levels of ADH with increased plasma osmolality and hypernatremia will allow diagnosis of the condition.

COMPLICATIONS

- Severe dehydration may occur if large volumes of drinking water are unavailable.

TREATMENT

- Drugs are available that mimic the action of ADH. The most commonly used drug of this category, desmopressin, previously offered only as a nasal spray for home use, has recently become available in pill form.
- For nephrogenic diabetes insipidus, thiazide diuretics are administered. These seem to work by decreasing glomerular filtration rate, allowing increased amounts of fluid to be reabsorbed at the proximal, rather than collecting, tubule.

Selected Bibliography

Bhata, E., Jain, S. K., Gupta, R. K., & Pandey, R. (1998). Tuberculous Addison's disease: lack of normalization of adrenocortical function after anti-tuberculous chemotherapy. *Clinical Endocrinology* 48, 355–359.

Brent, G. A. (1994). Mechanisms of disease: the molecular basis of thyroid hormone action. *New England Journal of Medicine* 331, 847–853.

Guyton, A. C. & Hall, J. A. (1997). *Textbook of medical physiology (9th ed)*. Philadelphia: W.B. Saunders.

Kampen, D. L. (1994). Estrogen and verbal memory in healthy postmenopausal women. *Obstetrics and Gynecology* 83, 979–983.

New, M. I. (1998). Diagnosis and management of congenital adrenal hyperplasia. *Annual Review of Medicine* 49, 311–328.

Payton, R. G. & Gardner, R. (1997). Pharmacologic considerations and management of common endocrine disorders in women. *Journal of Nurse Midwifery* 42, 186–206.

Porth, C. M. (1998). *Pathophysiology concepts of altered health states (5th ed)*. Philadelphia: J.B. Lippincott.

Romeo, J. H. (1996). Hyperfunction and hypofunction of the anterior pituitary. *Nursing Clinics of North America* 31, 769–778.

Smith, E. P. (1994). Estrogen resistance caused by a mutation in the estrogen-receptor in a man. *New England Journal of Medicine* 331, 1056–1061.

Theints, G. E., Howald, H., Weiss, U., & Sizonenko, P. C. (1993). Evidence for a reduction of growth potential in adolescent female gymnasts. *Journal of Pediatrics* 122, 306–313.

Witchel, S. F. & Lee, P. A. (1998). Identification of heterozygotic carriers of 21-hydroxylase deficiency: sensitivity of ACTH stimulation tests. *American Journal of Medical Genetics* 76, 337–342.

Wallymahmed, M. (1997). Practice: growth hormone deficiency in adults. *Nursing Times* 93, 50–51.

9 HOMEOSTASIS AND THE STRESS RESPONSE

To experience stress is part of what it means to be human. Stress may cause or result from sorrow, or it may accompany joy. Stress is a subjective experience that may be evaluated objectively. The physiologic and pathophysiologic effects of stress are described.

● ● ●

PHYSIOLOGIC CONCEPTS

Definition of Stress

In physics, stress is defined as a force put on a system that causes it to strain or give. In physiology, stress refers to a physical or psychological force imposed on an individual that causes a response. The goal of the response is usually to adapt to or eliminate the force. Physical and psychological forces that cause stress are called **stressors**.

TYPES OF STRESSORS

Stressors include positive (eustress) and negative (distress) stimuli. A stressor becomes pathologic when it exceeds an individual's capacity to handle it. Common pathologic stresses include infection, trauma, and physical disease. Mental anguish that comes from a need to perform, an experience of failure, or a great loss is also a known stressor, as are anticipation and worry. While occasional experiences of stress provide stimulation and intellectual challenge, prolonged stress challenges the body's ability to maintain physical and emotional homeostasis and is associated with negative bodily responses.

Homeostasis

Homeostasis was defined by Walter B. Cannon, a noted physiologist of the early 20th century, as the maintenance of the internal environment. Stressors threaten the body's ability to maintain homeostasis. The body responds to any change in internal conditions with reflexes designed to return itself to the previous state. Homeostasis is usually accomplished by activation of a negative feedback cycle. An initiating stimulus causes the activation of a response, which then directly or indirectly leads to a lessening of the initiating stimulus. This allows the body to remain in a dynamic steady state, whereby it continually adjusts to maintain its internal composition and function. Figure 9-1 shows a negative feedback cycle for a physical or mental stressor.

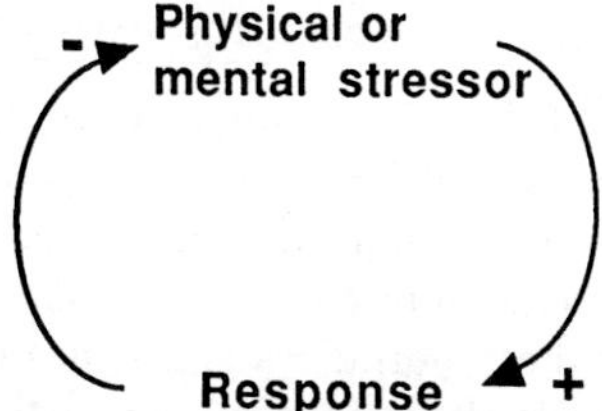

Figure 9-1. A stressor causes a response that acts in a negative feedback manner to reduce the original stressor.

PATHOPHYSIOLOGIC CONCEPTS

General Adaptation Syndrome

The general adaptation syndrome was first proposed in 1936 by Hans Selye to describe the pattern of physical responses seen after a variety of different stressor events. These responses have been shown to include: l) an increase in plasma glucocorticoids and enlargement of the adrenal glands, 2) a decrease in the size of the lymphoid organs and a decrease in the number of circulating white blood cells, and 3) ultimately an increase in the risk of developing certain diseases. Stressors used by Selye to develop his theory were all physiologic; since then the adaptation syndrome has been shown to occur also with psychological stressors as well. There are three stages of the general adaptation syndrome: the alarm stage, the stage of resistance, and the stage of exhaustion.

The **alarm stage** begins with activation of the reticular activating system, a part of the brain spread diffusely throughout the cerebral hemispheres that controls arousal. During this stage, the body becomes alerted to the presence of the stressor and the body's defenses are mobilized to fight or flee the stressor (the "fight or flight" response). The fight or flight responses depend on the release of hormones from the hypothalamus and the activation of the sympathetic nervous system.

The **stage of resistance** begins after the first alarm has quieted. From the hormonal and neural defenses mobilized during the alarm stage, certain responses are selected that can best cope with the particular stressor. This stage includes physical and psychological defenses focused on overcoming the stressor.

The **stage of exhaustion** is the final stage of the general adaptation syndrome. This stage develops only if the stressor was not adequately defeated or avoided during the resistance stage. In stage 3, the body's defenses fail and homeostasis cannot be maintained. It is during stage 3 that an individual may show the onset of certain disease states.

The Hormonal and Nervous Response to Stress

Several hormones and neurotransmitters are released in response to stress. These hormones and transmitters prepare the body to resist the stressor and are important for the mental and physical survival of the host (Fig. 9-2). Deleterious effects may occur with the prolonged, excessive release of these hormones and neurotransmitters, or with depletion of their levels after continual stimulation.

THE HYPOTHALAMIC-PITUITARY HORMONES

The hypothalamus is the primary structure in the brain responsible for maintaining homeostasis. It is affected by physical and psychologic stressors. Considered the master endocrine (hormonal) gland of the body, the hypothalamus controls the secretion of several important hormones. It also is connected through a wide neural network to other

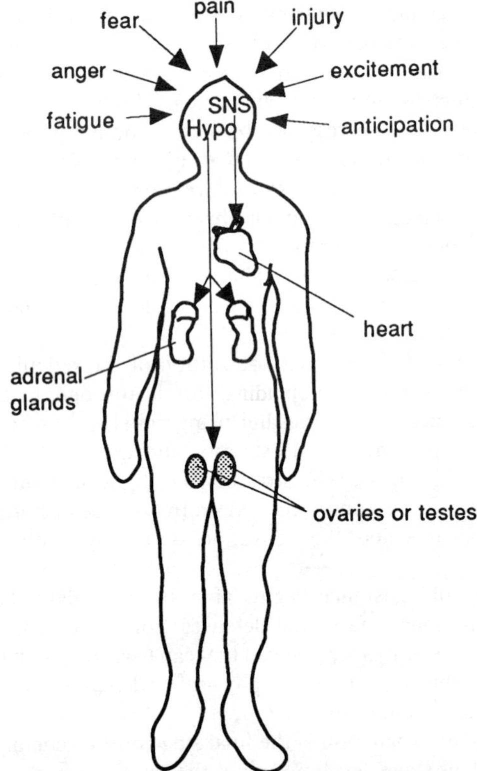

Figure 9-2. In response to a stressor the sympathetic nervous system (SNS) and hypothalmic-hormonal system (Hypo) are activated.

structures throughout the cerebral cortex and the limbic system. The hypothalamus is the part of the brain that is important in controlling water balance, body temperature, body growth, and hunger (Chapter 8). It is also involved in monitoring and responding to feelings of rage, passion, and fear. Also in the hypothalamus are integrated the responses of the sympathetic and parasympathetic systems. Stress affects the hypothalamus and therefore the release of several important hormones and neurotransmitters.

CORTISOL

The hypothalamus produces and releases corticotropin-releasing hormone (CRH) into the hypothalamic-pituitary portal blood flow system. CRH causes the anterior pituitary to secrete the adrenocorticotropin hormone (ACTH). This hormone circulates in the bloodstream to the adrenal cortex and causes the release of the glucocorticoid hormone, cortisol. CRH is always released at some baseline level. Emotional and physical stressors cause an increase in the hypothalamic release of CRH, which in turn increases ACTH levels and thereby stimulates cortisol release. Cortisol has multiple effects on the body.

Effects of Cortisol

Cortisol functions in several ways, many of which allow an individual to survive a stressor. The effects of cortisol include the following.

- Cortisol stimulates new formation of glucose (gluconeogenesis). Gluconeogenesis increases the availability of glucose as an energy source in times of immediate need.
- Cortisol stimulates the breakdown of stored energy molecules such as fat, protein, and carbohydrate to allow for the mobilization of energy if immediate fight or flight is required.
- Cortisol primes the body to respond to all stressors by promoting sympathetic responses, including those geared toward enhancing cardiac output and maintaining blood pressure.
- Cortisol appears to affect the central nervous system. When confronted by a stressor, arousal is initiated and maintained, and the individual becomes cognitively and emotionally equipped to respond.
- A high level of cortisol has many effects on the immune and inflammatory reactions, all of which are geared toward reducing inflammation and immune function. For instance, cortisol inhibits the production and release of all white blood cells, blocks B-cell and T-cell functions, and blocks the production of interleukins, which allow for communication among white blood cells.
- Cortisol reduces white blood cell accumulation at sites of injury or infection, causing a reduction in the usual inflammatory reactions. Because of these effects, cortisol can cause an increased susceptibility to infection and may delay or block healing.

Because of these negative effects, it is often wondered why cortisol release is stimulated during states of infection or tissue injury. It is possible that the short-term release of cortisol may help the body limit damage to tissues caused by inflammation, and it is only with chronic stress that harmful effects of prolonged immunosuppression become obvious.

- Cortisol stimulates gastric acid secretion, which may lead to a breakdown of the gastric mucosa.
- Cortisol affects the release of other hypothalamic-releasing factors and hormones. It inhibits the gonadotropin-releasing factors that control ovulation in women and sperm production and testosterone synthesis in men.
- Cortisol also appears to stimulate the release of the hypothalamic hormone somatostatin, an inhibitor of growth hormone release. It is possible that these effects of cortisol contribute to the reproductive dysfunction and growth deficiencies seen in some individuals with long-term stress.

THE ENDORPHINS

Endorphins are small peptides released from the hypothalamus or anterior pituitary, as well as from other tissues, in response to physical or mental stress. Endorphins may be released directly in response to stress or as a result of stimulation by CRH from the hypothalamus.

Effects of Endorphins

Endorphins are considered endogenous opiates because they have been shown to increase in response to painful stimuli. Endorphins:

- Reduce the perception of pain.
- Improve mood and increase feelings of well-being.

Prolonged exposure to pain or other stressors has been shown to deplete the store of endorphins, leading to increased pain perception and despair.

ANTIDIURETIC HORMONE

Antidiuretic hormone (ADH) is a hormone released from an extension of the hypothalamus called the posterior pituitary. ADH is an important hormone controlling salt and water handling by the kidney, and is also involved in the control of blood pressure. ADH is released in response to physical and psychological stress and appears to augment the effects of CRH. More specific roles for ADH in the response to stress are unclear.

GROWTH HORMONE

Growth hormone (GH) is released from the anterior pituitary in response to a balance of stimulatory and inhibitory hormones from the hypothalamus. GH release is initially stimulated by stress, and results in metabolic responses aimed at conserving energy. With prolonged stress, the release of GH is inhibited. Inhibition of GH with prolonged stress supports the clinical finding of failure to thrive in children exposed to physical or psychological abuse or neglect.

REPRODUCTIVE HORMONES

The reproductive hormones—estrogen, progesterone, and testosterone—are released primarily from the ovary or testicle in response to stimulation by gonadotropic hormones from the anterior pituitary. The gonadotropic hormones, in turn, are controlled by hormones from the hypothalamus. With prolonged stress, circulating levels of reproductive hormones may decrease, leading to reductions in fertility and libido. Similarly, the pituitary hormones prolactin and oxytocin, essential for breastfeeding, may be reduced during prolonged stress.

THE SYMPATHETIC NERVOUS SYSTEM

The sympathetic nervous system responds to stressful stimuli with the release of the catecholamines, epinephrine and norepinephrine, from sympathetic neurons and the adrenal medulla, an outgrowth of the sympathetic nervous system.

Effects of Catecholamines

The effects of catecholamines are similar whether they are released from nerves or from the adrenal medulla. However, catecholamines released from the adrenal gland are rapidly metabolized, and thus show more limited effects. Effects of the catecholamines include the following:

- Circulating or neurally released norepinephrine binds to receptors called alpha-receptors, identified as alpha$_1$ (α_1) and alpha$_2$ (α_2) types. Binding to α_1 receptors present on most vascular smooth muscle cells causes the muscles to contract, leading to a decrease in blood flow to organs supplied by those vascular beds. By this means, sympathetic activation leads to a decrease in blood flow to the organs of the gastrointestinal (GI) tract, the skin, and the kidneys. This maximizes blood flow to the brain, heart, and skeletal muscles in times of stress.
- Norepinephrine binds to receptors on the smooth muscle of the GI tract, causing relaxation of the muscle and thereby slowing digestion and GI motility.

- Norepinephrine release causes an increase in plasma glucose levels by increasing the breakdown of glucose storage forms in the liver and skeletal muscles, and causing the liver to release more glucose to the plasma.
- Norepinephrine released by sympathetic nerves innervating the eye causes dilation of the pupil, preparing the body for any type of attack or surprise.
- Circulating or neurally released epinephrine acts by binding not only to alpha-receptors, but also to beta-receptors, identified as β_1 and β_2. By binding to β_1 receptors on the heart, epinephrine causes an increase in heart rate and an increase in cardiac contractility, both of which serve to increase the cardiac output during stress.
- Epinephrine binding to β_2 receptors in the liver and skeletal muscle causes an increase in glucose release, resulting in increased glucose available for all cells to use if fight or flight is necessary.
- Epinephrine binding to β_2 receptors present on bronchiolar smooth muscle increases airflow to the lungs by relaxing the muscle, thereby opening up the air passages and providing more oxygen to tissues that may be called on during a stressful situation.

CONDITIONS OF DISEASE

Stress-Related Illnesses

Stress may influence the function of several systems and processes of the body, including the immune, cardiovascular, and reproductive systems, and the digestion and metabolism of foodstuffs. The skin may also exhibit signs of stress, and the central nervous system is an integral link in recognizing and responding to all stressors.

Because all parts of the body are affected by exposure to stressors, it is apparent why prolonged or intense physical or psychological stress can lead to changes in every organ or system. Examples of diseases or conditions that have been suggested to be stress related are shown in Table 9-1. How and if any one individual is affected by a particular stressor depends on a unique combination of genetics, current state of health and nutrition, family and social support systems, and previous experiences. Those in clinical practice see symptoms of stress in patients presenting with a variety of GI upsets, headaches, skin outbreaks, hypertension, and depression.

CLINICAL MANIFESTATIONS

Specific clinical manifestations of the conditions mentioned in Table 9-1 are presented in chapters pertinent to the organ systems involved. Only the general clinical manifestations seen in response to a stressful situation are presented here. Clinical manifestations present during

Table 9-1. Stress-Related Disorders

HEART DISEASE/CORONARY ARTERY DISEASE Irregular Heart Rate and Palpitations Angina Pectoris Mocardial Infarct	**MUSCULOSKELETAL DISORDERS** Headache Bachache Reduced Growth/Failure to Thrive
PERIPHERAL OR CENTRAL VASCULAR DISORDERS Hypertension Stroke	**SKIN DISORDERS** Psoriasis Acne
RESPIRATORY DISORDERS Asthma Hyperventilation	**IMMUNE SYSTEM DISORDERS** Frequent Infections Autoimmune Disease Cancer (?)
GASTROINTESTINAL DISORDERS Anorexia or Obesity Constipation or Diarrhea Ulcer Inflammatory Bowel Disease	**REPRODUCTIVE DISORDERS** Amenorrhea Impotence Sterility
NERVOUS SYSTEM DISORDERS Sleeplessness Fatigue Anxiety Depression	

acute stress are different from the clinical manifestations present in response to chronic stress.

- Acute stress is associated with increased heart rate and respiratory rate, sweating, dilated pupils, and a heightened state of awareness.
- Chronic stress may not be associated with any changes in cardiovascular or respiratory patterns, although blood pressure may be increased and asthmatic attacks may occur. With chronic stress, the person often appears distracted and distressed, is unable to sleep, and shows difficulty coping with the intense demands of the stressor. Family and professional relationships may suffer.

COMPLICATIONS

- All the conditions described in Table 9-1 can be complications of stress. In regard to the immune system specifically, high levels of acute stress, and even moderately intense chronic stress, have been associated with an increased susceptibility to viral infections and other illnesses.

- Besides the effects of cortisol on the immune system, recent studies have demonstrated the presence of nerve cell endings in contact with immune cells in the skin, the Langerhans' cells. This suggests a mechanism whereby neural excitation also may alter immune function.

TREATMENT

Treatment is frequently aimed at reducing the various symptoms of each disease or condition mentioned in Table 9-1. These types of treatments are provided in each pertinent chapter. Perhaps better therapy is to help the individual with a stress-related condition to avoid or remove the stressor. If the stressor cannot be eliminated, the individual may be advised on how to deal more effectively with it. Therapies to reduce the impact of stressors include:

- If the stressor has a psychological component, the individual is encouraged to talk about his or her concern with family, friends, or a therapist. Studies have shown that having even one person to count on and talk to can reduce the health effects of acute or prolonged stress.
- If the stressor is physical, interventions to reduce pain and prevent infection are essential. Pain and infection are themselves stressors; without interruption or relief, they compound the effects of the original stimulus.
- For physical or psychological stressors, relaxation techniques, biofeedback, and visualization therapy may help the individual reduce the impact the stressor is having on his or her life. Regular exercise is known to increase endorphin release, which may relieve the impact of stressors.

Selected Bibliography

Cannon, W. B., Britton, S. W., Lewis, J. T., & Groeneveld, A. (1927). The influence of motion and emotion in medulloadrenal secretion. *The American Journal of Physiology* 79, 433–465.

Cohen, S. (1991). Stress and the common cold. *New England Journal of Medicine* 325, 654–656.

Goleman, D. & Gurin, J. (1996). *Mind/body medicine: how to use your mind for better health.* New York: Consumer Reports Books.

Guyton, A. C. & Hall, J. A. (1997). *Textbook of medical physiology (9th ed).* Philadelphia: W.B. Saunders.

Hosoi, J., Murphy, G. F., Egan, C. L., Lerner, E. A., Grabbe, S., Asahina, A., & Granstein, R. D. (1993). Regulation of Langerhans' cell function by nerves containing calcitonin gene-related peptide. *Nature* 363, 159–162

Porth, C. M. (1998). *Pathophysiology: concepts of altered health states (5th ed).* Philadelphia: Lippincott-Raven Publishers.

Selye, H. (1946). The general adaptation syndrome and the diseases of adaptation. *Journal of Clinical Endocrinology* 6, 117–230.

10 NEUROENDOCRINE-IMMUNE INTERACTION

Joseph Cannon

A rapid decline in health or even the death of elderly persons after the loss of a spouse is a familiar situation. Many younger individuals have also noticed that their own resistance to infectious illness seems particularly labile during stressful periods. Recognizing the harmful effects of stress, caregivers intuitively strive to provide a supportive, stress-free environment for patients. The mechanistic explanations for these real-life empirical observations can be found in the anatomic and functional connections between the central nervous system, endocrine system, and immune system. This field of research is sometimes called "psychoneuroimmunology."

• • •

The exact biologic mechanisms that tie the central nervous system, the endocrine system, and the immune system together continue to be clarified. It appears that the common stimulus that integrates these systems is stress; the more intransigent aspect of this research may be understanding stress itself. The difficulty in reaching an understanding of stress is related to its subjective and inconsistent nature. For example, common experience has shown that conditions perceived as oppressive by some have no effect on others. Likewise, in the laboratory, exposing mice to inescapable shock causes suppression of certain immune parameters. However, if the mice have a means to escape the shock, they do not become immunosuppressed, even if the duration of exposure to the shock and the shock frequency is kept constant. Thus "stress" is subjective. Providing the means for a patient to avoid or to escape stress may represent the potential for therapy and for improved caregiving.

PHYSIOLOGIC CONCEPTS

Neuroendocrine Control of the Immune System

One of the seminal experiments that moved psychoneuroimmunology from the realm of anecdote to that of controlled observation was the report by Ader and Cohen in 1975 that conditioned (Pavlovian) immune responses could be induced in rats by pairing administration of an immunosuppressive drug (cyclophosphamide) with a neutral conditioning stimulus (saccharine in the drinking water). After sufficient paired conditioning, rats given the saccharine alone developed a significantly reduced antibody titer when exposed to antigen, compared with unconditioned animals. This was the first experiment that clearly demonstrated a psychological influence on immune function unrelated to an infectious or inflammatory condition, thereby suggesting a neural or an endocrine effect.

An effect on the immune system in humans by neural or endocrine activation also has been shown in controlled studies. Psychological stress has been associated with suppression of certain immune parameters. For example, the ability of lymphocytes to respond to mitogens (substances that initiate cell division) was depressed in blood samples taken from students just before oral fellowship exams. Lymphocyte responsiveness returned to normal several weeks after the examinations.

NEURONAL CONNECTIONS TO THE IMMUNE SYSTEM

If immune function is controlled by the brain, then interrupting (lesioning) neuronal pathways should disrupt normal immune function. Experiments have proved this. For example, lesioning the preoptic anterior hypothalamus (the structure that controls body temperature, eating, sleeping, and other "vegetative functions") reduces the number of leukocytes in the spleen and thymus, reduces natural killer-cell function, and suppresses antibody production. Lesions to the limbic system (which is involved in emotion and motivation) have the opposite effect on the spleen and thymus. Interestingly, lesions to the cerebral cortex exhibit *lateralized* influences: lesions on one side of the cortex increase T-cell number and function in the spleen and thymus, and lesions on the other side have the opposite effect.

Electron microscopy studies have confirmed that the secondary lymphoid tissues (thymus, spleen, lymph nodes) are innervated by the autonomic nervous system. In addition, all the elements necessary for synaptic signal transmission have been identified at the interface between nerve terminals and leukocytes in these tissues. As outlined in Table 10.1 and Figure 10.1, several neuropeptides have been identified in the neurons innervating lymphoid tissue. Corresponding receptors for these neuropeptides have been found on leukocytes, and leukocyte function is altered *in vitro* in response to these peptides. As with any synapse, a mechanism needs to be in place to break down the neuropeptides and thus terminate the individual signal; leukocytes possess appropriate enzymes to accomplish this. In addition, neurons have cytokine receptors (chemicals released by leukocytes) that make them susceptible to feedback control by leukocytes. And finally, leukocytes themselves make neuropeptides that can presynaptically influence neuronal function and signaling, further emphasizing the feedback loop. Examples of neuropeptides that bind to immune tissue and their effects include

- **Substance P**: Increases T-cell proliferation and B-cell antibody synthesis, the production of various cytokines (including interleukin[IL]-1, tumor necrosis factor [TNF], and reactive oxygen metabolite) by monocytes and macrophages, and neutrophil chemotaxis and phagocytosis. Substance P also increases histamine release from mast cells.

Table 10-1. Leukocyte-Hypothalmic-Pituitary-Adrenal Feedback

SYNAPTIC SIGNAL	PRESYNAPTIC NEURON	LEUKOCYTES
Signal initiation	Release of substance P, norepinephrine, or somatostatin from presynaptic neuron	
Signal transmission to receptor		Receptors present on leukocytes for substance P, norepinephrine, and somatostatin
Signal termination		Enzymes made by leukocytes to break down substance P, norepinephrine, or somatostatin
Presynaptic feedback	Receptors for cytokines on presynaptic neuron	Cytokine synthesis and release by leukocytes

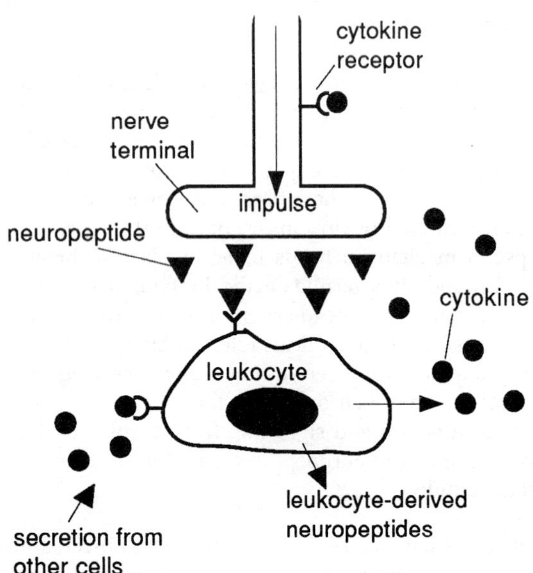

Figure 10-1. Synaptic characteristics of neuron-leukocyte communication.

- **Somatostatin:** Inhibits lymphocyte proliferation and antibody production.
- **Norepinephrine:** Enhances lymphocyte proliferation (by means of alpha-adrenergic receptors) when used in low concentrations, whereas it diminishes proliferation (by means of beta-adrenergic receptors) when used in high concentrations.
- **Circulating epinephrine:** Mobilizes preformed neutrophils and lymphocytes from storage depots (existing in the bone marrow and loosely adhering to the walls of large veins). In addition, low- or high-dose epinephrine alternately stimulates or inhibits monocyte function.

CYTOKINE CONNECTIONS

The other critical linkage between the neuroendocrine and the immune systems involve the cytokines, specifically neuroendocrine influences on cytokine synthesis, and conversely, cytokine-mediated alterations of neuronal function and endocrine secretion. Cytokines are small proteins that compose the communication network *between* leukocytes. As such, they control the proliferative, cytotoxic, and synthetic activities of all the different leukocyte populations. All cytokines have multiple and varied effects on multiple target cells. For example, interferon-gamma and one type of IL, IL-2, stimulate T-cell-mediated cytotoxicity (cell-destruction), whereas IL-4 and IL-10 promote antibody synthesis. IL-1 and TNF induce inflammation. IL-1 also enhances lymphocyte proliferation and antibody synthesis and has important influences on nonimmune cells. As a result, neuroendocrine modification of cytokine synthesis or cytokine receptor expression can have a more profound influence on immune function than direct neuroendocrine action on individual leukocytes. Cytokines, in turn, modify neuroendocrine function during times of infection or stress.

Hypothalamic-Pituitary-Adrenal Axis

The effector mechanisms that fight infection (proteolytic enzymes, reactive oxygen species, membrane-disrupting factors) are very destructive, and if these mechanisms are not controlled, they cause damage to a host's own cells. Cortisol, a hormone released from the adrenal gland, has pervasive immunomodulatory influences that provide this essential control at many levels. Cortisol is released both with stress and as part of the normal feedback control of immunologic and inflammatory processes. The functions of cortisol that keep the immune system under control include:

- Inhibition of macrophage phagocytosis, reactive oxygen species generation, and proteolytic enzyme release.
- Enhancement of antibody synthesis, lymphocyte proliferation, and cytokine production at **low** physiologic concentrations.

- Inhibition of antibody synthesis, lymphocyte proliferation and cytokine production at **high** physiologic and pharmacologic concentrations.
- Down-regulation of expression of substance P receptors.
- Stimulation of expression of enzymes that break down substance P and other neuropeptides at the synapse.
- Stimulation of beta-adrenergic receptor expression.

Because of its ability to control so many aspects of inflammation, synthetic preparations of cortisol often are given clinically to reduce inflammation.

The connection between infection and stress and the release of cortisol involves the feedback loop among the hypothalamus, the pituitary gland, and the adrenal gland, and it goes as follows: Infectious microorganisms or antigens stimulate secretion of IL-1 and other cytokines from macrophages. These cytokines travel to the hypothalamus and stimulate the release of corticotrophic-releasing hormone (CRH). From here, the normal endocrine circuit begins with successive release of adrenocorticotropic hormone (ACTH) from the pituitary and cortisol secretion by the adrenal cortex. Cortisol then feeds back on the macrophages and inhibits further cytokine release completing the loop. This cycle is shown in Figure 10.2. As such, cortisol is an integral part of a normally functioning immune system. If this cytokine–cortisol loop is disrupted by adrenal cortical insufficiency or the actions of drugs, then exaggerated and damaging inflammatory responses can occur.

Hypothalamic-Pituitary-Gonadal Axis

Women have substantially more responsive immune systems than men. This means that women are more resistant to infections, but

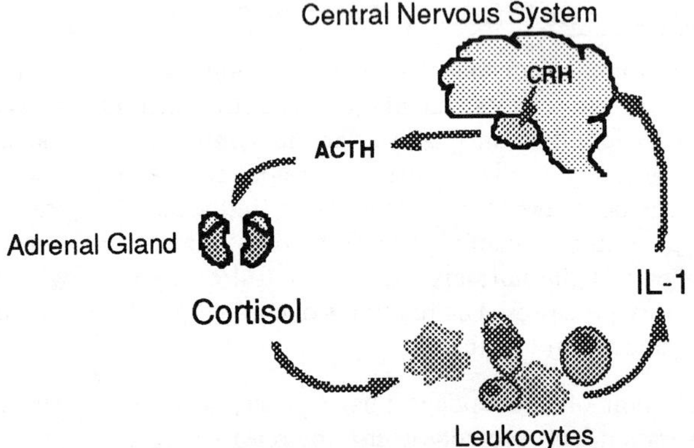

Figure 10-2. Negative feedback control of leukocyte function by means of the hypothalmic-pituitary-adrenal axis.

they are also more susceptible to autoimmune diseases. Androgens, estrogen, and progesterone all have profound influences on immune function, but only estrogen receptors have actually been found on lymphocyte subpopulations. There is evidence that receptors for the other steroid hormones are located on the thymic epithelium and the bone marrow stromal cells that nurture leukocyte development from stem cell precursors. In addition, progesterone may influence mature leukocytes through glucocorticoid (cortisol) receptors that are expressed on all leukocytes.

Estrogen and progesterone have complicated influences on cytokine production that are concentration dependent. Low concentrations of estrogen stimulate IL-1 production (compared with no estrogen at all). But the increase of concentrations through the normal range—expereinced during a menstrual cycle—leads to dose-related inhibition of IL-1 secretion. IL-1 synthesis is stimulated in a dose-related manner through the normal menstrual range of progesterone concentrations. However, high concentrations of progesterone, such as those reached during pregnancy, are inhibitory. This inhibitory influence of progesterone on the immune system is considered vital to the development of the immune tolerance that prevents the foreign tissue of the fetus from being rejected.

Although steroid hormones have received the most attention, the pituitary hormones involved in reproduction also have significant influences on immune function. Prolactin appears to have a supportive role in lymphocyte proliferation and can counteract cortisol-mediated inhibition. Stress can decrease circulating prolactin concentrations. Follicle-stimulating hormone also may stimulate IL-1 production.

PATHOPHYSIOLOGIC CONCEPTS

Hyporesponsive and Hyperresponsive Immune Reactivity

A *hyporesponsive* immune system can lead to pathologic conditions because the host is unprotected from infectious microorganisms or tumors. A *hyperresponsive* immune system can be pathologic owing to nonspecific damage to host tissues caused by overproduction of proteolitic enzymes and reactive oxygen species or by specific damage to host cells triggered by autoantibodies.

Stress-Related Immunosuppression

Physiologically and emotionally stressful situations stimulate autonomic, limbic, and, possibly cerebral cortical inputs to the hypothalamus that lead to the release of CRH and, subsequently, of cortisol. During prolonged or particularly severe stress, chronic elevations of cortisol are suspected of mediating immune dysfunction, or in some cases, immunosuppression. However, this is not at all a straightforward relation. For example, plasma cortisol concentrations increase during exercise, but exercise also *decreases* the sensitivity of leukocytes to cortisol. Thus, leukocyte inhibition is not an automatic consequence of increases in cortisol concentration. Stress-related immunosuppression is more likely caused by a combination of factors (including, for example, decreased prolactin concentrations) than strictly by a consequence of increased cortisol concentrations.

Age-Related Immunosuppression

Aging is associated with increased risk of cancer and reduced resistance to infectious disease. The critical lymphoid organ for T-cell development—the thymus—involutes with advancing age. This involution is characterized by reduction of the overall size of the thymus, but more important, by a proportionally greater loss of functional cells, with the mass replaced by inert fatty tissue. T-cell proliferation, T-killer-cell function, and T-cell enhancement of antibody synthesis all decline as well. These changes parallel age-associated declines in growth hormone. In animals, thymus involution can be reversed by growth hormone treatment (possibly in concert with other pituitary factors). These results raise hopes that "hormone replacement therapy" for senescent human immune systems can be devised that will improve immune surveillance against tumors and will bolster resistance to infectious microorganisms.

Immune Activation and Reproductive Dysfunction

Increased concentrations of IL-1 in the brain can inhibit the luteinizing hormone (LH) surge, and therefore prevent ovulation. This may be an important protective mechanism that prevents conception during periods of infection or illness. On the other hand, recurrent spontaneous abortions have been associated with abnormally high uterine concentrations of cytotoxicity-promoting cytokines such as TNF and interferon-gamma. These cytokines are thought to help drive an inappropriately robust immunologic response that leads to rejection of the fetus as a foreign intruder.

CONDITIONS OF DISEASE

Autoimmune and Hyperimmune Disease

Neuroendocrine influences on the immune system are most drastically represented by diseases that have a strong gender bias or that wax and wane with stressful events. All of the disease conditions identified below are discussed in detail elsewhere in this book. A brief enumeration of them is as follows:

- Asthma (Chapter 13) is a condition of airway hyperresponsiveness characterized by bronchoconstriction (wheezing) caused by mast cell release of histamine into the pulmonary tissues and by a subsequent inflammatory reaction. Although many factors are probably involved in an asthmatic response, inappropriate or exaggerated neuronal release of substance P, which stimulates mast cell degranulation, has been implicated, possibly in conjunction with insufficient production or release of another peptide, vasoactive intestinal peptide (VIP), which inhibits histamine release.
- Crohn's disease and ulcerative colitis are inflammatory bowel diseases (Chapter 16). Intestinal biopsies from patients indicate a possible neurogenic component in the inflammatory process such that abnormally high substance P and substance- P receptors concentrations exist and VIP concentrations seem lower than normal. Exacerbations are stress-related.
- Systemic lupus erythematosis (SLE) is an autoimmune inflammatory disease of connective tissue that can include skin rashes, joint pain, and fatigue (Chapter 3). The disease is more common in women than in men by a factor of 10:1. Androgens alleviate symptoms of SLE, and estrogen exacerbates the condition. Symptoms worsen during the luteal phase of the menstrual cycle but are not influenced to any great degree by pregnancy.
- Rheumatoid arthritis (RA) is an autoimmune disorder that results in the destruction of the synovial lining of the joints (Chapter 11). RA has a 3:1 prevalence in women, but it is relieved during the luteal phase of the menstrual cycle and during pregnancy—the high concentrations of progesterone at these times are thought to inhibit several of the inflammatory processes involved. Many cell types and inflammatory mediators have been implicated in this disease, but some possible neural–cytokine interactions deserve special note. IL-1 and TNF concentrations are high in the synovial fluid of patients who have RA. These cytokines stimulate release of substance P, which, in turn, stimulates several proinflammatory processes, including increased production of IL-1 and TNF. Thus, a destructive positive-feedback cycle is established.

CLINICAL MANIFESTATIONS

Clinical manifestations of the above disease states are described in the chapters identified.

DIAGNOSTIC TOOLS

Mechanisms for diagnosis of the above disease states are described in the chapters identified.

TREATMENT

- A better understanding of the relation between neuroendocrine factors and immune or inflammatory effectors should lead to improved therapies for these and other pathologic conditions.
- Steroid hormone activity can be modulated by receptor antagonists and other drugs.
- Neuropeptide release can be influenced pharmacologically as well as behaviorally by avoidance of exposure to stressors or, when exposure is unavoidable, by adoption of relaxation techniques and coping strategies.

Selected Bibliography

Ader, R., Felton, D. L., & Cohen, N., eds. (1991). *Psychoneuroimmunology (2nd ed)*. San Diego: Academic Press, 1218.

Berczi, I., Chow, D. A., Baral, E., & Nagy, E. (1998). Neuroimmunoregulation and cancer (review). *International Journal of Oncology* 13, 1049–1060.

Baker, J. R., Jr. & Zylke, J. W., eds. (1997). Primer on allergic and immunologic diseases. Special issue of the *Journal of the American Medical Association* 278, 1799–2034.

Cannon, J. G. & St Pierre, B. A. (1997). Gender differences in host defense mechanisms. *Journal of Psychiatric Research* 31, 99–113.

Chrousos, G. P. & Harris, A. G. (1998). Hypothalamic-pituitary-adrenal axis suppression and inhaled corticosteroid therapy. 2. Review of the literature. *Neuroimmunomodulation* 5, 288–308.

Miller, A. H. (1998). Neuroendocrine and immune system interactions in stress and depression (review). *Psychiatric Clinics of North America* 21, 443–463.

Payan, D. G. (1992). The role of neuropeptides in inflammation. In: Gallin, J. I., Goldstein, I. M., & Snyderman, R., eds. *Inflammation: Basic principles and clinical correlates (2nd ed)*. New York: Raven Press, 177–192.

Sternberg, E. M. (1997). Neural-immune interactions in health and disease. *Journal of Clinical Investigation* 100, 2641–2647.

11 THE MUSCULOSKELETAL SYSTEM

Skeletal muscles and bones support and move the body. Bones protect the internal organs and are moved by the muscles. Muscles are responsible for vascular tone, gut contractions, genitourinary function, and the beating of the heart. Some muscles function relatively independently of neural or hormonal stimulation, whereas other muscles are active only in response to neural stimulation. Diseases or injuries to the muscles and bones make movements difficult or painful. Life is impossible if the cardiac or respiratory muscles are destroyed.

● ● ●

PHYSIOLOGIC CONCEPTS

There are three types of muscles: skeletal, cardiac, and smooth. The basic processes of contraction are similar in all three types, but important differences exist. Although the focus of this chapter is the skeletal-muscular system, the unique characteristics of the cardiac and smooth muscles will be presented briefly.

Skeletal Muscle

Skeletal muscles are connected to bones through tendons. By contraction of the skeletal muscles, tendons move the bones. The contraction of skeletal muscles is controlled by lower motor neurons from the spinal cord. One motor neuron may innervate several muscle fibers. A motor neuron and the fibers it innervates are called a **motor unit**. In general, the muscles over which we have fine control are composed of a small number of motor units. Muscles that do not need fine control (i.e., the support muscles of the back) are composed of many motor units.

SKELETAL MUSCLE STRUCTURE

Each skeletal muscle is made up of many muscle cells, called **muscle fibers**. A given muscle may have a few hundred or several thousand fibers. The more muscle fibers present in a muscle, the greater the potential strength of that muscle.

Skeletal muscle is called striated muscle because of the banding that can be seen throughout the muscle with a light microscope. The striations reflect the subunits of each muscle fiber: the myofibrils. A single muscle cell is made up of many myofibrils. The myofibrils are composed of smaller subunits called myofilaments; myofilaments are the functional units of the muscle cell. They are composed of thick and thin contractile proteins, grouped together into a repeating pattern, called a **sarcomere**.

THE SARCOMERE

Three sarcomeres are aligned together in Figure 11-1. Each sarcomere contains thick and thin filaments. The thick filaments are located in the central region of the sarcomere, and are composed of several hundred copies of the contractile protein, **myosin**. The thin filaments are attached to the edges of the sarcomere. Thin filaments are composed of the proteins, **actin, tropomyosin**, and **troponin**.

The area of the sarcomere where only thick filaments are present is called the H zone. The area where only thin filaments are present is the I zone. The A band is the section where the thin and thick filaments overlap. The Z lines are the borders of the sarcomere where the actins attach. Each sarcomere spans from one Z line to the next.

CROSS-BRIDGES

Each myosin molecule is composed of six peptide chains: two heavy chains that twist together to form a long tail with two globular heads, and four light chains that group, two to a head, with the myosin heads. The heads form small projections that extend from the myosin filament. These projections are called **cross-bridges**. When a muscle is relaxed, the myosin cross-bridges are unattached in the sarcomere. During this relaxed state, an adenosine triphosphate (ATP) molecule binds to myosin and is split to ADP and a high-energy phosphate (P). The ADP and P remain bound to the myosin, without releasing the energy generated by the splitting of ATP.

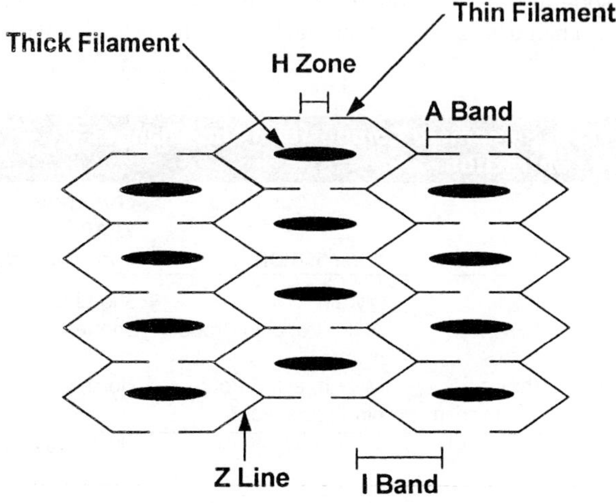

Figure 11-1. The sarcomere.

MUSCLE CONTRACTION

Contraction of a muscle occurs when the myosin cross-bridges bind to specific sites on the actin proteins. When this occurs, energy that has been stored in the myosin head from the previous splitting of an ATP molecule, is released. The released energy is used to swing the cross-bridges, causing the actin and myosin filaments to slide over each other. This shortens—contracts—the muscle. With cross-bridge swinging, the remaining ADP and P release from myosin.

During muscle contraction the lengths of the actin and myosin filaments do not change, but the I band and the H zone shorten. The different regions of the sarcomere are described in Table 11-1; the thick filaments, myosin heads, and thin filaments are shown in Figure 11-2. Each muscle contraction involves several repeated cycles of filament sliding. Each contraction provides tension for the muscle to do work.

EXCITATION-CONTRACTION COUPLING

Given that myosin and actin are ready to bind, and energy is available to be released to swing the cross-bridges, the question becomes: What prevents contraction of the skeletal muscle from happening all the time? The answer is that a skeletal muscle contraction only occurs in response to neural stimulation and activation of the motor units to the muscle.

When an action potential is delivered by a motor neuron to a skeletal muscle fiber, the neuron releases acetylcholine (ACh) into the neuromuscular junction. ACh diffuses to a specialized area of the muscle cell, called the end plate. Muscle cell end plates are concentrated with receptors for ACh. ACh binds to the receptors, causing the opening of sodium channels present in the muscle cell. With the opening of these channels, sodium ions rush into the cell, depolarizing it

Table 11-1. Sarcomere Composition and Changes During Contraction

REGION	FILAMENT	COMPOSITION	CONDITION WITH CONTRACTION
H zone	Thick	Myosin	Shortens
I zone	Thin	Actin, troponin, tropomyosin	Shortens
A band	Thick and thin overlap	Myosin, actin, troponin, tropomyosin	No change
Z line	Borders of sarcomere	actin attachments	No change

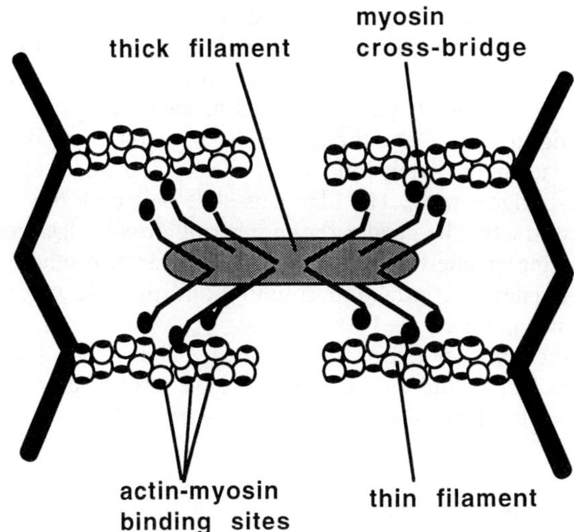

Figure 11-2. Diagrammatic representation of myosin molecules lined up in thick filaments with globular heads extending in to form cross-bridges with overlying and underlying actin molecules.

(making the cell positive on the inside) and initiating an action potential. The action potential passes along the entire muscle fiber, depolarizing the fiber. Depolarization spreads into the fiber through small tubules, called transverse (T) tubules, which run along the juncture between the A and I bands. When the inside of the cell becomes positive, calcium ion is released from intracellular bags of calcium (called "lateral sacs") that lie adjacent to the T tubules and extend from a calcium storage compartment; the **sarcoplasmic reticulum**. High levels of intracellular calcium initiate muscle contraction.

THE ROLE OF INTRACELLULAR CALCIUM IN INITIATING MUSCLE CONTRACTION

When a skeletal muscle fiber is at rest, myosin heads are prevented from binding to the actin filaments. Without binding to actin, energy from ATP cannot be released, cross-bridges cannot swing, and the muscle cannot contract. At rest, the myosin heads are prevented from binding to the actin molecule by the presence of the other two proteins of the thin filaments: tropomyosin and troponin. Elevated intracellular calcium changes the interaction of these proteins, as described later, and causes contraction.

At rest, tropomyosin is attached to the actin molecules in such a way that it blocks the sites on actin where the myosin cross-bridges would bind. Troponin attaches to the actin and the tropomyosin molecules. It also has a binding site for calcium. When calcium concentration inside the cell increases, calcium binds to troponin, causing troponin to shift its position on the tropomyosin molecule. This causes tropomyosin to shift its position on actin, uncovering the active site for binding myosin. Once the active site on actin is uncovered, the myosin heads immediately bind actin, release their stored energy, and the cross-bridges swing. The filaments slide past each other and the muscle contracts. The greater the number of cross-bridges connected and swinging at one time, the greater the tension produced by the muscle. Excitation-contraction coupling and the role of calcium is outlined in Figure 11-3.

After each cross-bridge swinging, a new ATP molecule binds to the myosin molecule (the old ADP and P have already been released). This causes the myosin cross-bridges to separate from actin and the

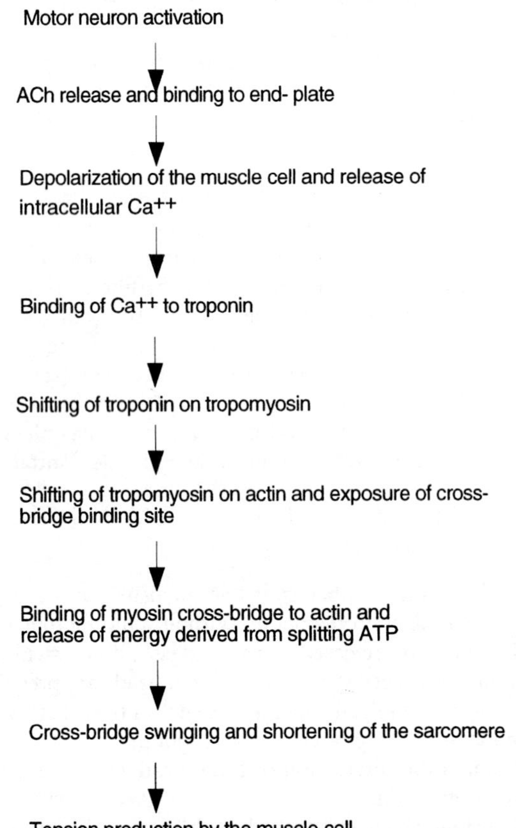

Figure 11-3. Flow diagram showing excitation-contraction coupling in a muscle cell, initiated by release of ACh from a motor neuron.

fiber to relax. Once relaxed, the new ATP molecule is split, and its energy is again stored in the myosin head. If calcium is still high intracellularly, the myosin cross-bridge will again bind actin, and this energy will be released, leading to a second contraction. Excitation-contraction coupling occurs when intracellular calcium levels increase from a resting molar concentration of less than 10^{-7} to approximately 10^{-5}. During a typical action potential, calcium concentration is approximately 2×10^{-4} molar; approximately 10 times the level required to maximally contract the muscle.

MUSCLE FIBER SUMMATION

Each calcium pulse lasts approximately 1/20 of a second and produces what is called a single muscle twitch. **Summation** occurs if calcium is maintained in the intracellular compartment by repeated neural stimulation of the muscle. Summation means individual twitches are added together, causing increased strength of the contractions. If stimulation is prolonged, the individual twitches blend together until the strength of contraction is at a maximum. At this point, the muscle is said to have reached **tetany**, which is characterized by a smooth, continued contraction. Summation and tetany in an individual muscle fiber is shown in Figure 11-4.

WHOLE-MUSCLE SUMMATION: MULTIPLE-FIBER SUMMATION

The total amount of tension produced by an entire muscle is the result of the summation of the tension produced by each muscle fiber. An increase in the number of fibers stimulated to contract will increase the amount of tension produced by the entire muscle. This is called

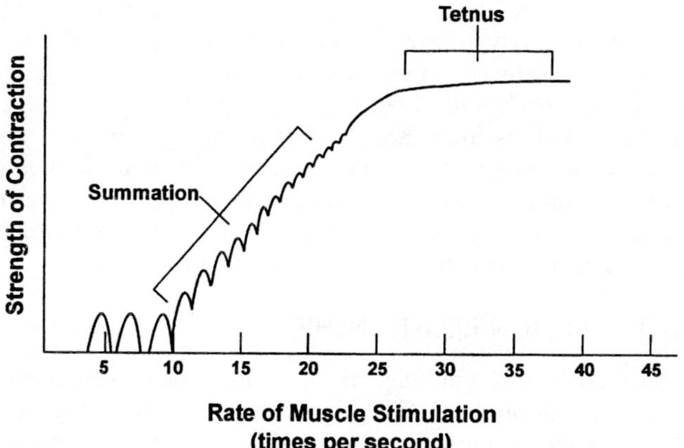

Figure 11-4. Summation and tetany.

multiple-fiber summation. Multiple-fiber summation occurs when additional motor units are activated, leading to the contraction of more muscle fibers.

RELAXATION OF THE MUSCLE

Muscle fibers relax when calcium is pumped out of the cytoplasm, back into the sarcoplasmic reticulum. Calcium pumping is an active process occurring in the membrane of the sarcoplasmic reticulum. This process uses energy derived from splitting a different ATP molecule. When calcium levels decrease to approximately 10^{-7} molar, troponin returns to its original position on the tropomyosin molecule, and tropomyosin again inhibits the binding of actin and myosin, which causes muscle contraction to stop.

MUSCLE METABOLISM AND MUSCLE FATIGUE

Muscle contraction depends on the production of ATP from one of three sources: 1) creatine phosphate (CP) stored in the muscle, 2) oxidative phosphorylation of foodstuff stored in or delivered to the muscle, and 3) anaerobic glycolysis. Muscle fatigue results when the use of ATP in a muscle becomes excessive.

When a muscle first starts contracting, it begins to use its stores of CP to drive contraction. CP contains a high-energy phosphate molecule that it transfers to ADP, to produce ATP (CP + ADP = C + ATP). This source of ATP is rapidly accessed, but is limited by the amount of CP present in the cell at the start of contraction. After several seconds, the muscle begins to rely mostly on oxidative phosphorylation. Sources of fuel for oxidative phosphorylation include, early on, glycogen stored in the muscle, and later, glucose and fatty acids delivered to the muscle in the blood supply. This source of energy is available for 30 minutes or so, depending on the intensity of contraction. If the intensity of exercise is very high, or the duration very long, the muscle begins to rely more and more on anaerobic glycolysis. Anaerobic glycolysis produces a limited amount of ATP, from the metabolism of muscle gylcogen and circulating blood glucose. A muscle using anaerobic glycolysis for a large part of its ATP production, rapidly fatigues. Muscle fatigue can be predicted experimentally by depletion of glycogen stored in the muscle. Lactic acid is a byproduct of anaerobic glycolysis and may accumulate in the muscle and blood with intense or prolonged muscle contraction, contributing to fatigue.

LENGTH-TENSION RELATIONSHIP

The resting length of a muscle fiber determines the maximum amount of tension it can produce. This relationship is shown in Figure 11-5. Muscle fiber length affects tension production as a result of stretching of the sarcomere. If a sarcomere is stretched beyond an optimum

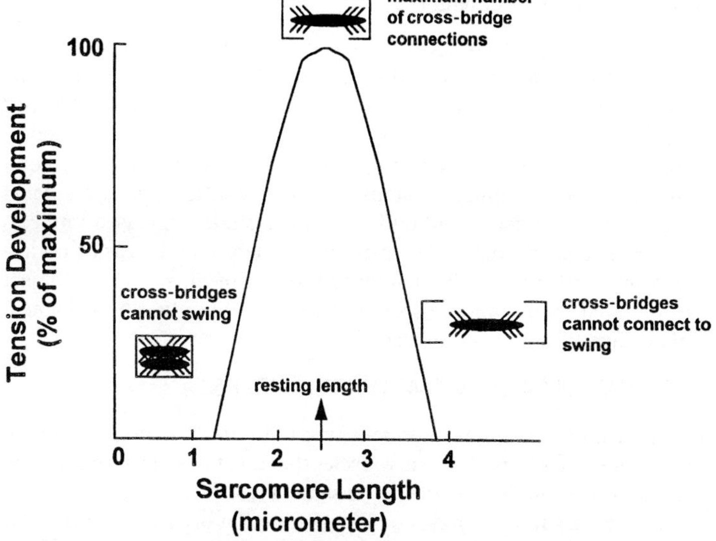

Figure 11-5. Length-tension curve.

length, as shown on the right side of the figure, some myosin cross-bridges will be unable to connect with the actin sites and some cross-bridges will not swing. This will reduce total tension. In contrast, if the sarcomere is less than optimally stretched, as shown on the left side of the figure, the cross-bridges will be unable to swing freely and sliding of the filaments will be limited, again reducing total tension. In a normal skeletal muscle, muscle length at rest will produce the maximum amount of tension.

ISOMETRIC CONTRACTION

Isometric contractions are those in which cross-bridge swinging occurs and tension is produced, without shortening of the muscle. An isometric contraction occurs when an individual is trying to lift a load that requires greater tension than can be produced by the muscle. No mechanical work is performed. Tension is produced, but the muscle does not shorten.

ISOTONIC CONTRACTION

Isotonic contractions occur when a muscle shortens against a constant load. Work is done to lift the load. An example of an isotonic contraction is when a weightlifter lifts a barbell. Most muscle contractions include isotonic and isometric periods.

SERIES ELASTIC ELEMENTS

There is typically a delay between excitation of a muscle and an isotonic contraction. A delay occurs because the elastic components of the muscle, including the tendons and the attachments of the sarcomeres, must be shortened before the muscle itself shortens. The elastic components of a muscle are called the **series elastic elements**. If a second contraction of the muscle occurs before the series elastic elements relax, there is no delay, and muscle tension can be increased immediately. This concept of the series elastic element may be easier understood by picturing a spring connected to an object. Before the object can be lifted by pulling the spring, the spring must first be stretched. This delays lifting of the object.

FAST-TWITCH AND SLOW-TWITCH FIBERS

Different muscles contain different types of muscle fibers, depending on the range of jobs performed. Muscles that must function continually, such as those of the respiratory system, must have long endurance and an ample supply of oxygen. Others function briefly and intensely, then relax; these muscles must be able to produce short bursts of high energy. Usually, a muscle will contain a mixture of fiber types, with one fiber type predominating but not exclusively. Two main divisions of muscle fibers are the fast-twitch and the slow-twitch fibers. Fast-twitch fibers may be glycolytic or oxidative.

Fast-twitch fibers release calcium rapidly from the sarcoplasmic reticulum, and rapidly split ATP to ADP on the myosin head. This causes the rate of cross-bridge swinging to be fast. Fast-twitch fibers may highly depend on oxidative phosphorylation, or may primarily use anaerobic glycolysis for energy.

Fast-twitch fibers that produce large amounts of energy for quick bursts of tension have large stores of glycolytic enzymes that can be used to produce ATP from anaerobic glycolysis. These are usually large fibers. They require less vascularization because they rely less on oxidative phosphorylation. This type of fast-twitch fiber appears white because of the reduced vascularity. These fibers are called *fast-glycolytic fibers*. Fast-glycolytic fibers tire rapidly and predominate in muscles of weightlifters and sprinters.

Fast-twitch fibers that rely mostly on oxidative phosphorylation, called *fast-oxidative fibers*, are well vascularized and contain elevated stores of the muscle protein myoglobin. Myoglobin combines in the muscle with oxygen, serving as an oxygen storage bank. Fast-oxidative fibers tire less rapidly and predominate in muscles of longer distance runners.

Slow-twitch fibers are small, highly vascularized fibers that depend predominantly on oxidative phosphorylation for the production of ATP. Muscles with slow-twitch fibers look red because of their high vascularity and presence of the protein myoglobin. Slow-oxidative fibers have long endurance and predominate in muscles required to produce tension for prolonged periods, such as back muscles.

STRETCH REFLEX

Many skeletal muscles contain special muscle fibers that act as stretch receptors, called **muscle spindle fibers**. Muscle spindle fibers are fibers wrapped by afferent nerve endings, which increase their rate of firing when the muscle is stretched. The impulses are transmitted to the spinal cord by an afferent neuron. In the spinal cord, the afferent neuron directly synapses on the motor neuron supplying the muscle (a monosynaptic reflex) or synapses on an interneuron, which then stimulates the motor neuron (multisynaptic reflex). Activation of the motor neuron causes the muscle to contract, thus removing the stretch on the muscle spindles, and their firing rate returns to normal. This process is called the stretch reflex. The opposite occurs if stretch on the spindles is suddenly reduced (called the negative stretch reflex). The result of either type of stretch reflex is maintenance of the muscle at a resting length. Voluntary muscle movement involves simultaneous contraction of regular muscle fibers and muscle spindle fibers of a muscle. This contraction allows movements to be fluid. The efferent neurons that innervate the muscle spindle fibers are called gamma neurons. The monosynaptic stretch reflex that results in the knee jerk response is shown in Figure 11-6.

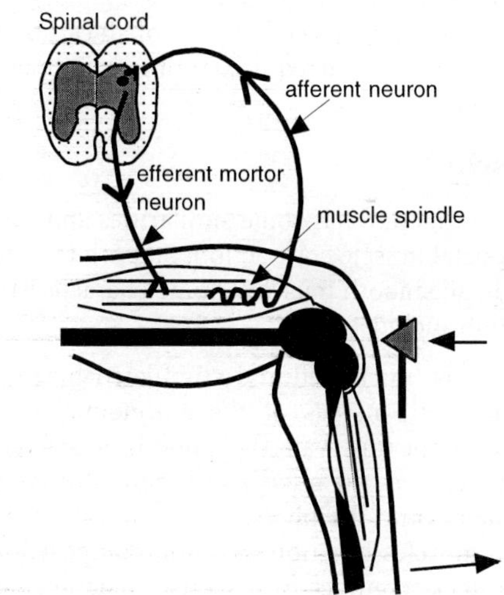

Figure 11-6. The knee-jerk reflex occurs when a muscle spindle fiber is stretched artificially. This sends a signal to the spinal cord leading to rapid contraction of the muscle.

Cardiac Muscle

Cardiac muscle contraction is similar to skeletal muscle contraction, with the following exceptions:

- Cardiac cells can contract spontaneously, that is, without neural stimulation. Neural stimulation can increase or decrease the rate of cardiac contraction.
- There are two sources of calcium involved in producing a cardiac muscle cell contraction. Calcium ions are released intracellularly from the sarcoplasmic reticulum, but also enter the cell from the extracellular fluid through sodium-calcium channels present in the T tubules. These channels are voltage sensitive and open during an action potential. Thus, the strength of cardiac contraction highly depends on the extracellular calcium level. In contrast, skeletal muscle contraction does not depend on extracellular calcium.
- Cardiac muscle cell contraction lasts approximately 10 times as long as skeletal muscle contraction. As a result, *cardiac muscle is unable to fire action potentials rapidly and does not undergo summation or tetany*. If the cardiac muscle were in a state of maintained contraction, the heart would be unable to fill with blood.
- At rest, cardiac muscle cells are stretched less than is required to produce maximum tension, which allows the heart to increase tension when it is stretched during times of increased filling (i.e., during exercise).
- Cardiac muscle fibers are connected to each other through areas of low resistance, called intercalated disks. Intercalated disks allow depolarization, beginning in one cell, to pass rapidly to neighboring cells, ensuring simultaneous contraction of all cardiac muscle cells. Simultaneous contraction is required for the maintenance of cardiac output and blood pressure.

Smooth Muscle

Smooth muscle contraction has some similarities and some important differences to skeletal muscle contraction. Smooth muscle contraction is not the same in all smooth muscles. Some characteristics of smooth muscle contraction include:

- Smooth muscle is innervated and stimulated by the sympathetic and parasympathetic nerves of the autonomic nervous system. These nerves do not innervate the smooth muscle at specific end plates, but branch over the muscle cells and diffusely release transmitter substances onto the fibers.
- Some smooth muscles function as a unit composed of millions of fibers. These fibers contract in response to action potentials produced from mechanical stretch, local chemical mediator release, or neural or hormonal stimulation. Spontaneous firing of action potentials can also occur. In this type of smooth muscle, action

potentials generated from any source pass from one cell to another across gap junctions. This type of smooth muscle is called **single-unit smooth muscle**. It is found in the gut, throughout the genitourinary tract, and in many blood vessels.

- Some smooth muscle fibers contract individually and only in response to neural stimulation. These fibers are usually innervated by one neuron that releases ACh or norepinephrine. These fibers depolarize and contract, but usually do not fire action potentials. This type of smooth muscle is called **multiunit smooth muscle**. It is found in the muscles of the eyes and in muscles that surround hair follicles. When contracted, these muscles cause the hair to stand up on the skin.
- Although smooth muscle contains actin and myosin, and splits ATP to produce tension, the thin filaments in smooth muscle fibers do not contain troponin. When intracellular calcium levels increase in smooth muscle fibers, calcium binds to a protein called calmodulin, resulting in phosphorylation of one of the light chains of the myosin heads. Phosphorylation of the light chain allows the myosin head to bind to actin and to split ATP.
- The sarcomeres of smooth muscle do not show striations under the microscope, but are more diffuse and less regular in pattern, allowing smooth muscle to contract over a wide range of lengths. There are many more actin molecules than myosin molecules in smooth muscle fibers, although maximal tension production is similar.
- In smooth muscle, most calcium enters from the extracellular fluid through voltage-sensitive calcium channels. Some calcium is released from the sarcoplasmic reticulum. In some smooth muscles, intracellular calcium levels always are sufficient to maintain a low level of cross-bridge connection. This results in a resting muscle tone in these muscles.
- The speed of cross-bridge cycling and muscle contraction is reduced in smooth muscle compared to skeletal muscle, most likely because myosin heads contain less ATPase. Therefore, it takes longer for ATP to be split, prolonging the amount of time myosin is attached to actin. A longer period of attachment results in increased production of tension. The slow speed of the calcium pumps in smooth muscle also prolongs contraction.
- A latch mechanism in smooth muscle allows muscle contraction to be maintained for long periods of time at a fraction of the energy expenditure of skeletal muscle. This mechanism is probably related to the length of time myosin remains attached to actin.

Tendons

Tendons are bundles of collagen fibers that attach the muscles to the bones. Tendons transmit force generated by the contracting muscle to the bone and thereby move the bone. The collagen fibers are considered connective tissue and are produced by fibroblast cells.

Ligaments

Ligaments are strong fibrous connections between two bones, usually at a joint. Ligaments allow and limit joint movement.

Bones

BONE STRUCTURE

Mature bone is composed of 30% organic (living) material and 70% salt deposits. The organic material is called the matrix, and is more than 90% collagen fibers and less than 10% proteoglycans (proteins plus polysaccharides). The salt deposits are primarily calcium and phosphate, with small amounts of sodium, potassium carbonate, and magnesium ions. The salts cover the matrix and are bound to the collagen fibers by the proteoglycans. The organic matrix gives bone its tensile strength (resistance to being pulled apart). The bone salts give bone its compressional strength (ability to withstand compression).

EXCHANGEABLE CALCIUM

Some calcium ion in bone is noncrystallized. This noncrystalline salt is considered exchangeable calcium, in that it can rapidly move between the bone, interstitial fluid, and blood.

BONE FORMATION

Bone formation is ongoing and can involve lengthening and thickening of the bone. The rate of bone formation changes throughout the life span. Bone formation is determined by hormonal stimulation, dietary factors, and the amount of stress put on a bone, and results from activities of the bone-forming cells, the osteoblasts.

OSTEOBLAST ACTIVITY

Osteoblasts are found on the outer surface and inside of bones. Osteoblasts respond to various chemical signals to produce the organic matrix. When the organic matrix is first produced, it is called the osteoid. Within a few days, calcium salts begin to precipitate on the osteoid and the bone hardens over the next several weeks or months. Some osteoblasts remain part of the osteoid, and are called osteocytes or true bone cells. As the bone forms, osteocytes in the matrix send out projections to each other, forming a system of microscopic canals (Volkmann's canals) in the bone.

FACTORS THAT CONTROL OSTEOBLAST ACTIVITY

Osteoblast activity is affected by diet, hormonal stimulation, and exercise. These factors interact and are dynamic, resulting in different rates of bone formation throughout a lifetime.

Exercise and Osteoblast Activity

Osteoblastic activity is stimulated by exercise and weight-bearing as a result of electrical currents produced when stress is applied to the bone. Bone fracture dramatically stimulates osteoblast activity, but the exact mechanism is unclear.

Hormonal Stimulation and Osteoblast Activity

Estrogen, testosterone, and growth hormone are strong promotors of osteoblast activity and bone growth. Bone growth is accelerated during puberty as a result of surging levels of these hormones. Estrogen and testosterone eventually cause the long bones to stop growing by stimulating closure of the epiphyseal plate (growing end of the bone). When estrogen levels decrease after menopause, osteoblastic activity is reduced. Deficiencies in growth hormone impede bone formation.

Diet and Osteoblast Activity

An adequate diet during childhood and adolescence is essential for maximal bone growth in length and thickness. Calcium ion deficiency during adolescence will result in bones less dense than optimum later in life. Most calcium deposited in bones for a lifetime is done so before the age of 20.

Vitamin D Control of Osteoblast Activity

Small amounts of vitamin D stimulate bone calcification directly by acting on the osteoblasts and indirectly by stimulating calcium absorption across the gut. Increased calcium absorption increases blood calcium concentration, which promotes bone calcification. Large amounts of vitamin D, however, may increase bone breakdown in an attempt to liberate calcium and so increase serum calcium levels. Thus, large amounts of vitamin D without adequate calcium in the diet can promote bone resorption.

BONE BREAKDOWN

Bone breakdown, called resorption, occurs simultaneously with bone formation and is also ongoing throughout life. Bone resorption results from the activity of cells called osteoclasts. Osteoclasts are multinucleated, large phagocytic cells derived from monocytes (white blood cells) present in the bone. Osteoclasts secrete various acids and enzymes that digest the bone and allow for its phagocytosis. Osteoclasts also secrete various cytokines that further stimulate resorption. Osteoclasts are usually present in only one small section of bone at a time, and phagocytize the bone section by section. Once they finish in one area, the osteoclasts disappear and osteoblasts arrive. The osteoblasts begin to fill in the clear section with new bone. This process allows old, weakened bone to be replaced with new, stronger bone.

REMODELING

The balance between osteoblast and osteoclast activity continually remodels, or renews, the bone. In children and teenagers, osteoblastic activity outpaces osteoclastic activity, leading to thickening and lengthening of the skeleton. Osteoblastic activity also outpaces osteoclastic activity in bones healing from fracture. In a young adult, osteoblastic and osteoclastic activity are typically in equilibrium, resulting in a constant total amount of bone mass. By middle age, osteoclastic activity outpaces osteoblastic activity and bone density begins to decrease. Osteoclastic activity is also accelerated in immobilized bones. By the seventh or eighth decade of life, dominance of osteoclastic activity may cause the bones to become brittle, leading to increased fractures. Osteoclastic activities are controlled by several physical and hormonal factors.

FACTORS THAT CONTROL OSTEOCLAST ACTIVITY

Parathyroid Hormone and Osteoclastic Activity

Osteoclast activity is primarily controlled by parathyroid hormone. Parathyroid hormone is released by the parathyroid glands located directly behind the thyroid gland. Parathyroid hormone release increases in response to decreased serum calcium levels. Parathyroid hormone increases osteoclastic activity and stimulates bone breakdown, liberating free calcium into the blood. Increased serum calcium acts in a negative feedback manner to reduce further release of parathyroid hormone. It has been hypothesized that estrogen reduces bone resorption by inhibiting the effect of parathyroid hormone on osteoclasts; the mechanism of this is unknown.

Other Effects of Parathyroid Hormone. Parathyroid hormone increases serum calcium by decreasing excretion of calcium by the kidneys. Parathyroid hormone increases renal excretion of phosphate ion, thereby decreasing blood phosphate levels. Renal activation of vitamin D depends on parathyroid hormone.

Calcitonin and Osteoclastic Activity

Calcitonin is a hormone secreted by the thyroid gland in response to high serum calcium. Calcitonin has a weak effect on inhibiting osteoclastic activity and formation. These effects increase bone calcification, thereby reducing serum calcium levels.

TYPES OF BONES

Bone is classified as long, short, flat, or irregular. Long bones are found in the extremities, whereas short bones are found in the ankles and wrists. Flat bones are found in the skull and rib cage. Irregular bones include the vertebrae, bones of the face, and the jaw.

Long Bones

Long bones consist of a long, thick shaft called the diaphysis, and two ends called the epiphyses. Proximal to each epiphysis is the metaphysis. In between the epiphysis and the metaphysis is an area of growing cartilage, called the epiphyseal or growth plate. Long bones grow by the accumulation of cartilage at the epiphyseal plate. Cartilage is replaced by the osteoblasts, and the bone elongates. By the end of the teen years, the cartilage is used up, the epiphyseal plate fuses, and the bones stop growing. Growth hormone, estrogen, and testosterone stimulate growth of long bones. Estrogen, in conjunction with testosterone, stimulates fusion of the epiphyseal plates. The shaft of a long bone is hollowed out along the medullar canal, which is filled with bone marrow.

Bone Marrow

Bone marrow consists of cells involved in blood cell formation (red marrow) and fat cells (yellow marrow). Marrow is found in long and flat irregular bones. Bone marrow biopsy is performed on flat bones.

Joints

Joints are areas of the body where two bones come together. A joint may be freely movable, called a **diarthrodial joint**, or may be immobile, called a **synarthrose joint**.

In a diarthrodial joint, the two ends of the bone are not connected directly, but come together in a fibrous joint capsule that surrounds and supports the joint. There are two layers of the joint capsule; an outer layer and an inner membrane layer called the synovium or *synovial membrane*. The synovial membrane secretes a slippery fluid, called *synovial fluid*, that lubricates the joint. The synovial membrane also covers the tendons that connect the bone to muscle, and the ligaments that connect the bones to each other. There is a well-developed vascular supply to the synovium, which may be damaged with joint trauma, leading to swelling, bruising, and pain surrounding the joint. In some joints, the synovial membrane forms a closed sac external to the joint, called a *bursa*. Bursa are found at areas where the bones are close together physically, or where a tendon runs over the bone. Bursa too may become inflamed, a condition called *bursitis*. Most joints in the body are diarthrodial joints, including the sacroiliac joint, the interphalangeal joints, the hip and knee joints, and the shoulder and elbow joints. Although all diarthrodial joints are considered movable, some of these joints move more than others (i.e., the sacroiliac joint is nearly fixed, whereas the shoulder joint is capable of moving in several different directions).

In synarthroses, the bones are held together by connective tissue, cartilage, ligaments, or other bones, thus fixing their position to a large degree. Examples of synarthroses are the joints of the skull bones, ribs, and intervertebral disks.

PATHOPHYSIOLOGIC CONCEPTS

Atrophy

Atrophy is the decrease in size of a cell or tissue. Muscle atrophy may result from muscle disuse or severing of the nerve supplying the muscle. With muscular atrophy, the size of the myofibrils is reduced. Although bones do not atrophy, bone density can decrease with disuse or metabolic deficiencies or disease.

Geriatric Consideration

Muscle mass, muscle strength, and bone density decrease in the elderly, usually as a result of disuse. However, decreased muscle mass, muscle strength, and bone density can be reversed, even in the very elderly (>85 years), with moderate, regular weight-bearing exercise.

Strains

A strain is trauma to a muscle or tendon, usually related to the muscle or tendon being stretched beyond its normal limit. Strains may involve tissue tears or ruptures. Inflammation occurs with injury to muscles or tendons, leading to pain and swelling of tissue. Healing may take several weeks.

Sprains

A sprain is trauma to a joint, usually related to a ligament injury. In a severe sprain, the ligament may be torn. Sprains lead to inflammation, swelling, and pain. Healing may take several weeks.

Joint Dislocation

Dislocation of a joint is the condition in which a bone is displaced from its position in the joint. A *subluxation* is a partial dislocation of the joint. Joint dislocation typically occurs after a severe trauma, which disrupts the ability of the ligament to hold the bone in place. Dislocations of a joint may also occur congenitally, for example, dislocation of the hip is sometimes seen in a newborn (developmental hip dysplasia). For a trauma-induced dislocation, there is associated marked pain, swelling, and loss of range of motion of the joint. Sometimes a "popping" noise may be heard or felt at the time of occurrence or during physical examination; in the newborn examination, manipulation of the joint to reproduce the sound or feeling of dislocation is used to diagnose the condition. Dislocation of a joint will usually be apparent on a radiograph and is treated by manipulation or surgical repair followed by immobilization until the joint structures are healed.

Rhabdomyolysis

Rhabdomyolysis, also called myoglobinuria, is the presence of large amounts of muscle protein, myoglobin, in the urine. Rhabdomyolysis usually occurs after major muscle trauma, especially a muscle crush injury. Long-distance running, certain severe infections, and exposure to electrical shock can cause extensive muscle damage and excessive release of myoglobin. Rhabdomyolysis may cause renal failure if the myoglobin gets trapped in the delicate capillaries or tubules of the kidney, interfering with renal blood flow.

Rigor Mortis

Rigor mortis is stiffening or contraction of muscles that occurs several hours after death. Rigor mortis is the result of ATP depletion in the muscle cells. Without ATP to bind to myosin, cross-bridges that are connected in the muscle at and soon after the time of death cannot release and the muscle stays contracted. Within a day, muscle proteins are destroyed by local enzymes released as cells degenerate, causing the muscles to relax.

CONDITIONS OF DISEASE OR INJURY

Muscular Dystrophy

Muscular dystrophy refers to a variety of diseases characterized by wasting of the muscles. The disorders are not caused by neural, hormonal, or blood flow abnormalities. All muscular dystrophies are inherited disorders involving an enzymatic or metabolic defect. With the defect, muscle cells die and are phagocytized by cells of the inflammatory system, leading to scar tissue buildup and loss of muscle function.

DUCHENNE'S MUSCULAR DYSTROPHY

The most common form of muscular dystrophy is Duchenne's muscular dystrophy, a sex-linked disorder passed on the X chromosome and seen almost exclusively in males. In approximately 50% of cases, the disease shows a clear family history and is passed from mother to son. The other 50% occur as spontaneous mutations on the X chromosome before or during conception. Because males only have one X chromosome, the defective gene that causes the disease is not compensated for by a healthy gene on another X chromosome.

Cause of Duchenne's Muscular Dystrophy

Duchenne's muscular dystrophy results from a defect in the gene that produces the protein dystrophin. Dystrophin appears to act as an anchor for the actin filaments; without it, the muscle fiber is literally pulled apart with repeated contractions. Without dystrophin, muscle cells die and are then phagocytized and replaced by fatty tissue.

Muscle cell weakness begins in the pelvic region by the time a child is approximately 2 or 3 years old. It then spreads to the legs and upper body within 3 to 5 years. When the muscle cells die, scar tissue and fat cells replace the dead cells, causing the muscles (especially the calf muscles) to appear strong and well muscled (called psuedohypertrophy) when they are weak and poorly functioning. Eventually, the skeleton begins to actually deform and the child becomes progressively immobile and finally restricted to a wheelchair. Cardiac muscle is often involved and approximately 50% of affected children develop heart failure. Respiratory effort is progressively compromised, related to the dysfunction of the diaphragm and other respiratory muscles as well as the inability to expand the chest because of severe kyphosis. Smooth muscle dysfunction may cause GI disturbance. Mental retardation may be present. Death usually occurs as a result of respiratory or cardiac complications in the 20s or younger.

CLINICAL MANIFESTATIONS

- Clumsiness, waddling gait, and frequent falls in toddlers.
- Walking on toes because of anterior tibial weakness.
- Decreased deep tendon reflexes.
- Pseudohypertrophy of the calf muscles.
- Gowers' maneuver, whereby the child uses his arms to push up on to his legs when standing up from the floor, is seen during the toddler years.
- Immobility and confinement to a wheelchair by the early teens.
- Curvature of the spine (kyphoscoliosis) caused by weakness of the postural muscles.
- Frequent respiratory infections from a failure to fully expand the lungs.

DIAGNOSTIC TOOLS

- Serum levels of the muscle enzyme creatinine phosphokinase (CPK) are elevated, even before symptoms develop. CPK may be elevated in female carriers who are asymptomatic for the disease.
- Muscle biopsy will demonstrate cell death, scar tissue, and fatty infiltration.

- Electromyography recordings (measurements of electrical signals in a muscle) will be reduced.
- Because the gene for dystrophin has been identified, prenatal testing for the disorder is possible.

COMPLICATIONS

- Family stress, feelings of guilt or blame, anger, and grief are common.
- Respiratory or cardiac failure and death are likely before adulthood.

TREATMENT

- Support groups and family counseling are important to improve family coping.
- Nonstrenuous exercises are recommended to maintain mobility and function as long as possible. Strenuous exercise may hasten muscle deterioration.
- Experimental studies involving intramuscular injection of dystrophin, or the gene for dystrophin, are under way in animal models. Insertion of the gene for dystropin may be accomplished by production of a genetically engineered virus that will carry the correct gene into host muscle cells.
- Experimental studies are under way in which healthy, immature muscle cells are taken from the fathers of young male children with muscular dystrophy and injected into the muscles of their sons. Whether significant improvement in muscle function will occur in the children is unclear.

Bone Fracture

A bone fracture is a break in a bone. Terms used to describe various types of bone fractures include:

- Complete fractures—fractures that extend through the bone.
- Incomplete fractures—fractures that extend partially through the bone.
- Simple (closed) fractures—fractures that do not cause a break in the skin.
- Compound (open) fractures—fractures that cause a break in the skin.

Open and closed fractures can be complete or incomplete. Other terms may be used to describe fractures, based on the angle of the break or whether the bone buckles or bends without breaking.

CAUSES OF BONE FRACTURES

The most frequent cause of bone fracture is trauma, especially in children and young adults. Falls and sports injuries are common causes of traumatic fractures. In a child, abuse must be considered when evaluating a fracture, especially if there is a previous history of fractures, or if the history of the current fracture is unconvincing.

Some fractures may result after minimal trauma or slight pressure if the bone is weak. These are called **pathologic fractures**. Pathologic fractures often occur in elderly persons who suffer from osteoporosis, or in an individual with a bone tumor, infection, or other disease.

Stress fractures may occur in normal bone as a result of prolonged or repeated low-level stress. Stress fractures, also called fatigue fractures, usually accompany a rapid increase in the training level of an athlete, or the beginning of a new physical activity. Because muscle strength increases more rapidly than bone strength, an individual may feel capable of performing beyond a previous level even though the bones may be incapable of supporting the added pressure. Stress fractures are most common in those who pursue endurance sports such as long-distance running. Stress factors may occur in weakened bone in response to only a slight increase in activity level.

Geriatric Consideration

Fractures resulting from even minor falls are a major cause of disability in the elderly. A large percentage of the elderly who suffer a fracture, especially of the hip, do not regain the same level of functioning as before the fall. Loss of independence frequently follows a fracture in the elderly, and frequently results in the individual being cared for in a nursing home, which results in high costs to the patient and to society. Many frail elderly never recover from a fracture. A fear of falling is a significant concern for many elderly individuals, even for those who have never fallen.

Pediatric Consideration

Stress fractures are becoming increasingly common in younger athletes, as the pressure to perform in sports at an early age is increasing. Girls and young women are especially affected, perhaps because of the combined pressure for thinness and athletic excellence.

EFFECTS OF A BONE FRACTURE

When a bone breaks, bone cells die. Bleeding typically occurs around the site and into the soft tissues surrounding the bone. The soft tissues are usually damaged by the injury. An intense inflammatory reaction follows the break. White cells and mast cells accumulate, causing increased blood flow to the area. Phagocytosis and removal of dead cell debris begins. A fibrin clot (fracture hematoma) forms at the break and acts as a meshwork on which new cells can adhere. Osteoblastic activity is immediately stimulated and immature new bone, called **callus**, is formed. The fibrin clot is soon reabsorbed, and the new bone cells are slowly remodeled to form true bone. The true bone replaces the callus and is slowly calcified. Healing takes several weeks to a few months (fractures in children heal faster). Healing can be delayed or impaired if the fracture hematoma or callus is disrupted before true bone is formed, or if the new bone cells are disrupted during calcification and hardening.

CLINICAL MANIFESTATIONS

- Pain usually accompanies a traumatic bone break and soft tissue injury. Muscle spasm may follow a bone break and contribute to the pain. With a stress fracture the pain typically accompanies activity and is relieved by rest. Pathologic fractures may not be associated with pain.
- An unnatural position of the bone or a limb may be obvious.
- Swelling around the site of a fracture will accompany the inflammatory processes.
- Impaired sensation or tingling may occur, signaling nerve damage. Pulses distal to the fracture should be intact and equal to the nonfractured side. A loss of distal pulse may indicate compartmental syndrome (see later), although the presence of a pulse does not rule out this disorder.
- Crepitus (a grating sound) may be heard with movement, as the broken ends of the bone move across each other.

DIAGNOSTIC TOOLS

- Radiograph can reveal a bone fracture.
- Bone scan can reveal a stress fracture.

COMPLICATIONS

- Nonunion, delayed union, or malunion of the bone may occur, leading to deformity or loss of function.
- Compartmental syndrome may occur. Compartmental syndrome is characterized by nerve and blood vessel damage or destruction that results from swelling and edema in the area of a fracture. With intense interstitial swelling, pressure exerted on blood vessels supplying the area may cause them to collapse. This leads to tissue hypoxia and may cause death of the nerves supplying the area. Typically, pain is intense. The individual may be unable to move the fingers or toes. Compartmental syndrome usually occurs in limbs that have tight volume restrictions, such as the arms. Risk of developing compartmental syndrome is greatest if muscle trauma has occurred with the break because swelling will be pronounced. Casting of a fractured limb too early or too tightly may cause increased pressure in the limb compartment, and permanent loss of function or loss of the limb may result. A cast must be immediately

removed and sometimes the skin of the limb must be split. To check for compartmental syndrome, the following are evaluated frequently in an injured or cast bone; pain, pallor, paresthesias, and paralysis. A pulse may or may not be felt.
- A fat embolus may occur after the break of a bone, especially a long bone. A fat embolus may be generated from exposure of the bone marrow, or may result from activation of the sympathetic nervous system leading to stimulation of free fatty acid mobilization after the trauma. A fat embolus after the break of a long bone frequently lodges in the pulmonary circulation where it may lead to respiratory distress and failure.

TREATMENT

- A fracture should be immediately immobilized to allow for formation of a fracture hematoma and to minimize damage.
- Realignment of the bone (reduction) is important to allow recovery of normal positioning and range of motion. Most reduction can be performed without surgical innervation (closed reduction). If surgery is required for fixation (open reduction), pins or screws may be inserted to maintain realignment. Traction may be required to maintain reduction and stimulate healing.
- Long-term immobilization after reduction is important to allow formation of callus and new bone. Long-term immobilization is usually accomplished by casting or the use of splints.

Acute Osteomyelitis

Osteomyelitis is an acute infection of the bone that may occur from the spread of a bloodborne infection (hematogenous osteomyelitis), or more commonly, after contamination of an open fracture or surgical reduction (exogenous osteomyelitis). A puncture wound to the soft tissue or bone resulting from an animal or human bite or a misplaced intramuscular injection may cause exogenous osteomyelitis. Bacteria are the usual cause of acute osteomyelitis, but viruses, fungi, and other microorganisms may be involved.

Osteomyelitis is a difficult disease to treat because local abscesses may develop. A bone abscess typically has a poor blood supply; therefore, delivery of immune cells and antibiotics is limited. Intense pain and lifelong disability may result if a bone infection is not treated immediately and aggressively.

CLINICAL MANIFESTATIONS

- Symptoms of hematogenous osteomyelitis in children may include fever, chills, and a reluctance to move a particular limb. In the adult, symptoms may be vague and include fever, fatigue, and malaise. A preceding urinary, respiratory tract, ear, or skin infection frequently precedes hematogenous osteomyelitis.

- Exogenous osteomyelitis typically presents with evidence of injury and inflammation at the site of pain. Fever and regional lymph node enlargement occur.

DIAGNOSTIC TOOLS

- Bone scan using injected radiolabeled nucleotides may show an inflammatory bone site. Magnetic resonance imaging (MRI) may allow for increased diagnostic sensitivity.
- Blood analysis may demonstrate elevation in complete blood count (CBC) and erythrocyte sedimentation rate, suggesting an active infection is in progress.

COMPLICATIONS

- Chronic osteomyelitis may develop, characterized by unrelenting, severe pain and decreased function of the affected body part.

TREATMENT

- Antibiotics may be prescribed to an individual suffering a bone break or puncture wound to the soft tissue surrounding a bone before a sign of infection develops. If a bone infection occurs, aggressive antibiotic therapy is required.

Osteoporosis

Osteoporosis is a metabolic bone disease characterized by a severe reduction in bone density leading to easy bone fracture. Osteoporosis occurs when the rate of bone resorption greatly exceeds the rate of bone formation. Bone that is produced is normal; however, there is too little of it, thus the bones are weak. All bones can be affected by osteoporosis, although osteoporosis usually develops in the bones of the hips, pelvis, wrists, and vertebral column.

CAUSES OF OSTEOPOROSIS

The rate of bone formation decreases progressively as an individual ages, beginning at approximately age 30 or 40. The more dense the bones are before that time, the less likely osteoporosis will occur. As people age into their 70s and 80s, osteoporosis becomes a common disease.

Although bone resorption begins to outpace formation by the fourth or fifth decade of life, in women the most significant thinning of the bones occurs during and after the menopause. It appears that the postmenopausal decrease in estrogen is primarily responsible for this development in the elderly female population. Although the mechanism by which estrogen acts to preserve bone density is unclear, it is thought that estrogen stimulates osteoblastic activity and limits the osteoclastic-stimulating effects of parathyroid hormones. Therefore, a loss of estrogen causes a pronounced shift toward osteoclastic activity. Thin women, fair-haired women, and women who smoke are especially prone to osteoporosis because their bones are less dense before menopause than are the bones of heavier, darker, and nonsmoking women. Elderly men are less prone to osteoporosis because they typically have denser bones (approximately 30% denser) than women, and reproductive hormone levels remain high until a man is in his 80s. However, elderly men have less dense bones than do younger men.

For men and women, other causes of osteoporosis include reduced physical activity and the ingestion of certain drugs, including corticosteroids and certain aluminum-containing antacids that increase calcium elimination. In regard to exercise, it has been shown that even very elderly men and women can significantly increase bone density by participating in moderate forms of weight-bearing activity. Family history also plays a role in determining an individual's future risk. Bone density has been shown to decrease in lactating women, although a return to near normal density occurs after weaning.

Pediatric Consideration

At particular risk for future development of osteoporosis are children and teenagers who do not consume adequate calcium or vitamin D during their bone-forming years. This is especially, but not exclusively, true of diet-conscious girls who frequently limit caloric and milk intake. Young women athletes in particular may have measurably less dense bone than their peers. This phenomena appears related to low estrogen levels, sometimes leading to amenorrhea (lack of or infrequent menstrual cycling), which often accompanies high or moderate physical exercise. Athletic women may also be thinner than their peers. These women may experience severe osteoporosis in later years.

CLINICAL MANIFESTATIONS

- Although insidiously advancing, osteoporosis may not be associated with any clinical manifestations unless a bone break occurs. Pain and deformity usually accompany a break.
- With weakness and collapse of the vertebral bodies, an individual may shrink in height or develop kyphosis (sometimes called dowager's hump).

DIAGNOSTIC TOOLS

- A careful family and personal history will identify patients at risk of developing osteoporosis. Physical examination identifying kyphosis and a demonstrable reduction in height will assist diagnosis.
- Patients who have previously experienced a fracture unrelated to significant trauma or overuse should be suspected of having osteoporosis, and observed accordingly.

- Bone-mineral content of the whole body, and bone-mineral density of specific bones such as the lumbar spine, femoral neck, and shaft of the femur, tibia, fibula and distal radius, are often assessed using dual-energy radiograph absorptiometry. This measurement offers an accurate reading of bone mass and allows a clinician to chart the rate of bone decay. Bone density testing that reveals a bone density of fewer than two standard deviations below normal (based on average of young women) is considered abnormal.

COMPLICATIONS

- Fractures of the hips, wrists, vertebral column, and pelvis.
- Hospitalization or placement in a nursing home, and loss of ability to perform activities of daily living may occur after an osteoporotic fracture.

TREATMENT

- Prevention of osteoporosis begins in childhood and the teen years with the beginning of lifelong habits of good nutrition and physical exercise to strengthen bones.
- Weight-bearing exercise, even in the very elderly (>85 years), has been shown to increase bone density and muscle mass, and improve balance and physical endurance.
- Estrogen-progesterone replacement therapy during and after menopause can reduce the development of osteoporosis in women. Contraindications for estrogen replacement include a family or personal history of breast cancer or a personal history of blood clots.
- Recently approved drugs known as bisphosphonates (e.g., pamidronate, etidronate, aledronate) have been shown to decrease bone resorption and prevent bone loss. These drugs are used for treatment and prevention of osteoporosis. The biophosphonates significantly increase bone density in the hip and spine especially, and can be used in postmenopausal and drug-induced (glucocorticoid) osteoporosis. They also are being evaluated as chemotherapeutic adjuvents for use in cancer therapy because of a potential to prevent bone metastasis.
- Calcitonin may also be prescribed for those suffering severe osteoporosis. Intranasal administration has recently become available, increasing patient usage.
- Testosterone therapy may reduce osteoporosis in men.
- Dietary supplements of calcium and vitamin D may reduce the development of osteoporosis in men and women.
- Cigarette smoking should be avoided.

Hyperparathyroidism

Hyperparathyroidism is a disorder of bone mineralization and muscle weakness caused by high levels of circulating parathyroid hormone.

Usually, the elevated parathyroid hormone results from a tumor of the parathyroid gland or another gland. With excess parathyroid hormone, bone resorption is stimulated, resulting in high serum calcium levels. Low serum phosphate accompanies high levels of parathyroid hormone. The bones become brittle and weak.

Secondary hyperparathyroidism can occur with states of hypocalcemia, caused by vitamin D deficiency or renal failure. Calcium levels remain low even with elevated parathyroid hormone.

CLINICAL MANIFESTATIONS

- Multiple pathologic fractures.
- Kyphosis of the spine and vertebral compression fractures.
- Fatigue and weakness because high serum calcium leads to decreased nerve and muscle cell excitability.

DIAGNOSTIC TOOLS

- Serum assay will demonstrate elevated serum calcium levels (>12 mg/dL; normal 8.6–10.5 mg/dL).
- Serum phosphate levels will be low (<2.0 mg/dL; normal 2.5–4.5 mg/dL)

COMPLICATIONS

- Calcium-based kidney stones may develop, causing pain and inflammation of the urinary tract.
- Electrocardiogram (ECG) (Chapter 12) abnormalities may develop, including premature ventricular contractions (PVCs) and sinus tachycardia, related to the effects of high serum calcium on cardiac muscle depolarization.

TREATMENT

- Treatment depends on the cause and severity of the disease.
- Fluids are essential in management.
- Oral phosphate may be administered.
- Specific drugs to treat hypercalcemia, including steroids and calcium-losing diuretics, may be used.
- Surgical excision of the parathyroid glands may be required.

Osteomalacia and Rickets

Osteomalacia is a metabolic bone disease seen in adults caused by decreased mineralization of the osteoid as a result of calcium or phosphate deficiency or both. Decreased mineralization results in soft, malleable bone. Osteomalacia usually occurs as a result of a vitamin D deficiency or insensitivity, or as a result of renal disease.

Vitamin D is required for the maintenance of calcium absorption in the gut. With vitamin D deficiency or insensitivity, decreased serum calcium develops, which in turn stimulates parathyroid hormone release. Increased parathyroid hormone stimulates bone breakdown to liberate calcium and increased renal excretion of phosphate. Without adequate mineralization of the bone, the bone becomes thinner. Abnormal amounts of noncrystallized osteoid accumulate and coat the channels of the inner bone, which leads to bone deformity.

Renal failure is associated with osteomalacia because of two factors: the inability of the kidney to activate vitamin D and the decreased ability to excrete phosphate in the urine. Increased serum phosphate also stimulates parathyroid secretion, and hence bone breakdown. Other causes of osteomalacia not directly related to dietary deficiency include the malabsorption of dietary calcium seen in Crohn's disease, malabsorption syndrome, or cystic fibrosis.

Rickets is a bone disease in children caused by vitamin D deficiency. Rickets causes disorganization of the bone, especially at the growth or ephiphyseal plates, retarding growth and distorting bone development. Frank rickets is uncommon in the United States, but may be seen in cases of extreme poverty or neglect, or may be subtle in presentation.

CLINICAL MANIFESTATIONS

- Osteomalacia may be symptomless until a fracture occurs. Vertebral collapse is common, with associated changes in posture and height.
- Rickets is characterized by permanent skeletal deformity including bowed legs, lumbar lordosis (convexity of the spine), and rib and skull deformity. Children may be unable to walk without support. They may also show poor dentition.

DIAGNOSTIC TOOLS

- Radiograph evaluation can demonstrate reduced bone ossification.
- Measurements of serum calcium and phosphate will be low in severe cases.

TREATMENT

- Vitamin D therapy with calcium supplementation is required.
- If osteomalacia or rickets is caused by another disease, that disease will require treatment.

Osteoarthritis

Osteoarthritis is a degenerative bone disease characterized by loss of articular (joint) cartilage. Without cartilage buffering, the underlying bone is irritated, leading to degeneration of the joint. Osteoarthritis may develop idiopathically (for no known reason) or may occur after trauma, repeated stress such as that experienced by a long-distance runner or ballerina, or in association with a congenital deformity. Individuals with hemophilia or other conditions characterized by chronic joint swelling and edema may develop osteoarthritis. Osteoarthritis is common in the elderly, affecting more than 70% of men and women older than the age of 65. Obesity can worsen the condition.

CLINICAL MANIFESTATIONS

- Pain and stiffness in one or more of the joints, commonly the hands, wrists, feet, knees, upper and lower spine, hips, and shoulders. Pain may be associated with tingling or numbness, especially at night.
- Swelling of the affected joints, with a decreased range of motion. Joints may appear deformed.
- Heberden's nodes may develop at the distal interphalangeal joints.

DIAGNOSTIC TOOLS

- Arthroscopy (visualization of the joint through a fiber-optic instrument), MRI, and CT scan may support the clinical diagnosis.

TREATMENT

- A balance between resting and exercising the joints, geared toward minimizing inflammation but preserving range of motion is helpful.
- Analgesics and anti-inflammatory drugs to reduce swelling and inflammation.
- Surgery may be required to correct a deformity or replace a joint.

Rheumatoid Arthritis

Rheumatoid arthritis (RA) is a chronic, inflammatory disease that causes degeneration of connective tissue. The connective tissue usually destroyed first is that which makes up the lining of the joints, the synovial membrane. In RA, the inflammation becomes unrelenting and spreads to surrounding structures of the joint, including the articular cartilage and the fibrous joint capsule. Eventually, the ligaments and tendons become inflamed. The inflammation is characterized by white blood cell accumulation, complement activation, extensive phagocytosis, and scarring. With chronic inflammation, the synovial membrane undergoes hypertrophy and thickens, occluding blood flow, and further stimulating cell necrosis and the inflammatory response. The thickened synovium becomes covered by inflammatory granular tissue called **pannus**. Pannus may spread throughout the joint, leading to further inflammation and scarring. These processes slowly destroy the bone and cause great pain and deformity.

CAUSES OF RHEUMATOID ARTHRITIS

Rheumatoid arthritis is an autoimmune disease that develops in susceptible individuals after an immune response against an unknown triggering agent. The triggering agent may be a bacterium, mycoplasma, or virus that infects the joints or resembles the joint antigenically. Typically, the original antibody response to the microorganism is IgG mediated. Although this response may successfully destroy the microorganism, individuals who develop RA begin to produce other antibodies, usually IgM or IgG, against the original IgG antibody. These self-directed antibodies are called rheumatoid factors (RFs). The RFs persist in the joint capsule, causing chronic inflammation and destruction of the tissue. RA is thought to result from a genetic predisposition to autoimmune disease. Women are more often affected than men. There is strong evidence to suggest that various cytokines, especially tumor necrosis factor alpha (TNF-α) contribute to the cycle of inflammation and joint destruction.

CLINICAL MANIFESTATIONS

- Onset of RA is characterized by general symptoms of inflammation including fever, fatigue, body aches, and joint swelling.
- Joint tenderness and stiffness develop, first because of acute inflammation and then from scar formation. The metacarpophalangeal joints and the wrists are usually first involved. Stiffness is worse in the morning and affects joints bilaterally. Episodes of inflammation are interspersed with periods of remission.
- Decreased range of motion. Joint deformity and muscular contractions.
- Extrasynovial rheumatoid nodules develop in approximately 20% of individuals with RA. These swellings consist of white blood cells and cell debris that present at areas of trauma or increased pressure. Usually, nodules develop in the subcutaneous tissue over the elbows and fingers.

DIAGNOSTIC TOOLS

- Elevated serum rheumatoid factor in 80% of cases.
- Radiograph changes including bony decalcification of the joints.
- Synovial fluid aspiration may show white blood cells in a sterile culture.

COMPLICATIONS

- Extrasynovial rheumatoid nodules may develop on cardiac valves, in the lungs, eyes, or spleen. Respiratory and cardiac function may be affected. Glaucoma may result if nodules that block outflow of ocular fluid develop in the eye.
- Vasculitis (inflammation of the vascular system) may lead to thrombosis and infarction.
- Loss of ability to carry out activities of daily living, depression, and family stress may accompany exacerbations of the disease.

TREATMENT

- Rest of the inflamed joints during exacerbations.
- Rest periods each day.

- Alternating hot and cold packs.
- Aspirin, other nonsteroidal anti-inflammatory drugs, or systemic steroids. Other therapies such as gold treatments may be tried.
- Anti-TNF medications are being used to block cytokine-mediated inflammation.
- Surgery to remove the synovial membrane or to correct deformity.

Osteogenesis Imperfecta

Osteogenesis imperfecta (OI) is a genetic disease characterized by a defect in the synthesis of connective tissue. It results in thin, poorly developed bones that fracture easily. There is a variety of genetic mutations that may result in this disease, all of which result in an abnormality in the production of procollagen proteins.

There are four general categories of OI, separated based on clinical manifestations and genetic analysis. OI is usually inherited as an autosomal-dominant disorder, meaning that an individual heterozygous for the trait will express the disease. The expression of the disease is variable. In other cases, the genetic disorder is inherited as an autosomal-recessive disease. In this case, the child is homozygous for the genetic error and the resultant pathology is more severe. These children typically die before, during, or soon after birth from fractures sustained in utero or during delivery.

CLINICAL MANIFESTATIONS

- For the autosomal-dominant condition, children may appear healthy until they begin to walk and fall as toddlers. At this time, frequent fractures with poor healing may occur. Some cases may be investigated as child abuse before the condition is diagnosed.
- Children will be of short stature and may have deformed cranial structure and limbs.
- Thin skin, with bluish sclera of the eye, indicates reduced collagen deposits.
- Tooth development and enamel is abnormal.
- Deafness frequently develops as the child ages because of bone deformity and scarring of the middle and inner ear.

DIAGNOSTIC TOOLS

- Elevation of serum alkaline phosphatase levels. Alkaline phosphatase is released with cell injury and is high during periods of rapid bone formation.
- Fibroblast analysis in a skin culture will demonstrate reduced quantity of connective tissue-producing cells.
- Prenatal diagnosis of osteogenesis imperfecta is possible.

COMPLICATIONS

- Infants homozygous for the autosomal-recessive condition are frequently stillborn or die within the first year of life.

TREATMENT

- Treatment is aimed at reducing the number of fractures that occur by teaching safety measures.
- Secure stabilizing of fractures with internal fixation is frequently performed.
- Moderate levels of growth hormone supplementation may improve growth outcome and reduce fracture occurrence.

Scoliosis

Scoliosis is curvature of the spine. It may result from an actual structural deformity of the vertebral column that is present at birth (congenital) or may develop as a result of a neuromuscular disease such as cerebral palsy or muscular dystrophy. Some structural scoliosis may develop for no known reason (idiopathic) or as a result of poor posture. Scoliosis results in deformity and occasionally pain. If the condition is untreated, respiratory and pulmonary function may be compromised.

CLINICAL MANIFESTATIONS

- Abnormality of the usual concave-convex-concave vertebral presentation seen in descent from shoulder to buttocks.
- Prominence of the ribs on the convex side.
- Unevenness in the height of the iliac crest that may cause one leg to be shorter than the other.
- Asymmetry of the thoracic cage and misalignment of spinal vertebrae will be apparent when the individual bends over.

DIAGNOSTIC TOOLS

- Physical examination and screening may allow for early diagnosis.
- Lateral deviation of the vertebrae can be confirmed by radiograph.

COMPLICATIONS

- Back pain may develop.
- Respiratory, cardiac, and GI complications may develop from thoracic or lumbar deformity.

TREATMENT

- Postural scoliosis is treated by passive and active exercises. An external brace may be used to encourage compliance and speed recovery.
- Structural scoliosis is treated with surgical intervention, which may

include placing a flexible rod down the back to reverse the curve of the vertebral column. Fusion of the spine at different levels to correct a deformity may be performed in severe cases.

Paget's Disease

Paget's disease is a bone disorder characterized by accelerated patterns of bone remodeling. Repeated episodes of rapid bone breakdown are followed by short periods of bone formation. The new bone is thickened and rough, and eventually leads to structural deformity and weakness. Blood flow to bones affected by Paget's disease is increased to support high metabolic demands. The long bones and bones of the cranium, spine, and pelvis are most commonly affected. Paget's disease is usually seen in those older than 70 years of age. There is no known cause of the disease.

CLINICAL MANIFESTATIONS

- Changes in the shape of the skull, with associated headaches, hearing abnormalities, and sometimes mental deterioration.
- Pain in the long bones, spine, or pelvis.
- Frequent pathologic fractures.

DIAGNOSTIC TOOLS

- Radiographs demonstrate bone deformity and will support a clinical diagnosis.
- Elevation of serum alkaline phosphatase supports the diagnosis.
- Bone biopsy can rule out infection or tumor.

COMPLICATIONS

- Heart failure may occur because of high blood flow demands of remodeling bones (high-output failure).
- Respiratory failure may occur if thoracic bones are affected and deformed.
- Paget's disease is a risk factor for sarcoma (bone cancer), perhaps related to the rapid rate of cell cycling seen with the disease.

TREATMENT

- Calcitonin may be administered to slow the rate of bone breakdown.
- Anti-inflammatory agents may reduce the pain associated with growing deformity. These drugs will reduce the constant inflammation that accompanies cell breakdown. The disease has no known cure.

Talipes Equinovarus

Talipes equinovarus, also called clubfoot, is a congenital abnormality characterized by deformity of the bones and soft tissue of the foot.

The front portion of the foot is abducted (turned in) whereas the rear of the foot is inverted. The foot is usually pointed down (in equinus). The individual typically walks on the tiptoes. Clubfoot results from abnormal development of the foot during gestation (fetal growth). This leads to abnormality of the muscles and joints and soft tissue contracture. There may be a genetic tendency for this disorder, and other associated structural malformations may be present.

CLINICAL MANIFESTATIONS

- Clubfoot is apparent at birth.

TREATMENT

- Casting of foot (or feet) immediately after birth with cast replacement weekly for several months.
- Corrective shoes may be necessary during the toddler years.
- Surgery may be performed, usually between 6 and 9 months of age.

Developmental Hip Dysplasia

Developmental hip dysplasia is dislocation of the hip present at birth (congenital) or occurring within the first year of life. The hip may be out of the hip joint or present in the joint but easily displaced. The acetabulum (joint cavity) may be abnormally shaped, which allows the head of the femur to slip. The cause of hip dysplasia is unknown, but a genetic tendency toward the disorder is apparent. Breech birth is a strong risk factor for hip dysplasia, as is any condition that limits space for the fetus in the uterus, such as multiple fetuses, abnormalities in the anatomy of the uterus, or amniotic fluid deficiency.

CLINICAL MANIFESTATIONS

- Asymmetry in leg length, leading to gait abnormality.
- Asymmetry in folds of the gluteus (buttocks).

DIAGNOSTIC TOOLS

- During each physical examination in the newborn period and up until 18 months of age, a thorough examination of the hips is performed at each well visit. This examination includes visual inspection of the limbs for differences in length and physical manipulation of the hip joints. In one procedure, the infant is placed on his or her back with his or her legs splayed outward. Pressure is then exerted downward on the knees, and the observer watches and feels for hip dislocation; a positive response is called Barlow's sign. A second maneuver follows in which the practitioner gently reduces the hip back into the joint, producing a telltale click, called Ortolani's sign.
- Ultrasound or radiograph is used to confirm the diagnosis.

COMPLICATIONS

- Limp and leg pain and deformity may result without treatment. In older children, undiagnosed hip instability may be a cause of delayed standing and walking.

TREATMENT

- Early treatment is essential and may involve bracing or casting depending on the child's age and the severity of the defect. Surgery may be required for late diagnosis or if casting or braces are ineffective.

Osgood-Schlatter Disease

Osgood-Schlatter disease is a condition that occurs during periods of rapid growth in early puberty, in which there is partial separation of the epiphysis of the tibia from the tibial tuberosity (joint area of the knee). This occurs as a result of physical stress placed on the knee during these growth periods. The stress is usually associated with sports such as running, biking, climbing, or hiking. This condition is especially common in teenage boys from the ages of 11 to 15, and girls from 8 to 13 years of age. Inflammation of the patellar tendon (tendonitis) and the development of ossified cartilage in the tibial tuberosity occurs. This condition is usually self-limited and symptoms resolve on closure of the tibial growth plate at the end of puberty. Occasionally minor symptoms may continue in adulthood.

CLINICAL MANIFESTATIONS

- Pain at the front of the knee, especially during physical activity or kneeling.

DIAGNOSTIC TOOLS

- A thorough history and physical examination is used to diagnose Osgood-Schlatter disease. An MRI or radiograph may be used to rule out other causes of pain.

COMPLICATIONS

- The condition is usually self-limited. Occasionally pain may continue past puberty.

TREATMENT

- Treatment is usually limited to the use of anti-inflammatory medications and ice packs after exercise. Rest and refraining from sports may be required during a flare-up. Knee supports or braces may be of some use.
- Occasionally, surgery may be performed if the condition is severe

or seems complicated by the development of bony fragments in the patellar tendon.

Bone Tumors

Bone tumors may be cancerous or benign. Bone cancer may occur as a primary disease (originating in the bone) or more commonly as a result of metastasis from another tumor.

Primary bone cancer may begin in any cell of the bone. Cancers of the bone marrow lead to leukemia or myeloma. Leukemia and myeloma are discussed in Chapter 5. Primary cancer of the osteoblast or osteocyte is called osteogenic sarcoma. Osteogenic sarcoma often occurs in a long bone, especially the femur (thigh), or in the knee. Cancers of the cartilage are called chondrosarcoma. Chondrosarcoma usually occurs in the femur or pelvis.

CLINICAL MANIFESTATIONS

- Pain related to inflammation with swelling in and around the bone.
- Pathologic fracture.

DIAGNOSTIC TOOLS

- MRI will identify tumors of the bones.
- Bone biopsy will identify the neoplasm and the involved tissue.

COMPLICATIONS

- Amputation of the limb is common.
- Anxiety, fear, and family stress often accompany the diagnosis of cancer, especially in children.

TREATMENT

For osteosarcoma and chondrosarcoma:

- Resection of the diseased part of the bone may allow successful treatment of the cancer without amputation.
- Amputation of the limb may be required.
- Chemotherapy is administered.
- Bone marrow cancers are treated with chemotherapy and radiation.

Selected Bibliography

Cummings, S. R., Browner, W. S., Baurer, D., Stone, K., Ensrud, K., Jamal, S., & Ettinger, B. (1998). Endogenous hormones and the risk of hip and vertebral fractures among older women. *New England Journal of Medicine* 339, 733–738.

Guyton, A. C. & Hall, J. A. (1997). *Textbook of medical physiology (9th ed)*. Philadelphia: W.B. Saunders.

Janas, J. (1996). Muscular dystrophy. *Nurse Practitioner Forum* 7, 167–173.

Kalkwarf, H. J., Specker, B. L., Bianchi, D. C., Ranz, J., & Ho, M. (1997). The effect of calcium supplementation on bone density during lactation and after weaning. *New England Journal of Medicine* 337, 523–528.

Kritz-Silverstein, D. & Barrett-Connor, E. (1993). Early menopause, number of reproductive years, and bone mineral density in postmenopausal women. *American Journal of Public Health* 83, 983–988.

Kessenich, C. R. (1996). Update on pharmacologic therapies for osteoporosis. *Nurse Practitioner* 21, 19–24.

Louis, D. (1991). Common vitamin-D deficiency rickets. In: Glorieux, F. H. (ed.). *Rickets.* New York: Vevey/Raven Press, pp. 107–122.

Majeska, R. J., Ryaby, J. T., & Einhorn, T. A. (1994). Direct modulation of osteoblastic activity with estrogen. *Journal of Bone and Joint Surgery (American)* 76, 713–721.

Rencken, M. L., Chesnut, C. H., & Drinkwater, B. L. (1996). Bone density at multiple skeletal sites in amenorrheic athletes. *Journal of the American Medical Association* 276, 238–240.

Saag, K. G., Emkey, R., Schnitzer, T., et al. (1998). Alendronate for the prevention and treatment of glucocorticoid-induced osteoporosis. *New England Journal of Medicine* 339, 292–299.

Schneider, M. F. (1994). Control of calcium release in functioning skeletal muscle fibers. *Annual Review of Physiology* 56, 463–484.

Slemenda, S. W., Reister, T. K., Hui, S. L., Millerm, J. Z., Christian, J. C., & Johnston, C. C. (1994). Influences on skeletal mineralization in children and adolescents: evidence for varying effects of sexual maturation and physical activity. *Journal of Pediatrics* 125, 201–207.

Theintz, D. E., Howald, H., Weiss, U., & Sizonenko, P. C. (1993). Evidence for a reduction of growth potential in adolescent female gymnasts. *Journal of Pediatrics* 122, 306–313.

Tosi, L. L. (1997). Osteogenesis imperfecta. *Current Opinion in Pediatrics* 9, 94–99.

12 THE CARDIOVASCULAR SYSTEM

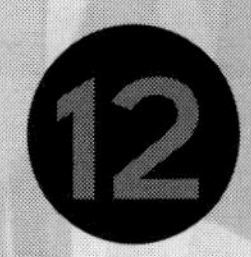

The cardiovascular system begins with the heart, a muscular pump that beats rhythmically and repeatedly 60 to 100 times a minute. Each beat causes blood to surge from the heart and travel throughout the body in a closed network of arteries, arterioles, and capillaries and return to the heart through venules and veins. The purpose of the cardiovascular system is to pick up oxygen in the lungs and nutrients absorbed across the gut and deliver them to all cells of the body. At the same time, the cardiovascular system removes metabolic waste products produced by each cell and delivers these to the lungs or the kidneys to be excreted.

● ● ●

PHYSIOLOGIC CONCEPTS

Anatomy of the Heart

The heart is a four-chambered, muscular organ that lies in the chest cavity, under the protection of the ribs, slightly to the left of the sternum. The heart sits within a loose, fluid-filled sac, called the pericardium. The four chambers of the heart include the left and right atria and the left and right ventricles. The atria sit next to each other above the ventricles. The atria and ventricles are separated from each other by one-way valves. The right and left sides of the heart are separated by a wall of tissue called the septum. There is normally no mixing of blood between the two atria, except during fetal life, and there is never mixing of blood between the two ventricles in a healthy heart. Connective tissue surrounds all chambers. The heart is extensively innervated by nerves.

Two Circulations of the Cardiovascular System

The left side of the heart pumps blood through the **systemic circulation**, which reaches all cells of the body except those involved with gas exchange in the lungs. The right side of the heart pumps blood through the **pulmonary circulation**, which delivers blood only to the lungs to be oxygenated.

SYSTEMIC CIRCULATION

Blood enters the left atrium from the pulmonary vein. Blood in the left atrium flows into the left ventricle through the atrioventricular (AV) valve, located at the juncture of the left atrium and ventricle. This valve is called the *mitral* valve. All cardiac valves open when pressure in the chamber or vessel above them is greater than pressure in the chamber or vessel below.

Blood from the left ventricle outflows into a large, muscular artery, called the aorta. Blood flows from the left ventricle into the aorta through the *aortic valve*. Blood in the aorta is delivered throughout the systemic circulation, through arteries, arterioles, and capillaries, which then rejoin to form veins. The veins from the lower part of the body return the blood to the largest vein, the inferior vena cava. The veins from the upper body return blood to the superior vena cava. The venae cavae empty into the right atrium.

PULMONARY CIRCULATION

Blood in the right atrium moves into the right ventricle through another AV valve, called the *tricuspid valve*. Blood leaves the right ventricle and travels through the fourth valve, the *pulmonary valve*, into the pulmonary artery. The pulmonary artery branches into left and right pulmonary arteries, which travel to the left and right lungs, respectively. In the lungs, the pulmonary arteries branch many times into arterioles and then capillaries. Each capillary perfuses past an alveolus, the unit of respiration. All capillaries reform to become venules, and the venules become veins. The veins join to form a large pulmonary vein.

Blood flows in the pulmonary vein back to the left atrium, completing the blood flow cycle. The heart and the systemic and pulmonary circulations are shown in Figure 12-1.

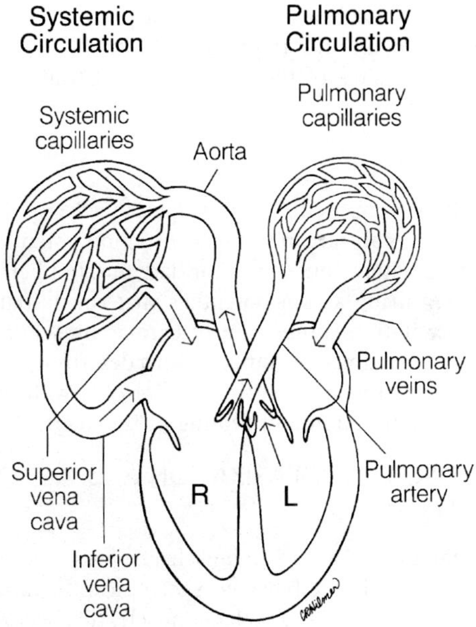

Figure 12-1. Anatomy of the heart.

FUNCTIONS OF THE SYSTEMIC AND PULMONARY CIRCULATION

As blood passes each cell of the body in the systemic circulation, carbon dioxide and other cellular waste products are added to the blood while oxygen and nutrients are delivered to the cells. In the pulmonary circuit, the opposite occurs: carbon dioxide is eliminated from the blood and oxygen is added. By continual cycling of the blood through the pulmonary and systemic circulations, oxygen supply and waste removal are ensured for all cells.

CORONARY ARTERY BLOOD FLOW

Two large arteries, called the left and right coronary arteries, branch off the aorta as soon as it leaves the left ventricle and supply blood to the heart. The left coronary artery quickly branches into the left anterior descending artery and the circumflex artery. The left anterior descending artery travels down the anterior portion of the septal groove between the right and left ventricles and branches several more times to supply blood to the anterior portion of the septum and to the anterior muscle mass of the left ventricle.

The left circumflex artery travels in the area between the left atrium and the left ventricle and supplies blood to the lateral wall of the left ventricle.

The right coronary artery travels in the groove between the right atrium and the right ventricle and branches off to supply blood to the posterior portions of the heart, including the posterior intraventricular septum. In most people, the right coronary artery supplies blood to important electrical sites of the heart: the sinoatrial (SA) node and the AV node.

Cardiac Muscle

Cardiac muscle is composed of highly specialized muscle fibers. Not only do these fibers contract in response to action potentials produced from neural stimulation, but many cardiac muscle fibers are capable of spontaneously firing action potentials that can initiate their own contractions. Excitation-contraction of cardiac muscle are described in the next several sections, beginning with a description of the cardiac action potential, and finishing with an outline of how the action potential leads to the contraction and beating of the heart.

CARDIAC MUSCLE DEPOLARIZATION AND ACTION POTENTIAL FIRING

Just like skeletal muscle, a cardiac muscle cell fires an action potential when the inside of the cell becomes significantly more positively charged than the outside. Like skeletal muscle, this occurs when voltage-sensitive sodium channels open in the cell membrane, resulting in a rush of positively charged sodium ions. Closure of the sodium channels quickly follows, again like skeletal muscle, but in cardiac muscle cells, **repolarization** (return of the membrane to resting levels) is delayed, which results in prolongation of the cardiac action potential. Delayed repolarization occurs because during the time sodium channels are opening, potassium channels close and reopen only sluggishly, thereby retaining the positive potassium charge inside the cell. In addition, and more importantly, voltage-sensitive calcium channels open with the initial depolarization, and calcium ions move into the cell, again maintaining intracellular positive charge. These calcium channels are called **slow channels** because their opening is delayed compared to sodium channels. Prolongation of the action potential is significant because it makes it impossible to fire a second action potential before the first is completed, and ensures that cardiac cells will not undergo summation and tetany of contractions: If cardiac cells underwent tentany, the heart could not relax and fill with blood between beats and would stop pumping out blood.

The Pacemaker

Most cardiac muscle cell have the capacity to fire action potentials on their own. However, certain cells are more permeable to sodium ions than others, and therefore start off more positively charged than other cells. These slightly depolarized cells reach threshold and fire sooner than other cells. The fast-firing cells pass their excitation easily to other cells because each cardiac muscle cell is connected to all other muscle cells of the heart. In effect, these cells control the rate, or pace, of contraction. Cells that normally depolarize fastest are the cells of the SA node. The SA node, located in the wall of the right atrium, is the primary pacemaker of the heart.

SPREAD OF ELECTRICAL DEPOLARIZATION THROUGH THE MYOCARDIUM

From the SA node, depolarization spreads rapidly through both atria and soon reaches the AV node, which is located in the lower right atrium near the juncture of the atria and ventricles. When the depolarization reaches the AV node, the electrical signal is delayed shortly before it is passed to the ventricles. During this delay, the atria reach action potential threshold and begin to contract, pumping their last bit of blood into the ventricles. While contraction of the atria is occurring, the electrical depolarization spreads through the AV node, down specialized muscle fibers to an area of the ventricles called the bundle of His. Depolarization then spreads rapidly down an extensive, wide-reaching group of specialized conducting fibers called Purkinje's fibers. In a normal heart, all ventricular muscle cells receive the electrical depolarization simultaneously from Purkinje's fibers and contract together. It is important that the entire ventricle contracts as a unit to have high pressure pumping of the blood out of the heart with each beat.

CARDIAC MUSCLE FIBERS

As described fully in Chapter 11, cardiac muscle fiber is made up of bands of protein filaments, called myofilaments, lying in series with each other. Each band is called a sarcomere. A cardiac sarcomere is shown in Figure 12-2. Sarcomeres in cardiac muscle are connected to each other at their borders to form intercalated disks. These are areas of low resistance across which electrical currents can pass.

MYOFILAMENTS

A sarcomere is made up of thick and thin filaments. The thick filaments consist of the contractile protein **myosin**. Cross-bridges extend from the myosin filaments to the thin filaments. The thin filaments include the second contractile protein, **actin**, and two regulatory proteins, **tropomyosin** and **troponin**. Tropomyosin is normally attached to each actin molecule in such a way that it partially blocks sites on actin to which the myosin cross-bridges need to bind for contraction to occur. Troponin is attached to tropomyosin and to the actin molecules.

CALCIUM INFLUX INTO THE CARDIAC MUSCLE CELL

When an action potential is delivered to the cardiac muscle cell, it passes into the cell through the T tubules, channels that are continuous with the extracellular fluid and adjacent to the intracellular sarcoplasmic reticulum. In response to the action potential, voltage-sensitive calcium channels open in the T tubules and allow a small amount of calcium to enter the cell from the extracellular fluid. This increase in calcium depolarizes the sarcoplasmic reticulum, causing many more calcium channels to open in this organelle, and a much larger amount of calcium to be released into the cytosol. The large increase in intracellular calcium then initiates muscle cell contraction.

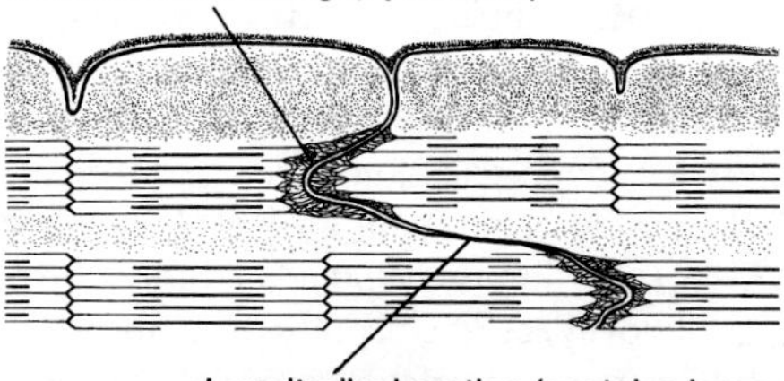

Transverse portion (myofibrillar junctions, desmosomes, and gap junctions)

Longitudinal portion (contains large gap junctions)

Figure 12-2. A sarcomere.

CARDIAC MUSCLE CONTRACTION

Once in the cytoplasm, calcium ions bind to the troponin molecules. Troponin and tropomyosin are shifted from the actin molecule, thereby allowing the myosin cross-bridges to join with the actin filaments. At this point, energy stored from a previous myosin-based reaction in which adenosine triphosphate (ATP) was split to adenosine diphosphate (ADP) plus a high-energy phosphate, is released and is used to swing the cross-bridges. This causes the myosin and actin filaments to slide past each other and muscle contraction to occur. Each contraction represents a heartbeat. Because all cardiac muscle cells are connected to each other at the edges of the sarcomeres, depolarization of one group of cardiac muscle cells spreads to neighboring cells and all cells contract as a unit.

CARDIAC MUSCLE RELAXATION

Adenosine diphosphate releases from the cross-bridge after it swings, and another ATP molecule binds to the myosin protein, causing the myosin cross-bridges to separate from actin. As long as calcium ion is available to bind troponin, this new ATP will be split, and its energy will be released when a new cross-bridge connection forms, thereby repeating the cycle and ensuring that the muscle will continue to contract. Many cross-bridge cycles and sliding of the filaments occur during one action potential. What ultimately stops the contraction is when calcium is pumped out of the muscle cell, back into the sarcoplasmic reticulum and the extracellular fluid. This is accomplished by a calcium-dependent ATPase present in the membrane of the sarcoplasmic reticulum, which again splits ATP, providing the energy needed to remove the calcium. Without calcium, tropomyosin again blocks the site on actin to which the cross-bridges bind and no further connection between myosin and actin can be made. Cross-bridge swinging (contraction) stops.

Unlike skeletal muscle, where there is always enough calcium released with each action potential to fully saturate all troponin sites and thus cause all cross-bridges to swing, in cardiac muscle less than maximal amounts of calcium are usually released with a single action potential. This means that under certain circumstances, cardiac contractile strength may be increased if necessary.

The Cardiac Cycle

Until the ventricles contract, the AV valves are open and blood flows from the atria into the relaxed, low-pressure ventricles. The aortic and pulmonary valves are closed because pressures in the aortic and pulmonary arteries are greater than in the relaxed ventricles. This allows blood to accumulate in the ventricles. This period of ventricular relaxation is called **diastole**. Blood volume in the ventricle immediately before ventricular contraction is called **end diastolic volume**.

When the ventricles contract, pressure inside the ventricles becomes greater than in the atria and the AV valves snap shut. For a brief period of time, pressure in the aorta and pulmonary arteries is still higher than in the ventricles, so the aortic and pulmonary valves remain closed. With increasing pressure in the ventricles, the aortic and pulmonary valves burst open and blood flows out of the ventricles at high speed and pressure. This period of ventricular contraction is called **systole**.

With the end of systole, the ventricles relax again. As pressure in the relaxing ventricles falls below pressures in the aortic and pulmonary arteries, the aortic and pulmonary valves snap shut. Blood entering the atria from the venae cavae and pulmonary veins causes pressure to rebuild in the atria, opening the AV valves. The cycle of filling and emptying begins again.

Arterial Pressures

The pulmonary artery and aorta are muscular vessels that expand with the surge of blood they receive from the ventricles. They hold this blood before releasing it to pass into the rest of the vascular system, not in big pulses followed by ebbs of flow, but in a steady stream. Pressure generated in the arteries at the peak of ventricular contraction is much greater than pressure in the arteries when the ventricles are relaxed. Both of these pressures are frequently measured. **Systolic pressure** is the arterial blood pressure generated during ventricular contraction. **Diastolic pressure** is the arterial blood pressure generated when the ventricles are relaxed.

Heart Sounds

Heart sounds are produced when the AV valves (mitral and semilunar valves) and the pulmonary and aortic valves snap shut. At least two (and sometimes four) heart sounds can be heard.

The first heart sound is heard when the AV valves snap shut during ventricular contraction. This sound is somewhat prolonged, low in pitch, and occurs with the onset of systole when pressure in the ventricles becomes greater than in the atria. The second heart sound is shorter and occurs when outlet valves from the ventricles, the pulmonary and aortic valves, snap shut. This happens during diastole, when the ventricles relax and pressures in the pulmonary artery and aorta—which have just received the surging blood—are greater than pressures in the right and left ventricles. Third and fourth heart sounds are sometimes heard and are related to the sound of blood reverberating in the ventricles (third sound) or entering the atria (fourth sound).

Cardiac Output

Repeated contractions of the myocardium are the heartbeats. Each beat pumps blood out of the heart. The amount of blood pumped per beat is the **stroke volume**. Cardiac output (CO), the volume of blood pumped per minute, depends on the product of the heart rate (HR; in beats per minute) and the stroke volume (SV; in milliliters of blood pumped per beat) as shown in Equation 12-1:

$$\text{CO (mL/min)} = \text{HR (beats/min)} \times \text{SV (mL/beat)} \qquad (12\text{-}1)$$

Cardiac output of an adult male ranges from 4.5 to 8 L/minute. Increased cardiac output is possible with increased heart rate or stroke volume.

The cardiac index is often calculated clinically and offers input on heart performance in an individual. The cardiac index is found by dividing the measured cardiac output by the body surface area of the individual.

CONTROL OF CARDIAC OUTPUT

Cardiac output can increase or decrease as a result of forces acting intrinsically or extrinsically to the heart, that is, with or without external input. Intrinsic control of cardiac output is determined by the length of the cardiac muscle fibers. Extrinsic control refers to the effect of neural stimulation on the heart.

INTRINSIC RELATIONSHIP BETWEEN FIBER LENGTH AND TENSION

The length of cardiac muscle fibers affects the tension they can produce because of the anatomic arrangement of muscle contractile proteins. When cardiac muscle fibers are stretched, more myosin cross-bridges can reach their actin binding sites, causing an increase in cross-bridge swinging and an increase in cardiac tension and cardiac contractility. This results in an increase in stroke volume and cardiac output (Equation 12-1). Increased stretch of the myofibrils occurs when there is increased filling of the heart. This means that the tension that is produced by the heart is proportional to the volume of blood in the heart immediately before ventricular contraction: the end-diastolic volume. Because of this response, the heart has reserve capacity to pump more forcefully when the volume of blood flow is increased, for example, as occurs with exercise and volume loading.

Because an increase in venous return will increase end-diastolic volume, the length-tension relationship of the heart ensures that *under most conditions*, increased blood flow into the heart will be matched by increased blood pumped out. This serves to return the end-diastolic volume back toward normal, making this response typically of short duration. The length-tension relationship of a normal heart under nonstimulated control conditions is shown in the lower curve of Figure 12-3. As shown, the resting heart has fibers stretched to a degree less than that required to produce maximum tension. This intrinsic response of the heart to its own muscle fiber stretch is called **Starling's**

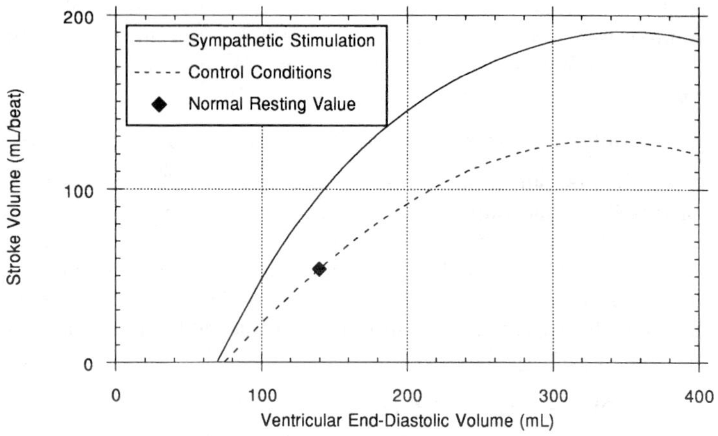

Figure 12-3. Length tension cure.

law of the heart, after the physiologist who first described it. Note that, unlike the skeletal muscle length-tension curve, the normal heart does not fall off the curve at higher fiber length.

The words "under most conditions" in the preceding paragraph refer to the fact that in damaged hearts, overstretch of the ventricles does not improve contractility, and the heart cannot pump out the extra blood, and thus continues to overfill and overstretch. This situation is characteristic of heart failure described later in this chapter.

A second reason why the stretch of cardiac muscle fibers determines cardiac output is that with increased venous return, the wall of the right atrium is stretched. This stretch causes an increased firing rate of the SA node and an increased heart rate of up to 20%. This increase in heart rate, coupled with an increase in stroke volume as a result of extra filling, can dramatically increase cardiac output. However, as mentioned earlier, because an increase in end-diastolic volume increases stroke volume, the intrinsic response to excess volume is usually temporary.

EXTRINSIC CONTROL OF CARDIAC OUTPUT

Heart rate and stroke volume are affected by the sympathetic and parasympathetic nervous systems and by circulating hormones.

Sympathetic nerves travel in the thoracic spinal nerve tracts to the SA node and release the neurotransmitter norepinephrine. Norepinephrine binds to specific receptors called β_1 adrenergic receptors, present on the cells of the SA node. On binding, activation of a second messenger system causes increased firing rate of the node, leading to an increase in heart rate. The heart rate is decreased if the activation of the sympathetic nerves and the release of norepinephrine are reduced. An increase or decrease in the heart rate is called a positive or negative **chronotropic** effect.

Sympathetic nerves also innervate cells throughout the myocardium, causing an increase in the force of each contraction (i.e., the contractility) at any given muscle fiber length. This causes an increase in stroke volume and is called a positive **inotropic** effect, as shown by the upper curve in Figure 12-3.

Parasympathetic nerves travel to the SA node and throughout the heart through the vagus nerve. Parasympathetic nerves release the neurotransmitter acetylcholine, which slows the rate of depolarization of the SA node and leads to a decrease in heart rate—a negative chronotropic effect. Parasympathetic stimulation to other sites in the myocardium appears to reduce contractility and therefore stroke volume, producing a negative inotropic effect.

Hormonal control of cardiac output mainly involves the adrenal medulla, an extension of the sympathetic nervous system. With sympathetic stimulation, the adrenal medulla releases norepinephrine and epinephrine into the circulation. These hormones travel to the heart and produce positive chronotropic and inotropic responses.

Arteries and Veins

All blood vessels except the capillaries are composed of three layers: the tunica adventitia, the tunica media, and the tunica intima.

The tunica adventitia is the outermost layer of the blood vessels, away from the lumen of the tube. It is primarily connective tissue and provides the vessels with physical support.

The tunica media is the middle layer of the vessel and is composed of vascular smooth muscle. This layer always has some basal tone, or tension, which can be increased or decreased. An increase in tension of the tunica media results in constriction of the vessel and a narrowing of its lumen. This increases the resistance to blood flow through the vessel. Relaxation of the smooth muscle causes dilation of the vessel and decreases the resistance to flow. Increases or decreases in the radius of the vessels occur through neural, hormonal, and local mediators of blood flow. Because of their capacity to change their resistance through contraction or relaxation of the smooth muscle, the arterioles in particular are called the **resistance vessels** of the circulatory system.

The third layer of the blood vessels is the tunica intima, the innermost layer. This single-cell layer is made up of endothelial cells and is surrounded on the outside by a basement membrane.

SPECIAL CHARACTERISTICS OF VEINS

The veins, although composed of the tunicae adventitia, media, and intima, have much less smooth muscle than the arteries and arterioles. They are thin vessels that can easily expand to accommodate large volumes of blood and are easily collapsed. Because of their capacity to hold large volumes of blood, the veins are called **capacitance vessels** of the circulatory system. This reservoir of venous blood can be called on in times of need when blood volume or pressure is low.

One-way valves are located periodically in the veins. These allow blood to proceed toward the heart, but not back the other way. Blood is returned to the heart through the veins as a result of the pressure gradient that exists between the veins and the heart. Surrounding skeletal muscles contribute to returning venous blood to the heart by squeezing the veins as the muscles contract. The valves prevent the blood squeezed up toward the heart from falling back down when the muscles relax. If one stands perfectly still for a long period of time, blood pools in the feet and ankles.

Capillaries

The capillaries are composed of endothelial cells. The diameter of the capillaries is 4 to 9 μm, barely large enough for a red blood cell to flow through. Lipid-soluble substances, such as oxygen and carbon dioxide, diffuse out of the capillary by passing across the endothelial cells. Substances that are not lipid soluble, such as small ions and glucose, may diffuse between the endothelial cells through intercellular clefts or pores. The exchange of oxygen and carbon dioxide, the supply of nutrients, and the removal of metabolic wastes all occur as a result of diffusion across the single-cell capillary.

The diameter of the capillary pores is smaller than the diameter of the plasma proteins and red blood cells. Because neither is lipid soluble, proteins and red cells are prohibited from moving out of the vascular system into the interstitial space.

PRECAPILLARY SPHINCTER

Immediately proximal to the capillaries are the the meta-arterioles, which deliver blood to the capillaries through a precapillary sphincter. The precapillary sphincter is a smooth muscle fiber encircling the entrance to the capillary. This fiber is not innervated by nerves, but responds to hormonal and local mediators of blood flow.

BULK FLOW ACROSS THE CAPILLARY

Bulk flow is the movement of a fluid as a result of a pressure gradient from high to low. In the vascular system, fluid moves back and forth from the capillary into or out of the interstitial fluid. Interstitial fluid is a plasma-like filtrate surrounding all cells. It is a vast volume and can store fluid in times of high plasma volume, or resupply the vascular system in times of plasma loss.

There are four forces affecting the bulk flow of fluid across a capillary into the interstitial space. They include capillary pressure, interstitial hydrostatic pressure, plasma colloid osmotic pressure, and interstitial fluid colloid osmotic pressure.

Capillary pressure is the remainder of the mean arterial pressure generated by the heart. For most capillaries, this pressure averages approximately 18 mmHg over the length of the capillary (see Fig. 12-4), with pressure at the arteriolar end significantly greater than the pressure at the venous end. Capillary pressure is a reflection of mean blood pressure. Therefore, if blood pressure increases, capillary pressure increases. If blood pressure decreases, capillary pressure decreases. Capillary pressure favors filtration of plasma out of the capillary into the interstitial space.

Interstitial hydrostatic pressure is the pressure exerted by fluid in the interstitial space. Interstitial hydrostatic pressure is primarily caused by water. If positive, it opposes filtration of plasma out of the capillary; if negative, it draws fluid out of the capillary. Recent research suggests that the pressure is negative in most tissues, averaging approximately 3 mmHg. In some tissues, it may be positive and oppose filtration.

Plasma colloid osmotic pressure refers to osmotic pressure exerted by plasma proteins. Plasma colloid pressure opposes filtration of plasma out of the capillary. This pressure develops when water is pushed out of the capillary by the hydrostatic pressure and the proteins are too large and too charged to follow. The concentration of protein left behind increases. As a large, nonsoluble particle increases in concentration, the osmotic pressure it exerts increases. This pressure serves to draw water back into the capillary. Plasma colloid osmotic pressure in most capillaries averages approximately 28 mmHg.

Interstitial fluid colloid osmotic pressure is normally a small force. Few proteins escape across the capillary into the interstitial compartment. Those that do are rapidly taken up into vessels of the lymph

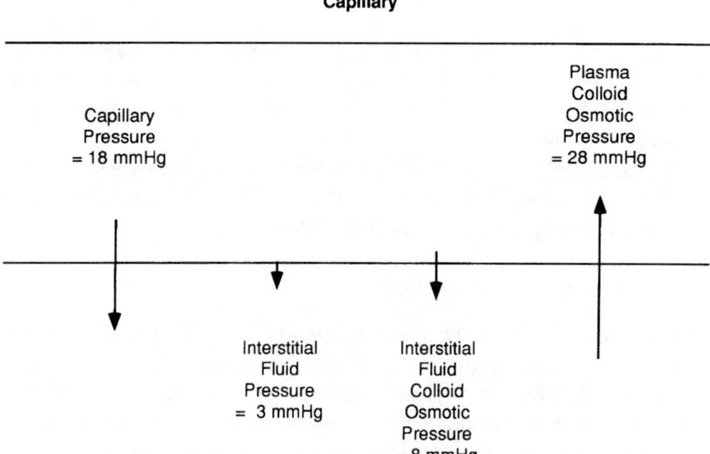

Figure 12-4. Forces of filtration and reabsorption across a capillary.

system. The lymph vessels return the proteins to the bloodstream by delivering them into the vena cava and the right atrium. Interstitial fluid colloid osmotic pressure averages approximately 8 mmHg.

Adding up the forces, filtration (18 mmHg + 3 mmHg + 8 mmHg) nearly balances reabsorption (28 mmHg) and little net movement of fluid across the capillary occurs (see Fig. 12-4). Extra fluid in the interstitial space is reabsorbed by the lymph flow.

Blood Flow

Blood travels in the vascular system by bulk flow; the movement of a fluid through a tube is based on the pressure difference between one end of the tube and the other. The pressure of the blood as it leaves the heart (P1) minus the pressure in a downstream vessel (P2), divided by the resistance offered by the blood vessels (R), determines the blood flow (F) through the vascular system, as expressed in Equation 12-2:

$$F = (P1 - P2)/R \tag{12-2}$$

BLOOD PRESSURE

Pressure at the beginning of the aorta is generated by the left ventricle. This pressure varies between approximately 120 mmHg during systole and 80 mmHg during diastole. The average, or mean, blood pressure is a pressure between systolic and diastolic. Because diastole lasts longer than systole, average blood pressure equals approximately 40% of systolic pressure plus 60% of diastolic pressure.

As blood moves through the large and small arteries, some pressure is lost. Much more is lost as blood traverses the arterioles and capillaries. By the time blood flow has reached the capillary, blood pressure at the arteriole end of the capillary, for most capillary beds, has decreased to approximately 35 mmHg. With movement through the capillary, this pressure decreases to 10 mmHg at the venous end, resulting in a mean blood pressure in the capillary of approximately 18 mmHg. By the time the blood reaches the vena cava, the pressure is zero.

Thus, the pressure gradient affecting flow is large between the aorta and the vena cava (90 mmHg to 0 mmHg). This is the force that drives the blood through the systemic circulation.

RESISTANCE

Resistance to flow through a vessel depends on the length of the vessel, viscosity of the fluid, and radius of the vessel. In the body, the length of the blood vessels is essentially fixed. Although potentially variable, blood viscosity is also fixed. Therefore, when discussing resistance to blood flow in the vascular system, one usually can consider only the radius of the blood vessels. Because of the dynamics of flow through a tube, a small decrease in the radius causes an enormous increase in resistance to flow. This is true both for blood flowing through a blood vessel and for water flowing through a hose or a pipe.

The smaller the vessel, the greater the effect narrowing that vessel has on blood flow. Varying the radius of the large arteries does not significantly affect blood flow. Likewise, because the veins are so distensible, they offer little resistance to flow. Instead, resistance to blood flow is determined by the radius of the arterioles. As mentioned earlier, this makes the arterioles the resistance vessels of the cardiovascular system.

Narrowing the arterioles decreases blood flow downstream into the capillaries and veins fed by that arteriole and backs up the blood upstream. Because blood pressure depends on blood flow, narrowing arterioles decrease blood pressure downstream and increase blood pressure upstream.

In contrast, if the arterioles are dilated, flow increases, resulting in increased downstream pressure and decreased pressure upstream of the arterioles. Control of arteriole diameter is an intricate balance between local effects and nervous and hormonal stimulation.

CAPILLARY RESISTANCE TO BLOOD FLOW

The capillaries offer a great deal of resistance to blood flow because they are so narrow. However, because they have no smooth muscle their diameter cannot be varied, so changes in capillary diameter cannot cause an increase or decrease in blood flow. The meta-arterioles immediately preceeding the capillaries do change diameter and affect capillary blood flow. Because of the extensive area that all the capillaries cover, blood flow through them is slow, which allows ample time for diffusion of oxygen and carbon dioxide.

TOTAL PERIPHERAL RESISTANCE

Resistance in the systemic vascular system is referred to as total peripheral resistance (TPR). It is impossible to directly measure resistance. Resistance in the cardiovascular system is calculated by measuring flow and pressure. The resistance equals pressure divided by flow. Resistance to flow in the pulmonary vascular system is much less than in the systemic system.

Mean Arterial Blood Pressure

From the previous discussion it should be apparent that in the vascular system it is difficult to discuss blood flow without referring to the blood pressure. The variable regulated by the body, and usually measured clinically, is the systemic arterial blood pressure (BP). Equation 12-3 is used to describe the variables controlling systemic mean arterial blood pressure:

$$BP = CO \times TPR \qquad (12\text{-}3)$$

where, for the cardiovascular system,

- BP is the mean arterial blood pressure,
- CO is the cardiac output (which equals HR × SV). Note: CO replaces F from Equation 12-2.
- TPR is the total peripheral resistance.

CONTROL OF BLOOD PRESSURE

Blood pressure control depends on sensors that continually measure blood pressure and send the information to the brain. The brain integrates all incoming information and responds by sending efferent (outgoing) stimulation to the heart and vasculature through the autonomic nerves. Various hormones and locally released chemicals add to the control of blood pressure.

SENSORS

Blood pressure is continually monitored by sensors called baroreceptors (pressure receptors). There are baroreceptors in the carotid artery arch (in the neck) and in the aortic arch where the aorta leaves the heart. These sensors are called the carotid and aortic baroreceptors. There are baroreceptors located in the arterioles supplying the kidney nephrons. Receptors in both atria and in the pulmonary artery also respond to changes in pressure. Because these receptors are in low-pressure areas of the vasculature, they are called low-pressure receptors.

All baroreceptors act as stretch receptors that respond to changes in blood pressure. Their stretch increases with increased blood pressure. This causes afferent neurons receiving information from the receptors to increase their rate of firing. These neurons travel to the brain and innervate the cardiovascular center in the brain. A decrease in blood pressure decreases the stretch of the baroreceptors, which reduces the firing of the afferent nerves innervating the cardiovascular center.

INTEGRATING CENTER FOR THE CONTROL OF BLOOD PRESSURE

The cardiovascular center in the brain is part of the reticular formation and is located in the lower medulla and pons. The signals concerning blood pressure are integrated here. If a change in blood pressure has occurred, the cardiovascular center activates the autonomic nervous system, leading to changes in sympathetic and parasympathetic stimulation to the heart and sympathetic stimulation to the entire vascular system. Resistance of the vasculature is altered and blood flow and blood pressure are affected.

EFFERENT NEURAL INNERVATION OF THE VASCULAR SYSTEM

Sympathetic nerves stimulate heart rate and contractility by binding to β_1 receptors in the heart. Parasympathetic nerves decrease heart rate by binding to cholinergic receptors. In addition, sympathetic nerves traveling in the thoracic and upper lumbar spinal tracts influence blood pressure by exerting control over virtually the entire peripheral vascular system (except the capillaries) through innervation of the tunica media (the smooth muscle).

At most blood vessels, sympathetic nerves release norepinephrine, which binds to specific receptors on the smooth muscle cells, called alpha (α) receptors. Stimulation of the α receptors causes the smooth muscle to contract, constricting the vessel, which increases TPR and therefore increases blood pressure.

Blood vessels supplying skeletal muscle have a different type of receptor, called β_2 receptors, that, when stimulated by norepinephrine, cause the vessels to relax. It appears that this sympathetic vasodilatory response plays a significant role only in the anticipatory response to exercise, perhaps serving to prime the skeletal muscle with oxygen and nutrient support before exercise onset.

Skeletal muscle blood vessels also possess receptors for acetylcholine. These receptors are called muscarinic receptors and do not appear to be innervated by parasympathetic neurons. However, they respond to acetylcholine released by certain sympathetic cholinergic neurons. These neurons also supply the vascular smooth muscle in skeletal muscle and cause relaxation of the vessels, thus increasing blood flow through these vessels.

HORMONAL CONTROL OF THE VASCULAR SYSTEM

There are several hormones that control the resistance of the vascular system. These hormones are released directly in response to changes in blood pressure, in response to neural stimulation, or both.

Norepinephrine and Epinephrine

Norepinephrine and epinephrine are released from the adrenal medulla in response to activation of the sympathetic nervous system. Both substances act like norepinephrine released from nerve terminals and bind to a receptors to cause vasoconstriction, or to β_2 receptors to cause vasodilation of arterioles supplying skeletal muscles. Norepinephrine and epinephrine also bind to β_1 receptors and increase heart rate.

RENIN-ANGIOTENSIN SYSTEM

Changes in blood pressure are sensed by the renal baroreceptors. If blood pressure is high, release of the hormone **renin** is decreased. If blood pressure decreases, renin release increases. Renin release is also stimulated by sympathetic nerves to the kidney. Renin controls the production of another hormone, angiotensin II.

Renin circulates in the blood and acts as an enzyme to convert the protein angiotensinogen to angiotensin I. Angiotensin I is a 10 amino acid protein, which is immediately split by angiotensin-converting enzyme into the 8 amino acid peptide, angiotensin II. Angiotensin-converting enzyme is the same enzyme that breaks down (and inactivates) the vasodilator hormone bradykinin. Blocking the action of angiotensin-converting enzyme blocks the production of angiotensin II and the breakdown of bradykinin.

Angiotensin II is a powerful vasoconstrictor that primarily causes constriction of the small arterioles. This causes an increase in resistance to blood flow and an increase in blood pressure. The increase in blood pressure then acts in a negative feedback manner to reduce the stimulus for further renin release. Angiotensin II also circulates to the adrenal gland and causes cells of the adrenal cortex to synthesize another hormone, aldosterone.

Aldosterone

Aldosterone circulates to the kidney and causes cells of the distal tubule to increase sodium reabsorption. Under many circumstances, reabsorption of water follows that of sodium, leading to an increase in plasma volume. An increase in plasma volume increases stroke volume, and hence cardiac output. It also causes increased blood pressure.

Renin-Angiotensin-Aldosterone Feedback Cycle

It should be emphasized that the stimuli causing the release of renin—decreased blood pressure and decreased plasma sodium concentration—are reversed by the actions of angiotensin II and aldosterone. This is an excellent example of a negative feedback cycle.

Antidiuretic Hormone

Antidiuretic hormone (ADH), or vasopressin, is released from the posterior pituitary in response to increased plasma osmolality (decreased water concentration) or decreased blood pressure.

Antidiuretic hormone is a potent vasoconstrictor with the potential to increase blood pressure by increasing the resistance to blood flow. Under all circumstances, except perhaps during severe hemorrhage, levels of circulating ADH are too low to affect the arterioles. However, ADH controls the reabsorption of water across the collecting ducts of the kidney back into the bloodstream. This effect has a clear influence on blood pressure by increasing plasma volume and therefore cardiac output. Without ADH, water does not follow sodium reabsorption in the kidney and severe dehydration may occur. Reabsorption of water in response to ADH reduces stimuli (increased plasma osmolality and decreased blood pressure) for ADH release.

Atrial Natriuretic Peptide

Atrial natriuretic peptide (ANP) is a hormone released from cells of the right atrium in response to an increase in blood volume. ANP acts on the kidney to increase the excretion of sodium ion (natriuresis). Because water will follow sodium in the urine, ANP serves to decrease blood volume and blood pressure.

SUMMARY OF BLOOD PRESSURE CONTROL

With a decrease in blood pressure, baroreceptor information is transmitted to the cardiovascular center in the brain. This causes a stimulation of sympathetic output to the heart and vascular system, increasing heart rate and TPR. Parasympathetic output is decreased, also increasing heart rate. Renin release increases, causing increased angiotensin II, which directly increases TPR and aldosterone synthesis. Increased aldosterone increases sodium reabsorption, and in the presence of ADH, water reabsorption. Increased plasma volume, stroke volume, and cardiac output result. Capillary pressure decreases directly with blood pressure and indirectly from sympathetic constriction of the arteriole feeding the capillary. This serves to decrease filtration of fluid out of the capillary. All of these responses serve to increase blood pressure toward normal, by increasing heart rate, stroke volume, and TPR (Fig. 12-5).

In contrast, if blood pressure increases, baroreceptor responses cause a decrease in sympathetic stimulation to the heart and vascular smooth muscle, and heart rate and TPR decrease. Increased parasympathetic stimulation to the heart contributes to the decrease in heart rate. There is a decrease in renin and ADH release, reducing TPR and plasma volume. ANP release increases. All these responses serve to decrease blood pressure toward normal.

Autoregulation

In general, blood pressure is controlled through neural and hormonal influences. However, individual tissues have mechanisms that regulate their own blood flow. This is accomplished by local vasodilation or vasoconstriction of meta-arterioles and precapillary sphincters. This local control of blood flow is called **autoregulation**, and is the means by which some organs can maintain constant blood flow over a wide range of blood pressure, from approximately 70 to 180 mmHg.

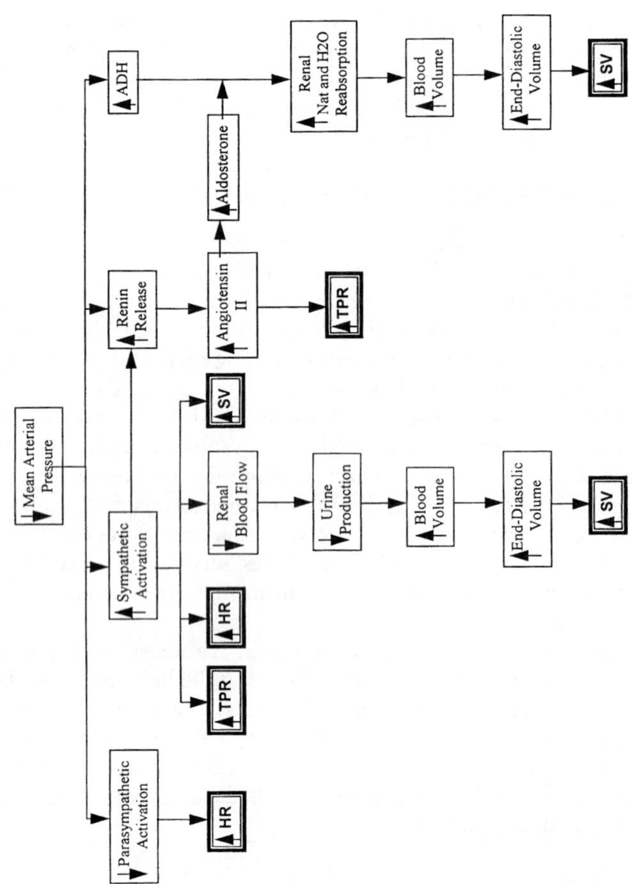

12-5. Flow diagram—reflex response to a fall in blood pressure.

THEORIES OF AUTOREGULATION

There are several theories to explain local control of blood flow. The most widely accepted theory suggests that chemical mediators are released by metabolizing cells that bind to meta-arterioles or precapillary sphincters, causing them to open or shut to blood flow.

Suggested chemical mediators that control local blood flow include adenosine, a metabolite of ATP, carbon dioxide, histamine, lactic acid, potassium ions, and hydrogen ions. All of these substances except histamine are byproducts of metabolism. Histamine is released by mast cells present throughout the interstitial space in response to immune stimulation or local injury. Adenosine appears to particularly regulate local blood flow in the heart.

An alternate theory concerning local control suggests that the meta-arterioles and capillary sphincters sense an oxygen or nutrient deficit that causes them to relax, thereby increasing blood flow to the surrounding cells.

OTHER CHEMICAL MEDIATORS INFLUENCING BLOOD FLOW

Various other chemicals are released by the blood vessels or by mediators of inflammation or healing, which affect blood flow to an area.

Nitric Oxide

Endothelial cells of the small arteries and arterioles respond to the binding of various vasoactive substances such as acetylcholine with the production of the vasodilator nitric oxide (previously called endothelial-derived relaxing factor). Nitric oxide diffuses through endothelial cells to underlying smooth muscle cells, causing relaxation of the smooth muscle. Nitric oxide release also occurs with increased blood flow through a vessel, allowing local dilation of the microvasculature to be matched by dilation of the small arteries and arterioles.

Serotonin

Serotonin (5-hydroxytryptamine) is primarily released by platelets drawn to an area of injury or inflammation. Effects of serotonin may be vasodilatory or vasoconstricting, depending on the site of release. Serotonin's ability to vasoconstrict and decrease blood flow appears to be one mechanism whereby platelets control or reduce bleeding.

Bradykinin

Bradykinin, like all members of the kinin family, is a small polypeptide that acts as a potent vasodilator of arterioles and increases capillary permeability.

Bradykinin is produced in the plasma or interstitial fluid by enzymatic splitting of a serum globulin in response to vascular or tissue injury or inflammation. The half-life of bradykinin (how long it is present in the circulation or interstitial fluid) is short. It is rapidly digested by angiotensin-converting enzyme or another enzyme, carboxypeptidase.

The effects of bradykinin are increased local blood flow, increased capillary permeability, and decreased vascular resistance. These effects allow delivery of mediators of the inflammatory and immune systems to a site of injury. Blockage of angiotensin-converting enzyme by various pharmaceutical agents prolongs the half-life of bradykinin and its effects.

Prostaglandins

There are many different groups of prostaglandins. Some cause dilation of the vascular system and some cause constriction. Prostaglandins are derived from arachidonic acid, which is present in all cell membranes and released with tissue injury. Prostaglandins work to control local blood flow. They may circulate to affect distant cells.

One main group of prostaglandins, those of the E series, cause local vasodilation and increased blood flow, making them important mediators of inflammation. Prostaglandins of the I series, especially PGI_2, called prostacyclin, also are vasodilatory. PGI_2 inhibits platelet aggregation and blood clotting. Thromboxane A_2 is an important prostaglandin that causes vasoconstriction and blood clotting.

Generally, prostaglandin synthesis can be blocked by aspirin and nonsteroidal anti-inflammatory drugs (NSAIDs). Low concentration of aspirin particularly appears to block production of thromboxane A_2. Glucocorticoids released from the adrenal cortex block prostaglandin synthesis and are considered potent anti-inflammatory agents.

Lymph Flow

The lymph system consists of closed-end vessels that course through almost the entire interstitial fluid space. Lymph fluid is derived from interstitial fluid and is therefore very similar in composition to plasma.

The lymph system consists of small capillaries that drain into larger lymph vessels. Like blood vessels, these larger vessels are composed of smooth muscle and endothelial cells. Lymph from the lower body flows up the thoracic duct and empties into the left jugular and subclavian veins. Lymph flow from the left arm, shoulder, and left side of the head travels in the thoracic duct and then into the left jugular and subclavian arteries. Lymph flow from the right arm and right side of the neck and head empty into the right jugular and subclavian veins.

Movement of lymph results from contraction of the smooth muscle lining the lymph vessels in response to its stretch, and the pumping action of the surrounding skeletal muscles. Valves present in lymph vessels prevent backflow.

ROLE OF THE LYMPH SYSTEM

The lymph system has three essential roles in the body, all of which depend on the greater permeability of lymph capillaries compared to blood capillaries.

Lymph capillaries retrieve any proteins that escape from the capillaries into the interstitial fluid. These proteins move easily into lymph vessels and are then returned to the blood circulation through the thoracic duct. This is essential because it allows interstitial colloid osmotic pressure to remain low. If proteins were allowed to accumulate in the interstitial space, interstitial colloid osmotic pressure would increase. This would result in increased forces favoring filtration into the interstitial fluid, which would soon cause massive interstitial edema. Death of the individual could occur from circulatory collapse.

The second essential role played by the lymph system is in the absorption of fats from the small intestine. In the small intestine, fats and fat-soluble vitamins are absorbed into small lymph vessels called lacteals, and are then delivered to the general circulation. Fat and the fat-soluble vitamins are required for life.

The third essential role played by the lymph system is in immune function. Because of the high permeability of the lymph capillaries, bacteria and other microorganisms enter the lymph system from infected areas and are transported to and through lymph nodes where they become trapped and removed from the circulation. Lymph nodes are an intertwining meshwork of vessels filled with tissue macrophages and T cells; bringing bacteria and other cellular debris to the lymph nodes allows the immune and inflammatory cells an opportunity to protect the host from widespread infection. Lymph nodes are spaced intermittently along the lymph vessels.

Fetal Circulation

There are several major differences between fetal circulation and the circulation of infants, children, and adults. While in utero, a fetus does not receive oxygen through its own lungs. Rather, maternal oxygen is delivered across the placenta into the umbilical vein. The umbilical vein delivers oxygen-rich blood to the right side of the fetal heart through the vena cava. Because of the maternal source of oxygen, the fetal lungs and most of the blood vessels supplying them are mostly collapsed, causing high resistance to blood flow through the fetal lungs, especially when compared to flow through the fetal systemic circulation, which offers low resistance because of the wide-open vessels of the placenta.

STRUCTURAL CHARACTERISTICS OF FETAL CIRCULATION

In the fetus, there are two connections (shunts) that exist and take advantage of the maternal oxygen source and the high resistance of the pulmonary circulation. The first of these connections is an opening between the right atrium and the left atrium, called the **foramen ovale**. Because resistance is so high in the pulmonary circuit leaving the right ventricle, fetal blood travels in the direction of lower resistance: from right atrium to left through the foramen ovale. Because blood entering the vena cava in the fetus has already been oxygenated by passage through the placenta, this right to left shunting is an economic move. Well-oxygenated blood is delivered to the systemic (left-side) circulation without needing to send blood through the collapsed, nonfunctioning pulmonary system.

Another shunting system between the right and left sides of circulation in the fetus is a vascular connection between the pulmonary artery and the aorta. This connection is called the **ductus arteriosus**. It allows oxygenated blood leaving the right side of the heart to bypass the fetal lungs and flow directly into the low resistance of the systemic circulation.

Newborn Circulation

With birth, the situation changes dramatically and suddenly. The newborn is no longer supplied with oxygen from the placenta because the low-resistance vessels of the placenta are no longer connected to the fetus. At birth, the newborn separates from the placenta, fluid in the lungs is squeezed out, and the newborn takes a deep breath, opening up the lungs and the blood vessels flowing through them. Immediately at birth, resistance of the pulmonary circulation falls while resistance of the systemic circulation increases. Blood flow no longer shunts right to left through the foramen ovale or the ductus arteriosus because those directions now offer higher resistance to flow. These shunt passages normally begin to close within a few hours after birth.

Tests of Cardiovascular Functioning

THE ELECTROCARDIOGRAM

The electrocardiogram (ECG) is the measurement of the electrical currents of the heart. Contraction of the atria and ventricles results from action potentials occurring simultaneously in all muscle cells of the atria and then all muscle cells of the ventricles. Electrodes placed in specific locations on the body can detect these action potential currents. The currents can then be graphically displayed and interpreted. The following is a brief overview of the currents measured by the ECG.

There are three currents produced in the normal ECG, as shown in Figure 12-6. The P wave corresponds to atrial depolarization. The QRS complex (beginning of Q wave to end of S wave) corresponds to depolarization of the ventricles. The T wave corresponds to repolarization of the ventricles. Repolarization of the atria occurs during the

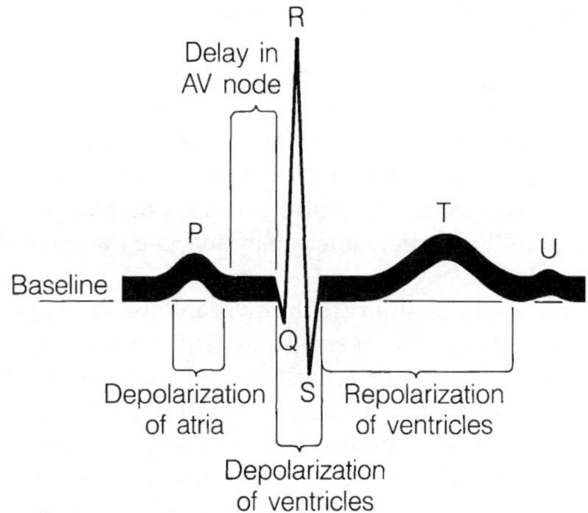

Figure 12-6. The electrocardiogram.

QRS complex and is nondistinguishable. Normal sinus rhythm is the expected rhythm of the heart driven by the SA node and passed along the normal, intact conduction system.

Patterns of the Electrocardiogram

Several patterns in the normal ECG stand out. First, the pattern of the three waves repeats itself with each beat. A time scale is usually shown on the recording, allowing one to determine the heart rate by counting any one of the waves over time. The P wave or the QRS complex can be counted.

Second, the QRS complex always follows the P wave in a normal beating pattern because the atria undergo an action potential and contract first. Their action potential subsequently spreads to the ventricles. The time between the end of the P wave and the beginning of the QRS complex reflects the time during which the action potential is delayed at the AV node.

Third, the size of the atrial depolarization, as measured by the height of the P wave, is less than the depolarization of the ventricles, as measured by the height of the QRS complex. This reflects the much greater muscle mass of the ventricles compared to the atria. The ventricular depolarization is a rapid spike, as shown by the narrow displacement of the QRS complex, indicating that conduction throughout the ventricle is rapid, and the entire ventricle contracts as one quick-firing unit. Increased horizontal spread of the QRS complex occurs with prolonged conduction of the electrical impulse through the ventricles, indicating ventricular hypertrophy. A bizarre QRS complex may indicate cardiac cell death.

MEASUREMENT OF CARDIAC ENZYMES

When cardiac muscle cells die during a myocardial infarct (MI), they release their intracellular contents. Specific proteins and enzymes normally present only inside cardiac cells can be measured in the blood. This allows one to accurately diagnose the existence and frequently the extent of myocardial cell death. Because different enzyme levels are elevated at different times after infarction, the timing of the infarct can be determined.

Proteins released after injury to the myocardial cells include myoglobin, normally found only in skeletal and cardiac muscle cells, and the cardiac specific contractile proteins, troponin T and troponin 1. Newly developed bedside laboratory kits capable of qualitatively measuring the presence of serum troponin molecules within minutes of a suspected infarct, have the capacity to revolutionize early detection of an MI. Enzymes released with cell death include myocardial creatine kinase (CK MB), the gold standard for determination of an MI, lactic acid dehydrogenase (LDH), and serum glutamic oxaloacetic transaminase (SGOT). The plasma concentration of these markers vary depending on the time of injury and the extent of the cell damage.

STRESS TESTING

Cardiac stress testing involves having an individual exercise up to his or her maximal capacity, while observers monitor physical symptoms and the ECG. In a simple exercise stress test, the patient is asked to either walk on a treadmill or ride an exercise bike. The pattern of the ECG is observed for alterations in rhythm, the presence of AV blocks, and evidence of ST-segment changes indicative of hypoxia. The onset of physical symptoms, such as chest pain and extreme shortness of breath, are monitored. Sometimes, an intravenous infusion of a radiolabeled isotope that has specific cardiac affinity is given during the exercise to monitor myocardial perfusion. An isotope commonly used is radioactive thallium-201. This isotope can be substituted for potassium by cells and is infused during the peak portion of the exercise test. After a short delay, a nuclear scan of the heart is performed. Areas of the heart that have been perfused by blood will be labeled with the thallium. Areas of the heart that are poorly or not perfused by blood during the exercise test will be identified as "cold spots," that is, without radiolabel. If the ischemia is temporary, the cold spots will disappear over time. Thallium-201 may also be used alone in patients unable to exercise.

ECHOCARDIOGRAPHY

Echocardiography is the use of ultrasound to visualize the heart. This test is highly sensitive, noninvasive, and provides visual information on the size and movement of the heart chambers, the function of the valves, and the flow of blood through the heart.

CARDIAC CATHERIZATION

In cardiac catherization, a flexible tube (catheter) is inserted through a peripheral vein (femoral or brachial) into the right side of the heart, or through a peripheral artery (femoral or brachial) into the left side of the heart. Through the catheter, the chambers of the heart can be visualized and chamber pressures and oxygen content measured. A radiolabeled dye may be injected through the catheter, and the ability of the dye to move through the heart chambers and vessels may be monitored using radiograph techniques. Valve movement can be observed.

PATHOPHYSIOLOGIC CONCEPTS

Thrombus

A thrombus is a blood clot that can develop anywhere in the vascular system, causing a narrowing of the vessel. With a decrease in vessel diameter, blood flow can be occluded (reduced or totally blocked). A thrombus can develop from any injury to the vessel wall because endothelial cell injury draws platelets and other mediators of inflammation to the area. Many of these substances stimulate clotting and activation of the coagulation cascade. Thrombus formation can occur when blood flow through a vessel is sluggish, which is why most thrombi develop in the low-pressure venous side of the circulation where platelets and clotting factors can accumulate and adhere to vessel walls.

Embolus

An embolus is a substance that travels in the bloodstream from a primary site to a secondary site, becomes trapped in the vessels at the secondary site, and causes blood flow obstruction. Most emboli are blood clots (thromboemboli) that have broken off from their primary site (usually deep leg veins). Other sources of emboli include fat released during the break of a long bone or produced in response to any physical trauma, and an amniotic fluid embolus that enters maternal circulation during the intense pressure gradients generated during labor contractions. Air and displaced tumor cells also may act as emboli to obstruct flow.

Usually emboli get trapped in the first capillary network they encounter. For instance, emboli traveling from deep leg veins are delivered in the venous system to the vena cava and the right side of the heart. From there, they enter the pulmonary artery and arterioles, encounter pulmonary capillaries, and become trapped. Arterial emboli usually develop in the heart, from a dislodged thrombus or as a result of an MI (heart attack) that causes the blood flowing through the heart to become sluggish, thereby increasing the risk of clotting. Irregular heart beats (palpitations) may also affect blood flow through the heart and cause embolus formation. Emboli from the heart can become trapped in the coronary vessels or any of the organs downstream, including the brain, kidneys, and lower extremities.

Aneurysm

An aneurysm is a dilation of the arterial wall caused by a congenital or developed weakness in the wall. Weakness in the wall may develop as a result of an infection, from trauma to the wall, or more commonly, from lesions produced by atherosclerosis. Aneurysms may burst with increased pressure, leading to massive internal hemorrhage.

Alterations in Capillary Forces of Filtration or Reabsorption

Occasionally, forces favoring filtration from the capillary into the interstitial fluid are greater than forces favoring reabsorption of fluid out of the interstitial fluid. The result is net filtration. Net filtration across the capillary results in interstitial edema.

The opposite occurs when forces favoring reabsorption of fluid from the interstitial space into the capillary are greater than those favoring filtration. This results in net reabsorption, which leads to increased plasma volume, stroke volume, and cardiac output. Blood pressure may be increased significantly.

CAUSES OF INCREASED CAPILLARY FILTRATION

Causes of increased capillary filtration include increased capillary pressure caused by high blood pressure and increased capillary leakage caused by injury or inflammation. An increase in protein concentration in the interstitial fluid caused by increased capillary breakdown or decreased lymph flow to the area would also cause net filtration, leading to edema and swelling of the interstitial space. Similarly, decreased production or increased loss of plasma proteins would reduce the reabsorption of fluid back into the capillary. This can occur with liver disease or loss of protein in the urine.

CAUSES OF INCREASED CAPILLARY REABSORPTION

Causes of increased reabsorption of fluid from the interstitial fluid include decreased blood pressure in the capillary due to a decrease in systemic pressure or constriction of the arteriole or precapillary sphincter. Increased plasma colloid osmotic pressure also draws fluid back into the capillary. Plasma colloid osmotic pressure increases with dehydration, leading to a return of fluid from the interstitium to the plasma, which helps return plasma volume toward normal. Finally, increased interstitial fluid pressure increases reabsorption by opposing further accumulation of fluid.

Stenosis

Stenosis is a narrowing of any vessel or opening. In the cardiovascular system, stenosis of the heart valves may occur. Stenosis of any valve usually occurs as a result of a congenital defect or an inflammatory process (i.e., after rheumatic fever).

RESULTS OF CARDIAC VALVE STENOSIS

Stenosis of a cardiac valve results in the chamber upstream of the stenosis pumping more forcefully to expel its blood through the narrowed orifice. After years of this extra work, cardiac muscle can hypertrophy (increase in size). If the chamber cannot pump forcefully enough to overcome the stenosis, blood flow out of the chamber will be reduced. Because of the chamber hypertrophy and the extra work it must do to pump through the narrowed orifice, the chamber increases its oxygen consumption and energy demands. The coronary arteries supplying the muscle may be unable to supply adequate oxygen to meet this demand.

As it becomes increasingly difficult for the upstream chamber to empty against the narrowed orifice, blood may accumulate in the chamber and stretch its muscle fibers. If this is significant or prolonged, a decrease in muscle contractility can result.

EXAMPLES OF CARDIAC VALVE STENOSIS

Any cardiac valve may become stenosed. Mitral stenosis is narrowing of the valve between the left atrium and left ventricle. Aortic stenosis is narrowing of the valve between the left ventricle and the aorta. Tricuspid stenosis is narrowing of the valve between the right atrium and the right ventricle. Pulmonary stenosis is narrowing of the valve between the right ventricle and the pulmonary artery.

Valve Incompetence

An incompetent valve is when the valve does not close completely (valve regurgitation). Any of the cardiac valves may be incompetent, which would allow blood to move in both directions through a valve when the heart contracts. Each chamber may hypertrophy.

Cardiac Shunts

In the cardiovascular system, a shunt is a connection between the pulmonary vascular system and the systemic vascular system. During fetal life, shunts between the right and left sides of the heart and between the aorta and pulmonary artery are normal. After birth, any shunting across the heart or between the pulmonary and systemic circulations is abnormal.

The direction blood flows through a shunt is determined by resistance to flow in each direction. Blood will flow in the direction of least resistance.

A RIGHT-TO-LEFT SHUNT

A right-to-left shunt is the flow of blood from the right side of the heart to the left, or from the pulmonary artery to the systemic circulation. After birth, right heart and pulmonary artery blood is poorly oxygenated. Therefore, a right-to-left shunt delivers poorly oxygenated blood to the systemic circulation. A right-to-left shunt is called a **cyanotic shunt** because delivery of poorly oxygenated blood to the systemic circulation causes cyanosis (bluish tinge to the skin). This is caused by deoxygenation of hemoglobin, as described in Chapter 13.

Fatigue results because cells of the muscles, brain, and other organs are not receiving adequate delivery of oxygen and nutrients. Respiratory rate increases as the body tries to compensate for the reduced oxygenation of the blood. Individuals with a cyanotic shunt may develop clubbing of the tips of the fingers, related to poor tissue perfusion.

Pediatric Consideration

An infant with a right-to-left shunt may assume a knee-to-chest position, which increases flow through the pulmonary system and results in improved blood oxygenation. In older children, this maneuver is performed by squatting.

A LEFT-TO-RIGHT SHUNT

A left-to-right shunt is the flow of blood from the left side of the heart to the right side, or from the aorta to the pulmonary circulation. Left heart blood is well oxygenated. Therefore, a left-to-right shunt overdelivers well-oxygenated blood directly into the right side of the heart, or immediately returns the blood to the pulmonary artery and lungs. Blood going to the lungs from the left side of the heart recirculates to the left atrium and left ventricle. Because the blood is well-oxygenated, this shunt is **acyanotic**.

A left-to-right shunt can be life-threatening because of the risk of hypertrophy of pulmonary vasculature as blood is continually recirculated through the lungs. Right heart failure may develop if there is a high volume of blood entering the right side of the heart from the left side of the heart. In addition, left heart failure may develop because of continual recycling of blood back into the left side of the heart from the lungs.

Alterations in the Electrocardiogram

Many conditions result in ECG alterations. Alterations in the ECG are associated with increased or decreased rate of contraction or changes in the force of contraction.

ECTOPIC PACEMAKER

An ectopic pacemaker is a site in the heart capable of automaticity that takes over control of the heart rate from the SA node. An ectopic pacemaker may occur if the SA node begins to depolarize very slowly, or if conduction of the signal from the SA node to the AV node is blocked. Usually, cells in the AV node or conducting cells of Purkinje's fibers assume the pacemaker role.

If the SA node no longer controls the heart rate, an ECG will usually demonstrate a reduced heart rate and *ventricular depolarization that does not follow atrial depolarization.*

SINUS NODE DYSRHYTHMIA

Sinus node dysrhythmia occurs when the SA node sets the heart rate too slow (sinus bradycardia), fewer than 60 beats/minute, or too fast (sinus tachycardia), from 100 to 160 beats/minute. Sinus bradycardia may occur in a well-trained athlete. Sinus tachycardia may occur with fever or exercise.

SINUS ARRHYTHMIA

Sinus arrhythmia is an irregular rate of beating, usually varying with respiratory patterns. It is common in children and young adults.

SINUS ARREST

Sinus arrest occurs when the SA node does not depolarize and fire an action potential. This would lead to an ectopic site taking control of the heart.

ATRIAL DYSRHYTHMIAS

Atrial dysrhythmias disrupt normal contraction of the atria. They may include ectopic pacemakers or irritation of the SA node. There are several types of atrial dysrhythmias.

Premature atrial contraction (PAC) is an atrial dysrhythmia that occurs when an area of the atrium other than the SA node fires an action potential earlier than expected. This discharge may pass down to the AV node and back up the conduction fibers to the SA node. A PAC interrupts the pattern of SA node firing. The ventricles usually depolarize after a PAC, but occasionally are in a refractory period and resist depolarization.

Atrial flutter is an atrial dysrhythmia that occurs when the atria begin to contract 160 to 350 beats/minute. The ventricles may not be able to keep up. With very rapid flutter, the ventricle may beat once for every five atrial beats. On an ECG, one would see many P waves, followed by an occasional QRS complex. Atrial flutter leads to hemodynamic instability.

Atrial fibrillation is an atrial dysrhythmia that occurs when the atria beat at more than 350 (up to 600) beats/minute. Ventricular depolarizations become irregular and may not follow atrial depolarization. Ventricular filling does not totally depend on organized atrial contractions, thus blood flow in and out of the ventricles is usually sufficient to meet normal energy needs, but not high demand times such as exercise.

ATRIOVENTRICULAR BLOCKS

Blocks of action potential spread from the AV node may occur anywhere in the conducting system of Purkinje's fibers or the bundle of His. The block may cause an extra long delay between the P wave and the QRS complex, or may totally uncouple the P wave from the QRS. Blocks are described as first degree (each QRS follows a P but with an extended delay), second degree (occasional P waves never cause a QRS complex), or third degree (complete block, in which the link between the P wave and the QRS complex is lost).

BLOCKS IN VENTRICULAR CONDUCTING BRANCHES

Conduction of the electrical signal from the AV node into and throughout the ventricle proceeds first through transitional fibers that join to form the bundle of His. The bundle of His enters the ventricles and immediately separates into left and right bundle branches. These branches supply the entire heart and terminate as very fine Purkinje fibers. Interruption of the signal anywhere in any of the conducting passages results in the entire ventricle taking longer to depolarize, spreading out the QRS complex. If some areas of the myocardium are completely blocked from receiving the excitation, the ventricular beat will be awkward and inefficient. Cardiac output will decrease.

VENTRICULAR DYSRHYTHMIAS

Ventricular dysrhythmia is an alteration in ventricular beating rate. A ventricular dysrhythmia is usually a more serious problem than is atrial dysrhythmia because a ventricular dysrhythmia can directly affect cardiac output. Although an increase in heart rate can increase cardiac output, cardiac output also depends on stroke volume. An abnormally high heart rate can cause a significant decrease in stroke volume because if the heart rate increases too much, filling time for the ventricle will be inadequate. There are several types of ventricular dysrhythmia.

Premature ventricular contraction (PVC) is a ventricular dysrhythmia that occurs when an ectopic site in the ventricle depolarizes spontaneously, causing ventricular contraction. This usually occurs when an area of the ventricle becomes irritated or injured, often because of lack of oxygen. Because the PVC can occur at any time in the cardiac cycle, usually the ventricle is not completely filled with blood before contraction occurs, so stroke volume will be reduced.

Ventricular tachycardia is a ventricular dysrhythmia that occurs when the ventricle is beating at a rate of 160 to 250 beats/minute. With this degree of limited filling time, stroke volume will be reduced or nonexistent.

Ventricular fibrillation is the most extreme example of ventricular dysrhythmia and occurs when the ventricle is depolarizing so erratically and rapidly that it does not contract at all as a unit, but rather quivers ineffectively. Cardiac output is zero and pulse and blood pressure are nonexistent. Without intervention, death will occur.

Some ECG changes are shown in Figure 12-7.

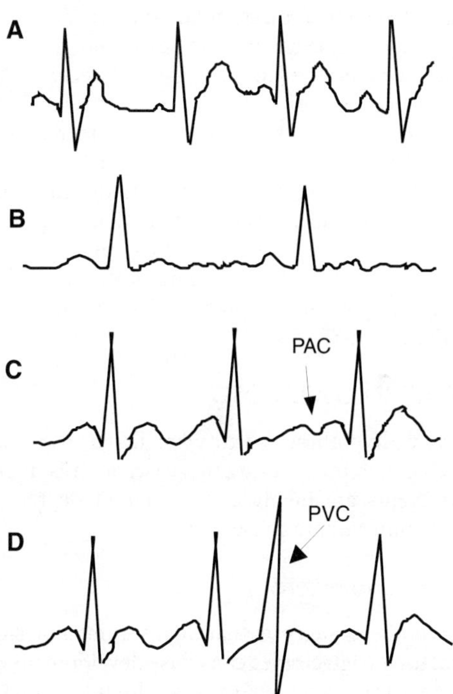

Figure 12-7. Electrocardiogram (ECG) depicton of a normal tracing (A); sinus bradycardia (B); premature atrial contraction (C); and premature ventricular contraction (D).

CONDITIONS OF DISEASE OR INJURY

Atherosclerosis

Atherosclerosis, or hardening of the arteries, is a condition of the large and small arteries characterized by accumulation of fatty deposits, platelets, macrophages, and other white blood cells throughout the tunica intima (endothelial cell layer) and eventually into the tunica media (smooth muscle layer). Arteries most often affected include the coronaries, the aorta, and cerebral arteries.

The first step in development of atherosclerosis appears to be injury to endothelial cells lining the lumen of the artery. With injury, endothelial cell integrity is breached and permeability of endothelial cells to various plasma components, including fatty acids and triglycerides, increases, allowing them access to the inside of the artery. Injury to the endothelial cells initiates inflammatory and immune reactions, causing the release of potent vasoactive peptides and the accumulation in and on the artery of macrophages and platelets. An early indication of damage is the presence of a "fatty streak" in the artery. In addition, many products of inflammation stimulate smooth muscle cell proliferation, causing smooth muscle cells to grow into the tunica intima. Additional plasma cholesterol and fats gain access to the tunica intima as permeability of the endothelial layer increases. With continued injury and inflammation, platelet aggregation increases and a blood clot (thrombus) begins to form. Scar tissue replaces some of the vascular wall, changing the structure of the wall. End results are cholesterol and fat buildup, scar tissue deposits, platelet-derived clots, and smooth muscle cell proliferation. All these factors cause a decrease in the diameter of the artery and an increase in its stiffness. The atherosclerotic area of an artery is called a **plaque**. The development of a plaque is shown in Figure 12-8.

CAUSES OF ATHEROSCLEROSIS

There are several hypotheses as to what first causes damage to the endothelial cells, thereby initiating this cascade. It is likely that different initiating events are involved, to different degrees, in different people. Five hypotheses are presented.

High Serum Cholesterol

The first hypothesis suggests that high serum cholesterol and high levels of circulating triglycerides can cause development of atherosclerosis. Fatty deposits, called foam cells, are found throughout and into the tunica media in persons with atherosclerosis.

Cholesterol and triglycerides are carried in the blood encased in fat-carrying proteins called **lipoproteins**. High-density lipoprotein (HDL)

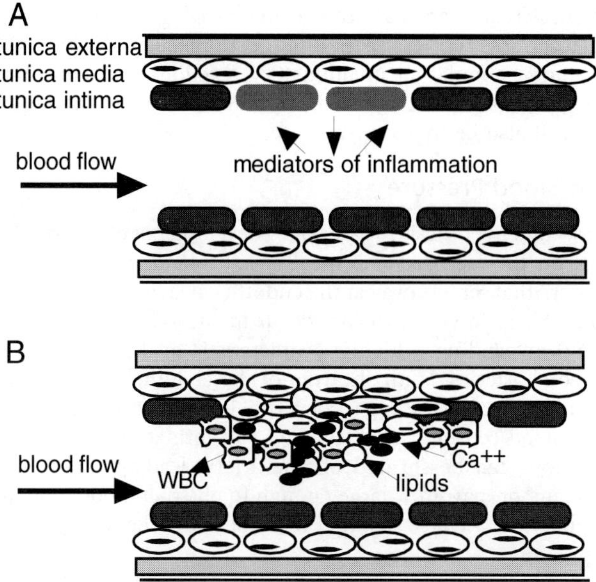

Figure 12-8. The formation of an atherosclerotic plaque with disruption of endothelial cell integrity (A) followed by WBC migration and deposits of fat (foam) cells and calcium (B).

carries fat away from cells to be degraded and is known to be protective against atherosclerosis. However, low-density lipoprotein (LDL) and very-low-density lipoprotein (VLDL) carry fat to cells of the body, including endothelial cells of the arteries. Especially at risk of atherosclerosis are persons who carry a specific mutation in the gene coding for the protein apolipoprotein B, which influences the binding of LDL to its receptor on the cell membrane. Individuals with errors in the LDL receptor are also at increased risk. In the arterial wall, oxidation of cholesterol and triglycerides leads to inflammation and production of free radicals known to damage delicate endothelial cells.

According to one hypothesis, the "oxidative-modification hypothesis of atherosclerosis," the initial oxidation of LDL in the subendothelial layer of the arteries turns on various inflammatory reactions, which ultimately attract monocyte and neutrophils to the site. These white blood cells further oxide LDL. Eventually, the monocytes mature into macrophages, which colonize the area, and internalize the LDL as fatty **foam cells**. Oxidized LDL is cytotoxic to vascular cells, further promoting inflammatory responses. According to this hypothesis, the higher the circulating level of LDL, the more frequently damage occurs.

An example of high cholesterol causing atherosclerosis is seen in patients with diabetes mellitus. Diabetes mellitus is a major risk factor for atherosclerosis. Persons with diabetes have high plasma cholesterol and triglycerides. Poor circulation to most organs causes hypoxia and tissue injury, stimulating inflammatory reactions that contribute to atherosclerosis. Because of extensive vascular pathology, many diabetic persons will also be hypertensive.

High Blood Pressure

The second hypothesis proposed for development of atherosclerosis is based on the fact that chronically high blood pressure produces shear forces that scrape away at the endothelial layer of the arteries and arterioles. Shear forces especially occur in sites of arterial bifurcation (splitting) or bending, which is characteristic of the coronary, aorta, and cerebral arteries. With shearing of the endothelial layer, damage can occur repeatedly, leading to a cycle of inflammation, accumulation of white blood cells and platelets, and clot formation. Any thrombus that develops can be sheared off the artery, leading to an embolus downstream, or may grow large enough to obstruct blood flow. It also may weaken the artery, causing it to burst under the maintained high blood pressure.

Infection

The third hypothesis proposed to explain how atherosclerosis develops suggests that some endothelial cells may become infected by a circulating microorganism. Infection produces cell-damaging free radicals directly and also initiates the cycle of inflammation (a process associated with free radicals). White blood cells and platelets arrive in the area and cause clots and scarring. A specific organism that has been implicated in this theory is *Chlamydia pneumoniae*, a common respiratory pathogen.

High Blood Iron Levels

A fourth hypothesis concerned with atherosclerosis of the coronary arteries is that high serum iron levels damage the coronary arteries or magnify damage from other insults. It is suggested that iron is rapidly oxidized and capable of producing artery-damaging free radicals. This theory is suggested by some to explain the striking difference in coronary artery disease incidence between men and premenopausal women. Men typically have much higher levels of iron than do menstruating women.

High Blood Homocysteine Levels

A fifth hypothesis suggests that persons with elevated plasma homocystine levels have increased vascular disease. Homocystine is an amino acid formed by the metabolism of methionine. Although it is unclear how elevated homocystine affects the vascular system, it is likely that homocystine may also increase oxidation of LDL. Epidemiologic evidence suggests a strong association between mild hyperhomocystinemia and coronary, cerebral, and peripheral vascular disease. Nutritional deficiencies in folic acid and the B vitamins are associated with elevated homocysteine.

SUMMARY OF CAUSES INDUCING ATHEROSCLEROSIS

Atherosclerosis occurs after damage to the endothelial cells lining the arteries, an occurrence that turns on inflammatory reactions and in many cases, free radical production. Damage may occur from physical injury, such as hypertension, or chemical injury, such as elevated LDL, infection, heavy metal exposure, or chemical insult.

Pediatric Consideration

Autopsy studies of children who have died in accidents have shown that fatty streaks on the arteries occurs in children 10 years of age or younger. Even though these early indications of atherosclerosis may be asymptomatic, they may be predictive of later coronary disease. Children with risk factors for atherosclerosis, including high body mass index, elevated systolic and diastolic pressures, and elevated cholesterol, show a larger percentage of fatty streaks than do children with few risk factors. Smoking in the teen years also increases incidence of fatty streaks.

CLINICAL MANIFESTATIONS

Clinical manifestations of atherosclerosis usually occur late in the course of the disease. They include:

- Intermittent claudication, an aching, cramping feeling in the lower extremities, occurring especially during or after exercise. Intermittent claudication is caused by poor blood flow through atherosclerotic vessels supplying the lower limbs. When oxygen demand of the leg muscles increases, the limited flow cannot supply the extra oxygen required, and pain from muscle ischemia develops. As atherosclerosis worsens, intermittent pain can progress to pain during rest because even normal demands for oxygen cannot be met.
- Cold sensitivity occurs with inadequate blood flow to the extremities.
- Skin color changes occur as blood flow decreases to an area. With ischemia, the area becomes pale. This is followed by local autoregulatory responses, resulting in hyperemia (increased blood flow) to the area, causing the skin to flush red.
- Reduced arterial pulses may be felt downstream from an atherosclerotic lesion. If blood flow is inadequate to support metabolic needs, cell necrosis and gangrene may develop.

DIAGNOSTIC TOOLS

- Elevated cholesterol and triglyceride levels may indicate a risk factor for atherosclerosis. Cholesterol levels higher than 180 mg/dL of blood in an individual 30 years of age or younger, or higher than 200 mg/dL in those older than 30, are considered elevated, and the individual is considered especially at risk of coronary artery disease.
- Radiographic studies of the arteries may allow visualization of atherosclerotic lesions. In these procedures, a dye is infused intraarterially, and its movement through the vascular system is observed.

COMPLICATIONS

- Hypertension may develop from long-standing atherosclerosis. Just as hypertension and high shear forces can cause atherosclerosis, atherosclerosis can cause hypertension. With thrombus formation, scar tissue, and smooth muscle cell proliferation, the lumen of the artery is reduced and the resistance to flow through the artery increases. The left ventricle must pump more forcefully to produce enough pressure to drive blood through the atherosclerotic vascular system, which can result in increased systolic and diastolic blood pressures.
- A thrombus may dislodge by breaking off from an atherosclerotic plaque. This may lead to obstruction of blood flow downstream, causing a stroke if the blood vessels of the brain are occluded or a myocardial infarction if the blood vessels of the heart are affected.
- Development of an aneurysm, a weakening of the artery, may occur from atherosclerosis. The aneurysm may burst, causing a stroke if it is located in the cerebral vasculature.
- Vasospasm may develop in atherosclerotic vessels. Normal endothelial cells act to block various vasoactive substances from directly binding to and acting on smooth muscle cells of the tunica media. If the endothelial layer is not intact, certain peptides such as serotonin and acetylcholine can diffuse directly to the underlying smooth muscle layer, causing the smooth muscle cells to constrict. This response may be involved in coronary artery spasm, or the spasm of cerebral arteries known as transient ischemic attacks. It may also be a cause of male impotence because vasodilation of the penile arteries is required for an erection to develop.

TREATMENT

- Diet modification *coupled with exercise* can lower LDL and improve HDL levels.
- Drug therapy is frequently used to lower total cholesterol and triglyceride levels and improve HDL. Drug goals should be individualized to meet specific patient needs.

- Aspirin or anticlotting drugs reduce thrombus formation.
- A well-planned exercise program may result in increased development of collateral vessels around occluded sites, may reduce the amount of circulating fat, and increase HDL.
- Good control of plasma glucose level is essential in diabetic patients.
- Cessation of smoking is essential for patients with atherosclerosis because of the damaging effects of smoke-related compounds on the endothelial cell wall.
- Antihypertensive medications will decrease shearing of the endothelial wall.
- Nitric oxide or nitroglycerine may be administered to patients experiencing vasospasm to relax the vessel wall.
- Antimicrobial therapy may offer protection against infectious injury to the endothelial layer.
- Blood donation by a man three times a year should reduce his iron levels to those seen in menstruating women.

Hypertension

Hypertension is abnormally high blood pressure measured on at least three different occasions from a person who has been at rest at least 5 minutes. Normal blood pressure varies with age, thus any diagnosis of hypertension must be age specific. The Joint National Committee on Prevention, Detection, Evaluation, and Treatment of High Blood Pressure has published revised guidelines on optimal, normal, high-normal, and hypertensive values of systolic and diastolic pressures. In general, optimal pressures are considered less than 120 mmHg systolic and 80 mmHg diastolic, while pressures considered hypertensive are higher than 140 mmHg systolic, and higher than 90 mmHg diastolic.

CAUSES OF HYPERTENSION

Because blood pressure depends on heart rate, stroke volume, and TPR, an uncompensated increase in any of these variables can cause hypertension.

Increased heart rate may occur with abnormal sympathetic or hormonal stimulation to the SA node. Chronically increased heart rate frequently accompanies conditions of hyperthyroidism. However, increased heart rate is usually compensated for by decreases in stroke volume or TPR, and thus does not cause hypertension.

Chronically increased stroke volume may occur if there is prolonged increase in plasma volume, as a result of renal mishandling of salt and water, or excess salt consumption. Increased renin or aldosterone release or decreased blood flow to the kidneys may alter renal handling of salt and water. Increased plasma volume would lead to increased end diastolic volume, and therefore increased stroke volume and blood pressure. Increased end diastolic volume is referred to as an increase in the **preload** of the heart. Increased preload is usually associated with an increased systolic pressure reading.

Chronically increased TPR may occur with increased sympathetic or hormonal stimulation to the arterioles, or an overresponsiveness of the arterioles to normal stimulation, both of which would cause a narrowing of the vessels. With increased TPR, the heart has to pump more forcefully, and therefore exert more pressure, to drive the blood through the narrow vessels. This is referred to as an increase in the **afterload** of the heart, and is usually associated with an increased diastolic pressure reading. With a prolonged increase in afterload, the left ventricle may begin to hypertrophy (increase in size). With hypertrophy, the ventricle's own oxygen demands increase further, which causes it to pump even more forcefully to meet those demands.

Each of the possible causes of hypertension mentioned may result from increased sympathetic nervous system activity. For many people, increased sympathetic nerve stimulation, or perhaps overresponsiveness of the body to normal sympathetic stimulation, may contribute to the development of hypertension. For some, this may happen with a prolonged stress response, which is known to involve sympathetic activation, or perhaps from a genetic excess of receptors for norepinephrine in the heart or vascular smooth muscle. Other genetic influences may be racially determined. For instance, there is evidence that blacks, who generally report more frequent and more severe hypertension, may have an alteration in sodium-calcium pumping such that calcium accumulates in the smooth muscle cells, increasing muscle contraction and resistance.

TYPES OF HYPERTENSION

Hypertension is often divided into primary or secondary hypertension, based on whether a cause can be identified. Most cases of hypertension have no known cause and are called primary or essential hypertension. When a clear cause of hypertension can be identified, it is called secondary hypertension.

Secondary Hypertension

An example of secondary hypertension is renal vascular hypertension, which develops as a result of renal artery stenosis. This condition may be congenital or a result of atherosclerosis. Renal artery stenosis reduces blood flow to the kidney, leading to activation of renal baroreceptors, stimulation of renin release, and production of angiotensin II. Angiotensin II directly increases blood pressure by increasing TPR, and indirectly by increasing aldosterone synthesis and sodium reabsorption. If repair of the stenosis is possible or the affected kidney is removed, blood pressure returns to normal.

Other causes of secondary hypertension include pheochromocytoma, an epinephrine-secreting tumor of the adrenal gland, which causes increased heart rate and stroke volume, and Cushing's disease, which causes increased stroke volume from salt retention and increased TPR as a result of hypersensitivity of the sympathetic nervous system. Primary aldosteronism (increased aldosterone of no known cause) and hypertension associated with oral contraceptives are also considered causes of secondary hypertension.

Pregnancy-Induced Hypertension

Pregnancy-induced hypertension (PIH) is a type of secondary hypertension because the hypertension reverses with birth of the infant. PIH appears to result in part from a combination of increased cardiac output and TPR. During normal pregnancy, blood volume increases dramatically. In healthy women, increased blood volume is accommodated by a decrease in vascular responsiveness to vasoactive hormones, such as angiotensin II. This causes TPR to decrease in normal pregnancy and blood pressure to be low. In women with PIH, normal decreased sensitivity to vasopeptides does not occur, so the large increase in blood volume increases cardiac output and blood pressure rises. PIH may occur as a result of an immunologic disorder that interferes with development of the placenta. PIH is dangerous for women and can result in seizures, coma, and death.

CLINICAL MANIFESTATIONS OF HYPERTENSION

Most clinical manifestations occur after years of hypertension, and include:

- Waking headache, sometimes with nausea and vomiting, caused by increased intracranial blood pressure.
- Blurred vision caused by hypertensive damage to the retina.
- Unsteadiness in the gait caused by central nervous system damage.
- Nocturia caused by increased renal blood flow and glomerular filtration.
- Dependent edema and swelling caused by increased capillary pressure.

DIAGNOSTIC TOOLS

- Diagnostic measurement of blood pressure using a sigmoid cuff manometer will show elevated systolic and diastolic pressures in an individual before any symptoms of the disease are present.
- Proteinuria and marked edema are present in women with PIH.

COMPLICATIONS

- Stroke may result from a high-pressure hemorrhage in the brain or from an embolus broken off a noncerebral vessel exposed to high pressure. Strokes may occur with long-standing hypertension if arteries supplying the brain become hypertrophied and thickened, thereby reducing blood flow to areas of the brain that depend on them. The cerebral arteries that are atherosclerotic may become weak, increasing the likelihood of an aneurysm.

- An MI may occur if the atherosclerotic coronary arteries cannot supply adequate oxygen to the myocardium or if a thrombus develops that blocks flow through a vessel. With chronic hypertension and the development of ventricular hypertrophy, the oxygen demands of the myocardium may not be met, and cardiac ischemia leading to an infarct may occur. Likewise, ventricular hypertropy may cause changes in the timing of the electrical conductance through the ventricle, leading to dysrhythmia, cardiac hypoxia, and an increased risk of clot formation.
- Renal failure may occur with progressive high-pressure damage to the renal capillaries, the glomeruli. With glomerular injury, blood flow to the functional units of the kidney, the nephrons, is impaired and these can become hypoxic and die. With damage to the glomerular membranes, proteins will be lost in the urine, decreasing the plasma colloid osmotic pressure and contributing to edema often seen with long-standing hypertension.
- Encephalopathy (brain damage) may occur, especially with malignant (swiftly progressing, dangerous) hypertension. The dramatically high pressure seen in this condition causes increased cerebral capillary pressure and drives fluid into the interstitial space throughout the central nervous system. Surrounding neurons collapse, and coma and death may result.
- Seizures may develop in women with PIH. The infant may be born small for gestational age because of poor placental perfusion, and may suffer hypoxia and acidosis if the mother develops a seizure before or during the birth process.

TREATMENT

To treat hypertension, one can lower heart rate, stroke volume, or TPR. Pharmacologic and nonpharmacologic interventions may help an individual reduce his or her blood pressure.

- Weight loss appears to reduce blood pressure in some people, perhaps by reducing the workload of the heart, and therefore heart rate and stroke volume.
- Exercise, especially coupled with weight loss, reduces blood pressure by reducing resting heart rate and possibly TPR. Exercise increases HDL levels, which may reduce the development of atherosclerosis-associated hypertension.
- Relaxation techniques may reduce heart rate and TPR by interrupting the sympathetic stress response.
- Quitting smoking is important in reducing the long-term effects of

hypertension because cigarette smoke is known to reduce blood flow to various organs and can increase the work of the heart.

- Diuretics act by several different mechanisms to reduce cardiac output by causing the kidney to increase its excretion of salt and water. Some diuretics (thiazides) appear also to decrease TPR.
- Calcium channel blockers decrease cardiac or arterial smooth muscle contraction by interfering with the calcium influx needed for contraction. Some calcium channel blockers are more specific for cardiac muscle slow calcium channels; some are more specific for vascular smooth muscle calcium channels. Calcium blockers, therefore, vary in their ability to preferentially reduce heart rate, stroke volume, and TPR. However, a **warning** concerning an increased frequency of negative cardiovascular events (fatal and nonfatal MI) associated with use of some types of calcium channel blockers, has resulted in a caution to their use.
- Angiotensin II converting enzyme inhibitors (ACE inhibitors) act to decrease angiotensin II by blocking the enzyme needed to convert angiotensin I to angiotensin II. This decreases blood pressure by directly decreasing TPR, and because angiotensin II is needed for aldosterone synthesis, by increasing loss of sodium in the urine, thereby reducing plasma volume and cardiac output. Because converting enzyme also breaks down the vasodilator bradykinin, converting enzyme inhibitors lower blood pressure by prolonging the effects of bradykinin.
- Beta-receptor antagonists (β-blockers), especially selective β_1 blockers, act on the β-receptors of the heart to decrease heart rate and cardiac output.
- Alpha-receptor antagonists (α-blockers) block the vascular smooth muscle α-receptors that normally respond to sympathetic stimulation with vasoconstriction. This reduces TPR.
- Direct arteriolar vasodilators may be used to decrease TPR.
- Some individuals may benefit from a sodium-restricted diet.

Raynaud's Disease

Raynaud's disease is a primary vascular disease characterized by a temporary spasm of the small arteries and arterioles, usually in the fingers, or less frequently, the toes. Spasm of the blood vessels leads to tissue hypoxia, which is characterized by pallor (whiteness) or cyanosis (bluish tinge) of the digits, followed by rubor (redness) as the local mechanisms of vasodilatation take over. Usually, there is no lasting damage with an episode of spasm. However, if the spasms are extensive or very frequent, tissue injury and scarring can occur. The cause of Raynaud's disease is unknown, but is ususally seen in young women in response to cold exposure.

Raynaud's phenomenon is a secondary disease that can occur following repeated exposure to vibration, such as would be experienced by a jackhammer operator. It may develop in an individual who has suffered damage from previous cold exposure. Raynaud's phenomenon might also develop in an individual suffering from a systemic disease such as lupus erythematosus or scleroderma.

CLINICAL MANIFESTATIONS

- Color changes of the digits with cold exposure.
- Numbness of the digits, then tingling and pain as the episode ends.

DIAGNOSIS

- A good physical examination and history will assist diagnosis.

COMPLICATIONS

- Gangrene if episodes are extensive.

TREATMENT

- Avoid exposure to the cold or vibrations.
- Treat underlying disease if present.

Varicose Veins

Varicose veins are tortuous (twisted) distended veins occurring where blood has pooled, often in the legs. Since blood flow in the veins is driven by contraction of surrounding skeletal muscles that squeeze blood back to the heart, long episodes of standing without muscle contraction can lead to pooling of blood in the legs. Varicose veins may also develop if valves that normally prevent backflow of blood are too weak to hold pooling blood and give way, thereby delivering even more blood to the next backstream valve. If this valve gives way, blood will continue to fill up the veins below.

Valve incompetence (weakness) can be a hereditary predisposition, or may occur following trauma to the valves. Obesity may contribute to the risk of developing varicose veins because of the associated sedentary lifestyle and the increased volume of blood pressing on the valves. Similarly, pregnant women are at increased risk of developing varicose veins because of their increased blood volume and body weight.

CLINICAL MANIFESTATIONS

- Bulging, distended veins, showing prominent bluish streaks and pools in the legs.

DIAGNOSIS

- Physical examination and family history will assist diagnosis.

COMPLICATIONS

- A blood clot may develop, since the risk of clotting increases when blood pools or is sluggish in its flow.
- Chronic venous insufficiency may occur if blood pooled in the vascular system is enough to significantly reduce cardiac output. Edema in the feet and ankles will be apparent.

TREATMENT

- Weight reduction.
- Elevation of the legs to assist blood flow return to the heart.
- Avoidance of tight-fitting clothes at the top of the legs or waist, which can restrict blood flow.
- Support hose for the lower legs to add support to the veins, assisting blood flow return to the heart.
- Walking and exercise to increase muscle strength and contraction of the leg muscles to increase blood flow return to the heart.
- Surgical stripping of the veins or cauterization may be performed.

Angina Pectoris

Angina pectoris is severe pain originating from the heart that occurs in response to an inadequate oxygen supply to the myocardial cells, compared to their oxygen demand. The pain of angina may radiate down the left arm, to the back, to the jaw, or into the abdominal area.

When the workload of any tissue increases, oxygen demand goes up. If the oxygen demand increases in healthy hearts, the coronary arteries dilate and bring more blood flow and oxygen to the muscle. However, if the coronary arteries are stiffened or narrowed with atherosclerosis and cannot dilate in response to an increased demand for oxygen, myocardial ischemia (inadequate blood supply) occurs, and the myocardial cells begin to use anaerobic glycolysis to meet their energy requirements. This form of energy production is very inefficient and results in the production of lactic acid. Lactic acid decreases myocardial pH and causes the pain associated with angina pectoris. If the energy demands of the cardiac cells are lessened, the oxygen supply becomes adequate and the muscle cells revert to oxidative phosphorylation for energy production. This process does not produce lactic acid. With removal of the accumulated lactic acid, the pain of angina goes away. Angina pectoris is, therefore, a short-lived experience.

TYPES OF ANGINA

There are three types of angina: stable, Prinzmetal's (variant), and unstable.

Stable angina, also called classic angina, occurs when atherosclerotic coronary arteries cannot dilate to increase flow when oxygen demand is increased. Increased work of the heart can accompany physical exercise such as sports participation or climbing stairs. Exposure to the cold, especially when coupled with work such as snow shoveling, increases the metabolic demands of the heart and is a strong stimulator of classic angina. Mental stress, including that caused by anger as well as mental tasks such as mathematics, may trigger classic angina. Pain of this type of angina typically goes away when the individual stops the activity.

Prinzmetal's angina occurs without any obvious increase in the workload of the heart, and in fact, frequently occurs during rest or sleep. In Prinzmetal's (variant) angina, a coronary artery undergoes a spasm, causing cardiac ischemia to occur downstream. Sometimes the site of spasm is related to atherosclerosis. Other times the coronary arteries do not appear to be sclerotic. It is possible that even if no visible lesions are apparent on the artery, subtle damage to the endothelial layer may be present. This allows vasoactive peptides access directly to the smooth muscle layer, causing its contraction. Dysrhythmias are common with variant angina.

Unstable angina is a combination of classic and variant angina, and is seen in an individual with worsening coronary artery disease. It usually accompanies an increased workload of the heart. It appears to result from coronary atherosclerosis, characterized by a growing, spasm-prone thrombus. Spasm occurs in response to vasoactive peptides released from platelets drawn to the area of damage. The most potent constrictors released by the platelets are thromboxane and serotonin, and platelet-derived growth factors. As the thrombus continues to grow, episodes of unstable angina increase in frequency and severity, and the individual is at increased risk of suffering irreversible damage.

CLINICAL MANIFESTATIONS

- Constricting or squeezing pain in the pericardial or substernal area of the chest, possibly radiating to the arms, jaw, or thorax. In stable and unstable angina, pain is typically relieved by rest. Prinzmetal's angina is unrelieved by rest but usually disappears in about 5 minutes.

DIAGNOSTIC TOOLS

- Alteration in the ST segment of the ECG may occur.
- Areas of reduced blood flow may be observed using radioactive imaging during an induced angina episode during an exercise stress test.

TREATMENT

Prevention

- Aspirin is sometimes prescribed to prevent anginal symptoms. Also, individuals prone to angina are encouraged to avoid working in the cold and other stressors known to precipitate an attack of classic angina.

- Invasive techniques such as percutaneous transluminal **coronary angioplasty** (PTCA) and **coronary artery bypass** surgery may reduce episodes of classic angina. With PTCA, the atherosclerotic lesion is dilated by a catheter inserted through the skin into the femoral or brachial artery and fed into the heart. Once in the affected coronary vessel, a balloon in the catheter is inflated. This cracks the plaque and stretches the artery. With bypass surgery, the diseased piece of a coronary artery is tied off, and an artery or vein taken from elsewhere in the body is connected to nondamaged areas. Flow is reinstated through this "new" vessel. The vessels most frequently transplanted are the saphenous vein or the internal mammary artery. Initial response to PTCA appears good, but vessels frequently (20–40%) become sclerotic again within a few months. Placing artificial tubes, or stents, into the artery to keep it open is becoming increasingly common, and appears to improve outcome. Coronary bypass relieves the pain of angina, but does not appear to affect long-term mortality.

Since the cause of angina is insufficient oxygen to meet the energy demands of the heart, once angina does occur, treatment is geared at reducing energy demands:

- Rest allows the heart to pump out less blood (decreased stroke volume) at a slower rate (decreased heart rate). This reduces the work of the heart, and therefore its oxygen requirements. Sitting is the preferable posture for rest. Lying down, in contrast, increases blood return to the heart, leading to increased end diastolic volume, stroke volume, and cardiac output.
- Nitroglycerin or other nitrates act as potent dilators of the venous system, decreasing venous return of blood to the heart. A decreased venous return decreases end diastolic volume, allowing the heart to decrease stroke volume. Nitrates dilate the arterial system as well, reducing the afterload against which the heart must pump, and increasing coronary blood flow. Dilation of a coronary undergoing spasm also may occur with nitrates.

All of these effects greatly reduce the inequalities of oxygen demand versus supply and nitroglycerin given sublingually (under the tongue) usually reverses angina.

- Beta-adrenergic blockers and calcium channel blockers reduce angina by reducing heart rate and contractility of the heart, therefore reducing its oxygen demands. Calcium channel blockers also reduce the afterload against which the heart must pump by dilating the arteries and arterioles downstream. Calcium channel blockers are particularly effective in reducing spasm of variant angina.

Again, a caution on the use of calcium channel blockers has been advanced.

- Oxygen therapy eases oxygen demands of the heart.

Myocardial Infarction

Myocardial infarction (MI) is the death of myocardial cells that occurs following prolonged oxygen deprivation. It is the culminating lethal response to unrelieved myocardial ischemia. Myocardial cells begin to die after about 20 minutes of oxygen deprivation. After this period, the ability of the cells to produce ATP aerobically is exhausted, and the cells fail to meet their energy demands.

Without ATP, the sodium-potassium pump quits, and the cells fill with sodium ions and water, eventually causing them to lyse (burst). With lysis, cells release intracellular potassium stores and intracellular enzymes, which injure neighboring cells. Intracellular proteins gain access to the general circulation and the interstitial space, contributing to interstitial edema and swelling around the myocardial cells. With cell death, inflammatory reactions are initiated. At the site of inflammation, platelets accumulate and release clotting factors. Mast cell degranulation occurs, resulting in the release of histamine and various prostaglandins. Some are vasoconstrictive and some stimulate clotting (thromboxane).

Effect of an MI on Cardiac Depolarization—With the release of the various intracellular enzymes, potassium ion, and the accumulation of lactic acid, the electrical conduction pathways of the heart are altered. This can result in interruption of atrial or ventricular depolarization, or in initiation of a dysrhythmia.

Effect of an MI on Cardiac Contractility and Blood Pressure—With the death of muscle cells, and as the electrical patterns of the heart change, the heart pumps in a less coordinated manner, causing contractility to decrease. Stroke volume falls, causing a fall in systemic blood pressure.

REFLEX RESPONSES TO A FALL IN BLOOD PRESSURE

Decreased blood pressure triggers the baroreceptor responses, leading to activation of the sympathetic nervous system, the renin-angiotensin system, and increasing the release of antidiuretic hormone. Stress hormones (ACTH and cortisol) are also released, which increase glucose production. Activity of the parasympathetic nervous system decreases.

With increased sympathetic and decreased parasympathetic nervous stimulation to the SA node, heart rate increases. Likewise, sympathetic and angiotensin stimulation of the arterioles causes an increase in TPR. Blood flow to the kidneys is reduced, reducing urine production and contributing to the stimulation of the renin-angiotensin system. Constriction of the arterioles causes a decrease in capillary pressure, reducing the capillary forces favoring filtration. Net reabsorption of interstitial fluid occurs, increasing the plasma volume and increasing venous return. Aldosterone synthesis stimulates sodium reabsorption, which in the presence of ADH, increases plasma volume further. Sympathetic simulation to the sweat glands and skin causes the individual to sweat and feel cool and clammy to the touch.

In summary, more blood (increased preload) is delivered to the heart, which is pumping at a faster rate against a narrowed arterial vasculature (increased afterload). The net result of activation of all the reflexes, which occur because of reduced cardiac contractility and fall in blood pressure, is to **increase the workload of the already damaged heart**. Oxygen demands of the heart increase. This can be disastrous because the initial problem causing the myocardial infarct was insufficient oxygen supply to heart cells. As the reflexes further increase the demands on the damaged heart, more and more cardiac cells become hypoxic. When oxygen demands of more cells cannot be met, zones of injured and ischemic cells increase around the central necrotic (dead) zone. These injured and ischemic cells are at risk of dying. The pumping ability of the heart falls further and hypoxia of all tissues and organs, including surviving areas of the heart, occurs.

Finally, as blood is erratically or ineffectually pumped, it begins to move sluggishly through the vessels of the heart. This, along with accumulation of platelets and other clotting factors, increases the risk of blood clot development.

CAUSES OF MYOCARDIAL INFARCT

Dislodgment of an atherosclerotic plaque from one of the coronary arteries, and subsequent trapping downstream that obstructs blood flow to the entire myocardium supplied by that vessel, can cause an MI. An MI might also occur if a thrombotic lesion adhering to a damaged artery becomes large enough to totally obstruct flow downstream, or if a heart chamber becomes so hypertrophied that it is unable to meet its oxygen demands. Hormonal inputs may also be involved. For example, estrogen has a cardioprotective effect on heart disease, while stress, with the release of the adrenocortical hormones (cortisol) is associated with an increased risk of MI.

CLINICAL MANIFESTATIONS

Although some individuals do not show any obvious signs of an MI (a silent heart attack), significant clinical manifestations usually occur:

- Abrupt (usually) onset of pain, often described as severe and crushing in nature. The pain may radiate anywhere on the upper body, but most often radiates to the left arm, neck, or jaw. Nitrates and rest might relieve ischemia outside the necrotic zone by decreasing the workload of the heart but will not completely relieve the pain of infarct.

- Nausea and vomiting, probably related to intense pain, are common.
- Feelings of weakness related to decreased blood flow to the skeletal muscles occur.
- The skin becomes cool, clammy, and pale due to sympathetic vasoconstriction.
- Urine output decreases related to decreased renal blood flow and increased aldosterone and ADH.
- Tachycardia develops, due to increased cardiac sympathetic stimulation and anxiety.
- A mental state of great anxiety and a feeling of doom often develop.

DIAGNOSTIC TOOLS

- Blood pressure may be decreased or normal depending on extent of myocardial damage and success of the baroreceptor reflexes. Heart rate is usually increased. A fourth heart sound may be heard.
- The ECG may show acute changes with elevation in the ST segment and T wave inversion. Within 1 or 2 days of the infarct, deepening of the Q wave occurs. Although the ST and T wave changes will disappear over time, the Q wave changes remain and can be used to detect a past infarct.
- Systemic signs of inflammation occur, including fever, elevated number of leukocytes, and increased sedimentation rate. These signs begin about 24 hours after the infarct and continue for up to 2 weeks.
- Cardiac enzyme levels (creatinine phosphokinase, serum glutamic oxaloacetic transaminase, and lactic dehydrogenase) in the serum increase as a result of myocardial cell death. The increases occur in a characteristic pattern, beginning immediately after an infarct and continuing for about a week.
- Troponin T and Troponin I levels become detectable in the blood, within 15 to 20 minutes. Myoglobin is detected within 1 hour, peaking within 4 to 6 hours of the infarct.

COMPLICATIONS

- Thromboemboli may develop as myocardial contractility falls. These emboli can block blood flow to other regions of the heart not previously damaged during the original infarct. They may also travel to other organs, blocking their blood flow and causing infarction in those organs.
- Congestive heart failure may occur when the failing heart cannot pump out all the blood it is receiving. Heart failure may develop soon after an infarct if the original infarct is very large, or may occur subsequent to activation of the baroreceptor reflexes. With activation of baroreceptor responses there is increased blood returned to the damaged heart and constriction of the downstream arteries and arterioles. This causes blood to accumulate in the heart

and leads to overstretch of the cardiac muscle cells. If the overstretch is severe enough, it can cause the contractility of the heart to decrease further as the muscle cells begin to fall down the length-tension curve.

- Dysrhythmia is the most common complication of an infarct. Dysrhythmia may develop due to alteration in electrolyte balance and decreased pH. Hypoxic areas of the heart may become irritable and initiate action potentials, also leading to dysrhythmia. The SA or AV nodes, or the transduction pathways (Purkinje's fibers or the bundle of His), may be part of the necrotic or ischemic zones, thereby affecting their signal initiation or passage. Fibrillation is the primary cause of death following a myocardial infarct outside the hospital setting.
- Cardiogenic shock (collapse of blood pressure) may occur with a prolonged, severe decrease in cardiac output. Cardiogenic shock may be fatal at the time of the infarct, or may cause death or disability days or weeks later as a result of subsequent pulmonary or renal failure following ischemia of those organs. Cardiogenic shock is usually associated with at least a 40% loss of myocardial muscle mass.
- Myocardial rupture may occur after a large infarct.
- Pericarditis, an inflammation of the heart, may occur, usually a few days after the infarct. Pericarditis occurs as part of the inflammatory reaction following cardiac cell injury and death. Some types of pericarditis may occur weeks after the infarct, and may represent an immune hypersensitivity reaction to the tissue necrosis.
- With healing after a myocardial infarct, scar tissue replaces dead myocardial cells. If this represents a large area of the myocardium, contractility of the heart may be permanently reduced. In some cases the scar tissue may be weak, leading to later myocardial rupture or development of an aneurysm.

TREATMENT

During the last decade, mortality following an MI has been significantly reduced, especially for white men and women. Mortality following an MI in African-American men and women has also declined in the last decade, although to a lesser extent. The main reasons for a decline in mortality appear to be related to improvements in the treatment of an MI, and better prevention of secondary complications. The poorer response to treatment in African-American men and women appears to be related to later diagnosis and more significant coronary artery disease at the time of presentation. Even more important than treatment of an MI after it has occurred, is the primary prevention of heart disease.

- Prevention of heart disease is vital. Preventing heart disease has been shown to occur with even moderate levels of exercise, including walking, cessation of smoking, and limitation of dietary fat and obesity. In addition, hormone replacement therapy in women after the menopause is associated with a reduced risk of MI, although perhaps not in the first few months after initiating therapy in women who have already experienced an MI.

If a heart attack does occur:

- Cessation of physical activity to reduce the workload of the heart helps to limit the area of damage.
- Cardiopulmonary resuscitation (CPR) may be required if the heart is in fibrillation. Electrical defibrillation may be required to restore rhythm.
- Immediate intravenous or intracoronary infusions of thrombolytic (clot-busting) drugs break up a causative embolus. Rapid use of these drugs (preferably within an hour of the infarct) is associated with a dramatically increased survival rate and with limiting the extent of further myocardial injury. Drugs to prevent new clot development, such as heparin, are also required. Instead of using clot-busting drugs, coronary angioplasty may be used to open coronary arteries.
- Oxygen is provided to increase oxygenation of the blood, reducing demands on the heart and increasing systemic perfusion.
- Pain medications (usually morphine and meperidine [Demerol]) are used for patient comfort and because acute pain stimulates sympathetic stimulation, raising heart rate and vascular resistance. In addition, pain increases mental stress and anxiety. Morphine is also a vasodilator that works to decrease preload and afterload.
- Nitrates are provided to decrease venous return and relax the arteries, decreasing preload and afterload and increasing coronary blood flow.
- Angiotensin-converting enzyme inhibitors are provided to decrease preload and afterload.
- Beta blockers should be provided to decrease heart rate, reducing the work of the heart.
- Diuretics are provided to increase renal blood flow. This preserves kidney function and prevents volume overload and development of congestive heart failure. Increased renal blood flow also reduces the release of renin.
- Positive inotropic agents (digitalis) are used to increase the contractility of the heart.
- Coronary artery bypass may be considered if the infarct was due to a thrombotic occlusion.
- Cardiac rehabilitation after an infarct involves a balance between rest and exercise and lifestyle modifications to reduce atherosclerotic risks and hypertension. Various cardiac drugs may be prescribed. Smoking cessation is essential. Weight loss and stress reduction may be beneficial. The family needs to be considered and involved.

Pericarditis

Pericarditis is inflammation of the fluid-filled pericardial sac surrounding the heart. Pericarditis can occur with any cardiac trauma, including a myocardial infarct, blunt or penetrating trauma to the chest, infection, or neoplasm. Kidney disease, rheumatic fever, and other systemic diseases may also cause pericarditis.

With trauma, disease, or infection, inflammation of the pericardial tissues causes fluid to accumulate in the interstitial space. This exudate may be purulent if a bacterial infection is present. Acute pericarditis usually resolves on its own in 2 to 6 weeks. Chronic pericarditis is diagnosed if the condition does not resolve. It is usually associated with other symptoms of heart disease or systemic inflammation.

CLINICAL MANIFESTATIONS

- Sharp chest pain, usually with a rapid onset, that worsens when the individual breathes, coughs, or changes position. Pain is lessened when the individual sits up and leans forward.
- Difficulty breathing and a dry cough.
- Fever is usually present.

DIAGNOSTIC TOOLS

- A friction rub can be heard with a stethoscope due to the inflamed sac rubbing over the heart with each beat.
- Systemic signs of inflammation (fever, elevated sedimentation rate, and increased leukocyte count) may occur.
- Echocardiography can indicate fluid accumulation in the pericardial sac.

COMPLICATIONS

Cardiac tamponade, compression of the heart due to extensive buildup of fluid or blood in the pericardial sac, may occur if the pressure in the pericardial sac increases to a level equal to or greater than the diastolic pressure of the heart. This causes diastolic filling of the heart to cease, collapsing stroke volume and cardiac output.

TREATMENT

- Bed rest, with elevation of the head of the bed to improve breathing.
- Oxygen therapy.
- Antibacterial, antifungal, or antiviral therapy if an infectious cause is suspected.
- Drainage of the pericardial fluid (pericardiocentesis) or removal of the pericardium (pericardiotomy) may be performed.

Myocarditis

Myocarditis is inflammation of the heart not related to coronary artery disease or myocardial infarct. Myocarditis most often is a result of a viral infection of the myocardium, but may be caused by a bacterial or fungal infection. Coxsackievirus is often implicated. Systemic disease such as lupus erythematosus may also cause the disorder.

Myocarditis results in weakening of the heart muscle and a decrease in cardiac contractility. The heart becomes flabby and dilated, with many foci of pinpoint hemorrhage developing in the endocardium, myocardium, and epicardial layers. Myocarditis is a major cause of heart transplantation in the United States.

CLINICAL MANIFESTATIONS

- Chest pain.
- Fatigue and dyspnea.

DIAGNOSTIC TOOLS

- Systemic signs of inflammation include elevated sedimentation rate and leukocytosis.
- Elevated levels of antiviral antibodies, frequently against the coxsackievirus.
- Echocardiography and coronary artery catheterization show normal arteries and cardiac valves. Biopsy of the muscle shows inflammation.

COMPLICATIONS

- Heart failure.
- Arrhythmia leading to sudden death.

TREATMENT

- Treatment of infectious cause or systemic disease.
- Control of heart failure.
- Heart transplantation.

Cardiomyopathy

Cardiomyopathy refers to any disease or injury of the heart not related to coronary artery disease, hypertension, or congenital malformations. Cardiac myopathy may occur following an infection of the heart, as a result of an autoimmune disease, or following the exposure of an individual to certain toxins, including many anticancer drugs and alcohol. Clinically, myopathies are divided into those resulting in ventricular dilation and those characterized by hypertrophy of the myocardium.

With dilated cardiomyopathy, the ventricle stretches, leading to heart failure. With hypertrophic myopathy, cardiac muscle thickens, especially along the intraventricular septum. This makes the ventricle stiff, resulting in reduced compliance and diastolic filling.

CLINICAL MANIFESTATIONS

- Dyspnea (difficulty breathing) and fatigue may occur if cardiac output is reduced.
- Dysrhythmia may occur as a result of atrial stretching.
- Emboli may develop as a result of sluggish coronary blood flow.
- Chest pain may be present.

DIAGNOSTIC TOOLS

- An ECG or echocardiogram will demonstrate a thickened myocardium.

COMPLICATIONS

- A myocardial infarct may occur if oxygen demand of the thickened ventricle cannot be met.
- Heart failure may occur in dilated cardiomyopathy if the heart cannot pump out as much blood as is entering.

TREATMENT

- Salt restriction and diuretics are used for dilated cardiomyopathy to reduce end diastolic volume. Other treatments for heart failure may be required.
- Anticoagulants are provided to prevent emboli formation.
- Beta-blockers are provided for hypertrophic cardiomyopathy in order to decrease the heart rate, allowing increased diastolic filling time. They also reduce ventricular stiffness.
- Surgical resection of some areas of hypertrophied myocardium may be attempted.
- Calcium channel blockers are not used since they may further decrease contractility of the heart.

Congestive Heart Failure

Congestive heart failure occurs when the heart is unable to pump enough blood out to maintain an adequate cardiac output. This can occur either as a result of diastolic dysfunction or systolic dysfunction.

Diastolic dysfunction usually occurs following prolonged hypertension. When the ventricle must pump continually against a very high afterload (increased resistance), muscle cells hypertrophy and become stiff. This causes a reduction in ventricular compliance; decreased ventricular filling, decreased end-diastolic volume, and decreased stroke volume follow. Blood pressure falls, activating the baroreceptor reflexes.

Systolic dysfunction as a cause of heart failure occurs as a result of injury to the ventricle, usually from a myocardial infarct. The damaged muscle is unable to contract forcefully, and again, stroke volume falls. With a progressive increase in end-diastolic volume, ventricular muscle cells become stretched beyond their optimum length, and less tension is produced as the ventricle becomes more distended with blood. Heart failure is a worsening cycle. The more overfilled the ventricle becomes, the less blood it can pump out, leading to further accumulation of blood and additional stretch of the muscle fibers. As a result, stroke volume, cardiac output, and blood pressure fall. The body's reflex responses initiated in response to the fall in pressure significantly worsen the situation.

REFLEXES INITIATED DURING HEART FAILURE

Decreased blood pressure is sensed by the baroreceptors. Most reflex responses initiated by baroreceptor activation significantly advance heart failure progression as shown in Figure 12-9. This occurs because the reflex responses either further increase ventricular filling (preload) or further reduce stroke volume by increasing the afterload against which the ventricle must pump. Increased preload and afterload serve to increase the workload and oxygen demand of the heart. If the increased oxygen demand cannot be met, the muscle fibers become increasingly hypoxic and contractility worsens. The downward spiral of heart failure continues.

As each of these reflexes further fill and stretch the heart and/or increase afterload, blood pressure continues to be below normal, causing these same reflexes to be maintained and heightened. Heart failure continues unless the cycle of overfill, decreased stroke volume, and decreased blood pressure is broken.

CAUSES OF HEART FAILURE

Heart failure may result from noncardiac causes such as long-standing systemic or pulmonary hypertension, or less commonly, anything that increases plasma volume to such a degree the ventricular fibers are stretched beyond their optimum length. Such causes can include kidney failure or water intoxication.

Cardiac causes of heart failure include myocardial infarct, cardiac myopathy, valvular defects, and congenital malformation. Pathways leading to heart failure, following myocardial infarct and chronic hypertension, are highlighted in Figure 12-9. As shown in the figure, if increased oxygen demand of a hypertrophied ventricle cannot be met by increased blood flow (usually because of coronary atherosclerosis), ventricular contractility will fall. In this case, diastolic and systolic dysfunction are both present.

PROGRESSION OF HEART FAILURE

Heart failure can begin on either the left or right side of the heart. For instance, long-standing systemic hypertension would cause the

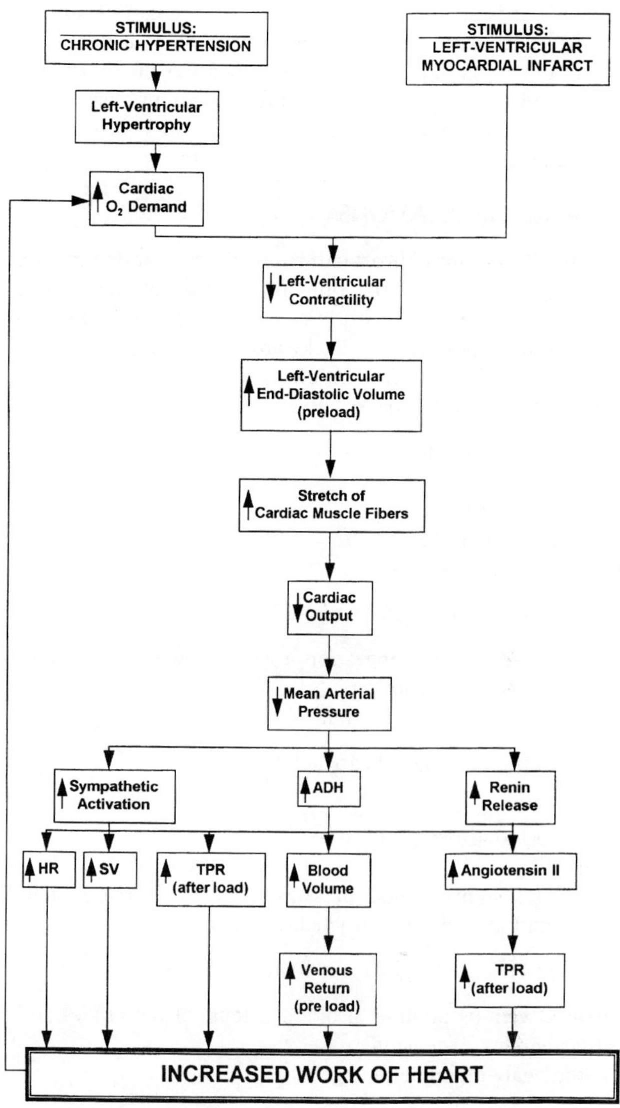

Figure 12-9. Flow diagram of heart failure.

left ventricle to hypertrophy and fail. Longstanding pulmonary hypertension would cause the right ventricle to hypertrophy and fail. The site of a myocardial infarct would determine which side of the heart is first affected following a heart attack.

Because a failing left ventricle would cause blood to back up in the left atrium, and then to the pulmonary circuit, right ventricle, and right atrium, it is apparent that left heart failure can eventually lead to right heart failure. In fact, the main cause of right heart failure is left heart failure. As blood is poorly pumped out of the right side of the heart, it begins to pool in the peripheral venous system. The end result is a further reduction in circulating blood volume and blood pressure, and a worsening cycle of heart failure.

CLINICAL MANIFESTATIONS

Clinical manifestations of heart failure are often separated into forward or backward effects, with the right or left side of the heart as the starting point of view. Forward effects are considered "downstream" from the failing myocardium. Backward effects are considered "upstream" from the failing myocardium.

Forward effects of left heart failure:

- decreased systemic blood pressure
- fatigue
- increased heart rate
- decreased urine output
- plasma volume expansion

Backward effects of left heart failure:

- increased pulmonary congestion, especially when lying down
- dyspnea (difficult breathing)
- if the conditions worsens, right heart failure

Forward effects of right heart failure:

- decreased pulmonary blood flow
- decreased blood oxygenation
- fatigue
- decreased systemic blood pressure (due to decreased left heart filling), and all the signs of left heart failure

Backward effects of right heart failure:

- increased venous pooling of blood, edema of the ankles and feet
- jugular venous distension
- hepatomegaly and splenomegaly

DIAGNOSTIC TOOLS

- A third heart sound may be present.
- Radiological identification of pulmonary congestion and ventricular enlargement may indicate heart failure.
- Magnetic resonance imaging (MRI) or ultrasound identification of ventricular enlargement may indicate heart failure.
- Measurement of ventricular end-diastolic pressure with a catheter inserted into the pulmonary artery (reflecting left ventricular pres-

sure) or into the vena cava (reflecting right ventricular pressure) can diagnose heart failure. Left ventricular pressure usually reflects left ventricular volume.

- Echocardiography can demonstrate abnormal dilation of the cardiac chambers and abnormalities in contractility.

TREATMENT

- Oxygen therapy to reduce the demands of the heart.
- Diuretics are administered to decrease plasma volume, thereby decreasing venous return and removing some of the stretch on the cardiac muscle fibers.
- Digoxin (Digitalis) is administered to increase contractility. Digoxin acts directly on the cardiac muscle fibers to increase the strength of each contraction regardless of the length of the muscle fibers. This increases cardiac output, relieving the ventricle of volume and lessening the stretch of the chamber.
- Angiotensin-converting enzyme inhibitors are administered to decrease production of angiotensin II. This reduces both afterload (TPR) and plasma volume (preload). Nitrates are also administered to reduce afterload and preload.

Rheumatic Fever

Rheumatic fever is a serious inflammatory disease that can permanently affect the structure and function of the heart, especially the heart valves. This illness occurs 1 to 4 weeks following an untreated throat infection with group A beta-hemolytic streptococcus bacteria. It is a relatively rare illness, however, affecting only 3% of those with an untreated streptococcal infection. Rheumatic fever is preventable with prompt antibiotic therapy.

Rheumatic fever can occur at any age, but mainly affects children between the ages of 5 and 15. It is likely that individuals who develop the disease have a genetic tendency to do so. This tendency may be related to an antigenic similarity between cardiac valves and group A beta-hemolytic streptococcus, or to a mistake in the presentation of the major histocompatibility antigens to white blood cells. Because of a genetic predisposition, a small number of individuals may experience repeated infections.

Approximately 10% of individuals who acquire rheumatic fever develop rheumatic heart disease. Rheumatic heart disease is the major cause of acquired cardiac valve disease. Damage to the heart following rheumatic fever can occur in any of the four cardiac valves, but is usually seen in the mitral and aortic valves.

THE COURSE OF RHEUMATIC HEART DISEASE

The course of the disease can be separated into acute and chronic stages. In the acute stage, the valves become swollen and red as the inflammatory reaction begins. Lesions may develop on the valve leaflets. As the acute inflammation subsides, scar tissue develops. This may deform the valves, and in some cases, cause the leaflets to fuse together, narrowing the orifice. A chronic stage of the disease may follow, characterized by repeated inflammation and continued scarring.

ASSOCIATED EFFECTS OF RHEUMATIC FEVER

Besides affecting the heart, rheumatic fever has other systemic effects. These include migratory (moving) joint inflammation and pain, occurrence of skin nodules, and occasionally a rash. The central nervous system is affected, causing behavioral changes, awkwardness in walking and speech, and a type of movement called chorea, characterized by spontaneous, jerky motions. These nervous system manifestations usually regress over the course of a few weeks or months.

CLINICAL MANIFESTATIONS

- A history of sore throat, positive for group A beta-hemolytic streptococcus is cultured. History of the infection usually includes headache, fever, swollen lymph nodes along the jaw, and stomach pain or nausea.
- Migratory polyarthritis occurs, with inflammation of the joints (swelling, redness, pain heat). The large joints of the elbows, knees, ankles, and wrists are often affected.
- Subcutaneous hard nodules develop that lie over the muscles of affected joints. These are painless and transitory.
- Erythema marginatum (a transitory rash) is seen, especially on trunk, inner arms, and thighs.
- Chorea (rapid, jerky movements) may occur, accompanied by clumsiness in movement.
- Behavioral changes may become apparent.

DIAGNOSTIC TOOLS

- Antistreptolysin O titer is increased in individuals after a streptococcal infection.
- Signs of inflammation during the acute phase include fever, arthralgia (joint pain), elevated sedimentation rate, and increased number of leukocytes.
- Elevated C-reactive protein is measurable in the serum. This protein is released by the streptococcal bacteria.
- An Aschoff body, a fibrous area of tissue necrosis, may be present on the heart.

COMPLICATIONS

- A heart murmur may develop in an individual without a previous murmur, or a worsening of a previous murmur may occur if rheumatic heart disease develops. Cardiomegaly (increased size of the heart), pericarditis, or congestive heart failure in a previously well individual may also occur.

TREATMENT

- The most important method available for reducing harmful effects due to rheumatic fever and rheumatic heart disease is to promptly identify the occurrence of a beta-hemolytic streptococcal infection and provide a full course of antibiotic therapy.
- If rheumatic fever develops, interventions to limit the disease include administration of antibiotics and anti-inflammatory drugs. Restriction of activities to reduce cardiac demand is also suggested.
- To prevent recurrence of rheumatic fever in susceptible individuals, prophylactic antibiotics are administered (usually a penicillin) for at least 5 years after the most recent occurrence. Education on the signs and symptoms of a streptococcal infection, and the need for prompt treatment, should be provided to the entire family.

Mitral Valve Stenosis

Mitral valve stenosis is a narrowing in the opening of the valve between the left atrium and the left ventricle. Mitral valve stenosis is usually due to a buildup of scar tissue following rheumatic fever or another cardiac infection. It may also result from a congenital defect in valve structure.

In order to pump blood through the narrowed orifice, the left atrium must contract more forcefully. If the left atrium is unable to pump through the narrow orifice, blood will pool in the atrium and back up into the lungs and right side of the heart. Right heart failure can result, especially if flow through the valve is so restricted that stroke volume and cardiac output are too low to maintain normal-range systemic blood pressure. If this occurs, baroreceptor reflexes initiating sympathetic and hormonal responses will be activatd, leading to increased plasma volume and increased TPR in an attempt to raise blood pressure. If plasma volume increases, further overfilling of the left atrium will occur, worsening the situation.

CLINICAL MANIFESTATIONS

- Clinical manifestations may be absent or severe, depending on the level of stenosis.
- Pulmonary congestion, with signs of dyspnea (difficulty breathing) and pulmonary hypertension, may occur.
- Dizziness and fatigue due to decreased left ventricular output may occur. Heart rate may be elevated due to sympathetic stimulation.

DIAGNOSTIC TOOLS

- A low-pitched murmur may be present during ventricular filling (diastole) as the blood reverberates through the constricted opening.

- Echocardiography may be used to diagnose abnormal valve structure and motion.

COMPLICATIONS

- Left atrial hypertrophy may cause atrial dysrhythmia or right heart failure.

TREATMENT

- Treatment for congestive heart failure may be required.
- Valve replacement or surgical correction of the stenosis may be attempted.

Aortic Valve Stenosis

Aortic valve stenosis is a narrowing in the opening of the valve between the left ventricle and the aorta. Like mitral valve stenosis, aortic stenosis usually follows rheumatic fever or is a congenital malformation. With aortic stenosis, the left ventricle must pump more forcefully to expel blood through the narrow orifice. This causes ventricular hypertrophy and eventually reduces compliance. As blood backs up in the ventricle, atrial pressure increases and blood backs up into the pulmonary system and the right side of the heart. If the stenosis is severe, systemic blood pressure may fall, initiating baroreceptor reflexes geared toward increasing plasma volume and TPR. Heart failure may occur.

CLINICAL MANIFESTATIONS

- Clinical manifestations may be absent or severe, depending on the level of stenosis.
- Pulmonary congestion, with signs of dyspnea and pulmonary hypertension, may occur if blood backs up into the pulmonary vascular system.
- Dizziness and fatigue may occur due to decreased cardiac output and decreased stroke volume. Heart rate may be elevated via sympathetic stimulation.

DIAGNOSTIC TOOLS

- A systolic heart murmur may be heard as blood rushes through the narrow orifice.
- Echocardiography may be used to diagnose abnormal valve structure and motion.

COMPLICATIONS

- Left ventricular hypertrophy may develop leading to congestive heart failure.

TREATMENT

- Treatment for congestive heart failure may be required.
- Valve replacement or surgical correction of the stenosis may be attempted.

Pulmonary Valve Stenosis

Pulmonary valve stenosis is a narrowing of the opening between the right ventricle and the pulmonary valve. Pulmonary valve stenosis most commonly occurs due to a congenital defect. With a narrow orifice, the right ventricle must pump more forcefully to expel blood. This can lead to right ventricular hypertrophy, backing up into the right atrium and causing dilation of the vena cava and blood accumulation in the systemic veins. Blood flow into the lungs and left side of the heart will be reduced if the stenosis is severe, leading to a decrease in blood pressure. Right heart failure may develop.

CLINICAL MANIFESTATIONS

- Clinical manifestations may be absent or severe depending on the level of stenosis.
- Decreased pulmonary flow causes poor oxygenation of the blood and feelings of weakness and fatigue.
- Venous distention and swelling of the ankles and feet is common.

DIAGNOSTIC TOOLS

- Echocardiography may be used to diagnose abnormal valve structure and motion.

COMPLICATIONS

- Right heart hypertrophy leading to right heart failure may occur.

TREATMENT

- Treatment for heart failure may be required.
- Valve replacement or surgical correction of the stenosis may be attempted.

Mitral Valve Regurgitation

Mitral valve regurgitation is the return of blood into the left atrium from the left ventricle through the mitral valve, occurring especially when the ventricle contracts. Mitral valve regurgitation results from an incompetent mitral valve. The mitral valve fails to snap shut completely upon initiation of ventricular systole. Mitral valve regurgitation is usually caused by rheumatic fever, other bacterial infection of the heart, or rupture of the valve with coronary artery disease.

With mitral valve regurgitation, some blood returns to the left atrium as the left ventricle contracts. This causes ventricular stroke volume and cardiac output to fall, leading to a decrease in blood pressure and activation of baroreceptor reflexes. Chronic dilation and filling of the ventricle and the atrium occur, leading to hypertrophy and potentially congestive heart failure. Blood backing into the pulmonary circulation causes pulmonary congestion and pulmonary hypertension.

CLINICAL MANIFESTATIONS

- Clinical manifestations may be absent or severe, depending on the level of stenosis.
- Pulmonary congestion, with signs of dyspnea and pulmonary hypertension, may occur if blood backs up into the pulmonary vascular system.
- Decreased cardiac output due to decreased stroke volume may cause dizziness and fatigue. Heart rate may be elevated via sympathetic stimulation.

DIAGNOSTIC TOOLS

- A systolic heart murmur may be heard as blood is pushed through the orifice.
- Echocardiography may be used to diagnose abnormal valve structure and motion.

COMPLICATIONS

Left ventricular and left atrial hypertrophy may develop, leading to congestive heart failure.

TREATMENT

- Treatment for congestive heart failure may be required.
- Valve replacement or surgical correction of the stenosis may be attempted.

Aortic Valve Regurgitation

Aortic valve regurgitation is the return of blood into the left ventricle from the aorta during diastole. Incompetence of the aortic valve usually follows rheumatic fever. With blood flowing backward into the left ventricle during diastole, diastolic pressure in the aorta is reduced. This leads to a characteristic increase in the pulse pressure: the difference between the measured systolic and diastolic pressures. Aortic regurgitation also increases left ventricular diastolic volume because blood is entering the left ventricle during diastole from both the left atrium and the aorta. This increases stroke volume and cardiac output. Aortic valve regurgitation leads to hypertrophy of the left ventricle, which can cause development of congestive heart failure.

CLINICAL MANIFESTATIONS

- A wide pulse pressure can be measured.
- Hyperkinetic (very strongly bounding) peripheral and carotid pulsations are typically present.
- Symptoms of heart failure may develop.

DIAGNOSTIC TOOLS

- A high-pitched diastolic heart murmur is frequently heard.
- Echocardiography may be used to diagnose abnormal valve structure and motion.

TREATMENT

- Treatment for congestive heart failure may be required.
- Valve replacement or surgical correction of the stenosis may be attempted.

Congenital Heart Defects

Congenital heart defects involve abnormal shunting between the left and right sides of the heart or between the aorta and pulmonary artery. The direction of blood flow in the shunt depends on the relative resistance of the pulmonary and systemic circulations.

Usually after birth, pulmonary vascular resistance falls and systemic vascular resistance increases. If a shunt is present under these conditions, the direction will be left to right. Well-oxygenated blood will flow from the left side of the heart into the right side or into the pulmonary circulation, resulting in overfilling of the pulmonary circuit and, since the blood is immediately delivered again into the left atrium, overfilling of the left side of the heart. This may lead to pulmonary congestion and left heart failure. If blood is delivered directly to the right side of the heart from the left through an opening in the septal wall, right heart failure may develop.

In a premature infant, immature development of the lungs may cause resistance to flow in the pulmonary circulation to be greater than resistance in the systemic circulation. The result will be a right-to-left shunt. In a right-to-left shunt, poorly oxygenated blood is delivered into the systemic blood supply, causing cyanosis. A shunting pathway that causes cyanosis is called a cyanotic defect.

TYPES OF CONGENITAL HEART DEFECTS

Congenital heart defects may involve the atria, the ventricles, any of the valves, or the great arteries.

Atrial Septal Defect

An atrial septal defect (ASD) is an abnormal opening between the left and right atria. It is a congenital disorder that occurs when the foramen ovale fails to close after birth, or when another opening between the left and right atria is present due to improper closure of the wall between the two atria during gestation.

Ventricular Septal Defect

A ventricular septal defect (VSD) is an abnormal opening between the left and right ventricles that occurs when the wall between the ventricles fails to close properly during gestation. It is the most common cardiac congenital defect. The size of the defect determines the severity of the symptoms.

Patent Ductus Arteriosus (PDA)

PDA is the maintenance after birth of an open ductus arteriosus, the connection between the pulmonary artery and the aorta. Normally the ductus closes soon after birth as a result of increased oxygenation in the pulmonary circulation. If the ductus does not close, blood will shunt between the two main arteries. The direction of blood flow will depend on the relative resistance to flow of the pulmonary and systemic circulation.

Transposition of the Great Vessels

This condition occurs when the openings of the aorta and pulmonary artery are switched; that is, the aorta originates in the right ventricle and the pulmonary artery originates in the left ventricle. This reversal results in separation of the left and right heart circulations.

Blood flows in the pulmonary vein to the left atrium. From there it flows to the left ventricle and back through the pulmonary artery to the lungs, to cycle again to the left atrium. This blood is oxygenated, but does not supply the systemic circulation.

At the same time, blood flows in the vena cava to the right atrium, to the right ventricle, through the aorta to the systemic circulation, and back again to the vena cava. This blood is not oxygenated. Obvious signs of cyanosis will be apparent.

Transposition of the great vessels is incompatible with life unless, as is frequently the case, a septal defect or a patent ductus arteriosus maintains communication between the two circulations. If no communication is present, surgical opening of the atrial septum is required until major surgery to redirect blood flow can be performed.

Coarctation of the Aorta

This congenital defect results in the narrowing of the aorta as it leaves the left ventricle. The narrowing can be proximal or distal to the ductus arteriosus.

Aortic coarctation that occurs proximal to the ductus arteriosus is called preductal coarctation. If the coarctation is severe, the major source of systemic blood flow will be pulmonary artery blood flowing through the ductus arteriosus. In order to keep infants with preductal coarctation alive until the stenosis can be surgically repaired, the ductus must remain open. This is accomplished by administering prostaglandin E intravenously or into the duct. Preductal coarctation is a cyanotic defect.

Postductal coarctation occurs if the narrowing is distal to the ductus arteriosus. In this case the duct usually closes. However, blood leaves the aorta via subclavian arteries, which branch off before the coarctation, and travels to the upper body. The result is an obvious disparity in the upper and lower body pulses, depending on the degree of coarctation. Systemic signs of poor blood flow will be apparent. Collateral vessels that deliver blood to the systemic circulation frequently develop around the coarctation.

Tetralogy of Fallot

This congenital heart defect is characterized by four presenting abnormalities: ventricular septal defect, pulmonary artery stenosis, right ventricular hypertrophy, and a shifting of the position of the aorta so that it opens into the right ventricle (an overriding aorta). Tetralogy of Fallot is a cyanotic defect.

CLINICAL MANIFESTATIONS

- With a right-to-left shunt, cyanosis, fatigue, and weakness occur. Knee-to-chest or squatting behavior may be used. Clubbing of the digits may develop.
- With a left-to-right shunt, pulmonary congestion and dyspnea may occur. Left heart failure may develop.

DIAGNOSTIC TOOLS

- With an atrial septal defect, a splitting of the second heart sound is frequently heard because closure of the pulmonary valve may be prolonged.
- With a ventricular septal defect, a systolic murmur is usually present.
- Postductal coarctation causes disparity in upper and lower body pulses and blood pressure.

TREATMENT

- Some defects may be small, require no treatment, or close spontaneously.
- Surgical correction of the defect is often required.
- Treatment for congestive heart failure may be necessary.
- Prostaglandin E is administered to maintain patency of the ductus arteriosus in preductal coarctation.
- Administration of the prostaglandin inhibitor indomethacin will initiate closure of the ductus in patent ductuctus arteriosus.

Shock

Shock is the collapse of systemic arterial blood pressure. With a severe fall in blood pressure, blood flow does not adequately meet the energy demands of tissues and organs. In addition, the body responds by diverting blood away from most tissues and organs to ensure that vital organs, that is, the brain, heart, and lungs, receive blood. The tissues and organs that are deemed expendable are severely jeopardized, especially the kidneys, the gut, and the skin. If the individual survives the shock episode, renal failure, gastrointestinal ulcers, and a sloughing of the skin often follow.

THE BARORECEPTOR RESPONSE TO SHOCK

With the beginning of shock, baroreceptor reflexes are activated and the body tries to compensate for the drastically reduced blood pressure. If the cause of shock continues, compensation will become inadequate and deterioration of all organs, including the lungs, heart, and brain, will progress. As the heart and lungs deteriorate, a deadly cycle is initiated. Oxygenation and cardiac output progressively fall and shock worsens, soon becoming irreversible. Irreversible shock results in death of the individual.

CAUSES OF SHOCK

Blood pressure depends on the product of the cardiac output (heart rate × stroke volume) and TPR. Therefore, anything that causes heart rate, stroke volume, or TPR to plummet can cause shock. There are six major causes of shock.

Cardiogenic shock can occur following collapse of the cardiac output, which often results from a myocardial infarct, fibrillation, or congestive heart failure.

Hypovolemic shock can occur if there is a loss of circulating blood volume, causing a severe drop in cardiac output and blood pressure. Hemorrhage and dehydration can cause hypovolemic shock.

Anaphylactic shock can occur following a widespread allergic response associated with mast cell degranulation and the release of inflammatory mediators, such as histamine and prostaglandin. These inflammatory mediators cause widespread systemic vasodilatation, which causes TPR and blood pressure to fall dramatically.

Septic shock can occur following a massive systemic infection and the release of vasoactive mediators of inflammation. These substances initiate widespread vasodilation, causing TPR and blood pressure to collapse. Septic shock may occur with a blood-borne bacterial infection, or from the release of gut contents with gastrointestinal perforation or a burst appendix. Some bacteria seem to be "superantigens" capable of rapidly stimulating septic shock.

Neurogenic shock occurs following sudden loss of vascular tone throughout the body. Neurogenic shock may be due to a brain injury involving the cardiovascular center of the brain, a spinal cord injury, or from deep general anesthesia. It may also occur as a result of a burst of parasympathetic stimulation to the heart that slows the heart rate and decreases sympathetic stimulation to the blood vessels. An example is sudden fainting with an emotional disturbance.

Burn shock occurs following a severe burn involving a substantial amount of total body surface area. Burn shock is an interesting combination of shock due to the systemic release of the vasodilatory mediators of inflammation causing a fall in TPR, and a collapse of the blood volume as plasma leaks across suddenly porous capillary membranes.

CLINICAL MANIFESTATIONS

Specific manifestations will depend on the cause of shock, but all, except neurogenic shock, will include:

- Cool, clammy skin.
- Pallor.
- Increased heart and respiratory rate.
- Dramatically decreased blood pressure.
- Individuals with neurogenic shock will have a normal or slow heart rate, and will be warm and dry to the touch.

DIAGNOSTIC TOOLS

- A measured severe decrease in blood pressure.
- Decreased or absent urine output.

COMPLICATIONS

- Multiorgan failure from prolonged decreased blood flow and tissue hypoxia.
- Adult respiratory distress syndrome from hypoxic destruction of the alveolar-capillary interface.
- Disseminated intravascular coagulation from extensive tissue death and hypoxia, causing overactivation of the coagulation cascade.

TREATMENT

- The cause of shock must be identified and reversed if possible.
- Plasma volume replacement is essential, except for cardiogenic shock. What is used for replacement depends on the cause of shock.
- Supplemental oxygen or artificial ventilation may be required.
- Vasopressor agents are given in order to return blood pressure toward normal.

Selected Bibliography

Berenson, G. S., Srinivasan, S. R., Bao, W., Newman, W. P. Tracy, R. E., Wattigney, W. A. (1998) Association between multiple cardiovascular risk factors and atherosclerosis in children and young adults. *New England Journal of Medicine* 338, 1650–1656.

Burt, M. J., Halliday, J. W., & Powell, L. W. (1993). Iron and coronary heart disease. *British Medical Journal* 307, 575–576.

Cutler, J. A. (1998). Calcium-channel blockers for hypertension—uncertainty continues. *New England Journal of Medicine* 338, 679–681.

Diaz, M. N., Frei, B., Vita, J. A., & Keaney, J. F. (1997). Antioxidants and atherosclerotic heart disease. *New England Journal of Medicine* 337, 408–416.

Estacio, R. O., Jeffers, F. W., Hiatt, W. R., Biggerstaff, S. L., Gifford, N., & Schrier, R. W. (1998). The effect of nisoldipine as compared with enalapril on cardiovascular outcomes in patients with non-insulin-dependent diabetes and hypertension. *New England Journal of Medicine* 338, 645–652.

Feit, L. R. (1997). The heart of the matter: evaluating murmurs in children. *Contemporary Pediatrics* 14, 97–122.

Furchgott, R. F. (1983). Role of endothelium in responses of vascular smooth muscle. *Circulation Research* 53, 557–573.

Gottlieb, S. S., McCarter, R. J., & Vogel, R. A. (1998). Effect of beta-blockade on mortality among high-risk and low-risk patients after myocardial infarction. *New England Journal of Medicine* 339, 489–497.

Graudal, N. A., Galloe, A. M., & Garred, P. (1998). Effects of sodium restriction on blood pressure, renin, aldosterone, catecholamines, cholesterols, and triglyceride. *Journal of the American Medical Association* 279, 1383–1391.

Greer, I. A., Lyall, F., Perera, T., Boswell, F., & Macara, L. (1994). Increased concentrations of cytokines interleukin-6 and interleukin-1 receptor antagonist in plasma of women with preeclampsia: a mechanism for endothelial dysfunction? *Obstetrics and Gynecology* 84, 937–940.

Grodstein, F., Stampfer, M. J., Manson, J. E., Colditz, G. A., Willett, W. C., Rosner, B., Speizer, F., & Hennekens, C. H. (1996). Postmenopausal estrogen and progestin use and the risk of cardiovascular disease. *New England Journal of Medicine* 335, 453–461.

Guyton, A. C. & Hall, J. (1997). *Textbook of medical physiology (9th ed)*. Philadelphia: W.B. Saunders.

Hakim, A. A., Petrovitch, H., Burchfiel, C., et al. (1998). Effects of walking on mortality among nonsmoking retired men. *New England Journal of Medicine* 338, 94–99.

Halliwell, B. (1994). Free radicals, antioxidant, and human disease: curiosity, cause, or consequence? *Lancet* 344, 721–724.

Hamm, C. W., Goldmann, B. U., Heeschen, C., Kreymann, G., Berger, J., & Meinertz, T. (1997). Emergency room triage of patients with acute chest pain by means of rapid testing for cardiac troponin T or troponin I. *New England Journal of Medicine* 337, 1648–1653.

Joint National Committee on Prevention, Detection, Evaluation, and Treatment of High Blood Pressure. (1997). *Archives of Internal Medicine* 157, 2413–2445.

Ludwig, E. H., Hopkins, P. N., Allen, A., Wu, L. L., Williams, R. R., Anderson, J. L., Ward, R. H., Lalouel, J. M., & Innerarity, T. L. (1997). Association of genetic variations in apolipoprotein B with hypercholesterolemia, coronary artery disease, and receptor binding of low density lipoproteins. *Journal of Lipid Research* 38, 1361–1373.

Porth, C. M. (1998). *Pathophysiology: concepts of altered health states (5th ed)*. Philadelphia: J.B. Lippincott Company.

Rosamond, W. D., Chambless, L. E., Folsom, A. R., et al. (1998). Trends in the incidence of myocardial infarction and in mortality due to coronary heart disease, 1987 to 1994. *New England Journal of Medicine* 339, 861–867.

Salonen, J. Y., Nyyssonen, K., Korpela, H., Tuomilehto, J., Seppanen, R., & Salonen, R. (1992). High stored iron levels are associated with excess risk of myocardial infarct in eastern Finnish men. *Circulation* 86, 803–811.

Stefanick, M. L., Mackey, S., Sheehan, M., Ellsworth, N., Haskell, W., & Wood, P. D. (1998). Effects of diet and exercise in men and postmenopausal women with low levels of HDL cholesterol and high levels of LDL cholesterol. *New England Journal of Medicine* 339, 12–20.

Straka, R. J., Swanson, A. L., & Parra, D. (1998). Calcium channel antagonists: morbidity and mortality—what's the evidence? *American Family Physician* 57, 1551–1559.

Welch, G. N. & Loscalzo, J. (1998). Homocysteine and atherothrombosis. *New England Journal of Medicine* 338, 1042–1050.

Yang, B. B. (1993). Cardiac effects of acetylcholine in rat hearts: role of endothelium-derived relaxing factor and prostaglandins. *American Journal of Physiology* 264, H1388–H1393

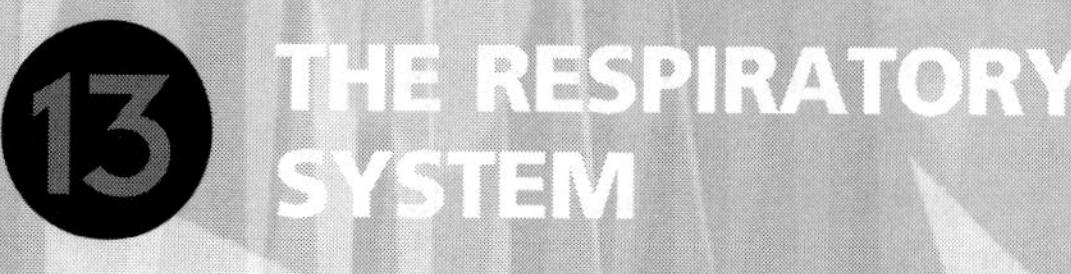

13 THE RESPIRATORY SYSTEM

The role of the respiratory system is to provide for the exchange of oxygen and carbon dioxide between the air and the blood. Oxygen is required by all cells so that the life-sustaining energy source, adenosine triphosphate (ATP) can be reproduced. Carbon dioxide is produced by metabolically active cells and forms an acid that must be removed from the body. For gas exchange to be performed, the cardiovascular and respiratory systems must work together. The cardiovascular system is responsible for perfusion of blood through the lungs. The respiratory system performs two separate functions: ventilation and respiration.

PHYSIOLOGIC CONCEPTS

Alveolus

The functional unit of the lungs is the alveolus (plural, alveoli). There are more than a million alveoli in each lung. Alveoli are small, air-filled sacs, across which oxygen and carbon dioxide and other gases diffuse. The large number of small alveoli ensures that the total area available for the diffusion of gas in each lung is enormous. If the airflow into an alveolus is blocked, it collapses and is unavailable for gas exchange. If airflow into several alveoli is blocked, exchange of gases may be impaired to the extent that the person becomes hypoxic or unconscious or dies.

Ventilation

The movement of air from the atmosphere into and out of the lungs is called ventilation. Ventilation occurs by bulk flow. Bulk flow is the movement of a gas or a fluid from high to low pressure.

Factors That Affect Ventilation

Ventilation is determined by the variables in Equation 13-1:

$$F = P/R \tag{13-1}$$

where F is the bulk flow of air, P is the difference in pressure between the atmosphere and the alveoli, and R is the resistance offered by the conducting airways.

Pressure Alveolar pressure varies with each inspiration and drives the flow of air. With the onset of inspiration, the thoracic cavity expands. As the thoracic cavity expands, the lungs also expand. According to Boyle's law, if the volume of an air-filled chamber increases, the pressure of the air in the chamber decreases. Therefore, as the lungs expand, pressure in the alveoli decreases to below atmospheric pressure, and air rushes into the lungs from the atmosphere (from high pressure to low). At the end of inspiration, the thoracic cavity relaxes, causing pressures in the alveoli, which are filled with the air of inspiration, to be higher than in the atmosphere. Air then flows out of the lung and down this pressure gradient.

Bronchial Resistance Resistance of the airways is usually low. Resistance is increased when the smooth muscle of the bronchiolar tubes constricts. Constriction of the bronchi results in a decrease in airflow into the lungs. Resistance is inversely proportional to the radius of a vessel to the fourth power. This means that if the radius of a bronchiolar tube decreases by one-half, the resistance to airflow in that tube increases by 16 (i.e., 2^4). Therefore, **when the air passages constrict even slightly, resistance to airflow goes up significantly.**

Bronchiolar resistance is determined by parasympathetic and sympathetic nervous system innervation of the smooth muscle of the bronchi and local chemical mediators.

Parasympathetic nerves are carried to the bronchial smooth muscle by way of the vagus nerve and cause contraction or narrowing of the airways, increasing resistance and reducing airflow. Parasympathetic nerves release the neurotransmitter acetylcholine (ACh). ACh acts by binding to cholinergic receptors on the smooth muscle of the bronchi.

Sympathetic innervation of the bronchial smooth muscle occurs by way of nerve fibers from the upper thoracic and cervical ganglia and causes relaxation of the bronchi. This reduces resistance and increases airflow. Sympathetic nerves release the neurotransmitter norepinephrine. Norepinephrine acts by binding to β_2 receptors on the smooth muscle of the bronchi.

Nervous Control of Respiration

Ventilation is controlled by the respiratory center in the lower brainstem areas of the medulla and pons. In the medulla, there are inspiratory and expiratory neurons that fire at opposite times in a preset pattern of rate and rhythm. Respiratory neurons drive ventilation by exciting motor neurons that innervate the main muscle of inspiration, the **diaphragm**, and the accessory muscles, the intercostal muscles.

Motor Neurons Driving Respiration The major motor neuron controlling respiration is the phrenic nerve. When activated by the central inspiratory neurons, the phrenic nerve causes the diaphragm muscle to contract and the chest to expand. As the chest expands, air begins to flow from the atmosphere into the lungs. Airflow into the lungs is called **inspiration.** As inspiration continues, firing of the central inspiratory neurons slows and firing of the expiratory neurons increases, causing cessation of motor neuron activity and relaxation of the diaphragm. Chest expansion reverses and air flows out of the lungs. Airflow out of the lungs is called **expiration.**

Central Chemoreceptors Central chemoreceptors in the brain respond to changes in the hydrogen ion concentration of the cerebral spinal fluid. Increased hydrogen-ion concentration increases the firing rate of the chemoreceptors. Decreased hydrogen-ion concentration decreases the firing rate of the chemoreceptors. Information from the central chemoreceptors is delivered to the respiratory center in the brain which, in response, increases or decreases the breathing pattern. Hydrogen-ion concentration usually reflects carbon dioxide concentration. Therefore, when carbon dioxide levels rise, hydrogen-ion levels rise, and the firing rate of inspiratory neurons is increased, causing an increase in respiratory rate. This is an example of negative feedback, because with an increase in the rate of breathing, the excess carbon dioxide and hydrogen ion will be blown off. With low carbon dioxide and low hydrogen-ion levels, the firing rate of the inspiratory neurons is reduced and respiration slows.

Peripheral Chemoreceptors Peripheral chemoreceptors exist in the carotid and the aortic arteries and monitor oxygen concentration in arterial blood. These receptors, called the carotid and the aortic bodies, send their impulses to the respiratory center of the medulla and pons primarily to increase the rate of ventilation when oxygen is low. They are less sensitive than the central chemoreceptors. The peripheral chemoreceptors also respond with an increase in firing rate to increased hydrogen ion dissolved in the blood. This is important because under certain circumstances free hydrogen ion increases without causing a change in carbon dioxide concentration (e.g., during conditions of metabolic acidosis caused by prolonged diarrhea or diabetes mellitus). Free hydrogen ion is relatively impermeable across the blood–brain barrier so would be unable to activate the central chemoreceptors directly.

Respiration

Respiration refers to the diffusion of gases between an alveolus and the capillary that perfuses it. Respiration occurs by diffusion, which involves the movement of a gas down its concentration gradient.

FACTORS THAT AFFECT RESPIRATION

The rate of diffusion of a gas (e.g., oxygen and carbon dioxide) is determined with Equation 13-2:

$$\dot{D} = \frac{(X_a - X_c) \cdot SA \cdot T}{d \cdot k} \qquad (13\text{-}2)$$

where $\dot{D}$ is the rate of diffusion, X_a is the concentration of gas in the alveolus, X_c is the concentration of gas in the capillary, *SA* is the surface area available for diffusion, *T* is the temperature of the solution, *d* is the distance across which diffusion must occur, and *k* is a physical constant that takes into account nonvariable characteristics of the gas such as its molecular weight and its specific solubility coefficient.

Concentration of Oxygen and Carbon Dioxide in the Alveolus and the Capillary

Alveolar oxygen concentration reflects atmospheric oxygen, whereas pulmonary capillary oxygen concentration reflects the oxygen concentration of systemic venous blood. Because systemic venous blood is blood returning from the peripheral circulation where much of the oxygen has been used by the cells of the body, it has a low oxygen concentration. The atmosphere is typically well supplied with oxygen. Therefore, oxygen is normally in higher concentration in the alveolus than it is in the pulmonary capillary. Values for oxygen concentration are directly proportional to the partial pressure of the gas and are usually expressed in millimeters of mercury.

At sea level, the partial pressure of oxygen is approximately 100 mm Hg in the alveolus and 40 mm Hg in the pulmonary capillary. Because alveolar oxygen concentration is greater than capillary, oxygen diffuses down its concentration gradient from the alveolus into the capillary. This is how deoxygenated blood is replenished with oxygen by respiration.

Carbon dioxide normally diffuses in the opposite direction. It is in low concentration in the atmosphere and thus in low concentration in the alveolus (40 mm Hg). Pulmonary capillary blood reflects systemic venous blood. Because carbon dioxide is a waste product of metabolizing cells, concentration of carbon dioxide in the capillary is high (46 mm Hg). Therefore, in the lungs, carbon dioxide diffuses down its concentration gradient, from the blood into the alveolus, where it will be expired.

Under some circumstances, concentration gradients of oxygen and carbon dioxide between the blood and the alveolus may be increased or decreased; magnified concentration gradients affect the diffusion rate of the gas. For example, during exercise, oxygen concentration in the blood entering the pulmonary capillaries may be less than 40 mm Hg because the exercising muscles have increased their oxygen usage. Carbon dioxide concentration would be greater in blood flowing to the lungs from exercising tissue because its metabolic production would be increased. In this situation, diffusion rates for both gases would be increased, allowing more oxygen to diffuse into the blood and more carbon dioxide to diffuse out of the blood.

Surface Area

Surface area (SA) refers to the field of alveolar and capillary membranes available for gas diffusion. Surface area is normally high in the lungs. Some diseases, including emphysema, tuberculosis, and lung cancer, can decrease the surface area available for diffusion, thus reducing the diffusion rates of oxygen and carbon dioxide.

Distance for Diffusion

The distance (*d*) across which oxygen and carbon dioxide must diffuse is normally quite small. Alveolar and capillary membranes are close to each other, separated only by a thin layer of interstitial fluid (Fig. 13-1).

Certain conditions, including pneumonia, can increase the distance of diffusion by causing edema and swelling of the interstitial space. This decreases the diffusion rate of the gases (Fig. 13-2). Interstitial fibrosis (scarring) can also increase the distance between the alveoli and the capillaries and so slow diffusion.

Temperature

A decrease in temperature (*T*) would decrease the diffusion rate of oxygen and carbon dioxide. An increase in *T* would increase the diffusion rate of both gases. An increase in temperature may play a role in meeting the increased metabolic demands during fever.

Permeability Coefficient

Carbon dioxide and, to a lesser extent, oxygen, have high permeability. Because the variable *k* in the equation is fixed for each gas, *k* does not play an active role in determining respiration.

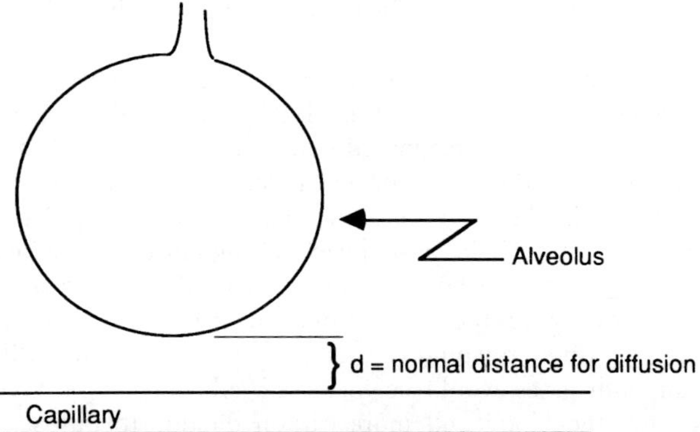

Figure 13-1. Normal alveolus–capillary distance allows for efficient diffusion of oxygen and carbon dioxide between the capillary and alveolus.

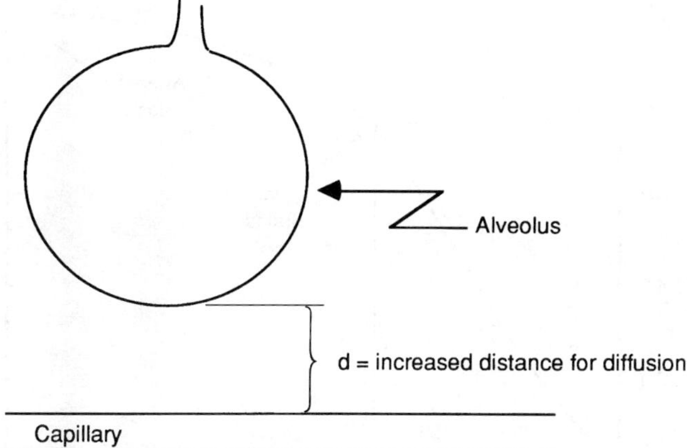

Figure 13-2. With interstitial edema, the alveolus–capillary distance is increased, resulting in reduced diffusion of oxygen and carbon dioxide between the capillary and the alveolus.

Oxygen Carrying in the Blood

Oxygen is carried both dissolved in the blood and bound to hemoglobin. The amount of oxygen dissolved in the blood depends on the partial pressure of oxygen in the air entering the alveoli and the solubility of oxygen. Normally the amount carried dissolved is small (only approximately 3 mL/L). Instead, most oxygen (98%) is carried bound to hemoglobin.

Hemoglobin is a protein molecule composed of four subunits, each combining a globulin molecule with a molecule of iron. Each iron molecule has a binding site for oxygen. Dissolved oxygen combines with hemoglobin until all four sites are saturated. At normal arterial oxygen concentration of 100 mm Hg, nearly 100% of hemoglobin molecules are saturated with oxygen. Even in venous blood, with a reduced oxygen concentration of 40 mm Hg, hemoglobin is still at least 75% saturated with oxygen (Fig. 13-3). The affinity of hemoglobin to bind oxygen is reduced by increased hydrogen-ion concentration, increased temperature, and increased amount of a substance produced by red blood cells during glycolysis, 2,3,diphosphoglycerate (DPG). A reduced affinity for oxygen means that hemoglobin releases oxygen to the tissues more readily. Increase in hydrogen ion, temperature, and DPG increased metabolism; therefore decreased hemoglobin affinity releases more oxygen to a cell and allows it to meet its metabolic demands.

Perfusion

For the respiratory system, perfusion refers to the movement of blood in the pulmonary vascular system, past the alveolar capillaries.

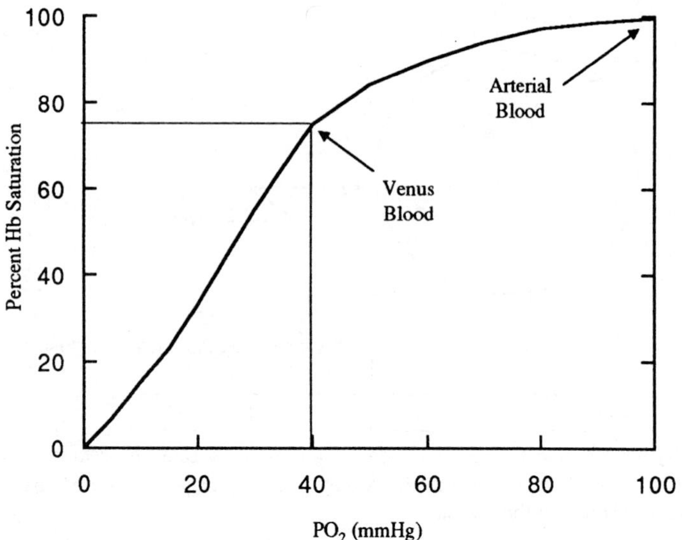

Figure 13-3. Oxygen-hemoglobin saturation curve. Notice at arterial O_2 levels (PO_2), nearly 100% of hemoglobin is saturated. Even at PO_2 of 60 mg Hg, 90% of Hb is saturated. In venous blood ($PO_2$40), 75% of Hb is saturated with blood.

Perfusion, like blood flow everywhere and like ventilation, occurs by bulk flow. In the lungs, perfusion and ventilation usually are well matched. This ensures that there is adequate oxygen available in each alveolus to replenish the blood flowing past it, and adequate blood flow to support each alveolus.

Circulations That Provide Blood Flow to the Lungs

Two separate blood circulations supply blood flow to the lungs from the heart. One is the pulmonary and the other is the bronchial circulation.

PULMONARY CIRCULATION

The pulmonary circulation consists of deoxygenated blood traveling in the pulmonary artery from the right side of the heart. This blood perfuses the respiratory portions of the lungs and participates in the exchange of oxygen and carbon dioxide across the capillaries and alveoli. After picking up oxygen and releasing carbon dioxide, it returns to the heart by way of the pulmonary vein. The pulmonary circulation accounts for approximately 8 to 9% of the total cardiac output. Pressure and resistance to flow in the pulmonary circulation are usually low, with a mean pulmonary pressure of approximately 12 mm Hg compared with a mean systemic pressure of approximately 90 mm Hg. The pulmonary circulation is compliant and can accommodate large variations in blood volume. Therefore, the pulmonary circulation can act as a reservoir for blood, that can be called upon in times of decreased systemic blood volume or pressure.

BRONCHIAL CIRCULATION

The bronchial circulation carries blood from the left side of the heart to the lungs through the thoracic aorta. This blood is well oxygenated and supplies oxygen to the structures of the lungs not involved in the exchange of gases, including the connective tissue and the large and the small bronchi. Blood returns to the left side of the heart through the pulmonary vein. Returning bronchial blood is deoxygenated because it has been used by metabolically active cells of the lungs but has not been involved in gas exchange. This blood mixes with the well-oxygenated blood coming from the pulmonary circulation back to the left side of the heart and slightly reduces the overall oxygen concentration of that blood.

Ventilation:Perfusion Ratio

Ventilation refers to air moving into and out of the lungs. Perfusion is the blood passing through the pulmonary circulation to be oxygenated. The ventilation:perfusion ratio, *V/Q*, is the ratio of airflow into the lungs divided by the pulmonary blood flow. In this expression, *V* is the volume of air moved with each breath, expressed as ml/min, and *Q* is the rate of blood flow in the pulmonary circulation, also expressed as milliliters per minute. Normally, perfusion is slightly greater than ventilation and the *V/Q* ratio is approximately 0.8. Therefore, the alveoli receiving oxygen are well perfused by blood, allowing optimal conditions for gas exchange.

Elasticity

Elasticity of the respiratory system refers to the degree to which the lungs resist inflation or stretching. The alveoli and other lung tissue normally resist stretching and recoil after the force causing the stretch or expansion is removed. This situation is partially caused by the surface tension of each alveolus and partially by the presence of elastic fibers throughout the lungs, which tend to recoil after stretch. Conditions such as emphysema reduce the elastic recoil of the lungs, resulting in chronic overinflation.

The reciprocal of elasticity of the lungs is **lung compliance.** Compliance refers to the ease of inflation or stretching of the lungs. Lung compliance is reduced by fibrosis, infection, or adult respiratory distress syndrome (ARDS).

Pleural Pressure

The lungs are surrounded by a thin membrane called the pleura. The outer layer of the pleural membrane is attached to the wall of the thoracic cavity. The inner layer of the pleura is attached to the lungs. With expansion of the thoracic cavity during inspiration, the outer layer is pulled out; this force is transmitted to the inner layer, which expands the lungs. In between the inner and outer layers of the pleura is the pleural space. This space is filled with a few milliliters of fluid that surround and lubricate the lungs. The pleural fluid is at negative pressure and opposes the elastic recoil (collapse) of the lungs. This helps keep the lungs expanded.

Surface Tension

Surface tension refers to the tendency of water molecules to pull toward each other and to collapse a sphere. Because each alveolus is lined with a thin water layer, the surface tension within each alveolus could be high, making it extremely difficult to expand an alveolus. With each breath, a certain pressure must be exerted to overcome the surface tension of the water layer. The amount of pressure needed to expand the alveolus is described by the Law of Laplace in Equation 13-3:

$$P = 2T/r \tag{13-3}$$

where P is the pressure needed to expand the alveolus, T is the surface tension of the water molecules, and r is the radius of the alveolus. As shown in this equation, the smaller the alveolus, the greater the pressure required to expand it. An inability to overcome the surface tension of an alveolus could lead to alveolar collapse. Normally, however, the surface tension of an alveolus is kept low by the presence of surfactant.

Surfactant

Certain cells inside the alveolus, called **type II alveolar cells,** produce an important substance called surfactant that helps reduce the surface tension of the alveolus, making it easier to inflate. Surfactant is a phospholipid that acts like a detergent to intersperse between water molecules in the alveolus, thereby weakening the bonds between them. This reduces surface tension and the tendency of the sphere to collapse.

When surfactant is present, a small alveolus actually requires less pressure to inflate than a large one because the surfactant is packed tightly together, greatly reducing the surface tension of the alveolus. This serves to compensate for the effect of small radius in the Laplace equation.

Tests of Pulmonary Function

LUNG VOLUMES

Spirometry is used to determine lung volumes. Spirometry is the measurement of the volume of air moving into and out of the lungs and is measured as an individual inhales and exhales into a closed chamber. Lung volumes usually measured include tidal, inspiratory reserve, expiratory reserve, and residual volumes, and, calculated from these, vital capacity (Fig. 13-4). Average values presented below for each of these volumes are for an adult male. Values for adult females are approximately 20 to 25% less.

Tidal Volume

The amount of air normally inspired (inspiratory volume) with each breath is the tidal volume. The amount of air inspired at rest usually equals the amount expired (expiratory volume). Tidal volume averages approximately 500 mL at rest.

Inspiratory Reserve Volume

The amount of air above the normal inspiration that can be maximally inspired with each breath is the inspiratory reserve volume. It averages approximately 3000 mL.

Expiratory Reserve Volume

The maximum amount of air that can be exhaled beyond normal exhalation is the expiratory reserve volume. This value averages approximately 1000 mL.

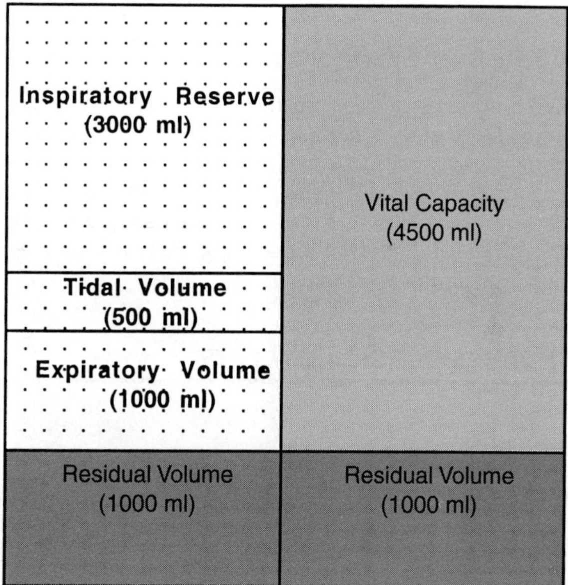

Figure 13-4. Approximate lung volumes per breath for a 70-kg male. Average lung volumes are proportional to body mass index.

Residual Volume

The air remaining in the lungs after maximum exhalation is the residual volume. The normal value is approximately 1000 mL.

Vital Capacity

The maximum amount of air an individual can inspire and expire during a single breath is the vital capacity. It includes inspiratory reserve, tidal, and expiratory reserve volumes. It is measured by having an individual take a maximum breath and then exhale as much as possible into the measurement chamber. In restrictive pulmonary disorders (e.g., resulting from neuromuscular disease, fibrosis, or loss of surfactant producing cells) vital capacity is reduced.

A common test of pulmonary function is to plot the percentage of the vital capacity an individual can expire in the first second of expiration, called the **forced expiratory volume** $(FEV)_1$. A healthy individual can expire approximately 80% of vital capacity as fast as possible in the first second. In obstructive pulmonary diseases such as asthma and emphysema, expiration is particularly affected, and the amount of air an individual can forcefully expire in the first second is reduced. In patients who have restrictive airway disease, expiration is usually normal. Therefore, whereas overall vital capacity is reduced in those who have restrictive airway disease, FEV_1 is normal.

Anatomic Dead Space

The amount of air in each breath that is measured as part of the tidal volume but that does not actually participate in gas exchange is the anatomic dead space. This air fills the conducting passages such as the trachea and the bronchioles. With rapid, shallow respirations, a greater percentage of each breath is wasted simply moving air in and out of the anatomic dead space compared with that seen with slow, deeper breathing.

PATHOPHYSIOLOGIC CONCEPTS

Atelectasis

Collapse of either a lung or an alveolus is called atelectasis. Collapsed alveoli are airless, and therefore do not participate in gas exchange. This results in a reduction in the surface area available for diffusion, and respiration is decreased. The collapse of previously expanded alveoli is called **secondary** atelectasis. Newborns may be born with alveoli collapsed at birth. This condition is called **primary** atelectasis.

Pediatric Consideration

As described later, primary atelectasis of the alveoli results in poor oxygenation of the newborn and is associated with significant morbidity and mortality. The cause of alveolar collapse is usually inadequate production of surfactant, resulting in high surface tension in the alveoli. The infant must work hard with each breath to overcome surface tension and expand the alveoli. This can lead to exhaustion and an ever-worsening exchange of gases.

Types of Atelectasis

The two main types of atelectasis are compression atelectasis and absorption atelectasis.

Compression Atelectasis Compression atelectasis occurs when a source outside the alveolus exerts enough pressure on the alveolus to collapse it. This occurs if the chest wall is punctured or opened because atmospheric pressure is greater than the pressure holding the lungs expanded (pleural pressure), and with exposure to atmospheric pressure, the lungs will collapse. Compression atelectasis can also occur if there is pressure exerted on the lungs or alveoli from a growing tumor, abdominal distention, or edema and swelling of the interstitial space around an alveolus.

Absorption Atelectasis Absence of air in the alveolus results in absorption atelectasis. If flow of air into an alveolus is blocked, the air currently inside eventually diffuses out and the alveolus collapses. Blockage usually occurs after mucus buildup and obstruction of airflow through a bronchus supplying a given group of alveoli. Any situation that results in mucus accumulation, such as cystic fibrosis, pneumonia, or chronic bronchitis, increases the risk of absorption atelectasis. Surgery is also a risk factor for absorption atelectasis because of the mucus-producing effects of anesthesia as well as a resultant hesitancy to cough up accumulated mucus after surgery. This is especially true if the surgery was in the abdominal or thoracic area where pain associated with coughing is intense. Prolonged bed rest after surgery increases the risk of developing absorption atelectasis because lying down causes a pooling of mucus secretions in dependent areas of the lung, decreasing ventilation to those areas. Mucus accumulation increases the risk of pneumonia because mucus can act as a breeding ground for microorganism growth.

Absorption atelectasis can also be caused by anything that reduces the production or concentration of surfactant. Without surfactant, surface tension in the alveolus is high, increasing the likelihood of alveolar collapse. Premature birth is associated with a reduction in surfactant and a high incidence of absorption atelectasis. Near-drowning may dilute out surfactant and so may be associated with absorption atelectasis as well.

Damage to the type II alveolar cells that produce surfactant also can lead to absorption atelectasis. These cells are destroyed by the breakdown of the alveolar wall that occurs during ARDS as well as by high oxygen therapy for a period longer than 24 hours. With loss of these cells, surfactant production is reduced.

Hypoxemia

The condition of reduced oxygen concentration in arterial blood is called hypoxemia. There are many causes of hypoxemia. Hypoxemia can occur if there is decreased oxygen in the air (hypoxia) or if hypoventilation occurs because of decreased lung compliance or atelectasis. Hypoxemia related to hypoperfusion (decreased blood flow past the alveoli) can occur from pulmonary hypertension, a pulmonary embolus, or a myocardial infarct. Hypoxemia may also occur if there is a problem with diffusion of oxygen across the alveolus into the capillary. This may occur with destruction of the alveolar–capillary interface or with edema of the alveolar–capillary interstitial space.

Because oxygen is carried in the red blood cell bound to hemoglobin, any decrease in hemoglobin concentration or carrying capacity can result in hypoxemia. Hemoglobin concentration is reduced in certain types of anemia. Binding sites for oxygen on the hemoglobin molecule may be occupied by other gases (e.g., carbon monoxide) that would also decrease the carrying capacity of hemoglobin for oxygen.

Cyanosis

Bluish discoloration of the blood that occurs if large amounts of hemoglobin in the blood are not completely bound with oxygen molecules is called cyanosis. There are four sites on hemoglobin where oxygen may bind. Hemoglobin fully bound with oxygen is called saturated. Desaturated or deoxygenated hemoglobin is not fully bound with oxygen.

If the hemoglobin concentration in the blood is normal, but the availability of oxygen to bind to hemoglobin is reduced, the hemoglobin molecules will be deoxygenated. Normally there are approximately 15 g of hemoglobin per 100 mL of blood. In arterial blood, more than 98%, or 14.7 g per 100 mL of blood, will be saturated with oxygen. Venous blood normally has an oxygen saturation of 75%; this comes to 11.3 g of hemoglobin per 100 mL of blood saturated with oxygen and about 4 g per 100 mL unsaturated. If arterial hemoglobin oxygen saturation falls below 70%, resulting in *5 g or more of unsaturated hemoglobin per milliliter of blood,* cyanosis will be apparent.

In hypoxemia caused by low hemoglobin concentration, such as with microcytic, hypochromic anemia, cyanosis will not develop because there will not be greater than 5 g of deoxygenated hemoglobin per 100 mL of blood. Cyanosis will not occur with carbon monoxide poisoning because the hemoglobin binding sites will still be saturated, although with the carbon monoxide molecule rather than oxygen. In both of these situations, hypoxemia would be present in the absence of cyanosis.

ALTERATIONS IN VENTILATION:PERFUSION RATIO

A decrease in ventilation may occur when delivery of air to some alveoli is obstructed, for example with mucus or by foreign-body aspiration. With decreased ventilation (*V*), the ventilation:perfusion ratio is decreased, because the blood flow (*Q*) will pass by underventilated alveoli. This mismatch in ventilation and perfusion is not beneficial for gas exchange, and is an example of right-to-left shunting of blood. Right-to-left shunting, described in Chapter 12, is characterized by delivery of deoxygenated blood to the systemic circulation. A decrease in the ventilation:perfusion ratio, however, will not last long in the lungs because of the pulmonary arteriolar response when exposed to low oxygen.

Pulmonary arterioles vasoconstrict in response to low oxygen concentration in underventilated alveoli. This serves to decrease blood flow to those alveoli, returning the ventilation:perfusion ratio back toward 1.0. This response is called **hypoxic vasoconstriction.** Hypoxic vasoconstriction is effective only if the extent of underventilated alveoli is limited. In conditions such as chronic bronchitis, alveolar obstruction is so widespread that a normal ventilation:perfusion ratio cannot be maintained. Hypoxic vasoconstriction of the pulmonary arterioles can lead to pulmonary hypertension as described in the following.

Under some circumstances, it is possible for ventilation of an alveolus to be adequate but capillary perfusion to be compromised. The result is a decrease in *Q* and an increase in the ventilation:perfusion ratio. This situation could occur as a result of a pulmonary embolus. A myocardial infarct would also cause decreased perfusion of the alveoli.

PULMONARY HYPERTENSION

Elevated blood pressure of the pulmonary vascular system is called pulmonary hypertension. It is a common condition in serious respiratory or cardiovascular disease.

Causes of Pulmonary Hypertension

The pulmonary circulation is usually a low-pressure, low-resistance circulation. Anything that causes 1) a prolonged increase in pulmonary blood flow, 2) an increase in pulmonary resistance to flow, or 3) an impediment in pulmonary vascular outflow, can result in pulmonary hypertension.

Increased Pulmonary Blood Flow If excessive blood volume is delivered to the lungs, increased pulmonary blood flow ocurs. For example, with a left-to-right shunt, blood from the left side of the heart goes back to the lungs rather than to the systemic circulation, thus overloading the lungs.

Increased Pulmonary Resistance to Flow Anything that obstructs the passage of blood into or through the lungs causes increased pulmonary resistance to flow. This includes pulmonary fibrosis (scarring) and the changes in the structure of the lungs that accompany chronic obstructive pulmonary disease (COPD). Long-term pulmonary hypoxic vasoconstriction is also a significant cause of increased pulmonary resistance and hypertension. Hypoxic vasoconstriction of the pulmonary arterioles occurs when the pulmonary circulation is exposed to low oxygen, causing the vascular smooth muscle of the pulmonary arterioles to constrict. This can be useful because it allows the ventilation:perfusion ratio to return toward 1.0. However, if the condition is chronic or extensive, hypertrophy of the arterioles and increased pulmonary resistance can result.

Impediment to Outflow This condition occurs with left-heart failure. Other causes of impediment to outflow are mitral or aortic stenosis or incompetence.

Consequences of Pulmonary Hypertension

Pulmonary hypertension can make it more difficult for the right side of the heart to pump. A type of heart failure called **cor pulmonale** can result. Cor pulmonale is right-sided heart failure caused by chronic lung disease. Pulmonary hypertension can also result in pulmonary edema because the capillary hydrostatic force favoring filtration is increased. Edema of the pulmonary interstitial space leads to a decreased diffusion rate of oxygen from the alveolus to the capillary owing to increased distance for diffusion.

Bronchiectasis

Bronchiectasis is abnormal dilation of a bronchus or bronchi. Bronchiectasis occurs from long-standing pulmonary obstruction of the lower airways by tumors, chronic infections, mucus accumulation as seen in cystic fibrosis, and exposure to toxins. The bronchi fill with mucus, resulting in atelectasis and development of abnormal connections between the bronchi. Ventilation of the alveoli is impaired.

Central Nervous System Depression

Central nervous system depression is a depressed respiratory drive resulting from alteration in function of the respiratory centers of the brain. Central nervous system depression can occur with hypoxemia or chronic elevation of carbon dioxide concentration, both of which occur when there is decreased pulmonary ventilation or perfusion. The respiratory center of the medulla and pons, which normally drives respiration, requires adequate oxygenation to function. Although the normal stimulus to breathe is carbon dioxide concentration of the cerebral spinal fluid (as reflected in hydrogen-ion concentration) high carbon dioxide levels can depress the respiratory center enough to cause a cessation of breathing.

CONDITIONS OF DISEASE OR INJURY

Upper Respiratory Tract Infections

Infections caused by any microorganism to the non–gas-exchanging upper structures of the respiratory tract, including the nasal passages, the pharynx, and the larynx are known as upper respiratory tract infections. Upper respiratory tract infections include the common cold, pharyngitis or sore throat, laryngitis, and uncomplicated influenza. Most upper respiratory tract infections are caused by viruses, although bacteria may also be involved either initially or secondary to a viral infection. All types of infections activate the immune and the inflammatory responses, leading to swelling and edema of the infected tissue. The inflammatory reaction leads to increased mucus production, contributing to the symptoms seen with upper respiratory tract infections, including congestion, excess sputum, and nasal discharge. Headache, low-grade fever, and malaise may also occur as a result of the inflammatory reaction.

RESPIRATORY DEFENSES AGAINST INFECTION

Although the upper respiratory tract is directly exposed to the environment, infections are uncommon and seldom progress to lower respiratory tract infections involving the lower airways and alveoli. Protective mechanisms abound throughout the respiratory tract to prevent infection. The **cough reflex** expels foreign bodies and microorganisms, and removes accumulated mucus. The **mucociliary blanket** consists of cells, located from the level of the bronchi up, which make mucus, and cilia cells that line the mucus-producing cells. The mucus-producing cells trap foreign particles, and the cilia beat rhythmically to propel the mucus and any trapped particles up the respiratory tree to the nasopharynx where they can be expelled as sputum, blown out the nose, or swallowed. This complex is sometimes referred to as the mucociliary escalator system. The cilia are delicate structures that can be paralyzed or injured by a variety of noxious stimuli, including cigarette smoke as described later.

If microorganisms evade these defense mechanisms and colonize the upper respiratory tract, a third important line of defense, the **immune system**, is in position to prevent their passage to the lower respiratory tract. This response is mediated by lymphocytes, but also involves other white blood cells such as macrophages, neutrophils, and mast cells brought to the area by the inflammatory process. If there is a breakdown of a defense mechanism of the respiratory system or if the microorganism is especially virulent, a lower respiratory tract infection might result.

EFFECTS OF CIGARETTE SMOKING ON RESPIRATORY DEFENSES

Cigarette smoke is known to alter the effectiveness of some respiratory defense mechanisms. Products of cigarette smoke are known to stimulate mucus production while paralyzing the cilia. This leads to the accumulation of thick mucus and any trapped particles or microorganisms in the airways, decreasing the movement of air and increasing the risk of microbial growth. A smoker's cough is an attempt to expel this thick mucus, which is difficult to propel, out of the respiratory tract. Lower respiratory tract infections are more common in smokers and in those exposed to secondhand smoke, especially infants and children.

Pediatric Consideration

Infants and children exposed to cigarette smoke before or after birth experience increased rates of upper respiratory tract infections, lower respiratory tract infections such as pneumonia, and childhood asthma compared with infants and children of parents who do not smoke. Urinary output of nicotine metabolites are grossly elevated in children whose parents smoke compared with those who do not. Several metabolites of nicotine are known carcinogens as well as pulmonary irritants.

CLINICAL MANIFESTATIONS

Clinical indications of upper respiratory tract infections depend on the infection site as well as the microorganism responsible for the infection. All clinical manifestations result from the inflammatory processes and any direct damage the microorganism inflicts. These include

- Cough
- Sneezing and nasal congestion
- Mucus production and drainage from the nose and down the throat
- Headache
- Low-grade fever
- Malaise (physical discomfort)

DIAGNOSTIC TOOLS

- A good history and physical will assist diagnosis.

COMPLICATIONS

- Sinusitis and otitis media may develop. Lower respiratory tract infections, including pneumonia and bronchitis may follow an upper respiratory infection.

TREATMENT

- The individual should rest to reduce the body's metabolic demands.
- Extra hydration, which helps liquefy the thick mucus, makes it easier to move out of the respiratory tract. This is important because mucus accumulation offers a breeding ground for secondary bacterial infection.
- Decongestants, antihistamines, and cough suppressants may provide some symptom relief. Some studies suggest zinc lozenges or increased vitamin C consumption may reduce the severity or likelihood of certain viral infections. Antibiotics are required if the infection is bacterial in origin or secondary.

Pediatric Consideration

In children, croup, a viral infection of the larynx or trachea, and epiglottitis, a bacterial infection of the epiglottis, may occur. Like adults, children develop significant inflammation and swelling of the respiratory tract with infections. In fact, children may demonstrate more drastic clinical manifestations with upper airway infections because the upper airways are much narrower to begin with, resulting in significant increase in resistance to airflow with even slight swelling and airway blockage. Symptoms of croup include a barking cough, hoarse voice, and stridor. Treatment for children who have croup may include a vaporizer, mist tent, or oxygen therapy. Those who have moderately severe croup are likely to benefit from intramuscular or nebulized glucocorticoids. The inflammation seen with epiglottitis may result in total obstruction to airflow, significant anxiety, and death. Children typically sit forward, and may drool. For children who have epiglottitis, hospitalization and perhaps intubation or tracheotomy may be required. Children who have epiglottitis should be kept as calm as possible (and so should their parents) to maintain airway patency until emergency support can be given.

Lower Respiratory Tract Infections

Pneumonia

Defined as an acute infection of the lung tissue by a microorganism, pneumonia is a lower respiratory tract infection. Most pneumonias are bacterial in origin, occurring as a primary condition or secondary to a previous viral infection. The most common cause of bacterial pneumonia is the gram-positive bacterium, *Streptococcus pneumoniae,* responsible for pneumococcal pneumonia. The bacteria *Staphylococcus aureus* and group A beta-hemolytic streptococci are also frequent causes of pneumonia, as is *Pseudomonas aeruginosa.* Other pneumonias are caused directly by viruses, such as that seen occasionally with influenza. Young children especially are susceptible to viral pneumonia, usually from infection with respiratory syncytial virus (RSV), parainfluenza, adenovirus, or rhinovirus. Mycoplasmal pneumonia, a relatively common pneumonia, is caused by a microorganism that is, in some respects, between a virus and a bacterium. Individuals who have acquired immunodeficiency syndrome (AIDS) frequently develop an otherwise rare pneumonia called Pneumocystis carinii. Individuals exposed to aerosols of previously standing water, for instance, from air-conditioning units or dirty humidifiers, may develop Legionella pneumonia. Finally, individuals who aspirate stomach contents after vomiting or who aspirate water in an experience of near drowning, may develop aspiration pneumonia. For these individuals, the aspirated material itself rather than a microorganism may cause pneumonia by stimulating an inflammatory reaction. Subsequent bacterial infection may also develop.

Risk of developing the pneumonias described above are greater for the young, the old, or for anyone immunocompromised or weakened by another disease or disability. Risks of death after pneumonia is also stratified based on age (over 50 or young, especially newborn) and the presence of coexisting illness such as congestive heart failure, neoplastic disease, or renal disease.

Much of the damage to the lung tissue after successful colonization of the lungs by a microorganism is the result of the usually vigorous immune and inflammatory reaction mounted by the host. In addition, toxins released by bacteria in bacterial pneumonia can directly damage cells of the lower respiratory system, including the surfactant-producing type II alveolar cells. Bacterial pneumonia results in the most striking immune and inflammatory response, the course of which has been well described for pneumococcal pneumonia.

STAGES OF BACTERIAL PNEUMONIA

For pneumococcal pneumonia, four stages of disease have been described. What occurs in these four stages is similar for the other types of pneumonia and is described in the following.

Stage 1, called hyperemia, refers to the initial inflammatory response occurring in the area of lung infection. It is characterized by increased blood flow and increased capillary permeability at the site of infection. It occurs as a result of inflammatory mediators released from mast cells after immune cell activation and tissue injury. These components include histamine and prostaglandin. Mast cell degranulation also activates the complement pathway. Complement acts with histamine and prostaglandin to vasodilate the pulmonary vascular smooth muscle leading to increased blood flow to the area and increased capillary permeability. This results in movement of plasma exudate into the interstitial space, causing swelling and edema between the capillary and the alveolus. Fluid buildup between the capillary and the alveolus increases the distance over which oxygen and carbon dioxide must diffuse, thereby decreasing the rate of gas diffusion. Because oxygen is less soluble than carbon dioxide, its movement into the blood is most affected, often leading to a decrease in hemoglobin oxygen saturation. During this first stage of pneumonia, infection spreads to neighboring tissue as a result of increased blood flow and breakdown of neighboring alveolar and capillary membranes as the inflammatory processes continue.

Stage 2 is called red hepatization. It occurs when the alveoli fill with red blood cells, exudate, and fibrin, produced by the host as part of the inflammatory reaction.

Stage 3, called gray hepatization, occurs as white blood cells colonize the infected part of the lung. Then, fibrin deposits accumulate throughout the area of injury and phagocytosis of cell debris occurs.

Stage 4, called the resolution stage, occurs when the inflammatory and immune responses wane; cell debris, fibrin, and bacteria are digested; and macrophages, the cleanup cells of the inflammatory reaction, dominate.

Pediatric Consideration

In the newborn period, pneumonia is most often caused by infection with group B streptococcal disease transmitted in utero. This disease can have a devastating effect, with an infant developing severe illness within hours of delivery. Treatment requires hospitalization, oxygen therapy, and intravenous antibiotics. This terrible disease may be reduced by prenatal screening of expectant mothers and treatment of women shown to be infected.

Geriatric Consideration

The most common cause of pneumonia in the elderly is pneumococcal pneumonia. The elderly are at the greatest risk of dying from pneumonia, usually related to preexisting disease, poor nutrition, and reduced immune responsiveness. Those in nursing homes are especially susceptible to outbreaks of pneumococcal pneumonia. The risk of acquiring pneumococcal pneumonia can be reduced or eliminated by immunization; it is recommended that those who are older than 65 years of age or who live in a nursing home be vaccinated. Reports indicate, however, that less than 30% of those over 65 have been vaccinated against pneumococcal pneumonia.

CLINICAL MANIFESTATIONS

Symptoms for pneumonia are similar for all types, but are usually most pronounced for those of bacterial origin.

- Significantly increased respiratory rate. Normal and abnormal respiratory rates vary with age, with young infants and children having more rapid normal rates of breathing than older children and adults.

- Fever and chills from the inflammatory processes and a cough that is often productive, purulent, and present throughout the day; infants may grunt in an attempt to improve airflow.
- Chest pain as a result of pleural irritation. The pain may be diffuse or referred to the abdominal area.
- Sputum that is rust colored (for *Streptococcus pneumoniae*), pink (for *Staphylococcus aureus*), or greenish with a particular odor (for *Pseudomonas aeruginosa*).
- Crackles, a poplike sound when the airways open suddenly, is indicative of lower airway infection. Wheezing, the high-pitched sound heard when air rushes through a narrow orifice, signifies obstruction to airflow.
- Fatigue, from both inflammatory reactions and hypoxia, if the infection is serious.
- Pleural pain from inflammation and edema.
- The subjective response of dyspnea is common. Dyspnea is a feeling of air hunger or a reported difficulty in breathing, which can be attributed in part to decreased gas exchange.

Geriatric Consideration

Geriatric patients may not demonstrate these typical signs of pneumonia. Instead, complaints of fatigue, disorientation, or both may be made by the patient or the caregiver.

DIAGNOSTIC TOOLS

- White blood cell count generally increases unless the patient is immunodeficient. This is especially true for bacterial pneumonia.
- Edema of the interstitial space is often apparent on chest radiograph (x-ray). Arterial blood gases may be abnormal.

COMPLICATIONS

- Cyanosis with accompanying hypoxia may develop. Ventilation may be reduced because of mucus accumulation, which may lead to absorption atelectasis.
- Hemoptysis, the coughing up of blood, may occur as a result of direct toxin injury to the capillaries or as a result of the inflammatory reaction and subsequent capillary breakdown.
- Respiratory failure and death may occur in extreme cases and may be related to either exhaustion or sepsis (spread of the infection in the blood).

TREATMENT

The causative agent as determined by a pretreatment sputum sample determines the treatment for pneumonia. Such treatement includes

- Antibiotics, especially for a bacterial pneumonia. Other pneumonias may be treated with anitbiotics to reduce the risk that a bacterial infection will develop secondary to the original infection.
- Rest.
- Hydration to help loosen secretions.
- Deep-breathing techniques to increase ventilation of alveoli and to reduce the risk of atelectasis.
- Other drugs specific for the type of microorganism identified in a sputum culture.

Tuberculosis

Tuberculosis is another example of a lower respiratory tract infection. It is caused by the microorganism *Mycobacterium tuberculosis,* which usually infects by inhalation of droplets, person to person, and colonizes the respiratory bronchioles or alveoli. It can also enter the body through the gastrointestinal tract, by means of ingestion of contaminated unpasteurized milk, or, occasionally, through a skin lesion.

If a significant amount of the tuberculin bacteria bypasses the defense mechanisms of the respiratory system and successfully implants in the lower respiratory tract, the host mounts a vigorous immune and inflammatory response. Because of this vigorous response, which is primarily T-cell mediated, only approximately 5% of people exposed to the bacillus develop active tuberculosis. Only those individuals who develop an active tuberculin infection are contagious to others and only during the time of active infection.

RISK FACTORS FOR TUBERCULOSIS EXPOSURE AND INFECTION

Those most at risk of exposure to the bacillus are those living in close quarters with someone who has an active infection. This includes homeless individuals living in shelters where tuberculosis is present, as well as family members of infected individuals. Children may be especially susceptible. Immigrants to this country from developing nations frequently arrive with active or latent infection.

Also at risk of exposure to and development of tuberculosis are health care workers caring for the infected, and those individuals using the same health care clinics or hospital units as people who have active infection. Of those exposed to the bacillus, individuals who have inadequate immune systems, including the undernourished, the old and the young, individuals receiving immunosuppressant drugs, and those infected with the human immunodeficiency virus (HIV) are most likely to become infected. The virulence of the strain also affects transmission, with certain highly infective strains identified.

IMMUNE RESPONSE TO TUBERCULOSOS

Because the mycobacterium tuberculosis bacillus is difficult to destroy once colonization of the lower respiratory tract occurs, the goal of the immune response becomes to surround and seal off the bacilli, rather than to kill them. The cell-mediated response involves T cells as well as macrophages. Macrophages encircle the bacilli, after which T cells and fibrous tissue wall off the bacilli–macrophage complex. This complex of bacilli, macrophages, T cells, and scar tissue is called a **tubercle.** The tubercle eventually becomes calcified and is called Ghon's complex, which can be seen on chest radiograph. Before engulfment of the bacteria is complete, the material liquefies. At this time, viable microorganisms can gain access to the tracheobronchial system and spread airborne to infect others. Even when adequately walled off, the bacillus is an anaerobic microorganism and may survive within the tubercle. It is believed that because of this viability, approximately 5 to 10% of individuals who do not initially develop tuberculosis may have a clinical demonstration of the disease at some other time in their lives, perhaps when they have become immunocompromised by age, other infection, or the need for anti-inflammatory medications.

Damage to the lung in those infected is caused by the bacilli as well as by a vigorous immune and inflammatory reaction. Interstitial edema and permanent scarring of the alveoli increase the distance for diffusion of oxygen and carbon dioxide, decreasing gas exchange. Also, the deposition of scar tissue and production of tubercles decrease surface area available for gas diffusion, decreasing diffusion capacity. Abnormalities in ventilation perfusion ratio occur that, if the disease is extensive, can lead to hypoxic vasoconstriction of pulmonary arterioles and pulmonary hypertension. Decreased lung compliance occurs with scar tissue.

CLINICAL MANIFESTATIONS

Clinical indications of tuberculosis may be absent with initial infection, and may never be present if active infection does not occur. If active tuberculosis develops, an individual usually demonstrates

- Fevers, especially in the afternoon.
- Malaise.
- Night sweats.
- Loss of appetite and weight loss.
- A productive, purulent cough accompanied by chest pain is common with active infection.

DIAGNOSTIC TOOLS

- A positive skin test for tuberculosis demonstrates cell-mediated immunity and is evidence only of previous exposure of the lower respiratory tract to the bacillus, but it is not evidence that active tuberculosis ever developed.
- Sputum culture of an actively infected individual will reveal the bacillus.

- Chest radiograph demonstrates current or previous tubercle formation.

COMPLICATIONS

- Severe disease may lead to overwhelming sepsis, respiratory failure, and death.
- Multidrug-resistant TB (see below) may develop.

TREATMENT

- Treatment of individuals who have active tuberculosis is lengthy because the bacillus is resistant to most antibiotics and rapidly mutates when exposed to antibiotics to which it is sensitive. Currently, treatment of individuals who have an active infection includes a combination of four drugs and lasts at least 9 months or longer. If the person does not respond to those drugs, other drugs will be tried and different protocols will be followed.
- Individuals who develop a positive tuberculosis skin test after having been previously negative, even though they show no symptoms of active disease, are usually put on a 6 to 9–month antibiotic course to support their immune response and to increase the likelihood that the bacillus will be eradicated completely.

Multidrug-Resistant Tuberculosis

A recent, *worldwide* and serious complication of tuberculosis is the development of tuberculin bacilli resistant to many drug combinations. Resistance develops when individuals do not complete the course of their therapy, and mutations of the bacillus make it nonresponsive to the antibiotics that were used for a brief time. The tuberculin bacillus mutates rapidly and often. Drug-resistant tuberculosis can also occur if an individual cannot mount an effective immune response, for instance, as seen in AIDS patients or in the malnourished. In these cases, antibiotic therapy is only partially effective. When health care workers or others are exposed to these strains of bacillus, they may develop drug-resistant tuberculosis as well, which can result in years of morbidity and frequently even in death. The treatment of those who have multidrug-resistant tuberculosis is more toxic and more expensive, as well as more likely to fail.

CLINICAL MANIFESTATIONS

- Maintenance of an active state of tuberculosis infection characterized by fever, chills, and cough.

COMPLICATIONS

- Death may occur. Passage to others of the drug-resistant strain may occur.

TREATMENT

- Different, usually more toxic drugs will be administered. The patient may be kept in the hospital or under some type of forced quarantine if compliance with the medical therapy is unlikely or impossible.

Pneumoconiosis

Defined as a restrictive pulmonary disease, pneumoconiosis results from occupational inhalation of dust—usually from stone, coal plants, or artificial fibers. Pneumoconiosis usually only develops after many years of dust inhalation.

Dusts that reach the lower respiratory tract stimulate an immune–inflammatory reaction resulting in the accumulation of dust-filled macrophages and the development of diffuse pulmonary fibrosis. Pulmonary fibrosis increases the distance across which diffusion of gases must occur, resulting in a decrease in gas exchange. Fibrosis also limits chest compliance and reduces ventilation. Additional influences such as cigarette smoking, which incapacitates the mucociliary escalator system, promote the likelihood of dusts reaching the lower respiratory system, increasing their damage.

Examples of diseases from dust inhalation include black lung disease, seen in coal miners; silicosis, which occurs in stone workers, including masons and potters; and brown-lung disease, seen in those exposed to cotton dust. Asbestos exposure also leads to fibrosis and may cause lung cancer.

CLINICAL MANIFESTATIONS

- Dyspnea.
- A generally nonproductive cough unless chronic bronchitis develops.
- A severe restriction of inspiratory volume.
- Cyanosis may develop from decreased ventilation coupled with decreased diffusion rate.

DIAGNOSTIC TOOLS

- A complete history and physical examination.
- Chest x-ray.

COMPLICATIONS

- Pulmonary hypertension leading to cor pulmonale may develop from severe fibrosis and decreased alveolar ventilation.

- Pneumonias may repeatedly occur as restrictive disease contributes to atelectasis and poor gas exchange.

TREATMENT

- A reduction of further exposure and avoidance of additive influences such as smoking.
- Prevention and treatment of pneumonia with antibiotic therapy is also important.

Pneumothorax

A pneumothorax is the collapse of all or part of a lung that occurs when air or another gas enters the pleural space surrounding the lungs. There are different types of pneumothorax: open, spontaneous, and tension.

OPEN AND SPONTANEOUS PNEUMOTHORAX

An **open** pneumothorax occurs when the chest wall has been opened and air is allowed into the pleural space from the atmosphere. Atmospheric pressure is greater than pleural pressure and collapses the lungs. A **spontaneous** pneumothorax occurs when the chest wall is intact, but the lungs spontaneously develop a leak (primary) or are injured and begin to leak air into the pleural space (secondary). Air entering the pleural space from the lungs can cause the underlying alveoli to collapse. Causes of open pneumothorax include stab and gunshot wounds, rib fractures, and penetrating and nonpenetrating trauma to the chest wall.

TENSION PNEUMOTHORAX

It is also possible to have a tension pneumothorax in which there is one-way movement of air from the lung into the pleural space through a small hole in the lung structure. In this case, air leaves the lung and enters the pleural space during inspiration. However, air cannot move back into the lungs with expiration because the small hole collapses as the lungs deflate. It is also possible for air to enter the pleural cavity from damage to the tracheobronchial tree. Any tension pneumothorax is a life-threatening situation as it results in increased pressure in the pleural space. As pleural pressure increases, widespread compression atelectasis can occur. Displacement of the heart and great vessels in the thoracic cavity may also occur, resulting in severe alterations of cardiovascular function.

CLINICAL MANIFESTATIONS

- Acute onset of pain in the thoracic area resulting from pleural trauma.

- Rapid, shallow breathing (tachypnea) and dyspnea are common.
- If the pneumothorax is extensive, or if it is a tension pneumothorax and air is accumulating in the pleural space, the heart and large blood vessels may be displaced toward the other lung, which would give the chest the appearance of asymmetry. Tracheal deviation may also be apparent.

DIAGNOSTIC TOOLS

- Blood gases and hemoglobin saturation will indicate hypoxia.
- Radiographs can identify a collapsed lung.

COMPLICATIONS

- A tension pneumothorax may collapse blood vessels, leading to reduced cardiac filling and causing a fall in blood pressure. The other lung may also be affected.
- A pneumothorax may lead to hypoxia, and severe dyspnea.

TREATMENT

- A tension pneumothorax is a life-threatening condition because the buildup of air in the pleural space can eventually collapse the underlying lungs and blood vessels. It must be treated immediately with insertion of a chest tube or a large-bore needle into the pleural space with subsequent suction of the air out of the space.
- A small spontaneous pneumothorax or a pneumothorax resulting secondarily to chest trauma is treated by insertion of a chest tube connected to a drainage tube until the pleural injury is healed. Any penetrating wound should be covered or closed.

Respiratory Failure

Inadequate exchange of gas that results in hypoxia, hypercapnea (increased arterial carbon dioxide concentration), and acidosis is called respiratory failure. It frequently develops when breathing becomes so difficult that exhaustion sets in and the individual no longer has enough energy to breathe. Respiratory failure becomes a vicious cycle; the more difficult it is to breath, the less the alveoli themselves are oxygenated, leading to death of the surfactant-producing cells, and an increased resistance to expansion. This means that the work of breathing is even harder than before and the cycle continues and worsens. Respiratory failure can develop after a variety of respiratory diseases, including widespread pneumonia, sepsis, and infection with certain viruses such as Hantavirus.

CLINICAL MANIFESTATIONS

- Cyanosis.
- Severe dyspnea.

DIAGNOSTIC TOOLS

- Respiratory failure is defined clinically as a partial pressure of oxygen in arterial blood of less than 50 mm Hg, and a partial pressure of carbon dioxide in arterial blood of greater than 50 mm Hg, with a pH of less than or equal to 7.25.

COMPLICATIONS

- Poor oxygenation of other organs may lead to multiorgan failure.
- Individuals in respiratory failure are at high risk of dying.

TREATMENT

- Oxygen support, including artificial ventilation, is required. In general, the sooner a person is put on ventilatory support, the better the prognosis.

Adult Respiratory Distress Syndrome (ARDS)

ARDS is a disease characterized by widespread breakdown of the alveolar and/or pulmonary capillary membranes. ARDS occurs after a major pulmonary, cardiovascular, or systemwide insult.

CAUSES OF ADULT RESPIRATORY DISTRESS SYNDROME

ARDS can occur as a result of direct injury to the capillaries of the lungs or to the alveoli. However, because the capillary and the alveolus are so intimately connected, extensive destruction of one typically leads to destruction of the other. This destruction occurs because of the release of lytic enzymes when cells die; it also occurs with inflammatory reaction subsequent to cell injury and death. Examples of conditions that affect the capillaries or the alveoli and can lead to ARDS are presented in the following.

Capillary Destruction

If breakdown is initially of the capillary membrane, movement of plasma and red blood cells into the interstitial space occurs. This increases the distance across which oxygen and carbon dioxide must diffuse, decreasing the rate of gas exchange. Fluid accumulating in the interstitial space moves into the alveoli, diluting surfactant and increasing surface tension. The exertion of pressure needed to inflate the alveoli is vastly increased. Increased surface tension coupled with edema and swelling of the interstitial space leads to widespread compression atelectasis, resulting in a loss of lung compliance, significantly decreased ventilation, and hypoxia. Causes of pulmonary capillary breakdown include septicemia, pancreatitis, venoms, and uremia. Pneumonia, smoke inhalation, trauma, and near drowning can also destroy the capillary membrane and initiate ARDS.

Alveolar Destruction

When the alveoli are the initial damage site, the surface area available for gas exchange is reduced, and, again, the rate of gas exchange is decreased. Causes of alveolar damage include pneumonia, aspiration, and smoke inhalation. Oxygen toxicity, which occurs after 24 to 36 hours of high-oxygen treatment, can also be a cause of alveolar membrane damage through the production of oxygen-free radicals and by damaging the surfactant-producing cells.

Without oxygen, vascular and pulmonary tissues become hypoxic, leading to further cell injury and death. Once the alveoli and capillaries are damaged, inflammatory reactions, including macrophage and neutrophil infiltration and the release of various cytokines, are initiated that lead to swelling and edema of the interstitial space and damage to the neighboring capillaries and alveoli. Within 24 hours of ARDS onset, hyaline membranes form within the alveoli. These are white, fibrin deposits that progressively accumulate and further decrease gas exchange. Eventually, fibrosis obliterates the alveoli. Ventilation, respiration, and perfusion are all compromised. Mortality associated with ARDS is approximately 50%.

CLINICAL MANIFESTATIONS

- Significant dyspnea.
- Decreased lung compliance.
- Rapid shallow breathing initially, resulting in respiratory alkalosis as carbon dioxide is blown off. Later, as the person fatigues, breathing may become slow and infrequent.

DIAGNOSTIC TOOLS

- Arterial blood-gas analysis demonstrates reduced arterial oxygen concentration. Oxygen therapy is ineffective in ARDS, regardless of the amount of oxygen supplied, because diffusion of the gas is limited owing to fibrin accumulation, edema, and capillary and alveolar breakdown.

COMPLICATIONS

- Respiratory failure may develop as the disease progresses and the individual has to work harder to overcome decreased compliance of the lungs. Eventually, exhaustion sets in and ventilation slows. This results in respiratory acidosis as carbon dioxide accumulates in the blood. Respiratory slowing and a fall in arterial pH are indications of impending respiratory failure and possible death.
- Pneumonia may develop after ARDS, because of fluid accumulation in the lungs and poor lung expansion.
- Renal failure and gastrointestinal stress ulcer can occur as a result of hypoxia.

- Disseminated intravascular coagulation may develop because of the large amount of tissue that can be destroyed during ARDS.

TREATMENT

Initially, treatment of ARDS is geared toward prevention, because ARDS is never a primary disease but always occurs after a major body catastrophe. When present, ARDS is treated as follows:

- Diuretics to decrease fluid load, and cardiostimulatory drugs to increase cardiac contractility and stroke volume. These interventions serve to reduce fluid buildup in the lungs and to reduce the likelihood of right-heart failure.
- Oxygen therapy and mechanical ventilation are often initiated.
- Anti-inflammatory drugs to reduce the damaging effects of inflammation are occasionally used, although their effectiveness is questionable.

Idiopathic Respiratory Distress Syndrome of the Newborn

Also called **hyaline membrane disease**, idiopathic respiratory distress syndrome (IRDS) of the newborn, is a condition of pulmonary hypoxia and injury resulting from widespread primary atelectasis. Primary atelectasis refers to the state of substantial alveolar collapse seen in a newborn. With alveolar collapse, ventilation is decreased. Hypoxia develops, leading to pulmonary injury and a subsequent inflammatory reaction with the accumulation of white blood cells and the release of various cytokines. The inflammatory reaction leads to edema and swelling of the interstitial space, further reducing gas exchange between capillaries and any functioning alveoli. Inflammation also results in the production of hyaline membranes, which are white fibrin accumulations lining the alveoli. Fibrin deposits further decrease gas exchange and reduce lung compliance. With a decrease in lung compliance the work of breathing is increased.

Decreased alveolar ventilation results in decreased ventilation:perfusion ratio and pulmonary arteriolar vasoconstriction. Pulmonary vasoconstriction can lead to an increase in right-heart volume and pressure, resulting in a shunting of blood from the right atrium through the still patent foramen ovale of the newborn, and directly to the left atrium. Likewise, high pulmonary resistance can result in deoxygenated blood bypassing the lungs and being delivered directly to the left side of the body via the ductus arteriosus. Both of these blood flow routes are considered right-to-left shunts in that they bypassed the lungs and so deliver poorly oxygenated blood to the systemic circulation. These examples of shunting worsen the condition of hypoxia, leading to significant cyanosis.

With each attempt to ventilate the collapsed alveoli, the infant must

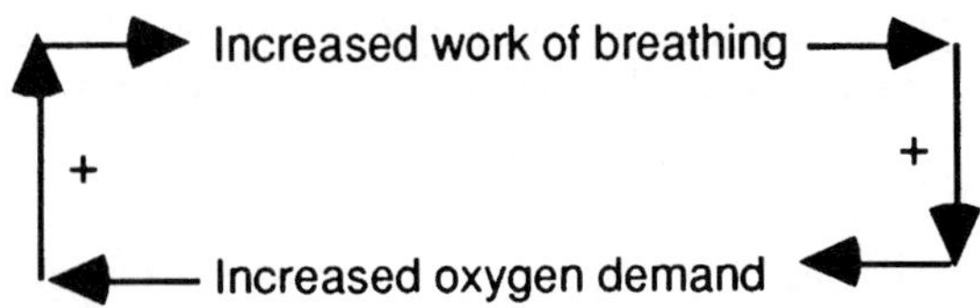

Figure 13-5. When the work of breathing is increased, oxygen demand increases, which further increases the work of breathing.

exert a large amount of energy. Such energy expenditure results in a correspondingly large oxygen demand, contributing to the evident cyanosis. With increased oxygen demand, the baby is caught in a positive-feedback cycle as shown in Figure 13-5.

At first the infant demonstrates rapid, shallow breathing in an attempt to meet this high oxygen demand, causing initial blood gases to indicate respiratory alkalosis as carbon dioxide is blown off. However, the infant soon tires from the extraordinarily difficult alveolar and lung expansion and is unable to keep up the respiratory effort. When this occurs, respiratory effort slows and blood gases reflect respiratory acidosis (buildup of carbon dioxide) and the onset of respiratory failure.

RISK FACTORS FOR IDIOPATHIC RESPIRATORY DISTRESS SYNDROME

The primary risk factor for the development of IRDS is prematurity. Between 5% and 10% of premature infants suffer from this syndrome. The more premature the infant, the more likely IRDS will develop. The mechanism whereby prematurity is associated with IRDS is threefold.

Most significantly, the type II alveolar cells that produce surfactant do not mature until between 28 and 32 weeks of gestation. Therefore, any infant born before surfactant is present in the alveoli encounters high alveolar surface tension with each breath. This contributes significantly to the primary atelectasis seen in IRDS and results in decreased alveolar ventilation and hypoxia. Second, alveoli of premature infants are small and unfolded. By Laplace's law, this factor also contributes to the increased pressure that must be exerted to overcome their surface tension. Third, premature infants have weak, immature chest muscles, making it almost impossible for an infant without surfactant to successfully expand his alveoli, breath after breath for hours.

Another group of newborns at risk of developing IRDS are infants born to insulin-dependent diabetic mothers. It appears that insulin provided by injection prevents the development of type II cells.

CLINICAL MANIFESTATIONS (usually present at birth)

- Increased respiratory rate.
- Duskiness of the skin caused by hypoxia.

- Intercostal or chest retractions with each breath.
- Nasal flaring with each breath.
- Many infants survive IRDS, and in these cases, the symptoms lessen and resolve, usually within 3 days.

DIAGNOSTIC TOOLS

- Diagnosis is usually made from the clinical appearance of the infant at birth coupled with the pregnancy history.
- Arterial blood gases may be drawn to assist in diagnosis and management.

COMPLICATIONS

- Some infants who survive IRDS go on to develop bronchopulmonary dysplasia (BPD), which is a chronic respiratory disease characterized by alveolar scarring, inflammation of the alveoli and the capillaries, and pulmonary hypertension. Effects of BPD may continue for years.
- Signs of dyspnea and hypoxia may continue and proceed to infant exhaustion, respiratory failure, and death, usually within 3 days.

TREATMENT

- Prevention is the first treatment of IRDS. This includes behavioral and pharmacologic attempts to delay or stop labor and accurate dating of pregnancy to minimize delivery of premature infants by cesarean section.
- Delay of parturition (delivery of an infant) for even 24 to 48 hours has been shown to reduce the incidence and severity of IRDS. This is because the stress of labor increases maternal and fetal cortisol release from the adrenal cortex. Cortisol has been shown to stimulate the type II cells to produce surfactant.
- Maternal injections of corticosteroids at least 24 hours before a premature infant is delivered can significantly reduce the incidence of IRDS.
- If an infant is born with IRDS, treatment is supportive and consists of oxygen therapy, maintenance of a quiet, warm environment to decrease oxygen requirements, nutritional support, and repeated evaluation of blood gases and acid-base status.
- A major treatment advance has been the development of artificial surfactant. Surfactant can be delivered directly into the lower respiratory tract of infants demonstrating signs of IRDS, and has been shown successful in reducing clinical manifestations of the disease. This treatment, combined with maternal steroid injections, offers the best hope for reducing the morbidity and mortality caused by IRDS.
- Diabetic women are closely monitored throughout pregnancy.
- Mechanical ventilation may be employed to treat IRDS. However, it is associated with increased risk of developing BPD.

Sudden Infant Death Syndrome

Characterized by the unexpected and the unexplained death of a previously healthy infant, sudden infant death syndrome (SIDS) typically occurs when the infant is between 1 week and 1 year of age. The highest incidence of SIDS is between 2 and 4 months of age, and occurs primarily during the night. At risk of developing SIDS are premature infants, infants born small for gestational age, and those born in multiple pregnancies. Males are at slightly increased risk. In some cases, there is also a history of an upper respiratory tract infection the week before death. Also at increased risk of developing SIDS are siblings of a child who has died of SIDS, and infants who have already experienced an episode of prolonged apnea, a "near-miss" occurrence of SIDS.

The incidence of SIDS has declined in recent years. This appears to be because of an understanding of behavioral risk factors as well as more restrictive diagnosing criteria. SIDS, however, remains the major cause of death in otherwise healthy infants during the first year of life.

CAUSES OF SUDDEN INFANT DEATH SYNDEOME

The cause of SIDS is unknown. Some evidence suggests that an immature central nervous system fails to respond appropriately to increasing levels of carbon dioxide. Normally, increasing carbon dioxide is a stimulation to breathe, until high levels eventually depress ventilation. Healthy infants show occasional periods of apnea, during which carbon dioxide levels rise, stimulating the infant to breathe. Infants who experience SIDS or who experience near-miss episodes of SIDS appear not to respond to rising carbon dioxide with a stimulation of ventilation. Instead, they may show only a depression of ventilation in response to carbon dioxide. In these infants, apnea would occur, carbon dioxide levels rise, and instead of stimulating breathing, the apneic episode would continue. Eventually, the high carbon dioxide levels would completely suppress ventilation and the child dies.

Another recently described phenomenon that may be involved in the development of SIDS in some infants is a prolongation of the cardiac QT interval (time before ventricular repolarization). It is suggested that this may lead to a fatal arrhythmia. Both respiratory and cardiac causes of SIDS are believed to have developmental as well as genetic influences.

OTHER CAUSES OF UNEXPECTED INFANT DEATH

The major behavioral intervention that has resulted in a significant reduction in the occurrence of SIDS has to do with the positioning of infants during sleep periods. Recently it has been suggested that many infants who were assumed to have died of SIDS actually suffocated while lying on mattresses or pillows that were too soft. When an infant lies face down, it has an increased risk of suffocation caused by its inability to move its head and face freely out of a confining position. This is especially true if the infant is weak because of prematurity or if the bed is too soft. In addition, if a baby's face is pressed into a small, soft depression on a mattress or pillow, it exhales into that depression and then rebreathes the same air. The carbon dioxide concentration in this pocket of rebreathed air increases, leading to central nervous system depression and cessation of breathing. Thus, it is recommended that infants should be propped on their side or back, not placed face down, and never left unattended on a water bed, soft mattress, pillow, or fur rug.

Another cause of infant death that is occasionally diagnosed as SIDS is child abuse. Injuries to the infant brainstem can occur with even moderate shaking, leading to respiratory depression and death. This condition is known as "shaken-baby syndrome."

CLINICAL MANIFESTATIONS

- Death by suffocation or heart failure caused by respiratory arrest.
- Symptoms of near-miss apneic episodes are cyanosis and, upon revival, gasping for air.

TREATMENT

- Treatment of SIDS is aimed at prevention. Children at high risk (as defined by having suffered a near-miss episode or having had a sibling who experienced SIDS) may wear monitors to signal apneic episodes. If a cardiac tendency to dysrhythmia is documented, antiarrhythmic drugs or monitors may be used.
- Prevention of other causes of infant death include care with where and in what position an infant is placed and vigilant prevention of child abuse.

Cystic Fibrosis

Cystic fibrosis is a hereditary disease characterized by alterations of exocrine gland function throughout the body. It results in production of large amounts of thick mucus and increased concentration of sodium and chloride in the sweat.

Cystic fibrosis is a relatively common genetic disease, affecting one out of every 2000 Caucasian children in the United States. It is much less common in other races. In most cases, cystic fibrosis occurs as a result of a defective gene located in the middle of chromosome 7. The gene on chromosome 7 normally produces a protein that controls the flow of chloride through all cells of the body. The gene has been named the transmembrane conductance regulator gene, and the protein it produces has been named the transmembrane conductance protein. Without this protein, secretions dry-out and become thick and obstructive. Cystic fibrosis is typically passed as an autosomal-recessive disease. Only individuals who carry two copies of the defective gene, one from each parent, will have the disease. Carriers of one cystic fibrosis gene and one normal gene are heterozygotic for the trait and do not demonstrate the disease.

EFFECTS OF CYSTIC FIBROSIS

When the transmembrane conductance protein is absent, copious amounts of mucus and heavily concentrated sweat are produced. The main body systems affected by the mucus accumulation are the pulmonary and the gastrointestinal systems. Other organs also are victims of the excess mucus, including the liver and the reproductive organs. Sweat glands oversecrete sodium chloride, and sweat accumulates on the skin.

Pulmonary Effects of Cystic Fibrosis

In the lungs, the thick mucus increases the risk of repeated pneumonias and chronic bronchitis. It also blocks alveolar ventilation, leading to absorption atelectasis. Chronic inflammation is present, which leads to edema of the capillary–alveolar interface. Bronchial scarring and fibrosis progressively destroy the bronchial passages. Lung compliance is reduced and ventilation impaired.

Gastrointestinal Effects of Cystic Fibrosis

In the gastrointestinal tract, thick mucus accumulates, blocking digestion and absorption of nutrients. The pancreatic duct becomes clogged, thereby preventing the pancreatic digestive enzymes from reaching the small intestine and further compromising digestion and absorption of nutrients. Failure to thrive is a common complication of the disease. Failure to thrive is defined as a downward deviation in weight of an infant or a child from a previously recorded maximum, crossing one or two percentile lines and persisting for longer than 1 month. Poor nutritional status contributes to the frequency and severity of pulmonary infections. Frequently the pancreas is destroyed, resulting in decreased insulin secretion and diabetes.

CLINICAL MANIFESTATIONS

- A protuberant abdomen apparent soon after birth, resulting from an inablility to pass meconium in the first stool.
- Salty taste when kissed caused by the salt buildup on the skin.
- Repeated bouts of respiratory tract infections throughout infancy and early childhood.
- Chronic rhinitis (or nasal drainage).
- Chronic cough and sputum production.
- Failure to thrive because nutrients are poorly absorbed.

DIAGNOSTIC TOOLS

- The diagnostic test for cystic fibrosis is a positive sweat test for excess chloride.
- Cystic fibrosis can be diagnosed prenatally by amniocentesis in couples who are known heterozygotes for the disease. Even eggs fertilized *in vitro* can be identified as being heterozygotic or homozygotic for the cystic fibrosis gene at the eight-cell stage. The option to implant the embryo or abort the fetus is available.

COMPLICATIONS

- Most individuals who have cystic fibrosis become progressively worse, and many die in their 20s or 30s, usually of bacterial pneumonia. Pulmonary hypertension can also develop as a result of decreased ventilation perfusion, leading to cor pulmonale.

TREATMENT

- The administration of prophylactic antibiotics is used to reduce repeated episodes of lung damage caused by lower respiratory tract infections such as pneumonia.
- Daily chest physiotherapy is essential to assist the individual in clearing the respiratory passages of mucus accumulations. Techniques include chest percussion and postural drainage, and frequent rest periods are advised to decrease energy demands.
- Increased nutrient intake is important to maintain a well-functioning immune system and to minimize growth deficiencies. Dietary education and digestive enzymes supplements can improve nutritional balance and growth.
- Experimental techniques are being performed in which the gene missing in cystic fibrosis is introduced into the lungs of an individual who has cystic fibrosis through a genetically engineered virus. The virus currently used is an attenuated cold virus, which when delivered into the lower respiratory tract proceeds to incorporate its DNA into the host's respiratory cell DNA. This is the normal pattern of viral infection in the lungs. However, when the virus adds its genetically altered DNA to the host's genome, in this case it also adds the missing cystic fibrosis gene. Preliminary results of these initial trials appear promising, although proof of success and safety are not yet available.
- Another option for patients who have cystic fibrosis may be lung transplantation.

Asthma

Asthma is an progressive respiratory disease characterized by inflammation of the respiratory track and spasm of airway bronchiolar smooth muscle. This results in excess mucus production and accumulation, obstruction to airflow, and a decrease in ventilation of the alveoli.

Asthma occurs only in certain individuals who aggressively respond to various airway irritants. Risk factors for this type of hyperresponsiveness include a family history of asthma or allergy, suggesting a genetic tendency. Repeated or intense exposure to some irritating stimuli, perhaps at a key developmental time, may also increase risk of this disease. Although most cases of asthma are diagnosed in childhood, adults may develop asthma without a previous history of the disease. Stimulation of adult-onset asthma often appears related to a worsening of previous allergies. Repeated upper respiratory infections may also trigger adult-onset asthma, as can occupational exposure to dusts and irritants.

Pediatric Consideration

Being exposed to cigarette smoke in utero or in early childhood is considered a risk factor for childhood asthma. Infection in infancy with RSV may also be a risk factor for childhood asthma. Children may outgrow asthma, although a tendency toward allergies often remains.

INFLAMMATORY REACTION IN ASTHMA

The pathophysiology of asthma involves a hyperresponsiveness of the airways after exposure to one or more irritating stimuli. Known stimuli for inducing an asthmatic reaction include viral infections, an allergic response to dust, pollen, mites, or pet dander; exercise; cold exposure; and gastrointestinal reflux. With airway irritability and hyperresponsiveness, both an **inflammatory reaction** and **bronchoconstriction** result. Although bronchoconstriction and a feeling that the air passages are closing may be the first symptom of an asthmatic attack, it is the delayed inflammatory reaction that makes asthma the serious disease it is.

The primary mediators of inflammation in an asthmatic reaction are the eosinophils, a type of white blood cell. Eosinophils concentrate in the area and release chemicals that stimulate mast-cell degranulation. They also draw other white blood cells to the area, including basophils and neutrophils; stimulate the production of mucus; and increase swelling and edema of the tissues. The inflammatory response begins with the initial stimulus, but it may take as long as 12 hours to become apparent.

More acutely felt is the effect of the chemical histamine on the bronchiolar smooth muscle. Histamine is released with mast-cell degranulation and quickly causes bronchiolar smooth muscle constriction and spasm. Histamine also stimulates mucus production and increased capillary permeability, further contributing to the more delayed congestion and swelling of the interstitial spaces.

Individuals who develop asthma may have either an overabundance of eosinophils or perhaps an overresponsiveness of the mast cells to stimuli initiating degranulation. IgE antibody, responsible for allergic attacks, may overreact in response to foreign antigens, turning on the inflammatory cascade. Regardless of the source of the hypersensitivity, the final result is bronchospasm, mucus production and accumulation, edema, and obstruction to airflow. Viral infection, allergy, and reflux appear to trigger a hypersensitivity response by means of irritating the airways. Exercise might also act as an irritant because large volumes of air are moved rapidly in and out of the lungs. This air has not been adequately humidified, warmed, or cleared of particulates and can trigger an attack.

PSYCHOLOGICAL STIMULI FOR ASTHMA

Psychological stimuli can worsen an asthmatic attack. Because parasympathetic stimulation constricts bronchiolar smooth muscle, anything that increases parasympathetic activity could trigger asthma. The parasympathetic system is activated with the emotions of anxiety and sometimes fear. Therefore, an individual having an attack may have worsening of symptoms as his anxiety peaks. In contrast, sympathetic innervation of bronchiolar smooth muscle leads to dilation of the bronchi. Typically, sympathetic stimulation is associated with conditions of fright and flight, during which increased ventilation is an important component of escape. Many of the therapeutic interventions traditionally used to treat asthma have relied on blocking parasympathetic or stimulating sympathetic responses. Newer treatment modalities have focused on blocking inflammatory response or mast-cell degranulation.

CLINICAL MANIFESTATIONS

- Significant dyspnea.
- Coughing, especially at night.
- Rapid, shallow breathing.
- Wheezing, audible with ascultation or by the unaided ear.
- An increase in the work of breathing, exemplified by chest retractions and with a worsening of condition, nasal flaring.
- Anxiety, related to the inability to get enough air.
- Air trapping because of the obstruction to airflow, especially seen during expiration in patients who have asthma. This is demonstrated as prolonged expiration time.

DIAGNOSTIC TOOLS

- Asthma is diagnosed by spirometry, a technique that measures and identifies reductions in vital capacity and reduced peak expiratory flow rates. Peak flowmeters are available for home use. With a peak flowmeter, the maximum amount of air that can be moved with each breath (vital capacity) is measured, both during an attack and during times between asthmatic episodes. Individuals who have asthma typically show a significant diurnal pattern, with peak flow readings significantly poorer in the early hours after midnight compared with late afternoon. During an asthmatic attack, maximum expiratory volume and maximum rate of expiration are further reduced. Worsening or improvement in a patient's condition can be followed by serial peak flow measurements.

- The saturation of hemoglobin with oxygen ("oxygen saturation") may be measured to determine how well the blood is being oxygenated in a person showing asthmatic symptoms. This technique involves placing a sensor over the finger and obtaining the information concerning the color of the blood flowing beneath it. Unsaturated hemoglobin is darker in color than saturated. This tool is easily used in the office and provides a rapid indication of a patient's ability to move air.
- Audible wheezing can be heard on auscultation of the lungs. Typically wheezing is heard only on expiration, unless the patient's condition is severe.
- Blood-gas analysis may demonstrate a decrease in arterial oxygen concentration and at first respiratory alkalosis as carbon dioxide is blown off in rapid breathing. If the condition persists and worsens, respiratory acidosis may develop as a result of status asthmaticus, as described in the following.
- Between asthmatic attacks, a person is usually asymptomatic. However, changes in lung function tests may be apparent even between attacks in patients who have persistent asthma.

COMPLICATIONS

- Status asthmaticus is a life-threatening condition of prolonged bronchiolar spasm that cannot be reversed with medication. In this case the work of breathing is greatly increased. When the work of breathing increases, oxygen demand also increases. Because individuals in an asthmatic attack are not meeting a normal oxygen demand, they certainly cannot meet the high-oxygen demands needed to inspire and expire against prolonged bronchiolar spasm, bronchiolar swelling, and thick mucus. This situation can lead to a pneumothorax from the enormous pressures exerted to ventilate. As the individual becomes exhausted with effort, respiratory acidosis, respiratory failure, and death can occur.

TREATMENT

- The first step in treatment involves evaluating a patient's stage of asthma. Staging is currently separated into four levels, depending on the frequency of symptoms and the frequency medications are needed to provide relief. Stages of asthma include 1) mild intermittent, 2) mild persistent, 3) moderate, and 4) severe. Treatment is based on staging.
- For all stages of asthma, prevention of exposure to known allergens is vital. This involves allegy-proofing the home, avoidance of ciga-

rette and wood-burning smoke, and the use of air conditioners to minimize the opening of windows, especially during high-pollen seasons.

- Monitoring peak flow frequently, especially during times of increased asthma incidence, such as the cold season (winter) or the pollen season (spring), is important as well, even for mild intermittent asthma. When a significant decrease in an individual's peak flow rate is first observed, added pharmacologic intervention can be started immediately instead of waiting until an attack is full blown.
- An important advance in prevention and treatment of an asthmatic attack has been the use of anti-inflammatory drugs early in the course of an attack or as preventive therapy. Inhaled steroids stop the inflammatory cascade. Similarly, inhaled drugs that stabilize mast cells are being used to prevent an asthmatic attack. The effects of these inhaled medications appear to be localized to the respiratory system, making their use safe and effective treatments for asthma. Because asthma is a progressive disease, it is important to maintain treatment even between episodes of asthmatic attacks. Any individual, regardless of stage of disease, may require anti-inflammatory drugs. For those who have persistent, moderate, and severe asthma, inhaled steroids are often used daily.
- Bronchodilators that act by stimulating the beta-adrenergic receptors of the airways are also a mainstay of asthma therapy. These drugs are inhaled (or given as a liquid in young children) at the onset of an attack and between attacks as needed. Bronchodilators do not prevent the delayed inflammatory response and so are not effective alone during a moderate or severe exacerbation of asthma, and too-frequent or sole reliance on them has led to a significant number of fatalities. The beta-adrenergic dilators may also be used before exercise in those who have exercise-induced asthma. Newly available long-lasting beta-adrenergic agonists may be able to reduced the need for frequent use of inhalers for some patients.
- The daily use of oral steroids may be necessary to control conditions of severe asthma, or they may be prescribed as a burst for 5–7 days to help return normal function more rapidly during an exacerbation in patients who have mild or moderate asthma. The chronic use of oral steroids for the treatment of childhood asthma is associated with a reduction in growth potential and with a thinning of the bones (osteoporosis).
- New drugs that inhibit important proinflammatory cytokines are now available. These drugs may permit some patients to rely less on the use of traditional inhalers.
- Anticholinergic drugs may be given to decrease parasympathetic effects and to relax the bronchiolar smooth muscle. However, these drugs have a narrow therapeutic range of safety and so are used infrequently in general practice.
- Behavioral intervention, aimed at calming the person to reduce parasympathetic stimulation of the airways, is important. When a

person who is crying stops, this allows for a slowing and a warming of the airflow, thereby reducing stimulation to the airways.

Acute Bronchitis

Bronchitis is a common, obstructive respiratory disease consisting of inflammation of the bronchi. It is usually associated with a viral or a bacterial infection or the inhalation of irritants such as cigarette smoke or chemicals present in air pollution. It is characterized by excess mucus production.

CLINICAL MANIFESTATIONS

- Cough, usually productive with thick mucus and purulent sputum.
- Dyspnea.
- Fever.
- Hoarseness.
- Crackles (discontinuous fine or course lung sounds) especially on inspiration.
- Chest pain occasionally may be present.

DIAGNOSTIC TOOLS

- Chest radiograph.

COMPLICATIONS

- Repeated episodes of acute bronchitis may result in the pathologic changes characteristic of chronic bronchitis.

TREATMENT

- Antibiotics for secondary or primary bacterial infections.
- Increased fluid intake and expectorants to loosen mucus.
- Rest to reduce oxygen demands.

Chronic Bronchitis

Chronic bronchitis is defined as an obstructive pulmonary disorder characterized by excessive mucus production in the lower respiratory tract. It must last for at least 3 consecutive months of the year for 2 consecutive years.

Excess mucus results from pathologic changes (dysplasia) of the mucus-producing cells of the bronchi. In addition, the cilia lining the bronchi become paralyzed or dysfunctional, and undergo metaplasia. These changes to the mucus-producing cells and the cilia cells derail the mucociliary escalatory system and cause the accumulation of large amounts of thick mucus that cannot be easily removed from the respiratory tract. The mucus acts as a breeding ground for infection and becomes highly purulent. Inflammation sets in, resulting in edema and swelling of the tissues and changes in the pulmonary architecture.

Ventilation, especially exhalation, is obstructed. Hypercapnea (increased carbon dioxide) develops, as exhalation is prolonged and difficult to accomplish through the mucus and inflammation. The decrease in ventilation causes a decrease in ventilation:perfusion ratio, with resulting pulmonary hypoxic vasoconstriction and pulmonary hypertension. Although the alveoli are normal, hypoxic vasoconstriction and poor ventilation result in decreased oxygen exchange and hypoxia.

The main risk factor for development of chronic bronchitis is cigarette smoking. Components of cigarette smoke stimulate changes in both the mucus-producing cells of the bronchi and the cilia. They also induce chronic inflammation, which is the distinguishing characteristic of chronic bronchitis.

CLINICAL MANIFESTATIONS

- A productive, purulent cough, easily worsened by inspired irritants, cold weather, or an infection.
- Air hunger and dyspnea.

DIAGNOSTIC TOOLS

- Blood gases show decreased arterial oxygen and increased arterial carbon dioxide.
- Polycythemia (an increase in red blood cell concentration) occurs as a result of chronic hypoxia, which, coupled with cyanosis, gives the skin a bluish coloration.
- Chest radiograph may document chronic bronchitis and fibrosis of the lung tissue.

COMPLICATIONS

- Pulmonary hypertension, resulting from chronic pulmonary hypoxic vasoconstriction, can occur, leading to cor pulmonale.
- Lung cancer progressing from cellular metaplasia and dysplasia may occur.

TREATMENT

- Education on decreasing further irritant exposure, especially cigarette smoke.
- Prophylactic antibiotic therapy, especially in the winter months, to reduce incidence of lower respiratory tract infections. This is important because any infectious process further increases the inflammatory outcomes of mucus production and swelling.
- Because many patients experience spasms of the respiratory tract with chronic bronchitis that are similar to spasms with chronic asthma, bronchodilators are frequently prescribed. Anti-inflammatory drugs also can reduce mucus production and relieve blockage.

- Expectorants and increased fluid intake to loosen the mucus.
- Oxygen therapy may be required.
- Vaccination against pneumococcal pneumonia is advised.

Emphysema

Emphysema is a chronic obstructive disease characterized by loss of lung elasticity and a reduction in alveolar surface area. Damage can be either restricted to the central part of the lobe, which results in the bronchiolar wall integrity being affected most, or it can be throughout the entire lung, which results in damage both to the bronchi and to the alveoli.

Loss of lung elasticity can affect both the alveoli and the bronchi. Elasticity is lost as a result of destruction of the elastin and collagen fibers found throughout the lung. The exact cause of emphysema is unclear, but the disease usually occurs after years of smoking. It appears that components of cigarette smoke directly change the structure of the elastic molecules. There may also be an effect on the elastic fibers related to repeated infectious ailments and the state of chronic inflammation that accompanies infection. As a result of the loss of elasticity, air passages and alveoli collapse, reducing ventilation. Airways collapse primarily on expiration because normal expiration occurs as a result of passive recoil after inspiration. Therefore, if there is no passive recoil, air is trapped in the lung and the airways collapse.

The walls between the alveoli, called the alveolar septa, can also be destroyed. This reduces the surface area of alveoli available for gas exchange and decreases the rate of diffusion.

Although the primary risk factor for emphysema is smoking, repeated exposure to secondhand smoke might also result in emphysema. In addition, there is a familial form of emphysema that occurs in individuals not necessarily exposed to cigarette smoke. This is a much less common cause of emphysema.

CLINICAL MANIFESTATIONS

- Air trapping, resulting from the loss of lung elasticity and leading to expansion of the chest (increased anterior-posterior diameter).
- Tachypnea (increased respiratory rate) caused by hypoxia and hypercapnia. Because of the effectiveness of increasing respiratory rate in this disease, most individuals who have emphysema do not show a significant alteration in arterial blood gases until late in the course of the disease when respiratory rate cannot mask hypoxia or hypercapnia. Eventually, all blood-gas values deteriorate, and frank hypoxia, hypercapnia, and acidosis are present. Central nervous system depression, resulting from high carbon dioxide levels (carbon dioxide narcosis), can occur.
- One key difference between emphysema and chronic bronchitis is the lack of sputum production in emphysema.

DIAGNOSTIC TOOLS

- As the disease progresses, blood-gas analysis will first demonstrate hypoxia. Late in the disease, carbon dioxide levels may also be elevated.
- Decreased measured FEV_1 and increased residual volume (air left in the respiratory tract after each breath) caused by loss of lung elasticity occurs.

COMPLICATIONS

- Pulmonary hypertension from chronic pulmonary hypoxic vasoconstriction, leading to cor pulmonale, may occur.

TREATMENT

Relieving the symptoms and preventing a worsening of the condition is the objective in emphysema treatment. There is no cure. Treatments include

- Encouraging the individual to stop smoking.
- Using breathing positions and patterns to reduce air trapping.
- Teaching the indivdual relaxation techniques and means of energy conservation.
- Oxygen therapy is eventually needed for many patients who have emphysema, so that they can complete tasks of daily living.

Chronic Obstructive Pulmonary Disease

Individuals who have long-standing emphysema also usually have chronic bronchitis and demonstrate indications of each disease. This condition is called COPD. Chronic asthma in association with either emphysema or chronic bronchitis may also result in COPD.

CLINICAL MANIFESTATIONS

- Symptoms of both emphysema and chronic bronchitis are usually present.
- Dyspnea is constant.

DIAGNOSTIC TOOLS

- History and physical examination.
- Chest x-ray.

COMPLICATIONS

- Pulmonary hypertension leading to cor pulmonale.
- Pneumothorax.

TREATMENT

- COPD treatment is as described for chronic bronchitis and emphysema, with the exception that oxygen therapy must be closely monitored. Individuals who have COPD have chronic hypercapnia that causes the central chemoreceptors, which normally respond to carbon dioxide, to adapt. What keeps these individuals breathing then is the low oxygen concentration of the arterial blood that continues to stimulate the less-sensitive peripheral chemoreceptors. These peripheral chemoreceptors only fire if the arterial partial pressure of oxygen decreases to less than 50 mm Hg. Therefore, if oxygen therapy were to result in a partial pressure of oxygen of greater than 50 mm Hg, this remaining drive to breathe would be extinguished. Individuals who have COPD typically have low oxygen levels and cannot be treated with high-oxygen therapy. This severely affects quality of life.

Lung Cancer

Defined as a cancer of the epithelial lining of the respiratory tract (bronchogenic carcinoma), lung cancer can occur anywhere in the lung. There are four general types of lung cancer.

Squamous cell carcinoma accounts for at least 30 to 40% of bronchogenic cancer. This cancer is clearly associated with cigarette smoking and exposures to environmental toxins, such as asbestos and components of air pollution. Squamous cell tumors are usually located in the bronchi at the site where the bronchi enter the lungs, called the hila, and from there extend down into the bronchi. Because the bronchi are to some degree obstructed, absorption atelectasis as well as decreased ventilatory capacity can occur. This tumor grows relatively slowly and has the best prognosis for a 5-year survival.

Small-cell carcinoma accounts for approximately 25% of all lung cancers. This type of tumor is also referred to as oat-cell carcinoma and usually occurs in the central areas of the lung. Small-cell carcinoma is an anaplastic, or embryonic, type of tumor, and therefore shows a high incidence of metastasis. It is often the site of ectopic tumor production and may cause early symptoms based on endocrine disturbances. Pulmonary manifestations that occur with this tumor also result from obstruction to airflow. This type of tumor is perhaps the one most often seen in cigarette smokers, and it has the worst prognosis.

Adenocarcinoma is a type of lung cancer arising from the glands of the lung. It usually occurs in the periphery of lung tissue, including the terminal bronchioles and the alveoli. This type of cancer accounts for approximately 30% of lung cancers. Adenocarcinomas are typically small and are usually slow growing, but they metastasize early and have a poor 5-year survival rate.

Large-cell undifferentiated cancer is highly anaplastic and associated with rapid metastasis. These tumors account for approximately 10–15% of all lung cancers and can occur peripherally or centrally in the lung. They are strongly correlated with cigarette smoking and can cause chest pain. This type of cancer has a poor prognosis for survival.

RISK FACTORS FOR LUNG CANCER

Lung cancer is on the rise in the United States, especially among women. The primary risk factor for lung cancer is the use of tobacco. Air pollution and exposure to chemicals and dusts, including asbestos, have also contributed to the rising rates. Lung cancer is often associated with chronic bronchitis, because of the overlap in risk factors as well as excess mucus possibly causing abnormal epithelial cell changes.

Exactly how cigarette smoking causes cancer is unclear. It appears that the metabolites of cigarette smoke affect the functioning of key genes regulating epithelial cell growth and development. Alterations in these key genes then allow a cancer to develop. Specific mutations in certain cancer suppressor genes have been shown to occur with prolonged exposure to nicotine and other components of cigarettes. Without properly functioning suppressor genes, uncontrolled cell division can occur.

Epithelial cells change progressively with the development of lung cancer, first showing subtle signs of metaplasia, then dysplasia, and finally neoplasia. These conditions preceding neoplasia are visible histologically in individuals who have chronic bronchitis and emphysema. The bronchial epithelial cells that appear to be most damaged by toxins are those at the bronchial bifurcations. It appears that mucus and toxins accumulate here, causing the most injury to these cells. The result is that the epithelial cells become thickened, the mucus-producing cells hypertrophy, and metaplasia and dysplasia occur. Alveolar cells may also be altered in structure and function.

CLINICAL MANIFESTATIONS

- A persistent cough.
- Hemoptysis (the coughing up of blood).
- Recurring lower respiratory tract infections frequently signal a lung cancer.
- Other symptoms seen with each particular type of lung cancer may vary, as described above.

DIAGNOSTIC TOOLS

- Chest x-ray followed by biopsy of suspicious lesions may diagnose the disease.

COMPLICATIONS

- Prognosis is poor. The 5-year survival rate for all types of lung cancer is only 13%. Some types of lung cancer have an even worse prognosis. For instance, oat-cell carcinoma has a less than 5% survival rate 2 years after diagnosis.

TREATMENT

- Any combination of surgery, radiation, and chemotherapy.

Selected Bibliography

Fine, M. J., Auble, T. E. Yealy, D. M., et al. (1997). A prediction rule to identify low-risk patients with community acquired pneumonia. *New England Journal of Medicine* 336, 243–250.

Guntheroth, W. G. & Spiers, P. S. (1992). Sleeping prone and the risk of sudden infant death syndrome. *Journal of the American Medical Association* 267, 2359–2362.

Guyton, A. C. & Hall, J. (1997). *Textbook of Medical Physiology (9th ed.)*. Philadelphia: W.B. Saunders.

Homer, C. J. (1997). Asthma disease management. *New England Journal of Medicine* 337, 1461–1463.

Hsia, C. C. W. (1998). Respiratory function of hemoglobin. *New England Journal of Medicine* 338, 239–247.

Jaffe, D. M. (1998). The treatment of croup with glucocorticoids. *New England Journal of Medicine* 339, 553–554.

Nuorti, J. P., Butler, J. C., Crutcher, J. M., et al. (1998). An outbreak of multidrug resistant pneumococcal pneumonia and bacteremia among unvaccinated nursing home residents. *New England Journal of Medicine* 338, 1861–1868.

Porth, C. M. (1998). *Pathophysiology Concepts of Altered Health States (5th ed.)*. Philadelphia: J.B. Lippincott Company.

Rongren, K. A. (1998). The step-wise approach to long-term asthma management: Review of the clinical guidelines. *The American Journal for Nurse Practitioner* 2, 7–16.

Schidlow, D.V. & Callahan, C. W. (1996). Pneumonia. *Pediatrics in Review* 17, 300–310.

Schwartz, R. M., Luby, A. M., Scanlon, J. W., & Kellogg, R. J. (1994). Effect of surfactant on morbidity, mortality, and resource use in newborn infants weighing 500–1500 gms. *New England Journal of Medicine* 330, 1470–B1480.

Schwartz, P. J., Stramba-Badiale, M., Segantini, A., et al. (1998). Prolongation of the QT interval and the sudden infant death syndrome. *New England Journal of Medicine* 338, 1709–1714.

Simons, F. E. & The Canadian Beclomethasone dipropionate-salmeterol xinafoate study group. (1998). *New England Journal of Medicine* 337, 1659–1666.

Snider, D. E. & Castro, K. G. (1998). The global threat of drug-resistant tuberculosis. *New England Journal of Medicine* 338, 1689–1690.

Valway, S. E., Sanchez, M. P., Shinnick, T. F., et al. (1998). An outbreak involving extensive transmission of a virulent strain of Mycobacterium tuberculosis. *New England Journal of Medicine* 338, 633–639.

Vander, A. J., Sherman, J., & Luciano, D. (1998). *Human physiology (7th ed.)*. Boston: McGraw-Hill.

Weitzman, S., Gortmaker, S., Walker, D. K. & Sobel, A. (1990). Maternal smoking and childhood asthma. *Pediatrics* 85, 505–511.

Welsh, M. J. & Smith, A. E. (1995). Cystic fibrosis. *Scientific American* Dec, 52–59.

Resources

Asthma and Allergy Foundation of America, 1125 15th St. N.W., Washington, DC 20005. Phone: 800-7-ASTHMA or 800-727-8462.

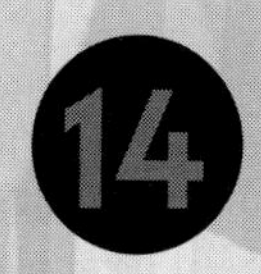

THE GENITOURINARY SYSTEM

Although the kidney is frequently thought of as simply being an organ for waste elimination, it is actually more than that. The kidney is essential in maintaining water, salt, and electrolyte balance and is an endocrine gland that secretes at least three hormones. The kidney helps control blood pressure and is especially susceptible to damage if blood pressure is too high or too low.

● ● ●

PHYSIOLOGIC CONCEPTS

Structure

The kidneys lie outside the peritoneal cavity in the upper posterior portion of the abdominal wall, one on each side of the body. Each kidney is made up of approximately one million functional units, each of which is called a **nephron**. As shown in Figure 14-1, the nephron begins as a capillary tuft, called the glomerulus. Plasma is **filtered** across the glomerulus by the process of bulk flow and enters the twisting, looping tubule of the nephron. Of the plasma that enters the tubule, only a small fraction is excreted as urine. The remaining plasma, compared with what entered the tubule across the glomerular capillary, has its final composition and volume drastically altered by the processes of renal **reabsorption** and **secretion**.

Each kidney is divided anatomically into an outer cortex containing all the glomerular capillaries and some short tubular segments and an inner medulla where most of the tubular segments are located. The progression of tubular segments from the glomerulus to the proximal and then the distal tubule and finally to the collecting tubule is shown in Figure 14-1. Each nephron's collecting tubule joins other collecting tubules to become several hundred large collecting ducts. The large collecting ducts are located in the papillae of the kidney, which is anatomically part of the innermost portion of the kidney, the renal medulla. The large collecting ducts feed into a central draining area, called the renal pelvis, and from there empty into the ureter. The ureter from each kidney is connected to the bladder (Fig. 14-2). The bladder stores urine until it is released outside the body in the process of micturition (urination). Micturition occurs through a single tube called the urethra.

Renal Blood Flow

The kidneys receive approximately 1 L of blood per minute—one-fifth of the cardiac output. This high rate of blood flow is not required for meeting extraordinary energy demands, but for allowing the kidney to adjust the blood composition continually. By adjusting the blood

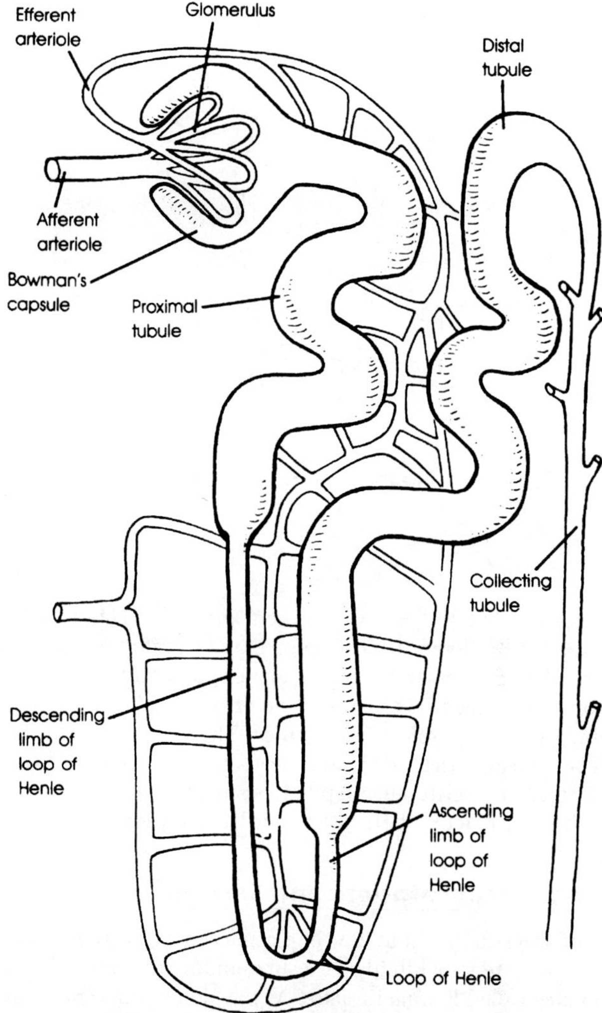

Figure 14-1. Nephron (used with permission from Vander, 1991).

composition, the kidney is able to maintain blood volume; ensure sodium, chloride, potassium, calcium, phosphate, and pH balance; and eliminate products of metabolism such as urea and creatinine.

Blood flows to the kidneys via the renal arteries, one renal artery to each kidney. In the kidney, the renal artery branches many times, ending as several afferent arterioles. Each afferent arteriole becomes the glomerular capillary that supplies a tubule with blood.

The glomerular capillary reforms not to become a venule as most

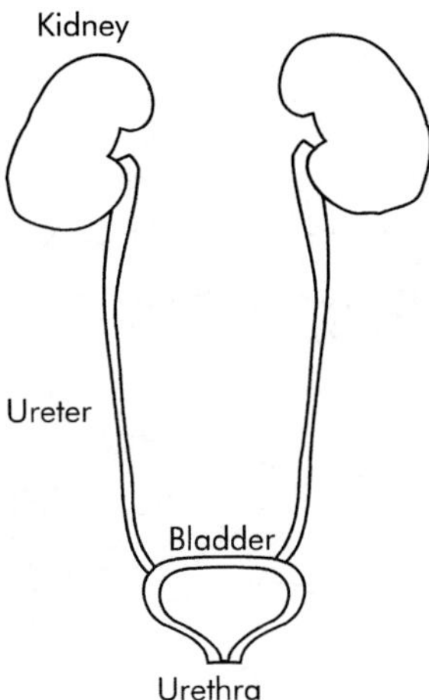

Figure 14-2. Urinary tract.

capillaries do, but to form the efferent arteriole. This is shown in Figure 14-1. The efferent arteriole soon branches into a second capillary network, the peritubular capillaries, which surround and support the nephron tubules themselves. At the end of each nephron, the peritubular capillaries finally reform to venules. The venules join to become veins. Blood leaves the kidney and heads back to the vena cava to be recirculated. The peritubular capillaries surrounding the long loop of the nephron (the loop of Henle) are called the **vasa recta**.

Filtration, Reabsorption, and Secretion

Filtration refers to the bulk flow of plasma across the glomeular capillary into the interstitial fluid space surrounding the start of the nephron, an area called *Bowman's space*. At the glomerulus, approximately 20% of the plasma is continually filtered into Bowman's space. This filtrate is of the same composition as the plasma, except that protein molecules are not usually filtered. The initial filtrate diffuses across Bowman's space and into the beginning section of the tubule, *Bowman's capsule*, to begin its journey through the rest of the tubule.

Some substances that enter the tubule at Bowman's capsule do not stay in the tubule. Instead, they move (or are moved) back into the blood across the peritubular capillaries by the process of **reabsorption**. Another group of substances is added to the urine filtrate, also across the peritubular capillaries, by the process of **secretion**. It is by reabsorption and secretion that each nephron manipulates the composition and volume of the initial urine filtrate to produce the final urine.

Glomerular Filtration

Glomerular filtration is the process through which approximately 20% of the plasma entering the glomerular capillary moves across the capillary into the interstitial space and from there into Bowman's capsule. Neither red blood cells nor plasma proteins are more than minimally filtered in healthy kidneys.

The process of filtration across the glomerulus is similar to that which occurs across all capillaries, as described in Chapter 12. What is different in the kidney is that the glomerular capillaries are permeable to small solutes and water. Also, unlike other capillaries, the forces favoring filtration of plasma across the glomerular capillary into Bowman's space are greater than the forces favoring reabsorption of fluid back into the capillary. Therefore, net filtration of fluid into Bowman's space occurs. This fluid then diffuses into Bowman's capsule and begins its journey through the rest of the nephron.

In the glomerulus, the primary force favoring filtration is capillary pressure. In most other capillaries, this pressure averages 18 mm Hg; in the glomerulus the average pressure is almost 60 mm Hg. This occurs as a result of decreased resistance to flow offered by the afferent arteriole feeding the glomerulus, compared with arterioles elsewhere. Therefore, the hydrostatic pressure reaching the glomerulus is greater, as shown in Figure 14-3.

Interstitial fluid pressure in Bowman's space is also much greater than in normal interstitial spaces (approximately 15 mm Hg versus approximately -3 mm Hg). This greater pressure is a result of the high fluid volume entering Bowman's space from the glomerulus, thus opposing further glomerular filtration. Capillary concentration of protein (plasma colloid osmotic pressure) is the same in the glomerulus as in other capillaries. The plasma colloid osmotic pressure increases throughout the length of the glomerulus as protein-free filtrate is pushed into Bowman's space, averaging approximately 28 mm Hg overall. This force opposes glomerular filtration. The interstitial fluid colloid osmotic pressure (the pressure exerted by interstitial proteins) is normally approximately 8 mm Hg. This pressure favors glomerular filtration.

Adding up the forces favoring filtration across the glomerulus (60 mm Hg + 8 mm Hg) and the forces favoring reabsorption (28 mm Hg + 15 mm Hg), a net force results of approximately 25 mm Hg favoring the filtration of plasma into Bowman's interstitial space. This filtrate enters Bowman's capsule, moves through the tubule, and becomes urine.

GLOMERULAR FILTRATION RATE

The glomerular filtration rate (GFR) is defined as the volume of filtrate entering Bowman's capsule per unit of time. GFR is nearly constant and gives a good indication of the health of the kidneys. GFR depends

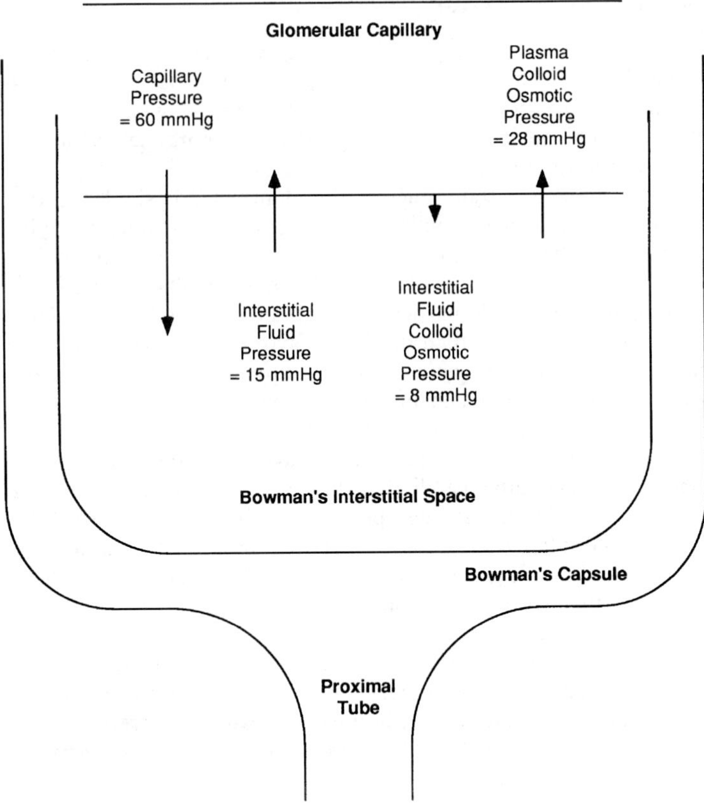

Figure 14-3. Forces favoring filtration and reabsorption across the glomerular capillary.

on the four forces determining filtration and reabsorption (capillary pressure, interstitial fluid pressure, plasma colloid osmotic pressure, and interstitial fluid colloid osmotic pressure). Therefore, any change in these forces can alter GFR. Likewise, GFR depends on the available surface area of the glomerulus for filtration. Therefore, a loss of glomerular surface area decreases GFR.

An average value for GFR in an adult male is 180 L/day (125 mL/min). A normal plasma volume is approximately 3 L (out of a total blood volume of approximately 5 L). This means that the kidney filters the plasma approximately 60 times each day! Equally remarkable is the fact that of the 180 L/day filtered into Bowman's capsule, only approximately 1.5 L/day are excreted from the body as urine. The rest is reabsorbed back into the blood across the peritubular capillaries.

MEASUREMENT OF GLOMERULAR FILTRATION RATE

GFR measurement is possible if one has a substance (call it x) that is freely filterable at the glomerulus and then is not reabsorbed, secreted, or changed in any way before it appears in the urine. To calculate the GFR from this substance, one would measure its concentration in a plasma sample (P_x), its concentration in a urine sample (U_x), and the urine volume over a certain period of time (V). Given these values, the equation for GFR, in milliliters per minute, can be solved as shown in Equation 14-1:

$$\text{GFR (mL/min)} = \frac{U_x(\text{mg/mL})V\,(\text{mL/min})}{P_x(\text{mg/mL})}. \qquad (14\text{-}1)$$

The classic substance that fits the criteria described above for substance x is the polysaccharide inulin. However, using inulin to measure GFR involves infusing it into an individual for an extended period. This offers a highly accurate but impractical method for measuring GFR. Instead, what is usually measured in plasma and urine is the concentration of creatinine, which is a naturally produced protein.

Creatinine is produced as a result of normal daily protein metabolism, a process that is assumed to occur at a nearly constant rate. (Note: Occasionally, this assumption may not hold true, e.g., after muscle trauma or intense exercise). To measure GFR using creatinine, a blood sample is drawn along with a timed urine sample, and creatinine concentrations in the blood and urine are measured.

GFR measured from creatinine concentration and urine volume is only an estimate of the true GFR, because a small amount of creatinine actually is secreted into the lumen of the tubule from the peritubular capillaries. Therefore, GFR estimated by creatinine will be slightly high, because more creatinine is excreted in the urine than was filtered at the glomerulus.

Measurement of GFR is important because it offers a clue to nephron function. In conditions of disease leading to renal failure, GFR falls.

Geriatric Consideration

GFR declines with age as a result of a 30 to 50% loss of functioning nephrons and as a reduction in renal blood flow. This means that when drugs that are normally cleared by the kidneys are given to an elderly individual, their dosage should be adjusted to reflect declining renal function. However, because muscle mass, and therefore plasma creatinine, also decline with age, there is not an increase in serum creatinine level to accompany the decrease in GFR. Because serum creatinine levels are frequently used to determine drug dosing, elderly individuals may receive inappropriately high doses of drugs in spite of their poor kidney function. This can have severe toxic consequences. In order to adjust for the effects of age on GFR, the following equation has been developed by Cockcoft and Gault:

$$\text{Creatinine clearance} = \frac{(140 - \text{age}) \times (\text{body weight in kg})}{72 \times \text{serum creatinine in mg/dL}} \quad (14\text{-}2)$$

Renal Clearance

The concentration of a substance totally cleared from the blood into the urine over time is known as renal clearance. The GFR described above for inulin is really the clearance of inulin, because all filtered inulin is cleared by the kidneys (it is neither reabsorbed nor secreted). For creatinine, clearance is actually greater than the GFR, because some creatinine is secreted into the urine as well as filtered.

Other substances not normally lost in the urine, such as glucose, have zero clearance. Although glucose is freely filtered across the glomerulus, it is normally totally reabsorbed by the tubules and none appears in the urine (none is cleared). Substances that are partially reabsorbed back into the plasma, for example, sodium and chloride ion, are cleared at a rate less than the GFR but greater than zero. Substances that are secreted from the blood into the tubule are cleared at a rate greater than the GFR.

MEASURING RENAL CLEARANCE OF ANY SUBSTANCE

Measuring the clearance of any substance is done by the same technique as measuring GFR. The concentration of the substance in the plasma and urine is determined, as is the urine volume over a given period. The equation expressing the clearance of any substance is UV/P, where U is the concentration of the substance in the urine (milligrams per millilter), V is the volume per time of urine (milliliters per minute), and P is the concentration of the substance in the plasma (milligrams per milliliter).

Only for a substance like inulin is the GFR equal to the clearance. For all other substances, clearance is either more or less than the GFR.

Measuring the clearance of a plasma substance that is 100% excreted by the kidneys allows one to estimate renal plasma flow, and from there, renal blood flow.

Measurement of Renal Plasma Flow and Renal Blood Flow

Measuring renal plasma flow involves measuring the clearance of a substance called para-aminohippurate (PAH). PAH is freely filtered at the glomerulus. It is not reabsorbed, but is actively secreted into the urine filtrate. Therefore, all PAH in the plasma (100%) is cleared by the kidneys. The clearance of PAH gives an estimate of renal plasma flow. Because the plasma is approximately 40 to 50% of the total blood volume, this allows one to estimate renal blood flow.

It is only possible to estimate renal blood flow from clearance of PAH because not all plasma entering the kidney goes through a glomerular capillary. Approximately 10 to 15% of renal blood flow feeds nonfiltering tissue such as fat and connective tissue. Therefore, clearance of PAH is said to give the **effective renal plasma flow** (ERPF), which is 10 to 15% less than total renal plasma flow, as shown in Equation 14-3:

$$C_{PAH} = U_{PAH}\ V/P_{PAH} = \text{ERPF} \qquad (14\text{-}3)$$

From the ERPF, the effective renal blood flow (ERBF) can be found with Equation 14-4:

$$\text{ERBF} = \text{ERPF}/1 - Vc \qquad (14\text{-}4)$$

where Vc is the measured hematocrit of the blood sample (the amount of blood occupied by red blood cells, not plasma).

Regulation of Renal Blood Flow

Maintenance of adequate renal blood flow is essential for kidney survival and for control of plasma volume and electrolytes. Changes in renal blood flow may increase or decrease the glomerular hydrostatic pressure, affecting GFR. The kidney has several mechanisms for controlling renal blood flow. These serve to maintain both kidney function and GFR constant in spite of systemic blood pressure changes.

Renal blood flow is controlled by intrarenal and extrarenal mechanisms. Intrarenal mechanisms include the inherent ability of the afferent and the efferent arterioles to dilate or constrict, thereby controlling blood flow through the kidney. This inherent ability is called **autoregulation**. Extrarenal mechanisms regulating renal blood flow include the direct effects of increased or decreased mean arterial pressure and the effects of the sympathetic nervous system. A third mechanism regulating renal blood flow that has both intrarenal and extrarenal components involves a hormone produced by the kidney that affects the entire systemic circulation. This hormone, called renin, exerts its effects through the production of a potent vasoconstrictor, angiotensin II.

AUTOREGULATION

Autoregulation is the intrinsic response of vascular smooth muscle to changes in blood pressure. Like many arterioles, smooth muscle cells of the afferent and the efferent arterioles respond to their own stretch with reflex constriction. When systemic blood pressure is increased, stretch on afferent arterioles is increased. Stretching the afferent arterioles causes them to constrict, reducing the blood flow and returning renal blood pressure back toward normal. In contrast, when systemic blood pressure is decreased, stretch on the afferent and the efferent arterioles is reduced, and the arterioles respond by relaxing and dilating to increase flow. As a result of autoregulation, renal blood flow remains nearly constant over a range of blood pressures between 80 and 180 mm Hg.

Autoregulation is especially effective during blood pressure increases. The bottom limit of autoregulation, 80 mm Hg, however, is reached more frequently than the upper limit. Therefore, GFR may decrease with severe hypotension.

SYMPATHETIC NERVOUS SYSTEM

Sympathetic nerves innervate both the afferent and the efferent arterioles of the kidney and can override autoregulation when stimulated. As is true in most of the cardiovascular system, stimulation of the sympathetic nerves causes constriction of the afferent arterioles, leading to increased resistance to flow. As a result, blood flow through the glomerulus decreases, causing a decrease both in capillary hydrostatic pressure and in GFR. Simultaneous sympathetic stimulation of the efferent arterioles, however, and their subsequent constriction, causes blood flow to "dam up" in the glomerulus. This can actually increase capillary hydrostatic pressure and glomerular filtration. The net result of sympathetic stimulation to the kidneys is a significant decrease in renal blood flow (because blood going in and out is reduced) but a lesser decrease in GFR. The sympathetic nervous system is stimulated when there is a decrease in systemic blood pressure.

Decreased renal blood flow in response to decreased systemic blood pressure is adaptive and helps the organism survive a hypotensive crisis. With hypotension, less water and salt is filtered at the glomerulus, causing less to be lost in the urine. This helps to increase blood volume and restore blood pressure.

In conditions of increased blood pressure, sympathetic stimulation to all arterioles is reduced. The afferent and the efferent arterioles dilate, and renal blood flow and GFR increase. This results in increased loss of water and salt in the urine, which helps to reduce blood volume and return blood pressure toward normal.

Note that sympathetic input dominates over autoregulatory mechanisms of the kidney. If sympathetic stimulation increases, renal blood flow decreases despite attempts by the kidney to autoregulate its flow.

Renin

Renin is a hormone released from the kidney in response to either a decrease in blood pressure or a decrease in plasma sodium concentration. Cells that synthesize and secrete renin and control its release are a particular group of cells of the nephron called the **juxtaglomerular (JG) apparatus**. This group of cells includes smooth muscle cells of the afferent arteriole and cells of the macula densa. The smooth muscle cells synthesize renin and act as baroreceptors monitoring blood pressure. Macula densa cells are part of the thick ascending limb of the nephron. These cells sense plasma sodium concentration. The macula densa cells and the afferent arteriolar cells are in close approximation to each other where the ascending limb of the distal tubule nearly touches the glomerulus. When the macula densa cells sense a change in plasma sodium, they pass that message on to the renin-secreting cells.

When blood pressure falls, the smooth muscle cells increase renin release. When blood pressure increases, the smooth muscle cells decrease their release of renin. If plasma sodium levels decrease, macula densa cells signal the renin-producing cells to increase their activity. If plasma sodium levels increase, macula densa cells signal the smooth muscle cells to decrease renin release.

Sympathetic nerves also stimulate the JG apparatus to secrete renin. Thus, decreased blood pressure causes increased renin both directly, via the JG baroreceptors, and indirectly, via the sympathetic nerves.

Once released, renin circulates in the blood and acts to catalyze the breakdown of a small protein, angiotensinogen, to a 10-amino-acid protein, angiotensin I (AI). Angiotensinogen is produced by the liver and is highly concentrated in the blood. Renin release is thus the rate-limiting step in the reaction. The conversion of angiotensinogen to AI occurs throughout the plasma, but primarily, it occurs in the pulmonary capillaries. AI has few effects of its own, but it is quickly acted upon by another enzyme readily available in the bloodstream—angiotensin-converting enzyme. Angiotensin-converting enzyme splits AI into an 8-amino-acid peptide, angiotensin II (AII).

Angiotensin II

AII is a potent vasoconstrictor that acts throughout the vascular system to increase smooth muscle contraction, thereby decreasing vessel diameter and increasing total peripheral resistance (TPR). An increase in TPR directly increases systemic blood pressure (Chapter 12). AII is also a potent hormone that circulates in the blood to the adrenal glands, causing the synthesis of the mineralocorticoid hormone, aldosterone.

Aldosterone

The hormone that circulates in the blood and binds to cells of the cortical-collecting duct is called aldosterone. The binding of aldosterone increases sodium reabsorption from the urine filtrate and causes sodium to return into the peritubular capillaries. Increased sodium reabsorption allows for increased water reabsorption, causing increased plasma volume. An increase in plasma volume increases venous return to the heart, thereby increasing the stroke volume and cardiac output. Increased cardiac output, like increased TPR, directly increases systemic blood pressure.

Other stimuli for aldosterone release, besides angiotensin II, are high plasma potassium level and a hormone of the anterior pituitary, adrenocorticotropic hormone (ACTH). In addition to affecting sodium reabsorption, aldosterone stimulates the secretion (and therefore the excretion) of potassium from the cortical-collecting duct into the urine filtrate. Aldosterone also affects sodium and potassium transport across the gut, in the same manner as it does across the collecting duct.

Renin-Angiotensin Reflex Response to Changes in Blood Pressure

With a decrease in blood pressure, the JG cells release renin, which in turn causes an increase in AII. AII constricts arterioles throughout the body, including the afferent and the efferent arterioles. This causes an increase in total peripheral resistance and a return of blood pressure back toward normal (Fig. 14-4). Renal blood flow is reduced, which causes less urine to be produced. This contributes to increased plasma volume and blood pressure.

The opposite occurs with increased blood pressure. With an increase in blood pressure, renin release decreases as does AII levels. This leads to dilation of systemic arterioles, a reduction of total peripheral resistance, and a decrease in blood pressure back toward normal. Decreased AII causes afferent and efferent arterioles to relax, leading

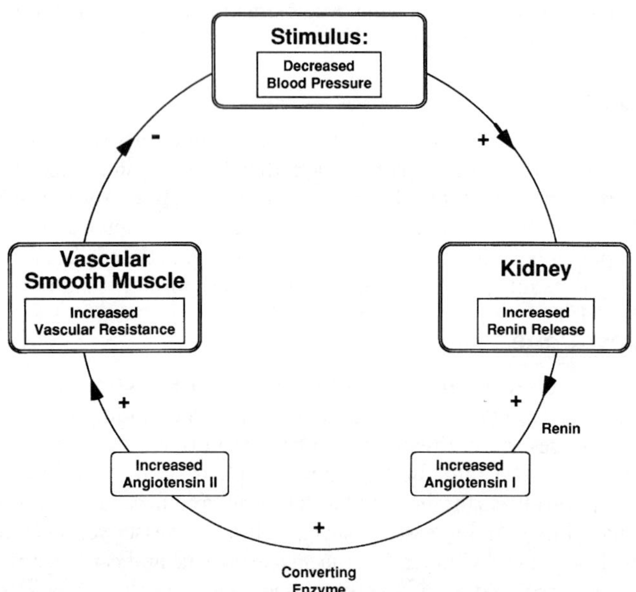

Figure 14-4. Response of renin, AI, AII to a decrease in blood pressure.

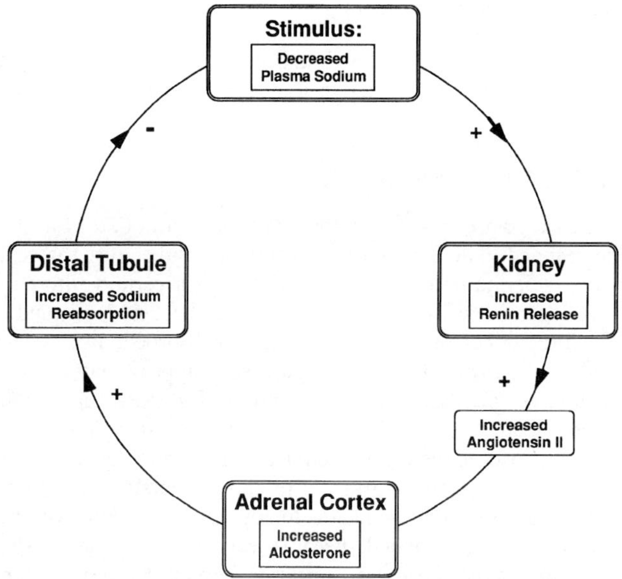

Figure 14-5. Response of renin, AI, AII to a decrease in plasma sodium.

to an increase in renal blood flow and urine output, which serves to decrease blood pressure.

Renin-Angiotensin-Aldosterone Response to Decreased Sodium

The second stimulus for renin release is plasma sodium concentration. Decreased sodium in the tubular fluid passing the cells of the macula densa causes increased renin release. As shown in Figure 14-5, increased renin leads to increased AII, which stimulates aldosterone synthesis and therefore increases sodium reabsorption. This reduces the stimulus for further renin release. The opposite is true if there is increased plasma sodium passing the macula densa cells.

Renal Reabsorption

Reabsorption is the second process by which the kidney determines the concentration of a substance filtered from the plasma. Reabsorption refers to the active (requiring energy and always being mediated by a carrier) or the passive (no energy required) movement of a substance filtered at the glomerulus back into the peritubular capillaries. Reabsorption may be total (e.g., glucose) or partial (e.g., sodium, urea, chloride, and water).

REABSORPTION OF GLUCOSE

Glucose is freely filtered at the glomerulus. All of the filtered glucose is normally reabsorbed by active transport, primarily in the proximal tubule.

TRANSPORT MAXIMUM FOR GLUCOSE

Because carriers are involved, a transport maximum (Tm) for glucose can be reached. The Tm is the amount of a substance that can be transported per unit of time. For glucose, at a certain filtered load (GFR × Plasma Concentration), all carriers become occupied. Any glucose filtered beyond that load is not reabsorbed, but is instead excreted in the urine. The Tm for glucose is approximately 375 mg/min of filtered glucose. The concentration of glucose that results in this filtered load, given a GFR of 125 mL/min, is 3.0 mg/mL of plasma (because glucose concentration clinically is frequently expressed as per 100 mL of blood, this works out to approximately 150 mg/100 mL of blood). However, glucose begins to appear in the urine even before this plasma level is reached, because each nephron has a slightly different Tm and the carrier transport rate may accelerate at the highest glucose concentrations. Plasma glucose seldom gets high enough that glucose Tm is reached unless an individual has diabetes mellitus (Chapter 17). Note that the kidney does not control blood glucose levels. It simply filters and reabsorbs all it can. The pancreas, via insulin release (Chapter 17), controls blood glucose.

In the kidney, glucose reabsorption is coupled with the reabsorption of sodium ions from the urine filtrate into the tubular cells. At some point this movement is driven by the splitting of adenosine triphosphate (ATP) by the sodium-potassium ATPase. It is a process that requires energy. It is this secondary use of energy that makes glucose transport an active (energy-requiring) process.

REABSORPTION OF SODIUM

Sodium reabsorption occurs throughout the tubule by a combination of simple diffusion and active transport. Approximately 65% of sodium reabsorption occurs across the proximal tubule and 25% across the loop of Henle. Therefore, only approximately 10% of the filtered sodium remains in the tubule by the time the filtrate reaches the distal convoluted tubule. The final concentration of sodium in the urine is usually less than 1% of the total amount filtered at the glomerulus.

Unlike glucose, the kidney regulates plasma sodium concentration. Although sodium is freely filtered and 98 to 99% is normally reabsorbed, the final 1 to 2% of its reabsorption can vary. Plasma sodium concentration is 145 mmol/L, and the amount of filtered sodium is approximately 18 mmol/min (supposing a GFR of approximately 180 L/day). This amounts to approximately 1500 grams of sodium filtered each day. Even 2% of this amount—30 g/day—is a considerable amount. This final 2% is affected by the presence or absence of the hormone aldosterone.

Transport of sodium back into the capillaries may either be coupled in the same direction to the reabsorption of another substance (cotransport), or it may be coupled in the opposite direction with another substance (countertransport). Substances cotransported with sodium include glucose, amino acids, and chloride. Hydrogen ion (H^+) is countertransported and thus secreted into the urine when a sodium ion is reabsorbed.

REABSORPTION OF CHLORIDE

Chloride reabsorption can be active or passive and is nearly always coupled to sodium transport. It is affected by the electrical gradient across the tubule. Like sodium, most chloride reabsorption (65%) occurs across the proximal tubule, less across the loop of Henle (25%), and the rest (10%) between the distal convoluted tubule and the collecting-duct system.

REABSORPTION OF POTASSIUM

Most potassium in the body is intracellular. Therefore, although plasma potassium is freely filtered across the glomerulus, its concentration in Bowman's capsule is low. Most potassium that is filtered is reabsorbed: 50% across the proximal tubule, 40% in the thick ascending limb, and the remaining 10% in the final part of the nephron, the medullary-collecting duct. Most potassium reabsorption is by passive diffusion.

Potassium is also *secreted* into the tubule by active transport across the cells of the proximal tubule, the descending limb of the loop of Henle, and the collecting ducts. The amount of secreted potassium is variable and depends on the amount of potassium ingested in the diet. An individual on a low-potassium diet only filters and reabsorbs, not secretes, potassium. An individual on a high-potassium diet filters, reabsorbs, *and* secretes potassium. Potassium secretion by the collecting ducts is stimulated by the hormone aldosterone released from the adrenal cortex.

REABSORPTION OF THE AMINO ACIDS

Amino acids filtered at the glomerulus are actively reabsorbed in the proximal tubule. All reabsorption of amino acids is carrier mediated. The Tm for the carriers is well above the amounts of amino acids normally filtered, so none are normally present in the urine.

REABSORPTION OF PLASMA PROTEINS

Very few plasma proteins are filtered across the glomerulus. Those that are filtered are actively reabsorbed across the proximal tubule.

Because the GFR is so high, the filtration of even a few molecules of plasma protein, such as albumin, would result in a significant daily loss of protein if reabsorption did not occur.

A few proteins filtered at the glomerulus are not reabsorbed. They are degraded by tubular cells and excreted in the urine. Examples of these proteins include the protein hormones, such as growth hormone and luteinizing hormone.

REABSORPTION OF UREA

Urea is produced in the liver as an end product of protein metabolism. It is freely filtered at the glomerulus. Because urea is highly permeable across most (but not all) of the nephron, it diffuses back into the peritubular capillaries. It follows water as water is reabsorbed from the urine filtrate moving through the nephron. By the end of the proximal tubule, approximately 50% of the filtered urea has been reabsorbed. From the end of the proximal tubule to the medullary-collecting ducts, the proximal tubule is impermeable to urea. Along this route, some portions of the tubule begin to secrete urea into the filtrate. Thus, at the point the filtrate reaches the medullary-collecting ducts, urea concentration has again reached what it was in the original glomerular filtrate. At the medullary-collecting ducts, urea once more becomes permeable and again follows water reabsorption out of the tubule. As the filtrate leaves the kidney, approximately 40% of the original filtered urea remains and is excreted.

Note that urea reabsorption depends on water reabsorption. If water reabsorption is low, more urea will be excreted, and vice versa.

Acid-Base Handling

The kidney plays a pivotal role in maintaining acid-base balance. Most metabolic processes in the body produce acid. These processes include oxidative phosphorylation, which produces the volatile acid carbon dioxide, and the metabolism of proteins that produce nonvolatile acids such as sulfuric and phosphoric acids. Although the lungs normally excrete all carbon dioxide produced by oxidation, the kidney is the only organ capable of eliminating nonvolatile acids. More important, the kidneys have the essential job of reabsorbing large quantities of the base bicarbonate, which is freely filtered at the glomerulus. Without this function, fatally low blood pH would occur. The kidneys assist in eliminating acid produced by cell metabolism in individuals who have lung disease by increasing the secretion and excretion of acid and by reabsorbing an increased amount of base.

REABSORPTION OF BICARBONATE

Reabsorption of bicarbonate is an active process that occurs primarily in the proximal tubule (and to a lesser extent in the collecting ducts).

As shown in Figure 14-6, reabsorption occurs when a molecule of water breaks down in the proximal tubular cell into an H^+ and a hydroxyl molecule (OH^-). The H^+ is actively secreted into the lumen of the tubule and joins with a bicarbonate molecule that has been filtered at the glomerulus. Hydrogen plus bicarbonate results in carbonic acid (H_2CO_3) which, in the presence of the enzyme carbonic anhydrase, breaks down to carbon dioxide and water. These diffuse back into the proximal tubular cell to be used again as this cycle repeats.

By this process, the filtered bicarbonate is saved from being excreted in the urine. The reaction of hydrogen with bicarbonate is reversible as shown in Equation 14.5:

$$CO_2 + H_2O \rightleftarrows H_2CO_3 \rightleftarrows H^+ + HCO_3^- \qquad (14.5)$$

The OH^- produced in the proximal tubule cell joins with an intracellular carbon dioxide molecule. In the presence of the enzyme carbonic anhydrase, it too proceeds to a bicarbonate ion. This bicarbonate also returns into the peritubular capillary as shown in Figure 14-6. The enzyme carbonic anhydrase is readily available.

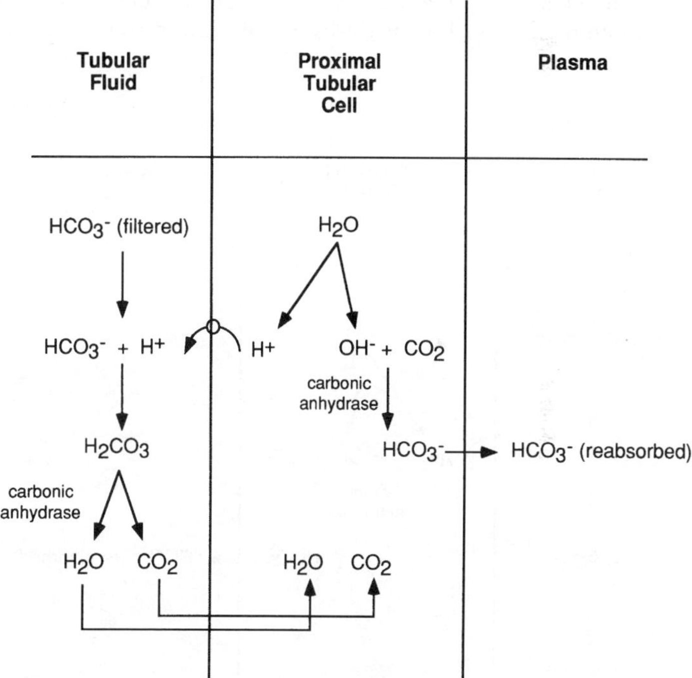

Figure 14-6. Reabsorption of filtered bicarbonate by the proximal tubular cells.

SECRETION AND EXCRETION OF ACID

The above reactions only serve to reabsorb filtered bicarbonate. They do not eliminate acid. The kidney does actively secrete and excrete H^+ in the urine as well, which allows it to rid the blood of metabolically produced nonvolatile acids. As shown in Figure 14-7, H^+ excretion occurs after most of the filtered bicarbonate has been reabsorbed. In this case, the H^+ produced in the proximal tubule cell from the breakdown of water moves into the lumen of the tubule and combines with filtered phosphate ions (or to a lesser extent, sulfate ions) and is lost in the urine.

The effect of excreting hydrogen bound to phosphate is not only the loss of acid in the urine but *a net gain of bicarbonate.* This is because a bicarbonate ion is still produced in the proximal tubule when carbon dioxide joins with OH^-. This bicarbonate is returned to the plasma.

A second mechanism by which the kidney excretes acid is by active secretion of ammonium ion (NH_4^+) into the tubular fluid (Figure 14-8). Ammonium ion is produced in the proximal tubular cell as a result of the metabolism of glutamine. Glutamine enters the cell from the peritubular capillary and from the tubular lumen, after being filtered across the glomerulus. Once in the tubule, ammonium ion cannot return into the proximal tubular cells; therefore, it is excreted in the

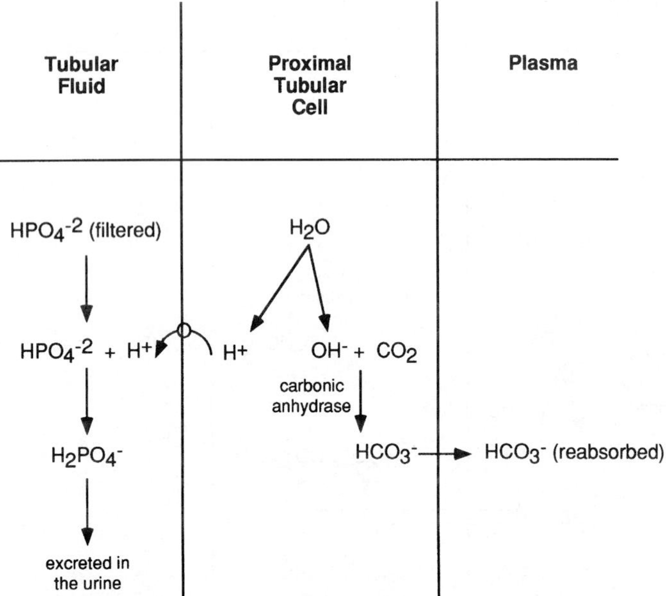

Figure 14-7. Excretion of H^+ bound to filtered phosphate.

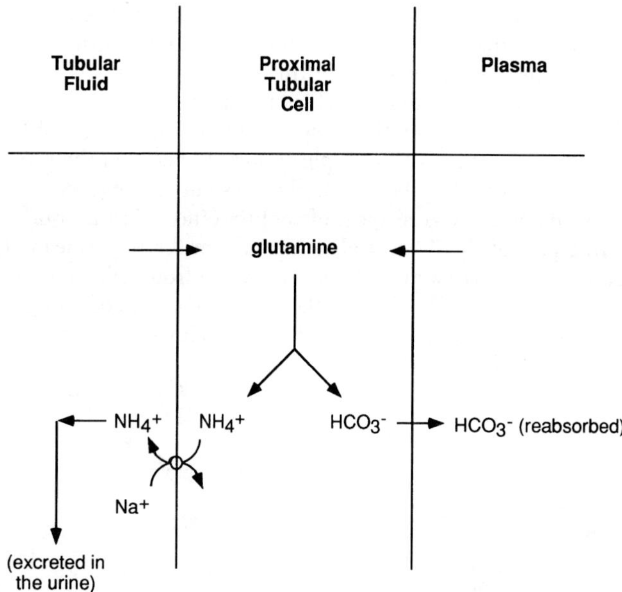

Figure 14-8. Excretion of H^+ as ammonium ion. Glutamine diffuses into the proximal tubular cell from the plasma and from the tubular fluid. The active transport of ammonium into the tubular fluid occurs as a result of a sodium-ammonium countertransport system.

urine. Bicarbonate produced from glutamine metabolism diffuses back into the peritubular capillary, thereby returning base to the blood. Finally, a small amount of H^+ is excreted free in the urine, causing the urine to normally have an acidic pH.

SECRETION OF BICARBONATE

Under conditions of alkalosis (excess base), the kidney can secrete bicarbonate, thus ridding the plasma of base and returning the pH toward normal. Secretion of bicarbonate is an active process occurring in the cortical-collecting duct. However, even under conditions of alkalosis, bicarbonate reabsorption in the proximal tubule is ongoing and essential. Loss of all filtered bicarbonate would be fatal.

Renal Concentrating Mechanism: The Countercurrent System

To survive periods without water, animals, including humans, must excrete a concentrated (hypertonic) urine. They must eliminate waste products, including urea, without losing much water in the process. In contrast, under conditions of water excess, animals must excrete large amounts of water in a dilute (hypotonic) urine. The kidney has adapted to handle day-to-day variations in water consumption by developing the **countercurrent multiplier system**. For this system to work, antidiuretic hormone (ADH) is required.

The countercurrent multiplier system exists in the loop of Henle, a long, curving portion of the nephron located between the proximal and the distal tubules. The multiplier system has five basic steps and depends on active transport of sodium (and chloride) out of the ascending part of the loop. It also depends on the impermeability of this part of the loop to water, which keeps water from following sodium out. Finally, this system relies on the permeability of collecting ducts to water. The five steps are outlined in the following section and are shown graphically in Figure 14-9.

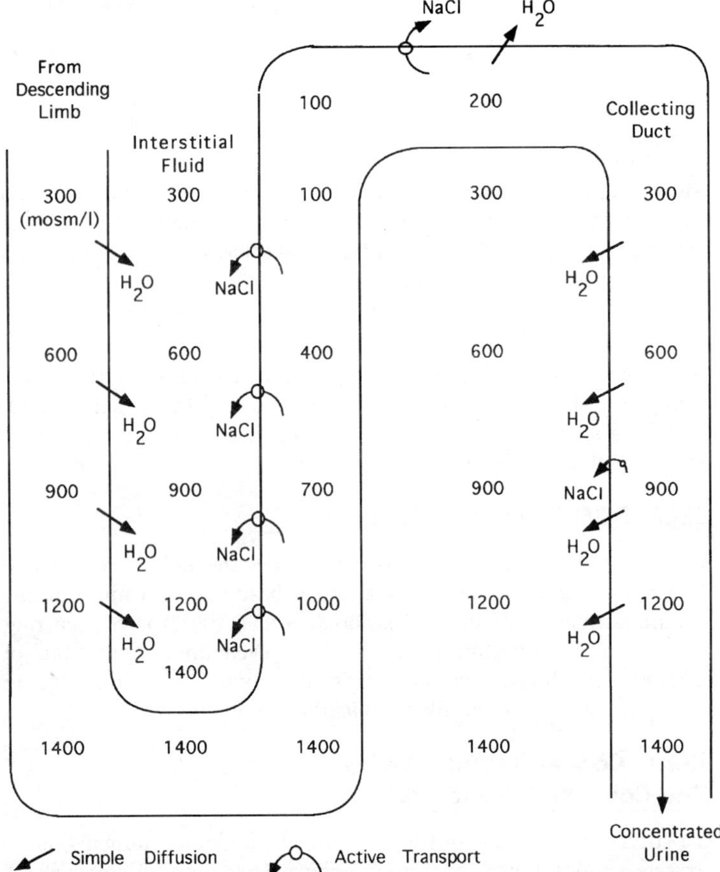

Figure 14-9. Formation of a concentrated urine in the presence of ADH. With ADH, water diffuses out of the collecting duct into the concentrated interstitium.

STEPS OF THE COUNTERCURRENT MULTIPLIER SYSTEM

1. When sodium is transported out of the ascending limb, the interstitial fluid surrounding the loop of Henle becomes concentrated.
2. Because water is impermeable across the ascending limb, water cannot follow sodium out of the ascending limb. The remaining filtrate becomes progressively diluted.
3. Water is permeable in the descending limb of the loop. Water leaves this section and flows down its concentration gradient into the surrounding interstitial space. This concentrates the descending limb fluid. As the fluid loops into the ascending limb, it is progressively diluted as sodium is pumped out.
4. The net result is the concentration of the interstitial fluid surrounding the loop of Henle. Concentration is highest surrounding the bottom of the loop, becoming more dilute as the ascending limb is followed up.
5. At the top of the ascending limb, tubular fluid is isotonic (equal in concentration to the plasma) or even hypotonic (more dilute compared with plasma).

RESULT OF THE COUNTERCURRENT MULTIPLIER SYSTEM

The goal of the countercurrrent system is to concentrate the interstitial fluid surrounding the loop of Henle (as described in step 4). This is vital because filtrate passes down the collecting ducts through this fluid. Permeability of the collecting ducts to water is variable. If permeability to water is high (as shown in Figure 14-9), as the water moves down through the concentrated interstitium, it will diffuse out of the collecting duct and back into the peritubular capillary. The result is little water excretion and concentrated urine. In contrast, if permeability to water is low, water will not diffuse out of the collecting duct and instead will be excreted in the urine. The urine will be dilute, as shown in Figure 14-10.

ROLE OF ANTIDIURETIC HORMONE IN CONCENTRATING THE URINE

Whether the collecting ducts are permeable to water is determined by the circulating level of the posterior pituitary hormone, ADH. Release of ADH from the posterior pituitary is increased in response to a decrease in blood pressure or an increase in extracellular osmolarity (decreased water concentration). ADH acts on the collecting tubules to increase water permeability. If blood pressure is low or plasma osmolarity is high, ADH release will be stimulated and water will be reabsorbed into the peritubular capillaries, increasing blood volume and pressure, and decreasing extracellular osmolarity. In contrast, if blood pressure is too high or extracellular fluid is too dilute (decreased osmolarity), ADH release will be inhibited and more water will be excreted in the urine, decreasing blood volume and pressure, and increasing extracellular osmolarity.

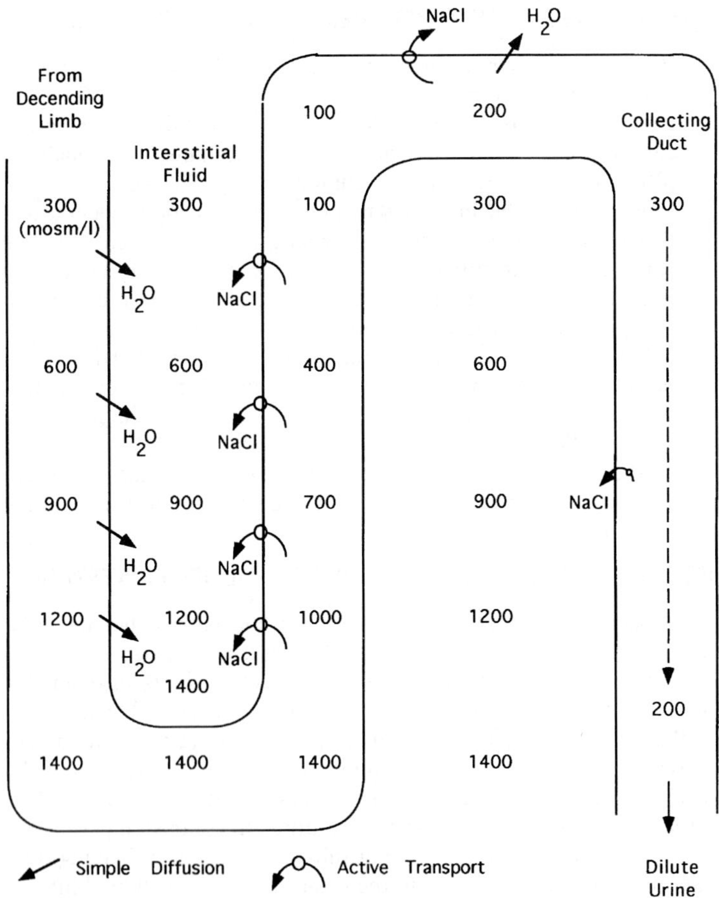

Figure 14-10. Formation of a dilute urine if ADH is absent. Note that because there is actually some NaCl transported out of the collecting duct, urine osmolity can be less than 300 mOsm/L.

Sensors that measure blood pressure and control ADH release include the carotid and the aortic baroreceptors and a group of receptors in the left atrium. Sensors that measure extracellular osmolarity lie in the hypothalamus, adjacent to the cells that actually synthesize ADH. After synthesis in the hypothalamus, ADH is stored in the posterior pituitary.

Approximately 1400 mOsmol/L is the most concentrated human urine can become. The most dilute concentration is less than 200 mOsmol/L.

Renal Endocrine Function

The kidney functions as an endocrine organ, not only with the production and release of renin but also with the production and release of two other hormones: 1,25-dihydroxyvitamin D_3, important for bone mineralization; and erythropoietin, required for red blood cell production.

1,25-DIHYDROXYVITAMIN D_3

The kidney acts in conjunction with the liver to produce an active form of vitamin D, called 1,25-dihydroxyvitamin D_3, from an inactive precursor consumed in the diet. The inactive form of vitamin D can also be produced in a reaction catalyzed by sunlight on a precursor present in the skin. Vitamin D is essential for maintenance of plasma calcium levels required for bone formation. The active form of vitamin D acts as a hormone by circulating in the blood and stimulating absorption of calcium—and to a lesser extent, phosphate—across the small intestine and across the kidney tubules. Vitamin D also stimulates bone resorption (breakdown). Bone resorption releases calcium, and thus plasma calcium is increased.

Parathyroid hormone is the stimulus for the kidney to play its role in activating vitamin D_3. Parathyroid hormone is released from the parathyroid gland in response to decreased plasma calcium. This is an example of a negative-feedback cycle: decreased plasma calcium leads to increased parathyroid hormone, which leads to increased renal activation of vitamin D_3. Activation of vitamin D_3 increases gut and kidney absorption of calcium, increasing plasma calcium and removing the stimulus for parathyroid release. Parathyroid hormone also directly stimulates bone resorption to release calcium into the plasma when necessary. Individuals who have renal disease frequently develop brittle, easily broken bones as a result of too little active vitamin D_3.

ERYTHROPOIETIN

The hormone that stimulates the bone marrow to increase the production of erythrocytes (red blood cells) is called erythropoietin. The cells of the kidney responsible for synthesizing and releasing erythropoietin respond to renal hypoxia. Individuals who have renal disease frequently demonstrate chronic and debilitating anemia.

Micturition

Micturition is the process of urination—the elimination of urine from the body. Micturition occurs when the internal and the external urethral sphincters at the base of the bladder are relaxed.

The bladder is composed of smooth muscle (the detrusor muscle), innervated by sensory neurons that respond to stretch, and parasympathetic fibers that travel from the sacral area to the bladder. An area of smooth muscle at the base of the bladder (the internal sphincter) is also innervated by parasympathetic nerves. An external sphincter composed of skeletal muscle is just below the internal spincter and at the top of the urethra. The external sphincter is innervated by motor neurons from the pudendal nerve. When urine accumulates, stretch of the bladder is sensed by afferent fibers that send the information to the spinal cord. Parasympathetic nerves to the bladder are activated, causing contraction of the smooth muscle and opening of the internal sphincter. At the same time, the motor neurons going to the external sphincter are inhibited and the external sphincter is relaxed, causing micturation to occur.

Micturation, however, can be voluntarily inhibited. This is possible because at the same time that the afferent nerves are conveying information on bladder stretch to the spinal cord, they are also sending information up the cord to the brainstem and cortex, allowing one to be conscious of the need to void. Descending neurons from the brain can inhibit or stimulate the spinal reflex to void. These descending pathways inhibit urination by causing contraction of the skeletal muscles of the pelvis as well as the external sphincter. Descending pathways also block the firing of parasympathetic nerves to the internal sphincter. For urination to be facilitated, skeletal muscles can be voluntarily relaxed. Voluntary control over micturition becomes functional in children by or before the time they become 3 or 4 years of age. However, it may become interrupted at any time by central nervous system disease or injury or from spinal cord trauma.

Tests of Renal Function

BLOOD UREA NITROGEN

Urea is a nitrogenous waste product of protein and amino acid metabolism. One important job of the kidney is to eliminate this potentially toxic substance from the body. With declining renal function, blood urea nitrogen (BUN) levels increase. Measuring BUN provides, therefore, an indication of kidney health.

BUN, however, is not only determined by renal function. It can also be affected by circumstances not associated with the kidney, such as increased or decreased dietary protein intake, or any unusual cause of an increased protein breakdown, such as a muscle injury. Likewise, liver disease may *decrease* BUN, because the liver is necessary to convert ammonia to urea. Because BUN levels are affected by these other factors, BUN is an indiscriminate indicator of renal disease. Therefore, instead of actually measuring BUN, the ratio of BUN to serum creatinine is often reported. Normally, this ratio is 10:1. Ratios greater than 15:1 suggest a nonrenal cause of urea elevation. Ratios less than 10:1 occur with liver disease.

SERUM CREATININE

Creatinine is a product of muscle breakdown. Creatinine is excreted by the kidney through a combination of filtration and secretion. Creatinine concentration in the plasma remains nearly constant from day to day. It varies slightly from approximately 0.7 mg/100 mL of blood in a small woman to 1.5 mg/100 mL in a muscular man. Levels greater than these suggest the kidney is not clearing creatinine and indicate renal disease. Serum creatinine is very indicative of renal function. As a rough guide, a doubling of serum creatinine levels indicates a 50% reduction in renal function. Likewise, a tripling of normal creatinine levels indicates a 75% reduction in renal function. The clearance of creatinine may be used to estimate GFR.

URINALYSIS

A urine sample may be easily obtained and evaluated for the presence of red blood cells, protein, glucose, and leukocytes, all of which are normally minimal to absent in the urine. Urine casts, which occur in the presence of high amounts of urine protein, may also be observed under some conditions of renal disease or injury. Urine osmolality (specific gravity) is measurable and should range between 1.015 and 1.025. Dehydration causes increased urine osmolality as more water is reabsorbed back into the peritubular capillaries. Overhydration results in decreased urine osmolality.

CYTOSCOPY

Cytoscopy is the process in which a lighted scope (cytoscope) is inserted up the urethra into the bladder. Bladder lesions, stones, and biopsy samples may be taken.

VOIDING CYSTOURETHROGRAPHY

Voiding cystourethrography involves bladder catheterization and infusion of a radioactive dye to study the shape and size of the bladder. It can be used to detect and grade the degree of vesicoureteral reflux. Negative effects of cystourethrography are that it is associated with gonadal radiation, and it may spread an unresolved bladder infection into the ureters or kidney if used inappropriately.

INTRAVENOUS UROGRAPHY

Intravenous urography is a technique in which a radiologic dye is injected intravenously, and x-ray films are taken sequentially as the dye filters through the kidney. Obstructions to flow in the glomeruli or tubules, vesicoureteral reflux, and stones may be visualized. A drawback to the use of this technique is the finding that some individuals are allergic to the dye and may suffer an anaphylactic reaction. High doses of radiation are involved.

RENAL ULTRASOUND

Renal ultrasound uses the reflection of sound waves to identify renal abnormalities, including structural abnormalities, kidney stones, tumors, and other masses. Because it is noninvasive and does not involve radiation exposure, this technique is frequently used to evaluate renal function in children who have had a urinary tract infection. It does not, however, offer sufficient detail to evaluate vesicoureteral reflux, renal scarring, or inflammation.

PATHOPHYSIOLOGIC CONCEPTS

Alterations in Glomerular Filtration

Glomerular filtration depends on the summation of forces favoring filtration of plasma across the glomerulus and forces favoring reabsorption of filtrate into the glomerulus. Anything that affects the forces of filtration or the forces of reabsorption affects net glomerular filtration. Forces favoring filtration are capillary pressure and interstitial fluid colloid osmotic pressure. Forces favoring reabsorption are interstitial fluid pressure and plasma colloid osmotic pressure.

ALTERATIONS IN CAPILLARY PRESSURE

Capillary pressure depends on mean arterial pressure. Increased mean arterial pressure increases capillary pressure, tending to increase glomerular filtration. A decrease in mean arterial pressure decreases capillary pressure and tends to decrease glomerular filtration. Autoregulation of afferent and efferent arterioles minimizes these changes unless the mean arterial blood pressure becomes too high (180 mm Hg) or too low (80 mm Hg).

Increased sympathetic activity and increased AII constrict afferent and efferent arterioles. These stimuli decrease the capillary pressure somewhat. However, because afferent and efferent arterioles are both affected, the responses tend to cancel each other out and GFR is nearly unaffected. Because the efferent arteriole response to sympathetic stimulation is especially sensitive, with heavy sympathetic stimulation, GFR may actually increase, as blood in the glomerulus is "dammed up" with greater constriction of the efferent compared to afferent arteriole.

ALTERATIONS IN INTERSTITIAL FLUID COLLOID OSMOTIC PRESSURE

Interstitial fluid colloid osmotic pressure is low because very few plasma proteins or red blood cells filter out of the glomerulus. With injury to the glomerulus or the peritubular capillaries, interstitial fluid colloid osmotic pressure may increase. If the interstitial fluid osmotic pressure increases, fluid is drawn out of the glomerulus and peritubular capillaries and swelling and edema occur in Bowman's space and the interstitial space surrounding the tubule. Swelling in Bowman's space or around the tubule can interfere with further glomerular filtration and tubular reabsorption because of increasing interstitial fluid pressure. Swelling and edema may also collapse the delicate glomeruli or peritubular capillaries, leading to hypoxia and death of the nephrons in extreme situations.

ALTERATIONS IN PLASMA COLLOID OSMOTIC PRESSURE

Plasma colloid osmotic pressure depends on the protein concentration of plasma. Plasma protein levels can decrease as a result of liver disease, protein loss in the urine, or protein malnutrition. Plasma colloid osmotic pressure is the major force favoring reabsorption of fluids back into the capillaries. If it decreases, less fluid reenters the capillaries. Fluid accumulates in the tubular and the peritubular (surrounding) areas. Again, swelling around the tubule can collapse the tubule and the surrounding peritubular capillaries, leading to hypoxia and death of the nephrons.

ALTERATIONS IN INTERSTITIAL FLUID PRESSURE

Interstitial fluid pressure in Bowman's space and surrounding the tubule can increase drastically if the glomerular or peritubular capillaries are damaged. Increased interstitial fluid pressure opposes further glomerular filtration. Increased interstitial fluid pressure can cause collapse of the surrounding nephrons and the peritubular capillaries, leading to hypoxia and renal cell injury or death. When cells die, they release intracellular enzymes that stimulate immune and inflammatory reactions (Chapter 3), which further contribute to swelling and edema. This worsens interstitial fluid pressure. With loss of glomerular filtration, blood volume and electrolyte composition cannot be regulated.

TUBULAR OBSTRUCTION

A common cause of increased interstitial fluid pressure is tubular obstruction. Obstruction causes fluid buildup in the nephron and back up into Bowman's capsule and space. Unrelieved tubular obstruction can collapse the nephrons and capillaries and can lead to irreversible renal damage, especially to the papillae, which are the final site for urine concentration. Causes of obstruction include renal calculi (stones) and scarring from repeated kidney infections.

Azotemia

Azotemia refers to abnormal elevation of nitrogenous waste products in the blood such as urea, uric acid, and creatinine. Azotemia indicates a decrease in GFR, occurring either acutely or with chronic renal failure. Azotemia is an early sign of renal damage.

Uremia

Uremia is a syndrome (a constellation of symptoms) that develop in an individual who has end-stage renal disease. Because the kidney is pivotal in maintaining water, acid-base, and electrolyte balance and for the removal of toxic waste products, the symptoms of uremia are widespread and affect all the organs and tissues of the body. Common symptoms include fatigue, anorexia, nausea, vomiting, and lethargy. Intractable itching (pruritus) may occur. Hypertension, osteodystrophy, and uremic encephalopathy develop as well, with central nervous system changes, including confusion and psychosis, characterizing end stages. The range of symptoms appears to be caused by acidosis, anemia from decreased erythropoietin, and the buildup of all waste products.

Nephrotic Syndrome

Nephrotic syndrome is the loss of 3.5 g or more of protein in the urine per day. Virtually no protein is normally lost in the urine. Nephrotic syndrome usually indicates severe glomerular damage. Diabetic nephropathy is the most common cause of nephrotic syndrome. In individuals who do not have diabetes, various glomerular diseases account for the disorder.

Loss of plasma proteins leads to sodium retention, hypoalbuminemia, and hypoimmunoglobulinemia. Thromboembolic complications are common. Clinical manifestations may include increased susceptibility to infections (caused by hypoimmunoglobulins) and generalized edema, called anasarca. Hyperlipidemia (elevated plasma lipids) is associated with hypoalbuminemia, perhaps as a hepatic response to low levels of albumin.

Treatment consists of mechanisms to reduce proteinuria. These include a soy-based protein, low-fat diet, with salt restrictions. Angiotensin-converting enzyme inhibitors reduce proteinuria and have become a mainstay of treatment. Diuretics may be prescribed to increase fluid loss. Protein supplements may be provided to prevent malnutrition unless renal failure is suspected (protein worsens renal failure).

Anasarca

Defined as a generalized edema in individuals suffering from hypoalbuminemia caused by nephrotic syndrome or other causes, anasarca is caused by a systemic decrease in capillary osmotic pressure. With a decrease in this major force favoring reabsorption of interstitial fluid back into the capillaries, edema of the interstitial spaces throughout the body occurs. The edema is usually soft and pitting and occurs early in the periorbital (surrounding the eye) regions, the ankles, and the feet.

Renal Osteodystrophy

Demineralization of bone occurring with renal disease is known as renal osteodysrophy. Renal osteodystrophy has many causes, including decreased renal activation of vitamin D_3, leading to decreased calcium absorption across the gut, and subsequent reduced serum calcium levels. In addition, decreased renal function leads to an accumulation of phosphate ions, and hyperphosphatemia causes the secretion of parathyroid hormone, which leads to bone breakdown (resorption). Decreased serum calcium levels also stimulate parathyroid hormone release. An elevated bone breakdown contributes to easy bone fracturing.

Renal osteodystrophy also occurs as a result of the role bone plays in acting as a buffer for plasma H^+. Bone buffering means bone takes up H^+ and removes it from the general circulation to help maintain plasma pH. In doing so, calcium (which is also positively charged) is leached from the bone to maintain electrical balance in the bone. With chronic acidosis of advanced renal disease, bone buffering of H^+ increases and the leaching of bone calcium becomes significant.

Treatment of renal osteodystrophy is aimed toward calcium and vitamin D supplementation. A phosphate-restricted diet is necessary.

Metabolic Acidosis/Renal Acidosis

Metabolic acidosis is a decrease in plasma pH not caused by a respiratory disorder. Chronic renal disease results in metabolic acidosis as a result of reduced H^+ excretion and altered bicarbonate reabsorption. The result is increased plasma H^+ and lowered pH.

Increased H^+ concentration contributes to bone resorption and causes neural and muscular function changes. The respiratory system is stimulated by the increase in hydrogen. Tachypynea (increased respiratory rate) occurs in an attempt to blow off the excess hydrogen as carbon dioxide. The respiratory response to renal acidosis is called respiratory compensation.

Uremic Encephalopathy

Uremic encephalopathy refers to neurologic changes seen in severe renal disease. Symptoms include fatigue, drowsiness, lethargy, seizures, muscle twitching, peripheral neuropathy (pain in the legs and feet), decreases in memory, and coma. Uremic encephalopathy appears to be caused by accumulation of toxins, alterations in potassium balance, and decreased pH. Treatment involves renal replacement with dialysis or transplantation if the condition is irreversible.

Renal Dialysis

The process of adjusting blood levels of water and electrolytes in a person who has poorly or nonfunctioning kidneys is called renal dialysis. In this procedure, blood is directed past an artificial medium containing water and electrolytes in predetermined concentrations. The artificial medium is the dialyzing fluid.

By simple diffusion across a selectively permeable membrane, water and electrolytes in the blood move down their individual concentration gradients, into or out of the dialyzing solution. As a result of simple diffusion, the final blood levels of these substances can be manipulated to be near normal. For example, sodium concentration in the dialyzing fluid can be adjusted to cause net loss or gain of sodium from the blood. Glucose is added to dialyzing fluid, at the same concentration present in blood, to ensure that glucose is not lost during dialysis. Urea is kept very low in the dialyzing fluid so that urea diffuses down its concentration gradient, out of the blood and into the artificial medium.

There are two types of dialysis: hemodialysis and peritoneal dialysis. Each is discussed in the following section.

HEMODIALYSIS

In hemodialysis, dialysis is done outside the body. The blood is passed from the body, through an arterial catheter, into a large machine. Two chambers separated by a semipermeable membrane are inside the machine. Blood is delivered to one chamber, dialyzing fluid is placed in the other, and diffusion is allowed to occur. Blood is returned to the body via a venous shunt.

Hemodialysis takes approximately 3 to 5 hours and is required approximately three times per week. By the end of the 2- to 3-day interval between treatments, salt, water, and pH balance are abnormal, and the individual usually feels unwell. Hemodialysis seems to contribute to problems of anemia because some red blood cells are destroyed in the process. Infection is also a risk.

PERITONEAL DIALYSIS

In peritoneal dialysis, which occurs outside the body, the individual's own peritoneal membrane is used as a natural, semipermeable barrier. Prepared dialysate solution (approximately 2 L) is delivered into the peritoneal cavity through an indwelling catheter placed under the skin of the abdomen. The solution is allowed to remain in the peritoneal cavity for a predetermined amount of time (usually between 4 and 6 hours). During this time, diffusion of water and electrolytes back and forth between the circulating blood occurs. The person can usually continue activity while the exchange takes place.

Peritoneal dialysis must be performed approximately four times per day. Because the procedure is performed daily—at home or at work—fluctuations in plasma composition seen between hemodialysis treatments are minimized and convenience is increased. Unlike with hemodialysis, individuals usually feel better on a daily basis. Problems with peritoneal dialysis include infections from the indwelling catheter or catheter malfunction.

Heart disease is common among patients who have renal failure for a variety of reasons, including increasing age and the high incidence of diabetes mellitus or hypertension in patients on dialysis. Recent studies have shown that patients on dialysis who suffer a myocardial infarct have high mortality and poor long-term survival.

Renal Transplantation

Defined as a form of renal replacement available to patients who have renal failure, renal transplantation involves placement of a donor kidney into the abdominal cavity of an individual suffering from end-stage renal disease. Transplanted kidneys can either come from living or dead donors. The more similar the antigenic properties of the donated kidney are to the patient, the more likely the transplantation will be successful.

Individuals receiving kidney donation must remain on a variety of immunosuppressant medications for life to prevent organ rejection. Ideally, immunosuppressive therapy should be individualized to match the characteristics of the donor kidney (donor source, age, status of the donor kidney) and the characteristics of the recipient (age, race, reactive antibodies present, transplant number, and tolerance toward immunosuppressive therapy). In addition, the degree of histocompatibility between donor and recipient must be considered. If rejection does occur, it may happen during the very early postoperative period, through the first 3 months, or it may be delayed months or years after the transplantation. All individuals on immunosuppression therapy are subject to increased risk of infection. Infections may be kidney related or independent of the renal system.

Pediatric Consideration

Children who receive renal transplantation frequently experience growth retardation. Whether this is a result of immunosuppressant therapy or a loss of a vital renal function such as erythropoietin production or vitamin D_3 activation is unclear. Recent studies suggest that erythropoietin replacement can reduce growth complications of renal transplantation. For all patients, medical therapy with erythropoietin can also drastically reduce the symptoms of anemia, especially fatigue, and can improve quality of life.

● CONDITIONS OF DISEASE OR INJURY

Hypospadias and Epispadias

Hypospadias is a congenital defect involving misplacement of the opening of the urethra in males from the tip of the penis to the ventral (under) side. This condition may be slight or extreme. Some infants demonstrate the urethral meatus (opening) in the scrotal or perineal area.

Epispadias is the congenital misplacement of the urethral opening to the dorsal side of the penis. This is less common than hypospadias.

CLINICAL MANIFESTATIONS

- Difficulty or inability to urinate adequately while standing may occur.
- Chordee (a bending of the penis) may accompany hypospadias.
- Inguinal hernia or undescended testes may accompany hypospadias.

DIAGNOSTIC TOOLS

- Diagnosis is made on physical examination of the newborn or infant. Because other abnormalities may accompany hypospadias and epispadias, chromosomal studies may be recommended.

COMPLICATIONS

- Ejaculatory dysfunction in the adult male may occur. If chordee is severe, penetration of the female may be impossible.
- If the dorsal urethral opening is extensive in epispadias, bladder exstrophy (exposure through the skin) is possible.

TREATMENT

- Surgical correction may be necessary, preferably before the child is 1 or 2 years old. Circumcision should be avoided in the newborn so that the foreskin may later be used for repair.

Renal Agenesis

Failure of the kidneys to develop is called renal agenesis. Renal agenesis may be unilateral or bilateral. Bilateral agenesis is incompatible with life.

Unilateral agenesis results in hypertrophy of the remaining kidney as it adapts to compensate functionally for the absent kidney. If the remaining kidney is malformed, successful compensation may not be possible.

CLINICAL MANIFESTATIONS

- Bilateral renal agenesis, called Potter's syndrome, is associated with facial anomalies and pulmonary disease. Infants born with Potter's syndrome die, *in utero* or soon after birth.
- With unilateral renal agenesis, no symptoms are apparent if the

remaining kidney is healthy. The remaining kidney may compensate and grow almost twice as big as otherwise expected. If the remaining kidney functions poorly, however, various disease manifestations may be present.

DIAGNOSTIC TOOLS

- Prenatal ultrasound can often detect renal agenesis. After birth, computerized axial tomography (CAT) scan or renal ultrasound are used to diagnose the condition.

TREATMENT

- No treatment is required if the remaining kidney is healthy.
- If structural or functional defects are present in the remaining kidney, surgery may be required.

Vesicoureteral and Urethrovesical Reflux

Vesicoureteral reflux is the retrograde (backward) flow of urine from the bladder into the ureters and the kidney. Urethrovesical reflux is the backward flow of urine from the urethra into the bladder. Vesicoureteral reflux usually occurs as a result of congenital misplacement of the ureters or urethra, which increase the likelihood of retrograde flow. Secondary causes include neurogenic bladder and repeated infections that cause structural scarring and impediment to the normal flow of urine. Urethrovesical reflux can occur during coughing or other activities that increase intra-abdominal pressure, especially in women because of the short length of the urethra.

CLINICAL MANIFESTATIONS

- Repeated urinary tract infections. These are especially suggestive of reflux in children younger than 5 years old.
- Irritability and poor feeding in infants.

DIAGNOSTIC TOOLS

- Intravenous urography and cystourethrography can help diagnose reflux. A dye is infused via a catheter, and its progression into the ureters, bladder, and urethra can be followed with a radiograph. Any retrograde movement can be identified. Grading of reflux is used to determine treatment.

COMPLICATIONS

- Renal obstruction and failure from repeated urinary tract infections may occur.

TREATMENT

- Spontaneous remission is common.
- Surgery may be necessary to correct the defect if it is severe anatomically or functionally.
- Prophylactic antibiotic therapy starting at birth (if the condition is known) may prevent repeated kidney infections.

Renal Calculi

Renal calculi refer to stones that occur anywhere in the urinary tract. Calculi are most commonly made up of calcium crystals. Less common causes include struvite or magnesium, ammonium, uric acid stones, or combinations of these different substances.

Renal calculi can be caused by increased urine pH (e.g., calcium carbonate stones) or decreased urine pH (e.g., uric acid stones). High concentration of stone-forming substances in the blood and urine and certain dietary habits or drugs can also result in stone formation. Anything that obstructs urine flow, leading to urine stasis (no movement) anywhere in the urinary tract, increases the likelihood of stone formation.

Calcium stones, usually formed with oxalate or phosphate, frequently accompany conditions that cause bone resorption, including immobilization and renal disease. Uric acid stones frequently accompany gout, a disease of increased uric acid production or decreased excretion.

CLINICAL MANIFESTATIONS

- Pain is often colicky (rhythmic), especially if the stone is in the ureter or below it. The pain may be intense. Pain location depends on the site of the stone.
- A stone in the kidney itself may be asymptomatic unless it causes obstruction or an infection develops.
- Hematuria, caused by irritation and injury of the renal structures, is common with calculi.
- Decreased urine output if obstruction to flow occurs.
- Dilute urine if obstruction to flow occurs, because ability to concentrate urine is interrupted by swelling around the peritubular capillaries.

DIAGNOSTIC TOOLS

- Blood and urine tests to look for stone-forming substances.
- Radiograph, ultrasound, or intravenous urography may locate a stone.

COMPLICATIONS

- Urinary obstruction can occur upstream from a stone anywhere in the urinary tract. Obstruction above the bladder can lead to hydroureter as the ureters swell with urine. Unrelieved hydroureter, or obstruction at or above the site where the ureter exits from the kidney, can lead to hydronephritis, which is the swelling of the renal pelvis and collecting-duct system. Hydronephritis can lead to an inability of the kidneys to concentrate the urine, leading to electrolyte and fluid imbalance.

- Obstruction causes increased interstitial hydrostatic pressure and can lead to a decrease in GFR. Unrelieved obstruction can cause collapse of the nephrons and the capillaries, leading to ischemia of the nephrons as the blood supply is interrupted. Renal failure can eventually develop if both kidneys are involved.
- Anytime there is obstruction to the flow of urine (stasis), the chance of a bacterial infection increases.
- Renal cancer may develop from repeated inflammation and injury.

TREATMENT

- Increased fluid intake increases urine flow and helps wash out the stone. High fluid intake in individuals prone to calculi may prevent their formation.
- If the stone content is identified, dietary modification may reduce the levels of the stone- forming substance.
- Appropriate alteration of urine pH may encourage stone breakdown.
- Extracorporeal (outside the body) lithotripsy (shock-wave therapy) or laser therapy may be used to break apart the stone.
- Surgery may be necessary to remove a large stone or to place a diversion tube around the stone to relieve obstruction.

Neurogenic Bladder

A neurogenic bladder is one that has experienced disruption of its neural connections. Neurologic disruption can be of the sensory or motor neurons; motor neurons affected may be located at the upper or lower level.

Interruption of sensory neurons leaves an individual unable to sense the need to void. Interruption of efferent nerves at the cortical or upper motor neuron level, causes voluntary control of micturition to be lost. Because higher centers also facilitate micturition, voiding will be incomplete. If the interruption is of the lower motor neurons at the sacral area or below, the spinal reflex controlling micturition will be blocked and the bladder will not empty spontaneously.

Causes of neurogenic bladder include multiple sclerosis, which affects the cortical level; spinal cord transection; trauma; or tumors anywhere in the spinal cord. Poliomyelitis especially injures lower motor neurons, whereas diabetes mellitus is a common cause of sensory neuron damage.

CLINICAL MANIFESTATIONS

- Sensory neuron interruption leads to dribbling and overflow incontinence because bladder fullness cannot be felt.
- Upper motor neuron and cortical interruption with an intact reflex arc lead to incontinence, small urine volume, and incomplete emptying. Infections may develop owing to urinary retention.
- Lower motor neuron interruption, below the level of the reflex arc, leads to overflow incontinence.

DIAGNOSTIC TOOLS

- History and physical examination will assist diagnosis.
- Neuromuscular studies may help locate lesion.

COMPLICATIONS

- Repeated urinary tract infections may occur.
- Chronic renal failure may develop from repeated infections and scarring.

TREATMENT

- Sensory neuron interruption is treated with bladder training. The bladder is emptied at predetermined (2–4 hours) intervals either naturally or with a catheter.
- Upper motor neuron and cortical interruption are treated by catheter drainage, or manual initiation of the reflex arc by stroking the abdominal or the perineal area.
- Lower motor neuron interruption is treated by catheter drainage or manual compression of the bladder.

Urinary Tract Infection

A urinary tract infection is an infection anywhere in the urinary tract, including the kidney itself, caused by proliferation of a microorganism. Most urinary tract infections are bacterial in origin, but fungi and viruses also may be implicated. The most common bacterial infection is by *Escherichia coli*, an organism commonly found in the anal area.

Urinary tract infections are especially common in girls and women. One cause is the shorter urethra in the female, which allows the contaminating bacteria to gain access more easily to the bladder. Other factors that contribute to the frequency of urinary tract infections in girls and women include the cultural tendency for girls to delay urination and the irritation to the skin of the urethral opening in women that occurs during sexual intercourse. The short urethra increases the likelihood that microorganisms deposited in the urethral opening during intercourse gain access to the bladder. Pregnant women have a progesterone-dependent relaxation of all smooth muscle, including the bladder and the ureters, so they tend to retain urine in these parts of the tract. The pregnant uterus might also obstruct urine flow in some situations.

A protective factor against urinary tract infections in women is the estrogen-dependent production of a mucus coating of the bladder, which has antimicrobial functions. With menopause, estrogen levels fall and this protection is lost. Protection against urinary tract infections in both sexes is offered by the usually acidic nature of urine, which acts as an antibacterial agent.

Although urinary tract infections are less common in males, they can occur. A frequent cause in older men is benign prostatic hyperplasia (BPH) or prostatitis. The prostate is a walnut-sized gland that sits immediately below the opening of the bladder. Hyperplasia of the prostate may cause obstruction to flow, which predisposes one to an infection. Normally, prostatic secretions have an antimicrobial, protective effect.

Individuals who have diabetes are also at risk of frequent urinary tract infections because of the high glucose content of the urine, poor immune function, and increased frequency of neurogenic bladder. Persons who have a spinal-cord injury or anyone using a urinary catheter to void are at increased risk of infection.

Pediatric Consideration

Even one urinary tract infection in a child younger than 5 years of age, of either sex, may indicate the presence of vesicoureteral reflux and should be evaluated with renal ultrasound, cystourethrography, or intravenous urography so that subsequent renal damage is prevented.

Geriatric Consideration

Age is a primary risk factor for urinary tract infections in both men and women and urinary tract infections are the most common cause of infection in nursing home residents. The elderly are especially susceptible because of prostatic hypertrophy; neurogenic bladder associated with long-term diabetes mellitus; poor muscle functioning, leading to incomplete voiding; and delayed voiding because of reduced mobility getting to a bathroom. Symptoms of infections in the elderly may be subtle; any elderly person who has abdominal symptoms such as nausea or vomiting should be worked up for urinary infection. Fever may or may not be present. Asymptomatic infections in the elderly are also very common; there does not appear to be a benefit in treating elderly patients who have asymptomatic infection.

TYPES OF URINARY TRACT INFECTIONS

Urinary tract infections may be divided into cystitis and pyelonephritis. Cystitis is an infection of the bladder, the most common site for an infection. Pyelonephritis is an infection of the kidney itself. Pyelonephritis can either be acute or chronic.

Acute pyelonephritis usually occurs as a result of an ascending bladder infection. Acute pyelonephritis may also occur as a result of a bloodborne infection. Infections may be in both or in one kidney.

Chronic pyelonephritis may result from repeated infections and is usually found in individuals who have frequent calculi, other obstructions, or vesicoureteral reflux. With all kidney infections, inflammatory and immune responses cause interstitial edema and possible development of scar tissue. The tubules are most often affected and may atrophy. With chronic pyelonephritis, extensive scarring and obstruction of the tubules results. Ability of the kidneys to concentrate urine decreases as the tubules are lost. The glomeruli are usually unaffected. Chronic renal failure may develop.

CLINICAL MANIFESTATIONS

Cystitis typically presents with

- dysuria (pain on urination).
- increased frequency of urination.
- a sense of urgency to urinate.
- white blood cells in the urine.
- lower back or suprapubic pain.
- fever accompanied by blood in the urine in severe cases.

Acute pyelonephritis typically presents with

- fever.
- chills.
- flank pain.
- dysuria.

Chronic pyelonephritis may have manifestations similar to acute pyelonephritis. However, it can also include hypertension and may eventually lead to signs of renal failure.

DIAGNOSTIC TOOLS

- Urine culture and sensitivity of the microorganism allow for identification and treatment.

COMPLICATIONS

- Renal or perirenal abscess formation may occur.
- Renal failure may develop after repeated infections if both kidneys are involved.

TREATMENT

- Antibiotic therapy, with a repeat urinalysis after or during drug therapy is required.
- If chronic pyelonephritis is caused by an obstruction or reflux, surgical treatment specific to relieve these problems is necessary.

Women and girls in particular should be

- encouraged to drink fluids frequently (cranberry juice has been shown to reduce the incidence of cystitis) and go to the bathroom as needed to wash out microorganisms that may ascend the urethra
- taught to wipe from front to back after urination to avoid contamination of the urethral opening with fecal bacteria
- encouraged to urinate after sexual intercourse to wash out ascending microorganisms.
- Bubble baths are discouraged in young girls because of the irritation of the urethral opening that may occur, leading to access of bacteria to the urethra. Likewise, girls should be discouraged from playing in the bathtub after shampooing.

Acute Glomerulonephritis

A sudden inflammation of the glomerulus is called acute glomerulonephritis. Acute inflammation of the glomerulus occurs as a result of deposition of antibody-antigen complexes in the glomerular capillaries. Complexes usually develop 7 to 10 days after a pharyngeal or skin streptococcal infection (poststreptococcal glomerulonephritis) but may follow any infection.

An inflammatory reaction is initiated in the glomerulus after deposition of antibody-antigen complexes. Inflammatory reactions in the glomeruli (or anywhere else in the body, see Chapter 3) cause complement activation and mast-cell degranulation, leading to increased blood flow, increased glomerular capillary permeability, and increased glomerular filtration. Plasma proteins and red blood cells leak through the damaged glomeruli. The eventual breakdown of the glomerular membrane causes swelling and edema of Bowman's interstitial space. This increases interstitial fluid pressure, which can collapse any functioning glomeruli in the area. Eventually, increased interstitial fluid pressure opposes further glomerular filtration.

Activation of the inflammatory reaction also draws white blood cells and platelets into the area of the glomerulus. Activation of coagulation factors occurs with inflammation, which can lead to fibrin deposits, scarring, and the loss of functional glomeruli. Glomerular membranes thicken and GFR decreases further.

Acute glomerulonephritis usually resolves with specific antibiotic therapy, especially in children. Some adults may not recover and may develop rapidly progressive glomerulonephritis or chronic glomerulonephritis.

Rapidly Progressive Glomerulonephritis

Rapidly progressive glomerulonephritis is an inflammation of the glomeruli that occurs so rapidly that there is a 50% decrease in GFR within 3 months of disease onset. Rapidly progressive glomerulonephritis can occur from a worsening of acute glomerulonephritis, from an autoimmune disease, or may be idiopathic (unknown) in origin.

Rapidly progressing glomerulonephritis is associated with diffuse proliferation of glomerular cells within Bowman's space. This gives rise to the appearance of a crescent-shaped structure obliterating Bowman's space. GFR decreases, leading to renal failure.

Goodpasture's syndrome type of rapidly progressing glomerulonephritis caused by antibodies produced against the glomerular cells themselves. Pulmonary capillaries are also attacked. Extensive scarring of the glomeruli result. Renal failure frequently occurs within weeks or months. The cause of Goodpasture's syndrome is unknown.

Chronic Glomerulonephritis

Chronic glomerulonephritis is the long-term inflammation of the glomerular cells. It may occur as a result of unresolving acute glomerulonephritis, or it might develop spontaneously. Chronic glomerulonephritis commonly occurs after years of subclinical glomerular injury and inflammation, associated with only slight hematuria (blood in the urine) and proteinuria (protein in the urine).

Common causes include diabetes mellitus and long-standing hypertension. Both of these diseases are associated with significant and repeated glomerular injury. The outcome is diffuse scarring and glomerular deterioration. Tubular atrophy frequently accompanies glomerular breakdown. Individuals with chronic glomerulonephritis who have diabetes or who are even mildly hypertensive have poor prognoses for long-term renal function. Chronic glomerulonephritis may also accompany long-standing lupus erythrematosus.

CLINICAL MANIFESTATIONS

All types of glomerulonephritis are associated with

- Decreased urine volume.
- Blood in the urine (brownish-colored urine), either gross or subtle.
- Fluid retention.

DIAGNOSTIC TOOLS

- Hematuria as measured by urinalysis.
- Red blood cell casts in the urine.
- Proteinuria greater than 3 to 5 g/day.
- Decreased GFR as measured by creatinine clearance.
- If the condition is caused by acute poststreptococcal glomerulonephritis, antistreptococcal enzymes, such as antistreptolysin-O and antistreptokinase, will be present.

COMPLICATIONS

- Renal failure may develop.

TREATMENT

- If the condition is caused by acute poststreptococcal glomerulonephritis, antibiotic therapy is required.
- Autoimmune destruction of the glomeruli may be treated with corticosteroids for immunosuppression.
- Anticoagulants to decrease fibrin deposits and scarring can be used in rapidly progressive glomerulonephritis.
- Strict glucose control in diabetics has been shown to slow or reverse the progression of glomerulonephritis. Research suggests that the angiotensin-converting enzyme inhibitors can reduce glomerular damage in diabetics even if frank hypertension is not evident.
- Angiotensin-converting enzyme inhibitors can reduce glomerular damage in individuals with chronic hypertension.

Myoglobinuria

Rhabdomyolysis or myoglobinuria is the presence of high levels of myoglobin in the urine. Myoglobin is an intracellular protein found in muscle. With muscle-cell damage, especially a crush injury or major body trauma, myoglobin levels in the blood can rise precipitously. A severe electrical burn may cause significant muscle damage and myoglobinuria as well. Normally, myoglobin is filtered in the urine and then is totally reabsorbed into the peritubular capillaries by active transport. However, with large amounts of myoglobin present in the blood, its threshold for reabsorption is exceeded and it spills in the urine. Large amounts of myoglobin in the urine filtrate clog the tubules, leading to obstruction, inflammation, and tubular and glomerular injury. Renal failure can result.

Individuals have reported myoglobinuria after intense episodes of athletics or long-distance running. It appears that besides muscle breakdown, the pounding or jarring effect on the kidney may contribute to the filtration of proteins in these circumstances. Sepsis and hyperthermia may also lead to myoglobinuria.

CLINICAL MANIFESTATIONS

- Hematuria.

DIAGNOSTIC TOOLS

- Red blood cells, protein, and protein casts are present in the urine.
- Elevated levels of plasma creatine phosphokinase, a product of muscle metabolism can be measured.

COMPLICATIONS

- Electrolyte imbalance, as a result of potassium and phosphate release from injured muscle cells, may occur.
- Renal failure may develop.

TREATMENT

- Treatment of a crush injury or trauma.
- Administration of sodium bicarbonate to facilitate renal elimination of myoglobin.
- Flushing the kidney with an osmotic diuretic (mannitol).
- Correction of electrolyte and volume imbalances.
- Short-term dialysis, allowing time for the kidneys to recover, may be necessary.

Hemolytic Uremic Syndrome

Hemolytic uremic syndrome is a condition of injury to the endothelial cells of the glomeruli as a result of a viral, rickettsial, or bacterial infection or, increasingly, from infection with the bacteria *E. coli* 0157 from inadequately cooked meat, especially hamburger. Damage to the glomerular endothelial cells results in swelling and edema and in a narrowing of the capillary to blood flow. This causes injury to passing red blood cells, which are then broken down in the spleen, resulting in hemolytic anemia. Damage to the glomerular cells stimulates inflammatory reactions, including complement activation, fibrin deposition, accumulation of white blood cells, and the release of a variety of vasoactive peptides. Platelets accumulate, leading to clotting and to a decrease in their circulating levels. Blood flow to the kidney may decrease, and scarring may occur.

CLINICAL MANIFESTATIONS

- Vomiting and abdominal pain.
- Bloody diarrhea.
- Bruising from thrombocytopenia (decreased platelets).
- Oliguria (decreased urine output).

DIAGNOSTIC TOOLS

- Urine culture may identify causative organism.
- Obstruction and inflammation may be visible using ultrasound or radiographs.

COMPLICATIONS

- Renal failure may occur. It may be either temporary or permanent.

TREATMENT

- Dialysis is required if renal failure develops.
- Blood transfusions may be used.
- Correction of fluid and electrolyte balance is required.

Pediatric Consideration

Especially susceptible to renal damage after infection with *E. coli* 0157 are children. Many children infected with this bacterium require dialysis or even die.

Renal Failure

The loss of function in both kidneys is known as renal failure. Because the kidneys have such a vital role in maintaining homeostasis, renal failure is associated with multiple systemic effects. All attempts at preventing renal failure are essential. If renal failure does occur, it must be treated aggressively.

Renal failure that occurs suddenly is called **acute renal failure**. Acute renal failure is usually reversible. Renal failure associated with progressive, irreversible loss of renal function is called **chronic renal failure**. Chronic renal failure usually develops after years of renal disease or damage, but it may occur suddenly in some situations. Chronic renal failure inevitably leads to renal dialysis, transplantation, or death.

ACUTE RENAL FAILURE

Causes of acute renal failure have been separated into three general categories: prerenal, intrarenal, and postrenal. Identifying the cause of acute renal failure is accomplished by a study of the patient's history and the quantity and quality of his or her urine.

Prerenal failure is the most common cause of acute renal failure. Prerenal failure occurs as a result of conditions unrelated to the kidney but that damage the kidney by affecting renal blood flow. Prerenal causes of acute kidney failure include anything that severely reduces systemic blood pressure, leading to shock, such as a myocardial infarct, an anaphylactic reaction, severe blood loss or volume depletion, or sepsis (a bloodborne infection). Surgical procedures resulting in a prolonged decrease in renal blood flow can also cause prerenal failure. Renal autoregulation is unsuccessful with a mean systemic blood pressure below 80 mm Hg.

Interruption of renal blood flow, and therefore oxygen delivery, can irreversibly damage the kidneys within 30 minutes. The tubules are most susceptible to the effects of hypoxia, and ischemic tubular necrosis (tubular cell death caused by decreased oxygenation) frequently develops.

Intrarenal failure is a type of acute renal failure that occurs as a result of primary damage to kidney tissue itself, and it can be caused by glomerulonephritis, acute pyelonephritis, and myoglobinuria.

With intrarenal failure, kidney cell damage usually occurs as a result of ischemic tubular necrosis. This tends to blur the distinction between prerenal failure and intrarenal failure because a main cause of ischemic tubular necrosis is decreased renal blood flow.

Tubular necrosis can also result from direct action of nephrotoxic (damaging to the nephron) drugs, such as various heavy metals and organic solvents. Aminoglycoside antibiotics, such as gentamicin, are also nephrotoxic. Radiopaque contrast media used for viewing the cardiac chambers or the gastrointestinal (GI) tract can be nephrotoxic in susceptible individuals. Ingestion of toxic amounts of analgesic mixtures, especially codeine and caffeine, may lead to acute tubular necrosis. Sporadic reports of elderly individuals, who use nonsteroidal anti-inflammatory drugs, having acute renal failure after an intense athletic event (e.g., a marathon run in heat) are concerning.

Postrenal failure is a type of acute renal failure that occurs as a result of conditions that affect the flow of urine out of the kidneys and includes injury to or disease of the ureters, bladder, or urethra. The usual cause of postrenal failure is obstruction. Obstruction can occur in response to many factors, including an untreated calculus, a tumor, repeated infections, prostatic hypertrophy, or a neurogenic bladder.

Most cases of renal failure are associated with low urine output. Occasionally, high output failure may occur. In this case, urine production continues. This is usually associated with a better outcome.

Recovery from acute renal failure typically occurs after a few weeks, but occasionally takes as long as 6 weeks after the onset of oliguria. Recovery begins with diuresis (increased urine output). Although urine is being produced, alterations in electrolyte balance continue. After the diuretic phase comes the recovery phase of acute renal failure, when renal function and electrolyte balance return. Full recovery usually occurs within 1 to 2 years. Some individuals may never recover total renal functioning.

CLINICAL MANIFESTATIONS

- Oliguria (decreased urine output), especially if the failure is caused by ischemia or by obstruction. Oliguria results from decreased GFR.
- Toxic tubular necrosis may be nonoliguric (high output) and is associated with the production of an adequate volume of dilute urine.

DIAGNOSTIC TOOLS

- A good history identifies precipitating causes of renal failure.
- Laboratory finding of azotemia (increased nitrogenous compounds in the blood), and elevated BUN and creatinine.
- Laboratory finding of hyperkalemia (increased potassium in the blood) and acidosis.

COMPLICATIONS

- Fluid retention from nonfunctioning kidneys may lead to edema, congestive heart failure, or water intoxication.
- Alterations in electrolytes and pH may cause uremic encephalopathy.
- If the hyperkalemia is severe (6.5 mEq/L), dysrhythmias and muscle weakness may occur.

TREATMENT

- Prevention of acute renal failure treatment is essential. Individuals experiencing shock should quickly treated with fluid replacement to support blood pressure. Individuals at risk of developing acute renal failure, for instance, those about to undergo heart surgery, may be given an osmotic diuretic before surgery to increase renal function. Adequate hydration before nephrotoxic drugs are administered may prevent acute renal failure from developing. For patients at high risk of suffering renal failure, the use of nephrotoxic drugs and intravenous radioactive dyes must be shown to be essential before they are employed, and their use may be contraindicated in some cases.

If renal failure does occur, recent data suggest that prevention of the oliguric phase results in a better prognosis. This involves:

- aggressive plasma volume expansion.
- diuretics to increase urine production.
- vasodilators, especially dopamine, may be given to increase renal blood flow.
- Dietary restrictions on potassium and protein are often implemented in acute renal failure. High-carbohydrate intake prevents the metabolism of proteins and reduces nitrogenous waste production.
- Antibiotic therapy to prevent or treat infections may be necessary because of the high rate of sepsis seen with acute renal failure.
- Continuous peritoneal dialysis is often employed during the oliguric stage of acute renal failure to give the kidneys time to recover. Dialysis also prevents the buildup of nitrogenous wastes, stabilizes electrolytes, and reduces fluid overload.

CHRONIC RENAL FAILURE

Chronic renal failure is the progressive, relentless destruction of renal structure. Chronic renal failure can result from virtually any of the diseases described in this chapter. Analgesic nephropathy, the destruction of the renal papillae related to the daily use for many years of analgesic medications, may also lead to chronic renal failure in susceptible individuals. Regardless of the cause, unremitting deterioration of the kidneys occurs.

Early in its course, fluid balance, salt handling, and waste accumulation are variable and depend on the part of the kidney in failure. Until renal function has decreased to less than 25% of normal, clinical manifestations of chronic renal failure may be minimal as surviving nephrons take over the functions of those lost. Surviving nephrons increase their rates of filtration, reabsorption, and secretion, and undergo hypertrophy in the process. As more nephrons progressively die, remaining ones have an increasingly difficult job, which leads to their own damage and eventual death. Part of this cycle of death appears related to the demands on remaining nephrons for increased protein reabsorption. With progressive loss of nephrons, scar tissue accumulates and renal blood flow may be reduced. Renin release may increase which, coupled with fluid overload, can lead to hypertension. Hypertension accelerates renal failure, perhaps by increasing the filtration (and therefore the demands for reabsorption) of plasma proteins.

STAGES OF CHRONIC RENAL FAILURE

Chronic renal failure is always associated with a progressive decrease in GFR. Stages of chronic renal failure are based on remaining GFR level and include:

- **Diminished renal reserve**, considered to occur when GFR is 50% of normal.
- **Renal insufficiency**, considered to occur when GFR decreases to 20 to 35% of normal. Remaining nephrons are highly susceptible to failing themselves as their load becomes overwhelming.
- **Renal failure**, considered to occur when GFR is less than 20% of normal. More nephrons continue to die.
- **End-stage renal disease**, considered to occur when GFR is less than 5% of normal. Few functioning nephrons remain. Scar tissue and tubular atrophy are present throughout the kidneys.

CLINICAL MANIFESTATIONS

- With diminished renal reserve, no symptoms may be apparent.
- With renal insufficiency, polyuria (increased urine output) may develop as the kidney is unable to concentrate the urine.

- With development of renal failure, urine output decreases as a result of low GFR.

DIAGNOSTIC TOOLS

- Radiographs or ultrasound demonstrates small, atrophied kidneys.
- Serum BUN, creatinine, and GFR are abnormal.
- Plasma pH is low. An elevated respiratory rate indicates respiratory compensation for metabolic acidosis.

COMPLICATIONS

- With development of renal failure, volume overload, electrolyte imbalance, metabolic acidosis, azotemia, and uremia occur.
- With development of end-stage renal disease, severe azotemia and uremia are present. Metabolic acidosis worsens, which significantly stimulates respiratory rate.
- Hypertension, anemia, osteodystrophy, hyperkalemia, uremic encephalopathy, and pruritis (itching) occur.
- Congestive heart failure and pericarditis can occur. Coma and death result without treatment.

TREATMENT

- Prevention of renal failure is the most important goal. Prevention includes lifestyle changes and drugs when necessary to control hypertension, good glycemic control in diabetics, and the avoidance of nephrotoxic drugs whenever possible. Long-term use of codeine-containing analgesics, and possibly nonsteroidal anti-inflammatory drugs should be avoided, especially in persons who have renal compromise. Early diagnosis and treatment of systemic lupus erythematous and other diseases known to damage the kidneys is essential.

Treatment for diminished renal reserve and renal insufficiency, renal failure, and end-stage renal disease include the following:

- For diminished renal reserve and renal insufficiency, the goals are to slow further nephron loss, primarily by the use of protein restriction and antihypertensive medications. Angiotensin-converting enzyme inhibitors are especially helpful in slowing progression.
- For renal failure, treatment is geared toward correcting fluid and electrolyte imbalances.
- For end-stage renal disease, treatment includes dialysis or renal transplantation.
- At all stages, prevention of infection is important.

Kidney Cancer

WILMS' TUMOR

Wilms' tumor is a cancer of any part of the kidney that typically develops in children younger than 4 years of age. Because of its early onset, it has been suggested that Wilms' tumor develops after one or more mutations in important tumor suppressor genes.

Wilms' tumor is a solid tumor that can grow to a large size. It may be encapsulated (contained within the capsule of the kidney). Staging and prognosis of the disease depends on encapsulation and spread; encapsulation is associated with a favorable prognosis, whereas spread of the tumor outside of the abdominal area to the lungs is associated with a poorer outcome. Overall, prognosis is good, with approximately 90% survival.

CLINICAL MANIFESTATIONS

- A large abdominal mass may be noted by parents or a health-care provider.
- Vomiting, abdominal pain, and hematuria may be present.

DIAGNOSTIC TOOLS

- Physical examination may identify the mass.
- CT scan or ultrasound may confirm the diagnosis.

TREATMENT

- Chemotherapy and surgery are used aggressively to destroy the tumor.

ADULT KIDNEY CANCER

Most adult kidney cancer is a result of renal cell carcinoma. This cancer is especially common in the sixth or seventh decade of life and is more common in males than in females. Risk factors for kidney cancer include repeated kidney stone irritation, smoking, and obesity. Occupational chemical exposures may also increase the risk.

Renal cell carcinoma is often symptomless in its early stages. When symptoms do occur they often include hematuria and the presence of a flank mass. At diagnosis, tumors are staged. Treatment and outcomes depend on staging, with outcomes ranging from 85% survival for stage I tumors to less than 10% survival for stage IV tumors.

CLINICAL MANIFESTATIONS

- Hematuria is the most common manifestation. It may be frankly visible, or may be microscopic and sporadic.
- A flank mass may be palpable. Flank pain may be present as well.

- Polycythemia may be present, reflecting alteration in the renal control of hematopoiesis.
- Fever may accompany the cancer.

DIAGNOSTIC TOOLS

- The use of CT scanning has improved the diagnosis of suspected renal cancer. Ultrasound, renal angiography, and MRI may confirm the diagnosis.

COMPLICATIONS

- Metastasis to the lungs or elsewhere may precede diagnosis.

TREATMENT

- Surgery to remove the affected kidney is usually performed. In patients who have only one functioning kidney, surgical techniques to preserve renal function in the affected kidney may be attempted.
- Chemotherapy and immunotherapy may be used as well.

Selected Bibliography

Ahmed, S. M. & Swedlund, S. K. (1998). Evaluation and treatment of urinary tract infections in children. *American Family Physician* 57, 1553–1560.

Barnett, B. J. & Stephens, D. S. (1997). Urinary tract infection: an overview. *The American Journal of the Medical Sciences* 314, 245–249.

Cecka, M. (1998). Clinical outcome of renal transplantation. *Surgical Clinics of North America* 78, 133–148.

De Broe, M. E.& Elseviers, M. M. (1998). Analgesic nephropathy. *New England Journal of Medicine* 338, 446–452.

Downie, L. L. & Lucarotti, C. L. (1996). My child has hypospadias. *Plastic Surgical Nursing* 16, 23–61.

First, M. R. (1998). Clinical application of immunosuppressive agents in renal transplantation. *Surgical Clinics of North America* 78, 61–77.

Guyton, A. C. & Hall, J. (1997). *Textbook of medical physiology (9th ed.)*. Philadelphia: W.B. Saunders.

Henrich, W. L., ed. (1994). *Principles and practice of dialysis.* Baltimore: Williams & Wilkins.

Herzog, C. A., Ma, J. Z., & Collins, A. J. (1998). Poor long-term survival after acute myocardial infarction among patients on long-term dialysis. *New England Journal of Medicine* 339, 799–805.

Hricik, D. E., Chung-Park, M., & Sedor, J. S. (1998). Glomerulonephritis. *New England Journal of Medicine* 339, 888–899.

Ifudu, O. (1998). Care of patients undergoing hemodialysis. *New England Journal of Medicine* 339, 1054–1062.

Kaplan, B. S., Trompter, R. S., & Muake, J. L., eds. (1992). *Hemolytic uremic syndrome and thrombocytopenic purpura.* New York: Marcel Dekker Inc.

Nissenson, A. R. (1998). Acute renal failure: definition and pathogenesis. *Kidney International* 53 (Suppl. 66), S7–S10.

Orth, S. R. & Ritz, E. (1998). The nephrotic syndrome. *New England Journal of Medicine* 338, 1202–1209.

Porth, C. M. (1998). *Pathophysiology concepts of altered health states (5th ed.)*. Philadelphia: J.B. Lippincott Company.

Vander, A. J. (1991). *Renal physiology (4th ed.)*. New York: McGraw-Hill.

Vander, A. J., Sherman, J., & Luciano, D. (1998). *Human physiology: the mechanism of body function (7th ed.)* Boston: McGraw-Hill. pps. 502–549.

Whelan, C. A. (1998). Chronic renal failure—non-dialysis care for the primary care provider. *The American Journal for Nurse Practitioners* 2, 21–31.

Zaontz, M. R. & Packer, M. G. (1997). Abnormalities of the external genitalia. *Pediatric Urology* 44, 1267–1297.

15 FLUID AND ELECTROLYTE AND ACID-BASE BALANCE

The maintenance of water, electrolyte, and acid-base balance is a daily job of all living organisms. In humans, water and electrolyte intake and output are regulated through hormonal and neural interactions that overlie behavioral and dietary practices. As for acid-base balance, most metabolic processes occurring in the body result in the production of acid. It is essential that these acids be removed from the body. The removal of carbon dioxide is performed by the lungs. The removal of other, nonvolatile (nongaseous) acids is performed by the kidneys. The lungs and the kidneys, together with various buffer systems in the body, maintain plasma acid concentration within narrow, physiologic limits.

● ● ●

PHYSIOLOGIC CONCEPTS

Water Balance

Water makes up approximately 60% of total body weight. Of this amount, two-thirds (66%) is intracellular and one-third (33%) is extracellular (i.e., in the plasma or interstitial space [Table 15-1]). Water is essential to life because of the role it plays in oxidative phosphorylation, the maintenance of osmotic pressure, and the transport of substances in the body and across cell membranes. Maintaining the balance of water in the body is equally essential; if an individual becomes over hydrated, dilution of plasma electrolytes and solutes, cell swelling, and possibly death can result. Likewise, if one becomes severely dehydrated, plasma solute and electrolyte overconcentration and cell shrinkage can lead to nervous system derangement and death. Water balance depends on water intake and water output. Stimuli to take in fluid may be physiologic or social. Outputs vary related to ambient temperature, exercise and clothing. Ultimately, it is the thirst drive

Table 15-1. Body Water Percentages

<table>
<tr><td colspan="3">Total body water
(60% of body weight)</td></tr>
<tr><td colspan="2">Extracellular fluid
(1/3 total body water)</td><td rowspan="2">Intracellular fluid
(2/3 total body water)</td></tr>
<tr><td>Plasma
(20%)</td><td>Interstitial fluid
(80%)</td></tr>
</table>

centered in the hypothalamus and the output of urine by the kidneys that maintain the harmony between intake and output.

NORMAL WATER INTAKE AND OUTPUT

Adults ingest between 1.5 and 2.5 L of fluid a day. Another 300 to 400 mL are produced in metabolic reactions daily. Daily outputs exactly balance these inputs in healthy individuals; 1.0 to 2.0 L excreted in urine, 100 mL excreted in the feces, 50 mL excreted in sweat, and approximately 1000 mL excreted through exhalation of air and surface evaporation. As highlighted in Figure 15-1, fluid ingestion and urine excretion are the only variables under the precise control of neural and hormonal stimuli.

CONTROL OF FLUID INGESTION

Although the amount of fluid we drink each day is influenced by dietary and social influences, the ultimate control over whether we ingest an adequate amount of fluid is exerted by the thirst center located in the hypothalamus at the level of the third ventricle. The sensation of thirst is sensed by hypothalamic osmoreceptors that increase their rate of firing with increased plasma osmolarity (i.e., decreased water concentration). When activated, these osmoreceptors,

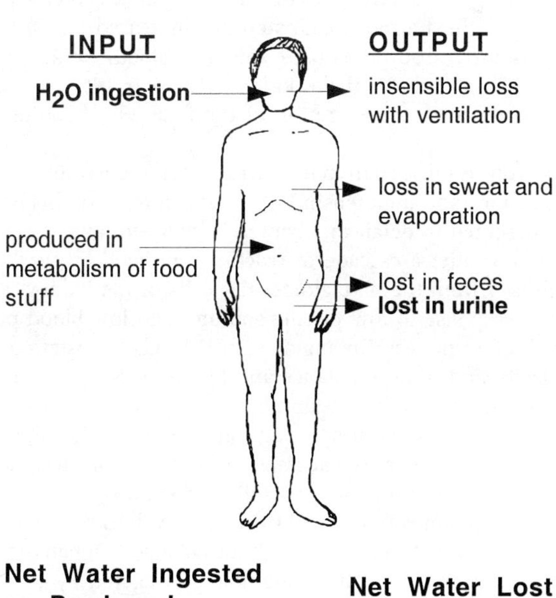

Figure 15-1. Fluid ingestion and excretion.

along with neighboring cells that sense blood pressure, signal the hypothalamus to increase the release of antidiuretic hormone (ADH) from the posterior pituitary gland (Chapters 10 and 14). ADH has two major effects. The first and most important being to increase the permeability of the renal collecting ducts of the kidney to water (Chapter 14). This allows water to be reabsorbed out of the urine back into the blood, thereby diluting the plasma back toward normal (and so reducing the stimulus for ADH release). The second effect of ADH is to act as a pressor agent; its other name is "vasopressin." In this role, ADH causes a constriction of vascular smooth muscle and an increase in blood pressure. This also reduces the stimulus for its continued release.

A second hormone, angiotensin II, also has a direct effect on the cells of the hypothalamus to increase the sensation of thirst. It, too, is an important dipsogenic (thirst-stimulating) hormone.

Electrolyte Balance

SODIUM

As the major extracellular ion in the body, sodium is responsible in large part for determining plasma osmolality and is also important in maintaining membrane potential and neural conductance. The regulation of plasma sodium is mainly achieved by the kidney, which freely filters and then reabsorbs at least 98% of filtered sodium. The remaining 2% is reabsorbed or excreted into the urine, depending on the presence or absence of the hormone **aldosterone**; increased aldosterone increases sodium reabsorption back into the blood, by acting at the level of the distal tubule of the kidney (Chapter 14). Low levels of aldosterone result in the excretion of the final 2% of sodium in the urine.

Aldosterone is released from the adrenal cortex as a result of stimulation by the hormone angiotensin II. A brief summary of this hormonal system, presented in detail in Chapter 14, is as follows: **Angiotensin II** is produced after a cascade of reactions initiated by the hormone **renin** released from the juxtaglomerular cells of the kidney. Renin is released in response to low plasma sodium, and low blood pressure. As a result of an increase in angiotensin II levels, aldosterone release is stimulated, and sodium balance and blood pressure return toward normal; this is an excellent example of a negative feedback cycle.

Sodium output also occurs through small amounts lost in the sweat and in the feces. In times of excessive sweating or diarrhea, depletion of sodium from these routes can be life-threatening.

Sodium ingestion is influenced by taste as well as by a homeostatic drive (salt appetite) to maintain sodium balance. Humans and other animals have a drive to ingest salt that is triggered by low plasma sodium. Humans and other animals also show a distinct preference for salt ingestion, a circumstance that for a minority of humans can lead to salt-sensitive hypertension.

POTASSIUM

Potassium, the major intracellular ion in the body, plays a vital role in determining cell membrane potential. Even though extracellular potassium is low, potassium concentration in the extracellular fluid is closely regulated because changes in extracellular concentration can result in life-threatening disturbances in neural and cardiovascular function. Potassium can shift between the intracellular and extracellular compartments, depending on various neural and hormonal influences, and the pH of the extracellular fluid. For example, beta-adrenergic nervous stimulation and insulin secretion both increase the movement of potassium intracellularly by stimulation of the Na^{++}/K^{+} pump. Increasing the pH of the plasma also increases the movement of potassium intracellularly.

The source of potassium in the body is that ingested in the diet. Excretion of potassium is primarily through the urine, with a small amount lost in the sweat and the feces. The major controlling factor over total body stores of potassium is the hormone aldosterone.

As described in Chapter 14, the maintenance of potassium balance is achieved by the kidney. Potassium is freely filtered across the glomerulus, and then at least 80% is reabsorbed. If there has been excess potassium ingested in the diet, the kidney can also secrete potassium into the urine to return to balance. If potassium is deficient in the diet, none is secreted into the urine and all is reabsorbed. Increased secretion (and so excretion) occurs in response to stimulation of the distal tubules of the kidney by the hormone aldosterone. Aldosterone is released from the adrenal cortex in response to angiotensin II, as described above. Aldosterone release is also, to a lesser extent, stimulated directly by low plasma potassium and by an increase in the pituitary hormone adrenocorticotropin (ACTH).

CALCIUM

Calcium is primarily an intracellular ion, with nearly 99% of its total body stores in bone and most of the remaining 1% intracellular in other tissues. A very small amount of extracellular calcium either circulates bound to albumin; is complexed to nonorganic substances such as citrate, phosphate, or sulfate; or exists in an ionized form. Calcium in the ionized form is important for muscle contraction and a variety of enzymatic reactions. It is also required for most steps of the coagulation pathway. Calcium is ingested in the diet, filtered, reabsorbed, and excreted by the kidney. It is not secreted.

The control of serum calcium primarily results from changes in the secretion of parathyroid hormone from the parathyroid gland: Decreased serum calcium stimulates increased parathyroid hormone secretion. Increased parathyroid hormone then acts in one of three ways to return serum calcium back toward normal. It 1) increases renal reabsorption of calcium; 2) stimulates bone breakdown to release bone calcium; or 3) stimulates the activation of vitamin D, thereby increasing calcium reabsorption across the gut. A second hormone, calcitonin, secreted from specialized cells of the thyroid gland, also exerts control over serum calcium levels. Calcitonin is released in response to increased serum calcium, and it acts to reduce serum calcium by causing a decrease in bone breakdown. It also decreases calcium reabsorption by the kidney, further lowering serum levels. Serum calcium is inversely related to serum phosphate.

PHOSPHATE

An important intracellular ion, phosphate is vital for most metabolic reactions and is an essential component of ATP, DNA, and RNA. Phosphate serves as a hydrogen-ion buffer in plasma and urine. Approximately 85% of phosphate is stored in bone, with 14% in all other cells; less than 1% is extracellular. Phosphate is ingested in the diet and, in proportion to its ingestion, is filtered and excreted in the urine. In the serum, it varies inversely with calcium. With renal failure, phosphate levels rise precipitously and result in low serum calcium levels.

MAGNESIUM

Primarily an intracellular ion, magnesium is stored in bone (50%), in body cells (approximately 49%), and in blood (1%). Magnesium is required for a variety of enzymatic reactions and is an important ion for DNA synthesis and RNA transcription, for translation, and for protein synthesis. Magnesium can bind to calcium receptors, either turning on the calcium response (mimicking) or blocking the effects of calcium. Magnesium is ingested in the diet and is filtered and excreted in the urine.

Acid-Base Balance

pH

The pH is a reflection of the ratio of acid to base in extracellular fluid. The pH in serum can be measured with a pH meter, or one can calculate it by measuring serum bicarbonate and the carbon dioxide concentrations and placing these values into the Henderson–Hasselbalch equation as shown in Equation 15-1:

$$\text{pH} = (pK + \log \text{HCO}_3^-)/\text{CO}_2 \qquad (15\text{-}1)$$

In this equation, HCO_3^- is the concentration of bicarbonate in the serum, and CO_2 is the concentration of dissolved carbon dioxide in the serum. The *pK* refers to the negative logarithm of the dissociation constant, *K*. The dissociation constant is a fixed value for the bicarbonate–carbon dioxide system at normal body temperature. It reflects the degree to which bicarbonate and carbon dioxide dissociate to accept or donate a hydrogen ion. For the bicarbonate–carbon dioxide system, *pK* is 6.1.

The pH reflects the hydrogen-ion concentration of the solution. The greater the hydrogen-ion concentration, the greater the acidity of the solution and the lower the pH. In contrast, the higher the pH, the lower the hydrogen-ion concentration, and the more basic the solution.

Acids

An acid is any substance capable of liberating a hydrogen ion. Examples of acids include the substances in bold in the following formulas, all of which are shown giving up a hydrogen ion:

$\mathbf{HCl} \rightleftarrows H^+ + Cl^-$
$\mathbf{H_2CO_3} \rightleftarrows H^+ + HCO_3^-$
Lactic acid $\rightleftarrows H^+ +$ lactate
$\mathbf{NH_4^+} \rightleftarrows H^+ + NH_3$

An acid can be strong or weak, depending on the degree to which it breaks down to liberate hydrogen ions. For example, hydrogen chloride (HCl) rapidly and totally breaks down into hydrogen and chloride ion; therefore, it is considered a strong acid. In contrast, few lactic acid molecules break down to hydrogen ion and lactate; therefore, lactic acid is considered a weak acid. The double arrow in each equation indicates that the reactions are reversible.

Bases

In each reaction above showing the dissociation (breakdown) of an acid, the substance produced along with the hydrogen ion is considered a base. A base is any substance that can accept a hydrogen ion, thereby taking it out of solution. Because each of these reactions is reversible, each substance produced with the hydrogen ion can rejoin with it and can move the reaction in the opposite direction. Thus, these substances can be considered bases. These reactions are rewritten in the following formulas with the base in bold:

$\mathbf{Cl^-} + H^+ \rightleftarrows HCl$
$\mathbf{HCO_3^-} + H^+ \rightleftarrows H_2CO_3$
lactate $+ H^+ \rightleftarrows$ lactic acid
$\mathbf{NH_3} + H^+ \rightleftarrows NH_4^+$

A base can be strong or weak, depending on the degree to which it accepts a hydrogen ion. Most acids and bases found in the body are weak.

Buffers

Weak acids and weak bases make good buffers. A buffer is a substance that can either take free hydrogen ions from a solution or release hydrogen ions to a solution, thereby preventing large fluctuations in pH. There are three important buffer systems in the body.

BICARBONATE–CARBONIC ACID BUFFER SYSTEM

The main buffer system in the body is the bicarbonate–carbonic acid buffer system. This system acts in the blood to buffer plasma pH. When free hydrogen ions are added to blood containing bicarbonate, the bicarbonate ions bind with the hydrogen ions, becoming carbonic acid (H_2CO_3). This ensures that there will be few free hydrogen ions remaining in solution, thereby preventing a significant decrease in blood pH. Carbonic acid is considered a weak acid; bicarbonate ion is considered its weak, conjugate (complimentary) base. As shown in Equation 15.2, carbonic acid can also dissociate to form carbon dioxide and water; therefore, the bicarbonate buffer system is primarily used to eliminate hydrogen ion from the body through the elimination of the volatile gas carbon dioxide. The breakdown of carbonic acid to carbon dioxide and water requires the enzyme **carbonic anhydrase**, which is present in red blood cells. The reaction of carbonic acid to carbon dioxide and water is reversible, and carbon dioxide and water can rejoin to form carbonic acid. This process also requires the action of carbonic anhydrase. This reversible reaction is shown in Equation 15-2.

$$CO_2 + H_2O \rightleftarrows H_2CO_3 \rightleftarrows H^+ + HCO_3^- \qquad (15\text{-}2)$$

PHOSPHATE BUFFER SYSTEM

The second buffer system used by the body is the phosphate buffer system. Phosphoric acid ($H_2PO_4^-$) is a weak acid. It dissociates in plasma to phosphate (HPO_4^{2-}) and hydrogen ion (H^+). Phosphate is a weak base. This buffer system is used by the kidney to buffer the urine as it excretes hydrogen ion. A sulfuric acid–sulfate buffer system is used to a lesser degree.

HEMOGLOBIN BUFFER SYSTEM

The third main buffer system in the body is provided by proteins in the blood, especially hemoglobin present in red blood cells. Hemoglobin binds to free hydrogen ions as the red blood cells circulate past metabolically active cells. As a result of the binding of free hydrogen ions by hemoglobin, increases in free hydrogen-ion concentration in the blood are minimized, and venous blood pH decreases only slightly compared with arterial blood. As the blood flows through the lungs, hydrogen ions dissociate from the hemoglobin and join with bicarbonate to become carbonic acid (Equation 15-2), which breaks down to carbon dioxide and water. Carbon dioxide is exhaled, resulting in the elimination of the metabolically produced hydrogen ions.

Respiratory Control of Acid-Base Balance

The lungs rid the body of carbon dioxide. Although carbon dioxide itself is not an acid, it becomes one when it joins with water to form carbonic acid (Equation 15.2). The minute-by-minute regulation of plasma pH is controlled by an increase or decrease in the rate of respiration, thereby increasing or decreasing the exhalation of carbon dioxide. This system is possible because of the sensitivity of the respiratory center in the brain to free hydrogen ions (Chapter 13), which usually vary in accordance with carbon dioxide.

Carbon Dioxide Production and Carriage in the Blood

Carbon dioxide is produced in all cells as a result of oxidative metabolism. From the cells, it diffuses into the bloodstream. Carbon dioxide is carried three different ways in the blood: dissolved, bound in the red cell, and as bicarbonate. Approximately 7% is carried dissolved in the blood. The amount of carbon dioxide dissolved in the blood depends on the product of its partial pressure in the blood and its solubility constant (how well it dissolves). The solubility constant of carbon dioxide in blood is 0.57. Although the partial pressure of carbon dioxide in the atmosphere at sea level is almost zero and thus is nearly zero in inspired air, venous blood carries carbon dioxide away from metabolizing cells and has a carbon dioxide partial pressure of 45 mm Hg. Partial pressure of carbon dioxide in arterial blood is nearly 40 mm Hg. Therefore, the amount of carbon dioxide dissolved in the blood differs between the arterial and venous circulations.

Twenty-three percent of carbon dioxide diffuses into the red blood cell and is carried bound to hemoglobin, as shown in Equation 15-3.

$$\text{Hemoglobin} + CO_2 = \text{Carboxyhemoglobin} \qquad (15\text{-}3)$$

Seventy percent of carbon dioxide is carried in the blood after reacting with water as shown in Equation 15.2. This reaction primarily occurs in red blood cells where carbonic anhydrase is plentiful. As a result of this reaction, a very large amount of carbon dioxide first forms carbonic acid, and then bicarbonate. The reaction is driven to bicarbonate because as each hydrogen ion is produced, it is rapidly buffered in the cell by hemoglobin. Therefore, free hydrogen concentration remains low, and the reaction continues to move to the right, until nearly all of the carbon dioxide has reacted to bicarbonate. Hemoglobin buffering of hydrogen ion ensures that there is no significant fall in pH. Carbonic anhydrase is present in the gut and kidney as well as in the red cells.

Elimination of Carbon Dioxide by the Lungs

As dissolved carbon dioxide diffuses into the lungs and is exhaled, the reactions shown in Equation 15.2 reverse and flow to the left.

When dissolved carbon dioxide diffuses out of the blood and into the lungs to be exhaled, carbon dioxide bound to hemoglobin becomes dissociated, dissolves in the blood, and is exhaled. Likewise, as carbon dioxide is blown off, bicarbonate ions react with hydrogen ions to form carbonic acid, which dissolves to carbon dioxide and water, and again, the carbon dioxide is exhaled.

Mass Action of Carbon Dioxide and Hydrogen

Mass action is the process in which a decrease in the product on one side of a reversible reaction causes all reactions to flow in that direction. Mass action also occurs in the opposite circumstance. For instance, if there is an increase in the amount of a substance on one side of a reversible reaction, the reaction is driven to flow away from that substance.

Mass Action: Equation 15-2

$$CO_2 + H_2O \rightleftarrows H_2CO_3 \rightleftarrows H^+ + HCO_3^-$$

When carbon dioxide is produced by the cells and diffuses into the blood to join with water, mass action serves to drive all reactions to the right. As long as carbon dioxide is still diffusing into the blood and hydrogen ion produced from its breakdown continues to bind to hemoglobin, preventing free hydrogen ions from accumulating, mass action pushes the reaction to the right. When free hydrogen ions begin to accumulate, mass action begins to drive the reaction in the opposite direction. Equilibrium for this reaction is reached when there is no longer a concentration gradient for carbon dioxide between cells and plasma or when all hemoglobin binding sites for hydrogen are filled and free hydrogen ions begin to accumulate.

Renal Control of Acid-Base Balance

URINE BUFFERS

Nonvolatile acids produced during metabolism are excreted in the urine as described in Chapter 14. Their excretion occurs as a result of active *secretion* of hydrogen ions by cells of the kidney into the urine filtrate. In the filtrate, hydrogen ions join with phosphate, sulfate, or ammonia (NH_3) buffers and are then excreted in the urine as salts of phosphoric acid, sulfuric acid, or ammonium ion (NH_4^+).

BICARBONATE HANDLING BY THE KIDNEYS

The kidney actively reabsorbs bicarbonate ion, which is easily filtered across the kidney capillaries back into the bloodstream so it is not lost in the urine. Extensive loss of bicarbonate—which is both a base and a primary buffer for the body—would cause severe acidosis (decrease in plasma pH). Under conditions of base excess, the kidney has the opposite capability; it actively secretes bicarbonate ion into the urine, thereby reducing pH as necessary.

Electrolyte Interactions and Exchanges

Cells of the body carefully balance the number of cations (positively charged ions) and anions (negatively charged ions) they contain. Therefore, if one cation increases intracellularly, another cation leaves the cell to keep the charge balance constant. Cations most often juggled include potassium, hydrogen, and, to a lesser extent, calcium ion. Anions juggled include chloride and bicarbonate.

CATION BALANCE

If plasma potassium concentration increases as a result of increased dietary intake or extensive cell death or trauma, more potassium diffuses into all cells of the body, including the kidney tubule cells. In response, hydrogen ion leaches out of the cells into the plasma. This leads to increased plasma hydrogen-ion concentration and a decrease in plasma pH. The high plasma potassium in the kidney cells causes those cells to increase potassium secretion into the urine filtrate. In response, less hydrogen ion is secreted into the urine by the kidney cells, further increasing hydrogen-ion levels in the plasma. Therefore, high plasma potassium can actually lead to a decrease in plasma pH, which can result in a metabolic acidosis.

The opposite situation occurs if plasma hydrogen-ion concentration increases for any reason. In this case, increased hydrogen ion diffuses into all cells, causing potassium to leach out into the plasma. Increased hydrogen-ion concentration in the kidney cells leads to an increased secretion of hydrogen into the urine, whereas potassium secretion and excretion in the urine decreases. Thus, chronic acidosis can cause hyperkalemia (increased potassium in the blood).

Increased plasma hydrogen also causes hydrogen ion to move into bone cells. Because of the presence of phosphate and other minerals, bone serves as an important buffer for free hydrogen ions. With accumulation of hydrogen ions in bone, bone cells leach calcium out into the plasma. Loss of bone calcium can weaken bones, increasing the risk of osteoporosis and fractures.

ANION BALANCE

The anions most frequently juggled between intracellular and extracellular compartments are chloride and bicarbonate ions. When chloride levels in the plasma fall, bicarbonate concentration in the plasma rises, causing alkalosis. This happens daily as chloride is extracted from blood passing through the stomach after a meal and is used by cells of the stomach to produce hydrochloric acid (HCl). HCl is secreted into the stomach to begin the digestive process. Plasma leaving the stomach is alkalotic (basic). However, chloride ions move back into the plasma as blood passes through the small intestine, lowering the bicarbonate levels and returning the plasma pH to normal before the blood leaves the gut.

Tests of Blood Electrolytes and Gases

Plasma osmolality is 275 to 295 mOsm/kg. Normal plasma electrolyte values in an adult are as follows:

Plasma sodium:	Normal: 135–148 mEq/L (also written, 135–148 mmol/L)
Plasma potassium:	3.5–5.0 mEq/L (3.5 to 5.0 mmol/L)
Serum calcium:	8.5–10.5 mg/dL
Serum phosphate:	2.5–4.5 mg/dL
Serum magnesium:	1.8–2.7 mg/dL

Normal blood gas values in an adult are as follows:

Partial pressure of carbon dioxide in arterial blood:	between 35 and 45 mmHg
Partial pressure of carbon dioxide in venous blood:	45 mmHg
Bicarbonate concentration in venous blood:	between 22 and 28 mEq/L (22–28 mmol/L)
The pH of arterial blood:	between 7.35 and 7.45
Partial pressure oxygen in arterial blood:	100 mm Hg
Partial pressure oxygen in venous blood:	40 mm Hg

PATHOPHYSIOLOGIC CONCEPTS

Fluid Volume Deficit

A fluid volume deficit is a reduction in extracellular fluid volume. A fluid volume deficit may occur after acute hemorrhage, diarrhea, prolonged vomiting, excessive sweating, or it may occur because of a shift of fluid from the extracellular to intracellular compartment. A fluid volume deficit may result from the loss of both salt and water, making it an isotonic deficit, or it may result from water deficiency only. A water-only deficiency would be characterized by hypernatremia (excessive sodium) in the blood. One measures fluid volume deficit by determining acute weight loss. Weight loss is calibrated, with 2% signifying mild deficit, between 2 to 5% signifying moderate deficit, and greater than 8% signifiying severe deficit.

Pediatric Consideration

Infants and children are at high risk of serious fluid volume deficit with prolonged diarrhea or vomiting. Worldwide, a main cause of infant mortality is infectious diarrhea leading to circulatory collapse. The use of replacement fluids for children at risk can significantly improve morbidity and mortality. Vaccination against a major cause of infant and early childhood diarrhea, rotovirus, is now available.

Fluid Volume Excess

A fluid volume excess is typically isotonic; that is, it is characterized by increased salt and water accumulation. The most common cause of fluid volume excess is renal dysfunction. Heart failure, liver disease or failure, and corticosteroid excess may also lead to volume excess. Fluid excess is characterized by an acute weight gain of over 5% of body weight. Lung congestion with respiratory rales, cough, and dyspnea may occur, as may dependent edema. Diuretic therapy may be required.

Hyponatremia

Plasma sodium concentration of less than 135 mEq/L, with plasma osmolality less than 280 mOsm/kg is called hyponatremia. Sodium loss can occur after vomiting, diarrhea, or excessive sweating. Hyponatremia may also occur if fluid loss is replaced with pure water instead of an electrolyte-containing fluid. Kidney disease characterized by excess reabsorption of water, as seen with Syndrome of Inappropriate ADH (SIADH; Chapter 10), may also lead to hyponatremia as may excessive use of sodium-losing diuretics.

Hyponatremia is characterized by alterations in central nervous system functioning, including confusion, depression, headache, stupor, and coma. Gastrointestinal complaints of cramping, diarrhea, and vomiting occur. Peripheral edema may result. Treatment is based on the cause and may include limiting water intake, discontinuing or changing a diuretic, and prescribing medications that block the function of ADH. Administration of a saline solution may be required.

Hypernatremia

Plasma sodium concentration greater than 148 mEq/L, with plasma osmolality greater than 295 mOsm/kg, is called hypernatremia. Hypernatremia usually occurs from a disproportionate loss of water compared with sodium (e.g., during watery diarrhea or sweating). Renal inability to reabsorb water (diabetes insipidus; Chapter 10) would also lead to hypernatremia as would neardrowning in salt water.

Clinical manifestations of hypernatremia include increased thirst and concentrated urine of low volume. Alterations in central nervous system functioning include decreased reflexes, seizures, and coma in extreme cases. Cardiovascular effects may include a decrease in blood pressure accompanied by an increase in heart rate. Treatment is oral rehydration. Serum osmolality must be carefully monitored so as not to disrupt central nervous system functioning.

Hypokalemia

Plasma potassium concentration less than 3.5 mEq/L is called hypokalemia. Hypokalemia may result from decreased dietary intake, increased loss either from the kidneys, gut, or through sweating, or from a shift of potassium from the extracellular to the intracellular compartment.

The clinical manifestations of hypokalemia depend on the degree of the disorder and the previous health status of the individual. Mild hypokalemia (serum potassium 3.0–3.5mEq/L) may not produce any symptoms in otherwise healthy persons. With more severe hypokalemia, symptoms of weakness, fatigue, nausea and vomiting, and constipation can occur. Muscle necrosis can occur with potassium less than 2.5 mEq/L, and with severe hypokalemia (potassium levels less than 2.0 mEq/L), paralysis can develop, leading to respiratory failure. Central nervous system dysfunction characterized by confusion or stupor may result. Hypokalemia also can lead to cardiac dysrhythmia, especially in patients who have preexisting cardiac disease or in those who take a wide range of drugs, including digoxin. Because hypokalemia stimulates aldosterone release, the kidneys are unable to concentrate the urine; this results in polyuria. Treatment is aimed at increasing dietary intake or at the use of supplements or infusion.

Hyperkalemia

Plasma potassium concentration greater than 5.0 mEq/L is called hyperkalemia. Hyperkalemia usually occurs with renal failure when the kidneys are unable to secrete potassium. It may also happen with major trauma or burns during which damaged cells release their intracellular potassium stores. Instances of hyperkalemia have been reported after accidental intravenous administration of highly concentrated potassium solutions or intravenous administration of potassium in patients who have low urine output.

Clinical manifestations of hyperkalemia include changes in muscle function, including cramping and weakness. Cardiac dysfunction may result in changes in the electrocardiogram (ECG), leading to cardiac arrest and death. Treatment depends on the cause and the extent. For excess ingestion, dietary changes are advised. Individuals who have kidney failure may require dialysis. Rapid movement of potassium out of the extracellular fluid may be accomplished by the administration of insulin, which increases intracellular transport of potassium.

Hypocalcemia

Hypocalcemia is a serum calcium concentration less than 8.5 mg/dL. Hypocalcemia may result from an inability to access bone calcium stores as a result of the dysfunction, suppression, or removal of the parathyroid gland. Hypocalcemia may also result from vitamin D deficiency leading to decreased absorption of dietary calcium. Increased protein binding of serum calcium as a result of decreased H^+ may lead to hypocalcemia as may elevation of phosphate levels resulting from renal failure.

The consequences of hypocalcemia include changes in neuromuscular function, including muscle spasms and cramping, and numbness and tingling of the extremities. The cardiovascular system may be affected, resulting in hypotension and decreased cardiac output. Bone pain, deformities, and fractures may result. Osteomalacia and childhood rickets can develop. Treatment of acute hypocalcemia involves intravenous infusion of a calcium compound. For long-term conditions, increased calcium and vitamin D in the diet are recommended.

Hypercalcemia

A serum calcium concentration greater than 10.5 mg/dL is known as hypercalemia. Hypercalcemia usually results from excess release of bone calcium. This typically happens with hyperparathyroidism or bone neoplasm. Other cancers may affect bone remodeling and result in hypercalcemia as well. Hypercalcemia may also occur after prolonged immobilization. Excess intake of vitamin D unaccompanied by increased dietary intake of calcium may lead to hypercalcemia. Lithium, used to treat manic-depressive disorder, increases serum calcium levels.

The clinical consequences of hypercalcemia include alterations in kidney function with an increased risk of kidney stones and polyuria related to an inability of the kidney to concentrate the urine. A variety of neuromuscular manifestations develop, including muscle weakness, loss of tone, and muscle atrophy. The cardiovascular system is affected leading to increased blood pressure and alterations in the ECG. Central nervous system dysfunction, including lethargy, stupor, and coma may occur. Treatment is aimed at reducing the further release of calcium from bone and at rehydration.

Hypophosphatemia

A concentration of serum phosphate less than 2.5 mg/dL is called hypophosphatemia. Hypophosphatemia may occur as a result of malnutrition and is common in those who abuse alcohol; it is at least partially related to poor nutrition in this population. Shifts of phosphate from the extracellular to the intracellular compartment may also lead to hypophosphatemia. Because phosphate transport intracellularly is stimulated by insulin, prolonged glucose administration or hyperalimentation may lead to depletion of extracellular phosphate. Similarly, insulin administration, either at too high a dose or in an attempt to treat an episode of diabetic ketoacidosis, may lead to hypophosphatemia. Decreased intestinal absorption of phosphate may accompany either prolonged diarrhea or the use of aluminum or calcium-containing antacids because these substances bind phosphate and increase its excretion in the stool.

Manifestations of hypophosphatemia include neuromuscular dysfunction characterized by tremors, muscle weakness, seizures, sometimes coma and death. Because phosphate is a vital component of ATP, all energy stores are affected. Red blood cell, white blood cell, and platelet function are diminished as well. Treatment is replacement therapy.

Hyperphosphatemia

A serum phosphate concentration greater than 4.5 mg/dL is called hyperphosphatemia. Most commonly, hyperphosphatemia is a result of diminished renal function, but it may also occur from a redistribution of intracellular phosphate, most commonly after a major trauma. Chemotherapy that destroys cancer cells may lead to hyperphosphatemia as the cancer cells are destroyed. Increased phosphate may occur from phosphate-containing laxatives or enemas.

Serious consequences of hyperphosphatemia include neuromuscular (tetany, weakness) and cardiovascular (dysrhythmia, hypotension) changes resulting from reciprocal hypocalcemia. Treatment is aimed at correcting the cause of the disorder. Dialysis may be required for clearing the blood.

Hypomagnesemia

A magnesium concentration less than 1.8 mg/dL is called hypomagnesemia. Hypomagnesemia may result from reduced intake related to malnutrition or alcohol abuse, or from gut malabsorption of magnesium related to laxatives or diarrhea. Overingestion of calcium may impair magnesium absorption across the gut because calcium and magnesium compete for the same transport site. Renal loss of magnesium may be excessive with the use of certain diuretics or with different magnesium-wasting kidney diseases such as diabetes mellitus, hyperaldosteronism, and hypoparathyroidism.

Clinical consequences of hypomagnesemia include personality changes, neuromuscular tetany or spasms, hypertension, and cardiac dysrhythmia. Treatment is replacement therapy.

Hypermagnesemia

Serum magnesium concentration greater than 2.7 mg/dL is called hypermagnesemia. This condition is relatively uncommon because the kidney can greatly increase magnesium excretion when required. Therefore, if hypermagnesemia does occur, it usually does so in individuals who have renal dysfunction. Overingestion of magnesium as a laxative, especially in those who have poor renal function, may also lead to the condition. Clinically, magnesium sulfate is provided to women who have toxemia of pregnancy, and a serious complication may be hypermagnesemia in this population.

Hypermagnesemia is associated with a variety of severe neurologic affects, including muscle weakness or paralysis, confusion, coma, and death. Because magnesium can compete for calcium binding sites in the smooth muscle and heart, hypermagnesemia may result in symptoms of hypocalcemia, including hypotension and cardiac dysrhythmia, leading to cardiac arrest in severe cases. Treatment is cessation of magnesium administration. The administration of calcium is also used to counter the effects of hypermagnesemia. Dialysis may be needed to clear the blood.

Acidemia

The decrease in arterial pH to less than 7.35 is called acidemia. Acidemia may result from respiratory, renal, or metabolic causes.

Acidosis

A systemic increase in hydrogen-ion concentration is called acidosis. Hydrogen-ion concentration can increase as a result of a failure of the lungs to eliminate carbon dioxide or if there is excess production of volatile or nonvolatile acids. Acidosis can also occur if there is a loss of bicarbonate base caused by persistent diarrhea or by a failure of the kidney either to reabsorb bicarbonate or to secrete hydrogen ions.

Alkalemia

Alkalemia is the increase in arterial blood pH above 7.45. Alkalemia may result from respiratory, renal, or metabolic causes.

Alkalosis

Alkalosis is a systemic decrease in hydrogen-ion concentration. Hydrogen-ion concentration can decrease as a result of excess loss of carbon dioxide during hyperventilation, excess loss of nonvolatile acids during vomiting, or excess ingestion of a base.

Compensation

The lungs and kidneys work together to maintain plasma pH within the range of 7.35 to 7.45. If acidosis or alkalosis results from a respiratory disorder, the kidneys respond by altering their handling of hydrogen ion and bicarbonate base to return the pH back toward normal. Renal actions aimed at reversing acidosis or alkalosis caused by a respiratory disorder are called renal compensation. Renal compensation begins to have an effect approximately 24 hours after a respiratory alteration in pH. Despite this delay, renal compensation is powerful.

If acidosis or alkalosis results from a metabolic or a renal disorder, the respiratory system responds by increasing or decreasing respiratory rate, to return the pH to normal. Respiratory actions aimed at reversing acidosis or alkalosis caused by a metabolic or renal disorder are called respiratory compensation. Respiratory compensation occurs immediately upon increased hydrogen-ion concentration, because hydrogen ion is the determining influence controlling the respiratory center in the brain.

CONDITIONS OF DISEASE

Many of the conditions and diseases that result in fluid and electrolyte disturbance are described elsewhere in this book, including diabetes insipidus and SIADH. Likewise, the effects of diarrhea and vomiting and renal, cardiac, and hepatic failure on fluid, electrolyte, and acid-base balance are presented in detail elsewhere. Therefore, only a few of the causes of fluid and electrolyte disturbance are reviewed in the following sections.

Psychogenic Polydipsia

Excessive water intake caused by a psychiatric abnormality, often schizophrenia, is called psychogenic polydipsia. This disorder occurs for no known reason, but it seems to worsen during times of exacerbation of psychotic symptoms. It may be worsened by medication-induced stimulation of ADH in this population.

CLINICAL MANIFESTATIONS

- Compulsive water ingestion coupled with high urine outflow characterize this disorder.

DIAGNOSTIC TOOLS

- Hyponatremia and hypo-osmolarity are apparent on laboratory analysis.
- Urine osmolarity is very low.

COMPLICATIONS

- Neurologic dysfunction leading to seizure or coma may result.

TREATMENT

- Behavioral intervention to decrease water intake may be effective.
- Drugs to reduce ADH may be prescribed.
- For severe intoxication, hypertonic saline my be infused carefully.
- Treatment of the underlying psychotic disorder may improve the condition.

Primary Hyperaldosteronism

Excessive synthesis and release of aldosterone from the adrenal gland is called primary hyperaldosteronism. Its causes may include an aldosterone-secreting tumor, or the condition may occur for no known cause (idiopathic). Other hormonal abnormalities, such as Cushing's disease due to elevated ACTH or adrenal hypoplasia may also lead to elevated aldosteronism.

Because aldosterone increases reabsorption of sodium but causes the secretion of potassium, electrolyte disturbance may result.

CLINICAL MANIFESTATIONS

- Symptoms of hypernatremia and hypokalemia develop.
- Blood volume expansion occurs.

DIAGNOSTIC TOOLS

- Laboratory analysis reveals the electrolyte abnormalities.
- Serum aldosterone levels measure high. Plasma renin activity is low.

COMPLICATIONS

- Neurologic dysfunction, cardiac irregularity, and hypertension may develop.

TREATMENT

- A salt-restricted diet or a potassium-sparing diuretic alleviates symptoms.
- Treatment of any underlying cause may cure the disorder.

Respiratory Acidosis

Respiratory acidosis is the decrease in arterial pH resulting from a primary respiratory disorder. It is the job of the lungs to eliminate metabolically produced carbon dioxide. If respiration is impaired and carbon dioxide levels increase, Equation 15.2 is driven to the right by mass action, causing an increase in hydrogen-ion concentration. Initially, the increase in hydrogen ion is buffered. However, if exhalation of carbon dioxide is significantly impaired, free hydrogen-ion levels increase, causing pH to decrease.

CAUSES OF RESPIRATORY ACIDOSIS

All obstructive pulmonary disorders (chronic obstructive lung disease, asthma, as well as hypoventilation of any origin, including drug overdose or airway obstruction) cause respiratory acidosis. Severe pulmonary congestion may lead to decreased diffusion of carbon dioxide into the lungs from the blood, reducing its elimination in expired air. Likewise, infant or adult respiratory distress syndrome from any cause is associated with reduced pulmonary blood flow and poor exchange of carbon dioxide and oxygen between the lungs and the blood, resulting in the accumulation of carbon dioxide.

COMPENSATION FOR RESPIRATORY ACIDOSIS

When acidosis is caused by a respiratory problem, renal compensation occurs. Renal compensation results in the kidney increasing its secretion and excretion of acid and increasing its reabsorption of base. Little or no bicarbonate is secreted into the urine. Renal compensation takes at least 24 hours to begin. Therefore, it occurs only in cases of respiratory acidosis lasting that long. If the compensation is successful, plasma pH will remain in the normal range.

CLINICAL MANIFESTATIONS

- Neurologic symptoms such as headache, behavioral changes, and tremors.
- Respiratory depression from increased carbon dioxide may occur.

DIAGNOSTIC TOOLS

- The partial pressure of carbon dioxide is greater than 45 mm Hg (because increased carbon dioxide is the cause of the problem).
- For respiratory acidosis lasting longer than 24 hours, plasma bicarbonate levels are increased (greater than 28 mEq/L), reflecting the fact that the kidney is excreting more hydrogen ion and reabsorbing more base.
- If renal compensation is successful, plasma pH will be low, but in the normal range. If compensation is unsuccessful or if the respiratory acidosis is more acute than 24 hours, plasma pH will reflect high hydrogen-ion concentration ($pH < 7.35$).
- Urine pH is acidic as the kidneys attempt to excrete more hydrogen ion and return pH toward normal.

COMPLICATIONS

- Paralysis and coma may result from cerebral vasodilatation in response to increased carbon dioxide concentration if levels become toxic.

TREATMENT

- Improvement of ventilation is essential. Mechanical ventilation may be required.

Respiratory Alkalosis

The increase in arterial pH resulting from any primary respiratory disorder is called respiratory alkalosis. Respiratory alkalosis results when carbon dioxide levels decrease to less than 38 mm Hg. With decreased carbon dioxide, Equation 15.2 is driven to the left, resulting in a decrease in free hydrogen-ion concentration and an increase in pH.

CAUSES OF RESPIRATORY ALKALOSIS

Hyperventilation is the main cause respiratory alkalosis. Causes of hyperventilation include fever and anxiety. Hypoxemia can stimulate hyperventilation if the partial pressure of oxygen in arterial blood decreases to less than 50 mm Hg (normal is approximately 100 mm Hg). Salicylate toxicity and brain infections can directly stimulate the respiratory center in the brain to increase respiratory rate, which can lead to respiratory alkalosis.

COMPENSATION FOR RESPIRATORY ALKALOSIS

Alkalosis caused by a respiratory problem stimulates renal compensation. Renal compensation involves the kidney returning pH toward normal by decreasing its secretion of hydrogen ion and actively secreting bicarbonate ion into the urine. Again, renal compensation requires 24 hours to become effective.

CLINICAL MANIFESTATIONS

- Central nervous system disturbances include dizziness, muscle contractions, and changes in consciousness.

DIAGNOSTIC TOOLS

- Blood gases reveal decreased partial pressure of carbon dioxide of less than 35 mm Hg (because decreased carbon dioxide is the cause of the alkalosis). The rapid respirations responsible for alkalosis are the major clinical manifestation.
- For respiratory alkalosis lasting longer than 24 hours, bicarbonate levels are decreased (less than 22 mEq/L), reflecting the fact that the kidney is reabsorbing less base or secreting base into the urine.
- If renal compensation is successful, plasma pH will be high, but it will be in the normal range. If compensation is unsuccessful or if the respiratory alkalosis is more acute than 24 hours, plasma pH will reflect the low plasma hydrogen-ion concentration and will be greater than 7.45.
- Urine pH is basic as the kidneys attempt to excrete more bicarbonate base and return pH toward normal.

COMPLICATIONS

- Convulsions and coma if the condition persists or becomes very severe.

TREATMENT

- Determining and treating the cause of hyperventilation is the most successful therapy.
- Increasing partial pressure of carbon dioxide by breathing into a bag and rebreathing the expired air may reverse the alkalosis in an acute situation.

Metabolic Acidosis

The decrease in arterial pH resulting from a nonrespiratory problem is called metabolic acidosis. Metabolic acidosis is characterized by the accumulation of nonvolatile acids.

CAUSES OF METABOLIC ACIDOSIS

Metabolic acidosis may occur if there is a decrease in the renal clearance of any nonvolatile acid, a loss of bicarbonate, or an increase in the production of nonvolatile acid.

Decrease in the Renal Clearance of Hydrogen Ion

During renal failure or if there is any interruption in renal blood flow, a decrease in the renal clearance of hydrogen ions occurs. As a result of these conditions, the kidney, which normally reabsorbs all filtered bicarbonate and actively secretes hydrogen ion into the urine, cannot function properly causing hydrogen ion accumulation. Nitrogenous waste accumulation, such as urea during renal failure or renal hypoxia, acidifies the blood.

Loss of Bicarbonate

With decreased renal function as the kidneys fail to reabsorb bicarbonate, loss of bicarbonate occurs. Bicarbonate levels also decrease with chronic diarrhea because bicarbonate is concentrated in intestinal secretions. High levels of extracellular chloride (hyperchloremia) cause metabolic acidosis because bicarbonate ions shift intracellularly. This is called hyperchloremic acidosis.

Increase in Nonvolatile Acids

Lactic acid produced during prolonged hypoxia, ketones produced as a byproduct of fat metabolism in diabetics, and acids resulting from overdose of drugs such as salicylates (a product of aspirin metabolism) are examples of nonvolatile acids. Excess protein metabolism during starvation or protein malnutrition also results in increased nonvolatile acid production.

COMPENSATION FOR METABOLIC ACIDOSIS

When acidosis is caused by a metabolic problem, respiratory compensation occurs. Respiratory compensation for metabolic acidosis involves the lungs expiring more carbon dioxide through increases in the rate and depth of respirations. Plasma pH returns toward normal. Respirations present during metabolic acidosis caused by diabetic ketoacidosis are called Kussmaul's respirations. Respiratory compensation can occur almost immediately with the onset of acidosis.

CLINICAL MANIFESTATIONS

- Weakness and fatigue occurring from poor muscle function.
- Anorexia, nausea, and vomiting.
- Warm flushed skin resulting from a pH-sensitive decrease in vascular response to sympathetic stimuli.
- If metabolic acidosis is caused by diabetic ketoacidosis, additional manifestations will include:
  - ketone smell (fruity) on breath
  - anorexia
  - nausea and vomiting
  - abdominal pain
  - Kussmaul's breathing
  - decreasing level of consciousness leading to coma
- If metabolic acidosis is caused by chronic renal failure, additional manifestations will include:
  - pruritis (itching).
- If metabolic acidosis is caused by diarrhea, additional manifestations will include:
  - signs of dehydration, including decreased blood pressure and decreased skin turgor
  - abdominal pain and cramping
  - frequent, loose stools

DIAGNOSTIC TOOLS

- Blood gases reveal decreased bicarbonate levels less than 22 mEq/L (because decreased bicarbonate either is the direct cause of the acidosis or reflects an increase in hydrogen-ion concentration).
- Because respiratory compensation occurs immediately, carbon dioxide levels decrease, reflecting that the lungs are increasing the rate of respiration to exhale more acid. The partial pressure of carbon dioxide is less than 35 mm Hg. Respirations are rapid and deep.
- If respiratory compensation is successful, plasma pH is low but in the normal range. If compensation is unsuccessful, plasma pH will reflect high plasma acidity and will be less than 7.35.

- Urine pH will be acidic if renal function is normal, because the kidneys will attempt to excrete more acid to return pH toward normal.
- If metabolic acidosis is caused by diabetic ketoacidosis, additional diagnostic tools will include:
  - increase in blood and urine glucose
  - ketonuria and decreased urine pH
- If metabolic acidosis is caused by chronic renal failure, additional diagnostic tools will include:
  - urine pH only slightly acidic or nonacidic
  - increased blood urea nitrogen (BUN)
  - decreased GFR

COMPLICATIONS

- If metabolic acidosis is caused by chronic renal failure, complications may include renal osteodystrophy and renal encephalopathy.
- If pH falls below 7.0, cardiac dysrhythmia can occur. This happens as a result of changes in cardiac conduction, which occur in direct response to a decrease in pH and because of the effects of increased hydrogen-ion concentration on plasma and intracellular potassium levels.

TREATMENT

- Treatment for metabolic acidosis is specifically based on treating the cause of the disorder. Administration of sodium bicarbonate may be necessary to raise pH rapidly if the person is at risk of dying. This procedure must be undertaken carefully because sodium bicarbonate infusion may cause brain swelling.

Metabolic Alkalosis

The increase in arterial pH resulting from a nonrespiratory problem is called metabolic alkalosis. There are several causes of metabolic alkalosis.

CAUSES OF METABOLIC ALKALOSIS

If there is excessive loss of acid or if base ingestion increases, metabolic alkalosis may occur. Dehydration and alterations in extracellular electrolyte levels, causing shifts in plasma electrolytes, can lead to metabolic alkalosis as well.

Loss of Acid

Because stomach contents are usually acidic, excessive vomiting can result in acid loss. This causes alkalosis directly and indirectly because of the loss of chloride in the vomit.

Increased Bicarbonate Levels

Ingestion of bicarbonate in the form of bicarbonate-containing antacids used to treat indigestion or heartburn can cause increased bicarbonate levels. Bicarbonate solutions may be used during cardiopulmonary resuscitation and can lead to metabolic alkalosis.

Decreased Extracellular Fluid Volume

Volume contraction or decreased extracellular fluid volume can lead to increased plasma bicarbonate levels and to metabolic alkalosis by causing less bicarbonate to be filtered across the glomerulus. A greater percentage of the filtered bicarbonate is reabsorbed back into the peritubular capillaries if the rate of blood flow is also reduced.

Alterations in Extracellular Electrolyte Levels

Alkalosis as a result of hydrogen ions shifting intracellularly is caused by alterations in extracellular electrolyte levels. For example, a decrease in extracellular chloride may cause metabolic alkalosis as chloride diffuses out of the cell and hydrogen ion shifts to the intracellular compartment. This is called hypochloremic alkalosis. Likewise, hypokalemia (decreased plasma potassium) may also cause metabolic alkalosis because of increased hydrogen excretion by the kidneys.

Compensation for Metabolic Alkalosis

When alkalosis is caused by a metabolic problem, respiratory compensation occurs. Respiratory compensation for metabolic alkalosis involves a decrease in the rate and depth of respirations. This serves to return plasma pH toward normal. Respiratory compensation can occur almost immediately upon alkalosis onset.

CLINICAL MANIFESTATIONS

- Neurologic manifestations are slow to develop, but may include confusion, hyperactive reflexes, spasms, and tetany (sustained muscle contraction).

DIAGNOSTIC TOOLS

- Blood gases reveal increased bicarbonate levels greater than 28 mEq/L (because increased bicarbonate either is the direct cause of the alkalosis or reflects a decrease in hydrogen-ion concentration).
- Because of respiratory compensation, carbon dioxide levels are increased, reflecting the fact that the lungs are slowing the rate of respiration to retain more acid, to return pH toward normal. The partial pressure of carbon dioxide is greater than 45 mm Hg. The rate and depth of respirations are reduced, possibly causing hypoxemia.

- If respiratory compensation is successful, plasma pH will be high but in the normal range. If compensation is unsuccessful, plasma pH will reflect the high plasma base concentration and will be greater than 7.45.
- Urine pH will be basic if renal function is normal, because the kidneys will attempt to excrete less acid and more base to return pH toward normal.

COMPLICATIONS

- With pH greater than 7.55, dysrhythmia and coma may result from alterations in neuronal and cardiac muscle cell depolarization.

TREATMENT

- If the cause is due to chloride or potassium deficiency, these ions must be replaced.
- If decreased extracellular volume is the cause, saline solution replacement is required.

Selected Bibliography

Adrogue, H. J. & Madias, N. E. (1998). Management of life-threatening acid-base disorders. *New England Journal of Medicine* 338, 107–111.

Bullock, B. L. (1996). *Pathophysiology: adaptions and alterations in function*. Philadelphia: J.B. Lippincott Company.

Gennari, F. J. (1998). Hypokalemia. *New England Journal of Medicine* 339, 451–458.

Guyton, A. C. & Hall, J. (1997). *Textbook of medical physiology (9th ed.)*. Philadelphia: W.B. Saunders.

Hood, V. L. & Tannen, R. L. (1998). Protection of acid-base balance by pH regulation of acid production. *New England Journal of Medicine* 339, 819–826.

Porth, C. M. (1998). *Pathophysiology concepts of altered health states (5th ed.)*. Philadelphia: J.B. Lippincott Company.

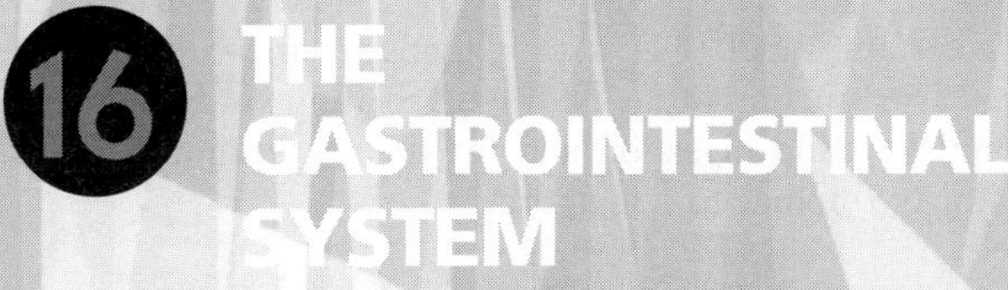

16 THE GASTROINTESTINAL SYSTEM

The gastrointestinal (GI) tract extends from the mouth to the anus. The function of the GI tract is to allow for food ingestion, propulsion, and digestion and for the absorption of nutrients necessary for our bodies to live and grow.

• • •

PHYSIOLOGIC CONCEPTS

Anatomy

As shown in Figure 16-1, the GI tract begins with the oral cavity, and continues into the esophagus and stomach. Food is stored in the stomach until it is released into the small intestine. The small intestine is divided into three sections, the duodenum, the jejunum, and the ileum. Digestion and absorption of food occur primarily in the small intestine. From the small intestine, food is passed to the large intestine, which consists of the colon and rectum. Accessory organs include the liver, pancreas, gallbladder, and appendix.

The entire GI tract is composed of several tissue layers: the innermost **mucosal** (secreting) layer; a **submucosal** connective tissue layer; circular and longitudinal smooth muscle layers, called the **muscularis externa**; and an outermost serous membrane, called the peritoneum (or adventitial) layer (Figure 16-2). These layers are connected to one another physically and through neural connections.

MUCOSA

The mucosal layer of the small intestine is the site of food absorption as described below. It consists of a lining of epithelial cells, a thin connective tissue layer called the lamina propria, and an underlying layer called the muscularis mucosa. It is across the epithelial cells that food particles leave the gut and enter the internal environment of the body.

SUBMUCOSA

The submucosal layer of the gut is a connective tissue matrix. It contains one of the two nerve networks of the gut, called the **submucous plexus**, and a system of blood vessels and lymphatics.

MUSCULARIS EXTERNA

The muscularis externa contains a thick **circular muscle** layer, and a thinner, **longitudinal muscle** layer. Contraction of the circular smooth muscle causes mixing of the food in the gut. Contraction of the longitudinal layer shortens the tube. In between the circular and longitudinal

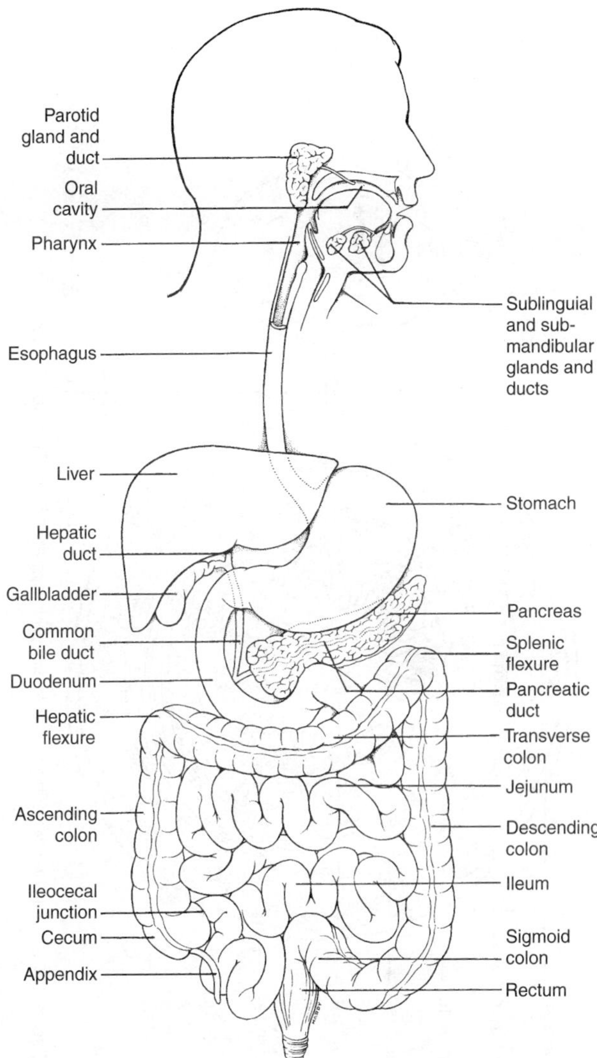

Figure 16-1. Digestive system (from Chaffee and Lytle, 1980).

smooth muscle layers is the second neural network of the gut, called the **myenteric plexus**.

Neural Regulation of the Gut

The two neural networks of the gut, the submucosal plexus and the myenteric plexus, make up the self-contained nervous system of the

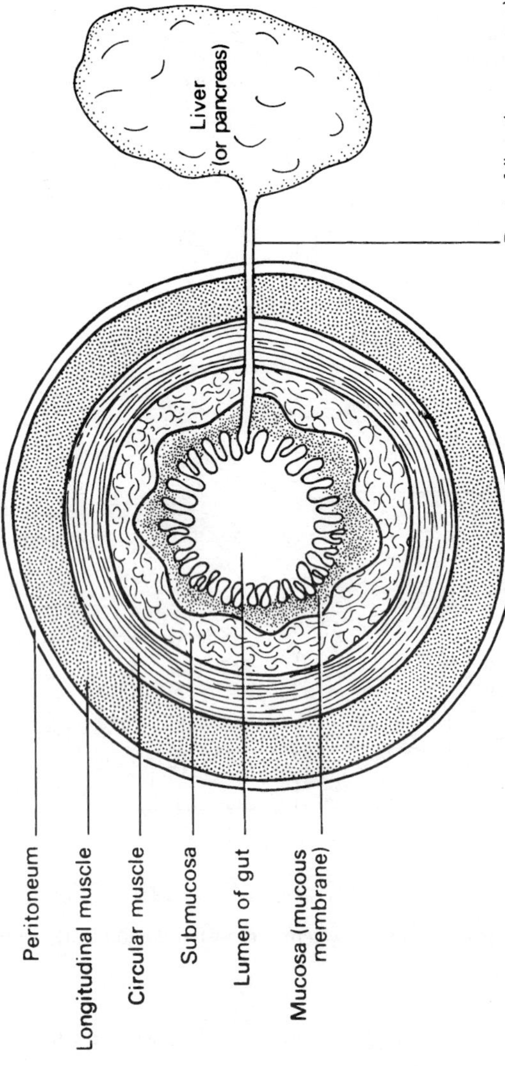

Figure 16-2. Transverse section of the digestive system (from Thompson, 1977).

gut, referred to as the **enteric nervous system**. The nerves of this system fire on their own without external stimuli. Because all the smooth muscle cells of the gut are connected, firing of the nerves in one area spreads the entire length of the gut. The neurons in the two plexuses synapse on each other, as well as on the surrounding smooth muscle cells, the exocrine glands throughout the GI tract, and the epithelial cells. They can affect contraction of the smooth muscle, the production of mucus, and the release of digestive enzymes. The neurons of the enteric nervous system include both adrenergic and cholinergic nerves, as well as nerves that release a variety of other neurotransmitters, including nitric oxide, endorphin, and various intestinal polypeptides. Although the firing of the enteric nervous system can occur without external input, the plexuses also receive external stimuli that can affect their rate of firing.

External Input to the Enteric Nervous System

Both the myenteric and the submucous nerve plexuses are innervated by sympathetic and parasympathetic nerves. Sympathetic fibers originate in the spinal cord between the levels of T8 and L3 and innervate the plexuses throughout the gut. They inhibit firing of the plexus, slowing the basic rhythm. Sympathetic nerves release norepinephrine in the gut. Parasympathetic nerves travel in the vagus nerve to the esophagus, the stomach, and the upper half of the large intestine. Other parasympathetic fibers travel in sacral divisions and innervate the distal half of the large intestine. Parasympathetic nerves release acetylcholine and stimulate firing of both the plexuses. This speeds peristalsis and mixing. Innervation of this distal part of the large intestine is important for stimulating defecation. The small intestine does not appear to be innervated by parasympathetic nerves.

In addition to external neural innervation, the cells of the enteric nervous system are also affected by GI hormones, as well as by a variety of irritants, including those present in some foodstuffs and in certain drugs and those released with infectious disease. These stimuli too can alter the firing rate of the enteric nervous system.

The Musculature of the Gut

As described above, the GI tract is composed of an outer longitudinal layer and an inner circular layer of muscle. A third muscle layer is thin, lying deep in the mucosal lining of the GI tract. The longitudinal and the circular muscle layers are responsible for mixing and moving the food throughout the entire GI tract.

The longitudinal and circular smooth muscles show an inherent rate of spontaneous muscle-cell depolarization at each segment of the GI tract. These inherent depolarizations cause action potentials, resulting in the muscle contractions. The contractions in each segment may vary in strength in response to internal or external nervous input, hormonal stimuli, and stretch. Although they vary in strength, gut contractions vary little in frequency. Gut contractions are slow, calcium-dependent contractions that occur over a wide range of muscle length. The contractions of the muscles at each gut segment determine the **motility** of that segment (i.e., the propulsion of food and secretions from one area to the next).

Gut Motility

ESOPHAGEAL MOTILITY

Movement of food in the esophagus occurs by the process known as **peristalsis**. When food enters the esophagus, the smooth muscle is stretched; this initiates a peristaltic wave that proceeds along the length of the esophagus, propelling the food with it. When the peristaltic wave reaches the end of the esophagus, the smooth muscle at the opening into the stomach relaxes and food moves into the stomach. The end of the esophagus, called the **lower esophageal sphincter**, is located in the abdominal cavity, below the level of the diaphragm. (Note: Although called a sphincter, this area is not anatomically different than the rest of the esophagus and so is not a true sphincter.) When a peristaltic wave is not passing down the esophagus, the esophageal sphincter is relaxed and in the closed position. This prevents reflux of stomach contents into the esophagus. Reflux is also prevented by the fact that the lower esophageal sphincter is in the abdominal rather than in the thoracic cavity; if this were not so, backflow of food from the high-pressure zone of the abdomen to the low-pressure thoracic area would easily occur. By having part of the esophagus in the abdominal cavity, the pressure difference is minimized.

STOMACH MOTILITY

When food enters the stomach, the stomach also responds with a peristaltic wave. As the wave of contraction reaches the lower end of the stomach, called the **antrum**, the wave picks up strength, which effectively mixes the food. This wave of contraction also causes the closure of the junction between the end of the stomach and the beginning of the duodenum—the **pyloric sphincter**. This is a true sphincter and is normally relaxed when food is not entering the stomach.

Gastric peristaltic waves occur as a result of the depolarization of the smooth muscle cells of the stomach. Pacemaker cells in the smooth muscle of the stomach depolarize continually at an inherent rate; this is called the **basic electrical rhythm** of the stomach. Normally, the depolarizations associated with the basic electrical rhythm are too slight to cause the muscle of the stomach to reach threshold and therefore do not lead to contractions. With increased stretch of the stomach or with neural and hormonal stimulation, the smooth muscle does depolarize to threshold and the strength of peristalsis increases.

As the peristaltic waves continue in the stomach, a small amount of material is forced through the pyloric sphincter into the duodenum. The more material in the stomach, the more rapid the initial emptying. Eventually, all of the stomach content empties into the small intestine.

SMALL INTESTINAL MOTILITY

Once the food, now called **chyme**, enters the small intestine, it continues to be mixed as a result of smooth muscle contraction there. In the small intestine, the contractions result in mostly stationary mixing, with slow forward propulsion down the gut. The slow propulsion occurs as a result of **segmentation**. Segmentation refers to the process by which slightly more frequent contractions in the upper gut, compared with the lower, eventually propel the chyme through the length of the small intestine. The thorough mixing during segmentation ensures that the chyme is acted upon by digestive enzymes and that it comes into repeated contact with the intestinal wall so that absorption is facilitated.

LARGE INTESTINE MOTILITY

The large intestine consists of the cecum, followed by the ascending, transverse, and descending colon; the sigmoid colon; and the rectum. The appendix is a blind pouch, growing off of the cecum. The rectum ends at the anus, the exit point from the body. Contraction of the large intestine occurs at a slow rate compared with the small intestine. This means that food entering the large intestine takes approximately a day to travel the entire length of the structure. A few times a day, usually after a meal, a wave of contraction, called a **mass movement** occurs. This is a powerful contraction that initiates the urge to defecate.

Hormones of the Gastrointestinal Tract

The GI hormones gastrin, secretin, cholecystokinin (CCK), and glucose-dependent insulinotropic peptide (GIP) play important roles in the function of the GI tract. These hormones and their roles are discussed in the text that follows.

Gastrin is released from endocrine cells in the stomach in response to parasympathetic stimulation, stretch of the smooth muscle, and the presence of protein in the food. Gastrin stimulates the secretion of histamine and gastric juices from the gut lining and of hydrochloric acid (HCl) from the parietal cells of the stomach. Histamine also stimulates HCl secretion. HCl in turn, activates the most important digestive enzyme in the stomach, pepsin. Pepsin and the gastric juices begin the digestion of protein in the stomach. Gastrin also stimulates intestinal motility. The further release of gastrin is inhibited by excess acid; this provides an excellent example of a negative feedback system.

Secretin is released from cells of the small intestine primarily in response to HCl present in the chyme coming into the small intestine from the stomach. Secretin stimulates intestinal secretions of base, as well as the pancreatic release of bicarbonate to neutralize the acid. This is essential because enzymes needed for digestion in the small intestine cannot work in an acidic environment. Secretin also slows the further passage of food from the stomach into the small intestine. This allows adequate time for digestion in the small intestine.

CCK is released from the small intestine primarily in response to fat and other food particles entering the intestine from the chyme. CCK causes gallbladder contraction; it also causes the release of pancreatic and intestinal digestive enzymes and of bile. The digestive enzymes and bile serve to promote the digestion and absorption of the food particles.

GIP is released from the small intestine in response to sugar in the chyme. GIP increases the release of insulin from the pancreas, which stimulates the transport of glucose across cell membranes. This assists in the absorption of sugar out of the gut.

Digestion of Food

Digestion of food begins in the mouth with the release of saliva, continues in the stomach, and is mostly accomplished in the small intestine. The process of digestion involves enzymes secreted in response to specific foodstuffs that act to break down carbohydrates into simple sugars, fats into free fatty acids and monoglycerides, and proteins into amino acids. It is only in these simple forms that these nutrients can be absorbed across the gut and used by the body.

PROTEIN AND CARBOHYDRATE DIGESTION

Protein digestion begins in the stomach with the enzyme pepsin and is completed in the small intestine by the action of the pancreatic enzymes trypsin and chymotrypsin. Carbohydrate digestion begins in the mouth with the activity of the enzyme salivary amylase, and is completed in the small intestine by the enzyme pancreatic amylase.

FAT DIGESTION

Fat digestion occurs in the small intestine, primarily as a result of the activity of the pancreatic enzyme lipase. Fats are digested by the action of lipase into free fatty acids and monoglycerides. Lipase, however, is a water-soluble enzyme: because fats are insoluble in water, their digestion by lipase would be extremely slow if it were not for the process of **emulsification**, which is the division of large fat complexes into smaller droplets. Emulsification increases the surface area of the fats available for digestion by pancreatic lipase. By increasing the surface area, lipase is a much more effective agent for digestion. Emulsification occurs by the mechanical mixing of the food in the intestine and by the presence in the intestine of bile. The emulsification and digestion of fat is shown in Figure 16-3.

Bile

Bile is a substance produced in the liver and contains bile salts, water, cholesterol, electrolytes, and bilirubin, which is a breakdown product of red blood cell metabolism. Although bile is continually released from the liver, it is stored and concentrated in the gallbladder. Bile is released from the gallbladder and travels to the small intestine via the common bile duct, in response to the hormone CCK. In individuals who do not have a gallbladder, bile is released directly from the liver in response to CCK.

Although bile contains no digestive enzymes, it does contain bile salts, the substance that serves to emulsify fats. Bile salts are phospholipids that act as detergents to break down (emulsify) fats into the small droplets. Once emulsified into droplets, lipase is then capable of digesting the fats into fatty acids and monoglycerides.

Absorption of Food

Although a small amount of lipid-soluble material may be absorbed across the stomach wall, most absorption of digested food occurs in the small intestine, across a multitude of fingerlike projections called

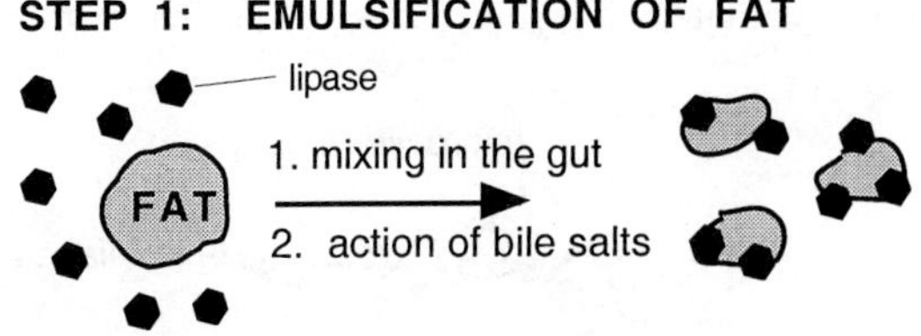

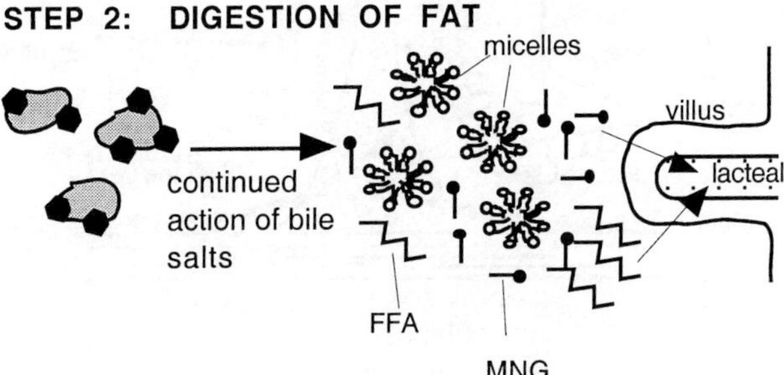

Figure 16-3. Emulsification (step 1) and digestion (step 2) of fat (free fatty acid, [FFA]; monoglyceride, [MNG]).

villi. Villi consist of the epithelial cells of the mucosal layer, a capillary network, and a central lymph vessel called a lacteal (Fig. 16-4). Many microvilli line the tops of the epithelial cells and further add to the enormous surface area provided by the villi for the absorption of food. Nerve fibers of the intrinsic plexuses and smooth muscle cells also are present in each villus. Certain digestive enzymes (brush border enzymes) are produced by cells of the villus as well.

Absorption of food occurs when digested food particles enter the villus from the lumen of the gut, and move either into the capillary or into the lacteal, thereby gaining access to the general circulation. The movement of food particles into the epithelial cells and across the capillary or the lacteal may either be by simple or facilitated diffusion or by active transport, depending on the substance.

ABSORPTION OF AMINO ACIDS

Amino acids, the result of protein digestion, are actively transported into the epithelial cells of the villi. Once in the villi, they move into the capillary by facilitated transport. In the bloodstream, they are delivered to body cells, especially the muscle cells, where they are used for protein synthesis. Amino acids not used for protein synthesis travel to the liver where they are converted to carbohydrates or fats and are either used for energy or stored throughout the body.

ABSORPTION OF SIMPLE SUGARS

The simple sugars that result from carbohydrate digestion are transported by either facilitated diffusion (fructose) or active transport

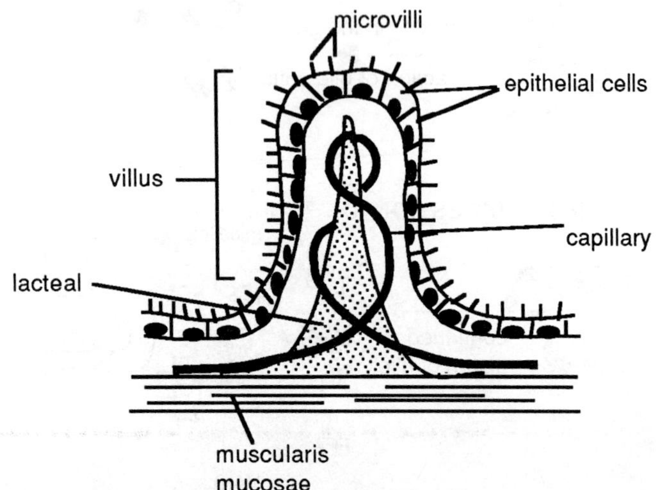

Figure 16-4. Villus showing a central lacteal, capillary network, microvilli, and the epithelial cells across which nutrients are absorbed.

(glucose) across the epithelial cells of the gut and into the capillary of the villus. From there, the sugars are delivered to all body cells and are used for energy production. Sugars not used immediately for energy production can be stored as fat or glycogen in all cells, especially liver cells.

ABSORPTION OF FREE FATTY ACIDS AND MONOGLYCERIDES

Even after being digested, the absorption of free fatty acids and monoglycerides would be extremely slow if it were not for the continued action of the bile salts. Bile salts further break the emulsified fat droplets into even smaller droplets called **micelles** (Fig. 16-3). The micelles contain fatty acids and monoglycerides, bile salts and other phospholipids, cholesterol, and several fat-soluble vitamins all combined together. The micelles stay in equilibrium with a *small amount* of free fatty acids and monoglycerides; these free fatty acids and monoglycerides are the substances actually absorbed into the circulation. As each molecule of free fatty acid or monoglyceride is absorbed, the micelles release replacements, thereby continuing the cycle of absorption. Without the micelles, the fat molecules would once again clump together and be unavailable for absorption.

Because the free fatty acids and monoglycerides are lipid soluble, they move by passive diffusion into the intestinal epithelial cells. In the cells they are changed back into triglycerides, a process requiring energy. Then, triglycerides join in the epithelial cell with cholesterol and phospholipids. This complex is encased in a protein coat, exits the epithelial cell, and moves by passive diffusion into the lacteal in the center of the villi. The complex of the triglyceride, cholesterol, and phospholipid is similar to a micelle and is called a **chylomicron**. Chylomicrons are carried in the lymph to the thoracic duct and then enter the general circulation.

The triglycerides can be used directly as an energy source by most cells of the body, or they can be changed into glucose in the liver and used as an energy source. Excess triglycerides are stored in adipose tissue.

Secretion of Mucus

Mucus is secreted along the entire length of the gut. Mucus is a thick substance that coats the wall of the gut and serves to protect it from being digested by the enzymes to which it is exposed. Mucus also serves to lubricate food, allowing for easier passage.

Without the production of mucus, gut wall integrity would be severely compromised, especially in the stomach where HCl is highly concentrated and is an essential component of protein digestion. In addition, stools would be hard without the lubricating effects of mucus.

Recirculation of Bile

After the bile salts deliver fatty acids and monoglycerides to the villi, some travel back to the chyme to pick up more molecules and repeat the process. Most of the remaining bile salts are eventually reabsorbed at the end of the small intestine and are recycled back to the liver via the portal vein to be used again. This process is called **enterohepatic circulation.**

Elimination of Waste Products

Absorption, primarily of water and electrolytes, continues to occur in the large intestine. Most absorption occurs in the upper half of the colon. Of the approximately 1000 mL of chyme that enters the large intestine each day, only 100 mL of fluid and virtually no electrolytes are excreted. Besides water, which makes up approximately 75% of feces, feces contain dead bacteria, some undigested fat and roughage, and a small amount of protein. Bilirubin byproducts give the feces its color.

The process of elimination, or defecation, occurs as a result of peristaltic contractions of the rectum. These contractions are produced in response to stimulation of the longitudinal and the circular smooth muscles by the myenteric plexus. The myenteric plexus is stimulated by parasympathetic nerves traveling in sacral segments of the spinal cord. Mechanical stretching of the rectum with stool is also a strong stimulator of peristalsis. When a peristaltic wave is initiated, the internal anal sphincter, a smooth muscle, relaxes. If the external anal sphincter is also relaxed, defecation occurs. The external anal sphincter is a skeletal muscle and thus is under voluntary control. In fact, relaxation of the internal sphincter causes reflex contraction of the external sphincter in all individuals except babies and some people who have spinal cord transection. This effectively stops defecation. If the defecation reflex occurs at an appropriate time after the internal sphincter relaxes, the reflex contraction of the external sphincter can be consciously reversed and defecation results.

Hunger and the Ingestion of Food

Hunger is controlled by an area of the brain in the lateral hypothalamus. Stimulation of this area causes a strong desire to seek out and to eat food. The lateral hypothalamus receives numerous inputs that can stimulate hunger. For instance, hunger can be stimulated by the occurrence in the stomach of hunger contractions. These contractions appear to increase in frequency and intensity the longer the stomach is empty. The exact mechanism by which they occur is unclear.

Hunger is also stimulated by a fall in blood nutrients, such as amino acids, fats, and glucose, and by a rise in the hormones that accompany nutrient deficit (e.g., glucagon). A decrease in the level of hormones present when food is plentiful may also stimulate hunger (e.g., insulin). Input to the hypothalamic hunger center can include input from other areas of the brain as well. For instance, higher brain centers can stimulate hunger in response to certain situations or experiences. Likewise, input from the emotional center of the brain, the limbic system, may also stimulate hunger, as may different smells activating from the olfactory center.

Conversely, the ventromedial nucleus of the hypothalamus appears to be the site where satiety, the opposite of a hunger drive, occurs. This center is influenced by the fullness of the stomach and blood levels of nutrients and hormones, but in the opposite direction as is required for hunger stimulation. Emotions and habits may also influence the satiety center.

Tests of Gastrointestinal Functioning

BARIUM CONTRAST X-RAY FILMS: UPPER AND LOWER GASTROINTESTINAL SERIES

In this test, a radiopaque solution is introduced into the upper or the lower GI tract and then x-ray films are obtained to follow its progress. This technique is able to identify position and size of GI structures and obstructions in the GI tract; however, its identification of ulcers, fissure, or early cancers is poor.

ENDOSCOPY

Endoscopy is the process whereby a thin, rigid or flexible scope is passed into the GI tract to visualize the esophagus (*esophagoscopy*), stomach (*gastroscopy*), upper small intestine (*duodenoscopy*), large intestine (*colonoscopy*), or sigmoid colon (*sigmoidoscopy*). With this instrument, the walls of the GI tract can be visualized, allowing identification of ulcerations, blockages, and other irregularities. Special tools at the end of the scope allow tissue to be sampled for biopsy and culture.

Whether patients should have colonoscopy or sigmoidoscopy for screening of colon cancer depends on personal risk factors, including age, family history of GI or other cancers, and personal history of polyps or cancer. With colonoscopy, the practitioner can fully visualize the entire large intestine. Patients are generally anesthesized for this procedure. Because many colon cancers develop in the sigmoid colon and because sigmoidoscopy is usually accomplished without general anesthesia, this procedure is recommended for general screening of low-risk populations.

ULTRASOUND

Ultrasound is a procedure whereby sound waves are reflected from tissue to provide an image. It is a highly sensitive technique and can be used to visualize the structure of the abdominal organs to identify abnormalities, abscesses, stones, and other structures.

COMPUTED TOMOGRAPHY

The process whereby a computer integrates images from several x-ray projections to provide a vivid cross-sectional image is called computed tomography (CT). CT is used to image all GI organs and to identify structural and other abnormalities.

MAGNETIC RESONANCE IMAGING

The process whereby shifts in the magnetic axis of atoms in response to externally applied electromagnetic fields are transformed by computer to produce a cross-sectional image of the structures of the GI tract is known as magnetic resonance imaging (MRI). MRI is used extensively to identify structural abnormalities, alterations in blood flow, and vessel patency.

PATHOPHYSIOLOGIC CONCEPTS

Anorexia

Defined as a loss of appetite or desire for food, anorexia often occurs as a symptom with other GI alterations, including nausea, vomiting, and diarrhea. It can also be present with conditions not associated with the GI tract, such as cancer.

Anorexia nervosa is a condition in which one chooses not to eat because of a morbid fear of being fat. The term anorexia nervosa is actually a misnomer because individuals who have this disorder still have a desire to eat and are still hungry, so by definition are not truly anorectic.

Pediatric Consideration

Most people who develop anorexia nervosa are adolescent or postadolescent females, frequently perfectionists for whom being thin is a sign of success, or athletes who may believe that their performance depends on a level of thinness only possible by the strict avoidance of food. Although less common, young men may also develop anorexia nervosa. In young men, the condition is frequently associated with depression or concerns about sexual orientation. Anyone who has anorexia nervosa needs intense and prolonged therapy to overcome the condition.

Nausea

Nausea is a subjective, unpleasant sensation that often precedes vomiting. Nausea is caused by distention or irritation anywhere in the GI tract, but it can also be stimulated by higher brain centers. Interpretation of nausea occurs in the medulla, which is either adjacent to or part of the vomiting center.

Vomiting

Vomiting is a complex reflex mediated through the vomiting center in the medulla oblongata of the brain. Afferent impulses travel to the vomiting center as both vagal and sympathetic afferents. Afferent impulses originate in the stomach or duodenum in response to excessive distention or irritation, or sometimes they originate in response to chemical stimulation by emetics (agents that cause vomiting), such as syrup of ipecac. Hypoxia and pain can also stimulate vomiting by means of activation of the vomiting center. Vomiting can also occur through direct stimulation of an area of the brain adjacent to the vomiting center in the brain. Certain drugs initiate vomiting by activating this center, called the chemoreceptor trigger zone, which lies in the floor of the fourth ventricle. Vomiting as a result of rapid motion change is believed to work through stimulation of this trigger zone. Activation of the chemoreceptor trigger zone can cause vomiting either directly or indirectly by its subsequent activation of the vomiting center. Input from higher brain centers in the cortex and increased intracranial pressure (ICP) can also stimulate vomiting, probably by directly stimulating the vomiting center. Projectile vomiting occurs when the vomiting center is directly stimulated, frequently by increased ICP.

When the vomiting reflex is initiated in the vomiting center, it is carried out by activation of several cranial nerves to the face and throat, and spinal motor neurons to the diaphragm and abdominal muscles. Excitation of these pathways results in the coordinated response of vomiting. Certain symptoms generally precede vomiting, including nausea, tachycardia, and sweating.

Diarrhea

Diarrhea is an increase in fluidity and frequency of stools. Diarrhea may be large or small volume and may or may not contain blood. Large-volume diarrhea can occur as a result of the presence of a nonabsorbable solute in the stool, called osmotic diarrhea, or as a result of irritation of the intestinal tract. The most common cause of irritation is a viral or bacterial infection of the large or the distal small intestine.

Irritation of the intestine by a pathogen affects the mucosal layer of the intestine, leading to increased secretory products, including mucus. Microbial irritation also affects the muscular layer, leading to increased motility. Increased motility causes large amounts of water and electrolytes to be lost in the stool because the time available for their reabsorption in the colon is reduced. An individual who has severe diarrhea can die from hypovolemic shock and electrolyte irregularities. Cholera toxin released from the cholera bacteria is an example of a substance that strongly stimulates motility and directly causes secretion of water and electrolytes into the large intestine, contributing to the devastating loss of these important plasma constituents. Other infectious agents can also cause diarrhea, either severe or mild. Infection with *Escherichia coli* 0157, found in undercooked ground beef, causes a severe bloody diarrhea. Large-volume diarrhea can also be caused by psychological factors, such as fear or some types of stress, mediated through parasympathetic stimulation of the gut.

Small-volume diarrhea is characterized by frequent loss of small amounts of stool. Causes of this type of diarrhea include ulcerative colitis and Crohn's disease. Both of these illnesses have physical and psychogenic components and are discussed later in this chapter.

Pediatric Consideration

Infants and children are especially susceptible to the severe effects of diarrhea and should be monitored closely for early signs of dehydration. In developing countries, diarrhea from infectious disease, especially cholera, is the number one cause of infant and early childhood death. Any child who has moderate or severe diarrhea should receive fluid replacement with osmotically balanced products.

Constipation

Constipation is defined as difficult or infrequent defecation. Because frequency of stool varies among individuals, the second half of this definition is subjective and rightfully should be interpreted as a relative decrease in the number of stools for an individual. In general, however, bowel movements fewer than once every 3 days are considered to indicate constipation.

Defecation can become difficult if the stool is hard and compact. This can occur if an individual is dehydrated or if a bowel movement is delayed, which allows more water to be absorbed out of the stool as it sits in the large intestine. Bulk or high-fiber diets keep stools moist by osmotically drawing water into the stool and by stimulating peristalsis of the colon by distention. Therefore, people who eat low-bulk diets or highly refined foods are at a greater risk for constipation. Exercise promotes defecation by physical stimulation of the GI tract. Therefore, individuals who lead sedentary lives are at higher risk of suffering from constipation.

Fear of pain during defecation can be a psychologic stimulus to withhold a bowel movement and can cause constipation. Other psychological inputs might also cause delay of defecation. Sympathetic stimulation of the GI tract decreases motility and can slow defecation.

Sympathetic activity is increased in individuals who have long-termstress. Certain drugs such as antacids and opiates can also cause constipation.

Spinal cord trauma, multiple sclerosis, intestinal neoplasm, and hypothyroidism can result in constipation. A disease characterized by a dysfunctional myenteric plexus in the large intestine, called Hirschsprung's disease (congenital megacolon), also causes constipation. This disease should be apparent soon after birth.

Peritonitis

Inflammation of the peritoneum, a membrane that lines the abdominal cavity, is called peritonitis. Peritonitis usually occurs as a result of the passage of bacteria through the GI tract or abdominal organs into the peritoneal space following perforation of the gut or rupture of an organ. Surgery or a penetrating wound to the gut also allows spillage into the peritoneal cavity. The severe infection that occurs with movement of gut contents into the peritoneal cavity emphasizes the fact that the GI tract is really external to the body, rather than part of the internal environment.

Peritonitis is characterized by pain, especially over the inflamed area. Pain may change in location, being centrally located at first, and then becoming more site-specific as the inflammation worsens. Pain may be rebound in nature; that is, the person may complain of more pain when pressure on the abdomen is removed quickly. This is related to the sudden wave of movement that occurs through the peritoneal fluid when a pressure is released.

Individuals who have peritonitis frequently demonstrate increased heart rate as a result of the hypovolemia occurring from the movement of fluid into the peritoneum, nausea and vomiting, and a rigid abdomen that indicates widespread inflammation. In addition, general signs of inflammation such as fever, an increase in white blood cell count, increased sedimentation rate, and tachycardia are present. Sepsis leading to multiorgan failure may occur without appropriate treatment. Treatment usually includes surgery, antibiotics, and fluid and electrolyte replacement.

CONDITIONS OF DISEASE OR INJURY

Gastroesophageal Reflux Disease

The condition of gastroesophageal reflux disease (GERD) is caused by the reflux of stomach contents into the esophagus. GERD is commonly called "heartburn" because of the pain that occurs when the acid normally present only in the stomach, burns or irritates the esophagus.

CAUSES OF GERD

Usually occurring after a meal, GERD is caused by conditions that either weaken the tone of the esophageal sphincter or increase the pressure in the stomach compared with the esophagus. By either of these mechanisms, stomach contents move into the esophagus.

The contents of the stomach are usually prevented from entering the esophagus by the esophageal sphincter. This sphincter normally opens only when a peristaltic wave delivering a bolus of food moves down the esophagus. When this happens, the smooth muscle of the sphincter relaxes and food enters the stomach. It is important that the esophageal sphincter always remains closed except at this time, because many organs are crowded together in the abdominal cavity, causing abdominal pressure to be greater than thoracic pressure. Therefore, the tendency is for contents of the stomach to be pushed up into the esophagus. If one has a weakened or incompetent sphincter, it will not remain closed to stomach contents. Reflux will occur from the high-pressure zone (the stomach) to the low-pressure zone (the esophagus). A weakened sphincter can be a congenital defect or the result of damage to the esophagus. Repeated episodes of GERD may actually worsen the condition by causing inflammation and scarring of the lower esophageal area.

In some circumstances, even if the sphincter has normal tone, reflux will occur if there is an unusually high pressure gradient at the sphincter. For example, if stomach contents are excessive, pressure may increase significantly. This may result from an extra large meal, pregnancy, or obesity. High abdominal pressures tend to push the esophageal sphincter into the thoracic cavity; this exaggerates the pressure gradient between the esophagus and the abdominal cavity. Lying down, especially after a large meal, also contributes to reflux.

A hiatal hernia may also cause reflux. A hiatal hernia is a protrusion of a part of the stomach through the opening in the diaphragm. If this occurs, high pressure in that part of the stomach results in stomach contents being pushed into the esophagus.

Reflux of stomach contents irritates the esophagus because of the high acid content in the stomach. Although the esophagus also has mucus-producing cells, they are not as active or as prevalent as they are in the stomach. The role of the bacteria *Helicobacter pylori* (*H. pylori*) in influencing symptoms of GERD is under study.

CLINICAL MANIFESTATIONS

- Burning pain in the epigastric area, called **dyspepsia**, which may radiate to shoulders, back, or neck.
- Belching and a sour taste may accompany the pain.
- Pain usually occurs within 30 to 60 minutes after a meal or during sleep when the individual is lying down.

DIAGNOSTIC TOOLS

- A good history identifies many individuals at risk of GERD.
- A pH probe, passed into the lower esophageal area reveals an abnormally low pH in individuals who have GERD (below 4.0).

COMPLICATIONS

- Esophagitis, or chronic inflammation of the esophagus, can occur with long-standing GERD. If this occurs, the mucosal layer of the esophagus can become ulcerated by acid. Damage to the mucosal layer can lead to chronic inflammation, spasm of the muscles, and scarring of the esophagus, which can block food passage. Vomiting and dysphagia (difficulty swallowing) with eating may occur.
- The risk of esophogeal cancer is increased in those who have chronic esophagitis.

TREATMENT

- Reduce abdominal pressure by eating more frequent small meals rather than big ones. If obesity is a problem, nutritional counseling and exercise may be advised.
- Sit up during and after eating.
- Sleep with head elevated.
- Drink extra fluids to wash refluxed material out of the esophagus.
- Use antacids to neutralize the acidic content of the stomach.
- Use antihistamines or, especially, proton pump inhibitors that reduce stomach acid secretion because these may relieve the pain of heartburn.
- Consider surgery, if reflux is caused by a hiatal hernia.

Peptic Ulcer

The term peptic ulcer refers to an erosion of the mucosal layer anywhere in the GI tract; however, it usually refers to erosions in the stomach or duodenum. Gastric ulcer refers only to an ulcer in the stomach.

CAUSES OF PEPTIC ULCER

There are two main causes of ulcers: too little mucus production or too much acid being produced in the stomach or delivered to the intestine. A variety of conditions may cause either or both of these disturbances.

Decreased Mucus Production as a Cause of Ulcer

Ulcers most commonly develop when the mucosal cells of the gut do not produce adequate mucus to protect against acid digestion. Causes of decreased mucus production can include anything that decreases blood flow to the gut, causing hypoxia of the mucosal layer and injury to or death of mucus-producing cells. This type of ulcer is called an ischemic ulcer. Decreased blood flow occurs with all types of shock. A particular type of ischemic ulcer that develops after a severe burn is called Curling's ulcer.

Decreased mucus production in the duodenum also can occur as a result of inhibition of mucus-producing glands, called Brunner's glands, located there. Brunner gland activity is inhibited by sympathetic stimulation. Sympathetic stimulation is increased by chronic stress, thus making a connection between chronic stress and ulcer development.

The main cause of decreased mucus production appears to be related to gastric infection with the bacteria *H. pylori*. *H. pylori* colonizes the mucus-secreting cells of the stomach and duodenum, reducing their ability to produce mucus. Approximately 90% of patients who have duodenal ulcer and 70% of patients who have gastric ulcer show *H. pylori* infection. *H. pylori* infection is endemic in some countries. Infection appears to occur by means of ingestion of the microorganism.

The use of various drugs, especially nonsteroidal antinflammatoy drugs (NSAIDs) is also associated with an increased risk of ulcer development. Aspirin, especially, causes irritation of the mucosal wall, as do the other NSAIDs and glucocorticosteroids. These drugs appear to work by inhibiting protective prostaglandins in the gut wall. Approximately 10% of patients taking NSAIDs develop an active ulcer. Serious gastric or intestinal bleeding can occur from NSAIDs, with little early warning. The elderly are especially susceptible to GI injury from NSAIDs. Other drugs or foods associated with ulcer development include caffeine, alcohol, and nicotine. These drugs seem to injure the protective mucosal layer also.

Excess Acid as a Cause of Ulcer

Acid production in the stomach is necessary for activation of stomach digestive enzymes. Hydrochloric acid (HCl) is produced by the parietal cells in response to certain foods, drugs, hormones (including gastrin), histamine, and parasympathetic stimulation. Foods and drugs such as caffeine and alcohol stimulate the parietal cells to produce acid. Some individuals might be overreactive in their parietal response to these substances or other foods, or they may simply have a greater number of parietal cells than normal and therefore release excess acid.

Because gastrin stimulates the production of acid, anything that increases the secretion of gastrin can lead to excess acid production. The main example of this condition is called Zollinger–Ellison syndrome, a disease characterized by tumors of the gastrin-secreting endocrine cells. Other causes of excess acid include excessive vagal stimulation to the parietal cells that is seen after severe brain injury or trauma.

Ulcers that develop under these circumstances are called Cushing's ulcers. Excess vagal stimulation during psychologic stress may also cause excess HCl production.

Increased Delivery of Acid as a Cause of Duodenal Ulcer

Too rapid movement of stomach contents into the duodenum can overwhelm the protective mucus layer there. This occurs with irritation of the stomach by certain foods or microorganisms, as well as by excess gastrin secretion or abnormal distention.

Rapid movement of stomach contents into the intestine also occurs in the condition called **dumping syndrome**. Dumping syndrome happens when the ability of the stomach to hold and slowly release chyme into the duodenum is compromised. One cause of dumping syndrome is surgical removal of a large part of the stomach. Dumping syndrome not only results in rapid delivery of acid to the intestine, but it can cause cardiovascular hypotension. Hypotension occurs because the delivery of multiple food particles to the intestine all at once results in a large amount of water moving from the circulation into the gut by osmosis.

CLINICAL MANIFESTATIONS

- Burning abdominal pain (dyspepsia), often occurs at night. The pain is usually located in the midline, epigastric area, and is often rhythmic in nature.
- Pain that occurs when the stomach is empty often signifies a duodenal ulcer. This is most common.
- Pain that occurs immediately after or during eating, suggests a gastric ulcer. Occasionally, the pain may be referred to the back or shoulder as well.
- The occurrence of pain often comes and goes; it sometimes occurs daily for several weeks and then disappears altogether until the next exacerbation.
- Weight loss is common with gastric ulcers. Weight gain may occur with duodenal ulcers because eating relieves the discomfort.

DIAGNOSTIC TOOLS

- Ulcers are diagnosed primarily by history and endoscopy. With endoscopy, not only can the gut lining be viewed for ulcers, but tissue samples can be taken for biopsy. The presence or absence of *H. pylori* can be determined.
- *H. pylori* infection may also be diagnosed by blood tests for antibody and by breath tests that measure metabolic waste production by the microbe.

COMPLICATIONS

- An ulcer may in some instances go through all mucosal layers, causing perforation of the gut. Because gut contents are not sterile, this can lead to infection of the abdominal cavity. The pain of perforation is severe and radiating. It is unrelieved by eating or antacids.
- Obstruction of the lumen of the GI tract may occur as a result of repeated episodes of injury, inflammation, and scarring. Obstruction is most often at the pyloris; the narrow passageway between the stomach and the small intestine. Obstruction causes feelings of stomach and epigastric distention, heaviness, nausea, and vomiting.
- Hemorrhage may occur when the ulcer has eroded an artery or vein in the gut. This can result in hematemesis (vomiting of blood) or in melena (passage of upper GI blood in the stool). If bleeding is extensive and sudden, symptoms of shock may occur. If bleeding is slow and insidious, microcytic hypochromic anemia may develop.

TREATMENT

- Identify and then instruct patients to avoid foods that cause excess HCl secretion; this improves symptoms for some individuals.
- Educate patients that avoidance of alcohol and caffeine improves symptoms and increases healing of a preexisting ulcer.
- Discontinue or reduce NSAIDs ingestion; this often relieves symptoms in mild cases.
- Strongly urge individuals who smoke to quit because tobacco both irritates the gut and delays healing.
- Prescribe antacids, antihistamines, or proton-pump inhibitors to neutralize stomach acid and to relieve symptoms of an ulcer.
- Individuals documented to have an ulcer caused by *H. pylori*—the majority of patients by far—are treated with the addition of an antibiotic to the standard antacid therapy previously used. Typically, patients are placed on two antibiotics plus a bismuth or on a proton-pump inhibitor and antibiotics. Adding antibiotics to the acid-lowering strategies used previously can truly cure many patients of their ulcers rather than just temporarily improving their symptoms.
- Stress management, relaxation techniques, or sedatives can be used to relieve psychological influences.

Malabsorption

Failure of the small intestine to absorb certain foodstuffs is called malabsorption. Inability to absorb can be 1) of one type of amino acid, fat, sugar, or vitamin, 2) of all amino acids, fats, sugars, or 3) of all fat-soluble vitamins. Malabsorption of everything absorbed in one segment of the small intestine can also occur, with other small-intestine segments being spared.

Causes of malabsorption include pancreatic digestive enzyme deficiency; microorganism infection; damage to the mucosal layer of the gut; or for fats and fat-soluble vitamins, impairment of bile production or lymph function. Genetic deficiencies in specific enzymes may also occur. Lactose malabsorption can result from the inability to break down lactose into absorbable monosaccharides. This can result from a congenital deficiency in the enzyme lactase or a decrease in lactase after an intestinal disease. Crohn's disease and bowel resection are common causes of malabsorption, as is sprue, a disease characterized by injury to the villi and that apparently is caused by a hypersensitivity to gluten. Gluten is a product of wheat, barley, rye, and oats.

CLINICAL MANIFESTATIONS

Clinical manifestations of malabsorption are specifically related to what is not being absorbed and whether other areas of the bowel can compensate. Specific symptoms are related to the dietary deficiency that occurs. Generalized symptoms usually include those related to the GI tract or to the loss of fat-soluble vitamins:

- Fat malabsorption results in steatorrhea (fat in the stool). Diarrhea, flatulence, bloating, and cramps often occur. Stools are bulky but of light weight and float, and are malodorous.
- Bile salt deficiency results in malabsorption of fat-soluble vitamins, causing
  - vitamin A deficiency—night blindness
  - vitamin D deficiency—bone demineralization and increased risk of fractures
  - vitamin K deficiency—poor coagulation with prolonged prothrombin time, easy bruising, and petechia (hemorrhagic spots on the skin)
  - vitamin E deficiency—perhaps resulting in poor immune function
  - lactose malabsorption results in osmotic diarrhea and flatulence (gas)

DIAGNOSTIC TOOLS

- The presence of over 7 g of fat per day in an adult consuming a typical American diet is considered malabsorption. Weight loss or failure to gain weight in infancy or young childhood may indicate malabsorption.

COMPLICATIONS

- Failure to thrive may occur in severe cases, leading to malnutrition, infection, and even death.

TREATMENT

- Identification of the cause of malabsorption.
- Provision of needed nutrients through other food sources or supplements.

Appendicitis

Inflammation of the appendix, which may occur 1) for no obvious reason, 2) after obstruction of the appendix with stool, or 3) from either the organ or its blood supply being twisted, is known as appendicitis. The inflammation results in a swollen, tender appendix, which leads to gangrene as the blood supply is compromised. The appendix may also burst; this typically happens between 36 and 48 hours after the onset of symptoms.

CLINICAL MANIFESTATIONS

- Abrupt onset of diffuse pain in the epigastric or periumbilical area.
- Over the next few hours, the pain becomes more localized and may be described as a pinpoint tenderness in the lower right quadrant.
- Rebound tenderness (pain that occurs when pressure is removed from the tender area) is a classic symptom of peritonitis and is common with appendicitis. Guarding of the abdomen occurs.
- Fever.
- Nausea and vomiting.

DIAGNOSTIC TOOLS

The diagnosis of apendicitis continues to be difficult for clinicians. In at least 20% of cases of appendictis, the diagnosis is missed; in another 15 to 40% of cases, the appendix is normal in patients sent to surgery for suspected appendicitis. Diagnostic criteria for identifying appendicitis include:

- Elevated white cell count greater than 10,000/mL.
- Fever greater than 37.50°C (99.5°F).
- The presence of pain in the right lower quadrant.
- CT scannning is an excellent tool for the diagnosis of appendicitis, especially appendiceal CT used in the emergency department by radiologists trained in its use. Ultrasound may also be effective.

COMPLICATIONS

- Peritonitis can occur if the swollen appendix bursts. Peritonitis significantly increases the risk of postoperative complications.

TREATMENT

- Surgical removal of the appendix.
- If the appendix bursts before surgery, antibiotics are necessary to reduce the risk of peritonitis and sepsis.

Pediatric Consideration

The peak age of incidence of appendicitis in children is between ages 10 and 12. In children, especially infants and toddlers, appendicitis is often misdiagonsed, with a perforation incidence in children less than 3 years of age greater than 90%.

Inflammatory Bowel Disease

Inflammatory bowel disease includes Crohn's disease and ulcerative colitis. Both of these conditions appear to be autoimmune diseases of unknown cause, with widespread activation of proinflammatory cytokines contributing to the scarring and inflammation of the tissue. They both have strong genetic influences and are exacerbated by stress.

CROHN'S DISEASE

Crohn's disease is a chronic inflammatory disease of the bowel characterized by inflammation of all layers of the GI tract. It especially affects the submucosal layer and the small and large intestines.

The inflammation of Crohn's occurs as sharply outlined granulomatous lesions that appear in skip pattern scattered throughout the affected area of the gut. Interspersed between areas of inflammation is normal gut tissue. With chronic inflammation, fibrosis and scarring occur and make the bowel stiff and inflexible. If the fibrosis occurs in the small intestine, it can significantly interfere with the absorption of nutrients. If the disease is primarily localized in the colon, water and electrolyte balance can be disturbed. Abnormal connections or fistulas sometimes develop between different parts of the digestive tract and between the GI tract and the vagina, bladder, or rectum. This can contribute to malabsorption and cause infection.

CLINICAL MANIFESTATIONS

- Intermittent, usually nonbloody, diarrhea.
- Colicky pain.
- Weight loss.
- Malabsorption.
- Fluid and electrolyte imbalance may result.
- Malaise.
- Low-grade fevers.

DIAGNOSTIC TOOLS

- Sigmoidoscopy reveals irregular, scarred bowel.

COMPLICATIONS

- Toxic megacolon, dilation of the colon resulting from interference with its neural or vascular integrity, may occur. This condition can be life-threatening.
- Obstruction of the intestine caused by scarring may occur. Fistulas between the colon and other abdominal organs may occur.
- Systemic manifestations of Crohn's disease include arthritis, skin lesions, and various blood disorders, including autoimmune anemia and hypercoagulability.
- Children afflicted with Crohn's disease may experience growth retardation, resulting from malabsorption as well as from the anti-inflammatory drugs used to treat the disease.

TREATMENT

- Anti-inflammatory drugs are used to interrupt the constant cycle of inflammation.
- Nutritional supplementation and diet education.
- Psychological support.
- Total parenteral nutrition, which involves food solutions being delivered intravenously, may be needed during exacerbations to allow the gut to heal.
- Given the role of proinflammatory cytokines in contributing to the course of Crohn's disease, recent use of antibodies against one proinflamamtory cytokine, tumor necrosis factor α (TNF-α) has been used to treat the disease in experimental studies. Results appear promising at this point.

ULCERATIVE COLITIS

Ulcerative colitis is an inflammatory disease of the rectum and colon that primarily affects the mucosal layer of the large intestine. It is spread continuously throughout the affected area. There is no skip pattern. Ulcerative lesions form crypts in the base of the mucosal layer, called Lieberkühn's crypts. These are characterized by pinpoint hemorrhages that can abscess. Thickening of the wall of the bowel can occur.

Ulcerative colitis typically goes through stages of exacerbations and remissions. The disease can be mild, moderate, or fulminating. Bloody diarrhea mixed with mucus is characteristic of each stage, but it is intensified with increasing severity of the disease.

CLINICAL MANIFESTATIONS

- Mild cases demonstrate small-volume, chronic, bloody diarrhea.
- With worsening cases, more and more of the colon is affected, resulting in increasing diarrhea, with loss of electrolytes.
- Fever.
- Weight loss.
- Abdominal pain increasing with severity of disease.

DIAGNOSTIC TOOLS

- Sigmoidoscopy reveals hemorrhagic mucosa with ulceration.
- Blood analysis demonstrates anemia and low serum potassium.

COMPLICATIONS

- Toxic megacolon may develop.
- Perforation of the gut wall with peritonitis may occur.
- There is an increased risk of colon cancer with ulcerative colitis.
- Systemic manifestations of ulcerative colitis include arthritis, skin lesions, and various blood disorders, including autoimmune anemia and hypercoagulability.
- Children afflicted with ulcerative colitis may experience growth retardation, resulting from the malabsorption and diarrhea, as well as from the anti-inflammatory drugs used to treat the disease.

TREATMENT

- Anti-inflammatory drugs.
- Nutritional supplementation.
- Bulk-free diet to decrease stool frequency.
- Psychological support.
- Surgical resection of the bowel may be necessary.

Diverticular Disease

Diverticular disease is characterized by one or multiple herniations of the mucosal layer of the colon through the muscular layers. Herniations of the mucosal layer are believed to occur when an individual frequently exerts high pressures inside the lumen of the colon while straining to pass a low-bulk stool. This disease is more common among people who eat low-fiber, low-bulk meals.

CLINICAL MANIFESTATIONS

Some individuals may be asymptomatic. However, clinical manifestations usually include

- A change in bowel habits
- Excess gas

DIAGNOSTIC TOOLS

- A good history and physical examination assist diagnosis.
- Barium enema may identify diverticuli. Barium enemas should be avoided if risk of perforation is high.

COMPLICATIONS

- Diverticulitis, an inflammation or infection of the diverticula, may occur. The diverticula may become infected if bacteria-rich pieces of stool become trapped in the diverticula. Systemic signs of an infection, including fever and elevated white cell count, occur.
- Perforation of the gut from severe diverticulitis may occur. With perforation, pain (usually in the lower left quadrant), nausea, and vomiting occur. Fever and elevated white cell count are present.

TREATMENT

- Dietary modification to increase stool bulk.
- Exercise to increase the rate of stool passage.
- Diverticulitis is usually treated with antibiotics and the withholding of solid food until healing occurs.
- Perforation requires surgery and antibiotic therapy.

Hirschsprung's Disease

Hirschsprung's disease is the congenital absence of autonomic ganglia innervating the myenteric plexus in the anorectal junction and some or most of the rectum and colon. Autonomic ganglia to the myenteric plexus normally stimulate motility and ensure the passage of stool. With Hirschsprung's, stool accumulates in the bowel.

CLINICAL MANIFESTATIONS

- Delayed passage of meconium after birth indicates a high suspicion of Hirschsprung's.
- Constipation in an infant may signify Hirschsprung's.
- Vomiting and irritability are common.

DIAGNOSTIC TOOLS

- Rectal biopsy that demonstrates an absence of ganglion cells confirms diagnosis.

COMPLICATIONS

- Electrolyte disturbances and perforation of the bowel if distension is unrelieved.
- Fecal impaction.

TREATMENT

- Surgical resection of the affected area.

Esophageal Cancer

Esophageal cancer is uncommon in the United States. It is primarily related to alcohol and tobacco use. Caustic injury to the esophagus and chronic gastroesophageal reflux also have been implicated in esophageal cancer. Prognosis for esophageal cancer has traditionally been poor, but it is improving with better diagnostic techniques.

CLINICAL MANIFESTATIONS

- Dysphagia (difficulty swallowing) is the most common symptom.
- Anorexia and weight loss follow.

DIAGNOSTIC TOOLS

- Endoscopy followed by tissue biopsy is used to diagnose esophageal cancer.

TREATMENT

- Surgical resection, radiation, and chemotherapy.

Stomach Cancer

Stomach cancer has decreased in the United States; however, it is still the seventh leading cause of death in this country. There appears to be a genetic predisposition to stomach cancer and an increased risk associated with consumption of preserved and smoked meats. There also appears to be a strong link between *H. pyloria* infection and stomach cancer. It has been suggested that the decreasing rates of stomach cancer in the United States may be because of the frequent use of antibiotics, and hence the eradication of *H. pylori*. Decreased use of nitrate preservatives with better refrigeration has also contributed.

CLINICAL MANIFESTATIONS

Stomach cancer is frequently asymptomatic until advanced. When symptoms are present they include

- Vague abdominal discomfort.
- Indigestion.

- Weight loss.
- Anorexia.
- A palpable abdominal mass may be present.

DIAGNOSTIC TOOLS

- Diagnosis follows a careful history and the use of endoscopy followed by tissue biopsy.

TREATMENT

- Surgical resection of all or part of the stomach.

Colorectal Cancer

Colorectal, or intestinal, cancer is common in the United States. Most colorectal cancers are carcinomas and usually begin in the secretory glands of the mucosal layer. Most colorectal cancers begin in preexisting polyps.

Dietary risk factors for colorectal cancer include high fat and low fiber. Withholding stools may also allow toxins present in the stool to initiate or promote cancer. There is a genetic risk factor for colorectal cancer and specific genes associated with colon cancer have been identified. High intake of fruits and vegetables may protect against the development of colorectal cancer by increasing dietary bulk and by providing antioxidants that may protect cells from damage by carcinogens. The presence of polyps in the colon and rectum indicates an increased risk of cancer development.

CLINICAL MANIFESTATIONS

- Changes in bowel habits, resulting in diarrhea or constipation may occur.
- Occult or frank blood in the stool is a strong warning sign.

DIAGNOSTIC TOOLS

- A palpable mass may be felt by digital examination.
- Tests for occult blood in the stool may indicate cancer.
- Early identification of polyps with digital examination, sigmoidoscopy, or colonoscopy (examination of the entire rectum and colon with a fiber-optic lens), and surgical removal of any visualized polyps may prevent cancer from developing.
- Genetic markers for colon cancer may predict who is at greatest risk of developing the disease, thus allowing appropriate preventive measures to be initiated.
- Blood tests for specific antigens associated with colorectal cancer, especially carcinoembryonic antigen (CEA), can be useful in the early identification of a recurring colorectal cancer. CEA levels are poor screening tools for cancer for the general population because

measurable levels of CEA are only present with advanced disease. In addition, false-positive results (prediction of cancer when it is not present) frequently occur.

TREATMENT

- Preventive measures are important and include dietary education on increasing roughage, fruits, vegetables, and grains to increase bulk, decrease fat, and provide protective antioxidants.
- Staging of the disease based on dissemination of tumor cells to regional lymph nodes is important in determining the prognosis and treatment of the disease. Identification of even micrometastases can influence outcome.
- If colorectal cancer is present, surgery is required with or without follow-up chemotherapy.

Geriatric Consideration

Colorectal cancer usually occurs in the elderly. Recommendations for digital examination and tests for occult blood in the stool usually begin after the age of 40, and visualization of the rectum and colon is recommended after the age of 50. Individuals who have a first-degree relative with colon cancer are advised to undergo colonoscopy before the age of 50.

Selected Bibliography

Bickston, S. J. & Cominelli, F. (1998). Treatment of Crohn's disease at the turn of the century. *New England Journal of Medicine* 339, 401–402.

Blaser, M. J. (1998). Helicobacter pylori and gastric disease. BMJ, 316, 1507–1510.

Chaffee, E .E. (1980). *Basic physiology and anatomy (4th ed.)*. Philadelphia: J.B. Lippincott.

Ferzoco, L. B., Raptopoulos, V., & Silen, W. (1998). Acute diverticulitis. *New England Journal of Medicine* 338, 1521–1525.

Fisher, R. S. & Parkman, H. P. (1998). Management of nonulcer dypepsia. *New England Journal of Medicine* 339, 1376–1381.

Guyton, A. C. & Hall, J. (1997). *Textbook of medical physiology (9th ed.)*. Philadelphia: W.B. Saunders.

Irish, A. S., Pearl, R. H. Caty, M. G., & Glick, P. L. (1998). The approach to common abdominal diagnoses in infants and children. *Pediatric Clinics of North America* 45, 729–772.

Lee, J. M. & O'Morain, C. A. (1997). Trends in the management of gastro-oesophageal reflux disease. *Postgraduate Medical Journal* 74, 145–150.

Liefers, G. J., Cleton-Jansen, A. M., van de Velde, C., et al. (1998). Micrometastases and survival in stage II colorectal cancer. *New England Journal of Medicine* 339, 223–228.

Porth, C. M. (1998). *Pathophysiology concepts of altered health states (5th ed.)*. Philadelphia: J.B. Lippincott Company.

Rao, P. M., Rhea, J. T., Novelline, R. A., et al. (1998). Effect of computed tomography of the appendix on treatment of patients and use of hospital resources. *New England Journal of Medicine* 338, 141–146.

Saiki, T., Mitsuyama, K. Toyonaga, A., et al. (1998). Detection of pro- and anti-inflammatory cytokines in stools of patients with inflammatory bowel disease. *Scandinavian Journal of Gastroenterology* 33, 616–622.

Vander, A. J., Sherman, J., & Luciano, D. (1998). *Human physiology (7th ed)*. Boston: McGraw-Hill.

Resources

Crohn's and Colitis Foundation, 386 Park Avenue, New York, NY 10016. Phone: (800) 343-3637.

17 THE PANCREAS AND DIABETES MELLITUS

The pancreas is a large, diffuse abdominal organ that functions as both an exocrine and endocrine gland. In this chapter, both roles are presented, followed by a detailed description of diabetes mellitus, a condition in which the pancreatic hormone, insulin, is either ineffective or absent. Pancreatitis and pancreatic cancer are discussed briefly.

● ● ●

PHYSIOLOGIC CONCEPTS

Exocrine Functions of the Pancreas

The exocrine functions of the pancreas involve the synthesis and release of digestive enzymes and sodium bicarbonate from specialized cells of the pancreas called **acini cells**. The acini cells release their contents into the pancreatic duct. From the pancreatic duct, the enzymes and bicarbonate solution travel through the sphincter of Oddi into the first section of the small intestine, the duodenum. The pancreatic enzymes and bicarbonate solution each play an essential role in the digestion and absorption of food in the small intestine.

SECRETION OF PANCREATIC ENZYMES

The secretion of the various pancreatic enzymes occurs primarily as a result of stimulation of the pancreas by cholecystokinin (CCK), a hormone released from the small intestine. The stimulus for the release of CCK is the presence of a mixture of food particles entering the duodenum from the stomach. The pancreatic enzymes include trypsin, amylase, and lipase and are responsible for the digestion of proteins to amino acids, carbohydrates to simple sugars, and fats to free fatty acids and monoglycerides, respectively. The food mixture from the stomach is called **chyme**.

SECRETION OF SODIUM BICARBONATE

Sodium bicarbonate is released from the acini cells into the pancreatic duct in response to a second small-intestine hormone, secretin. Secretin is released in response to the acidic chyme entering from the stomach. When delivered to the small intestine, sodium bicarbonate neutralizes acidic chyme. This function is essential because the digestive enzymes are inactivated in an acidic environment. Neutralization of the acid in the duodenum also protects this area against acid injury to the mucosal wall and subsequent ulcer development.

Endocrine Functions of the Pancreas

The endocrine functions of the pancreas involve the synthesis and release of the hormones insulin, glucagon, and somatostatin. These hormones are each produced by separate, specialized cells of the pancreas, called the **islets of Langerhans**.

SYNTHESIS AND SECRETION OF INSULIN

The synthesis of insulin in the pancreas comes from the enzymatic cleavage of a proinsulin molecule, which itself was the cleavage product of an even larger preproinsulin molecule. Proinsulin is composed of an A peptide fragment connected to a B peptide fragment, by a C peptide fragment and two disulfide bonds (Fig. 17-1). Enzymatic cleavage of the C peptide connections leaves the A and the B peptides connected to each other through only the two disulfide bonds. In this form, insulin circulates unbound in the plasma.

Insulin is released at a basal rate by the *beta cells* of the islets of Langerhans. The primary stimulus to increase insulin release above baseline is a rise in blood glucose. Fasting blood glucose level is normally 80 to 90 mg/100 mL of blood. When blood glucose increases to more than 100 mg/100 mL of blood, insulin secretion from the pancreas increases rapidly and then returns to baseline in 2 to 3 hours. Insulin is the main hormone of the **absorptive stage** of digestion that occurs immediately after a meal. Insulin levels are low between meals.

Insulin circulates in the plasma and acts by binding to insulin receptors present on most cells of the body. Once bound, insulin works through a protein kinase messenger system to cause an increase in

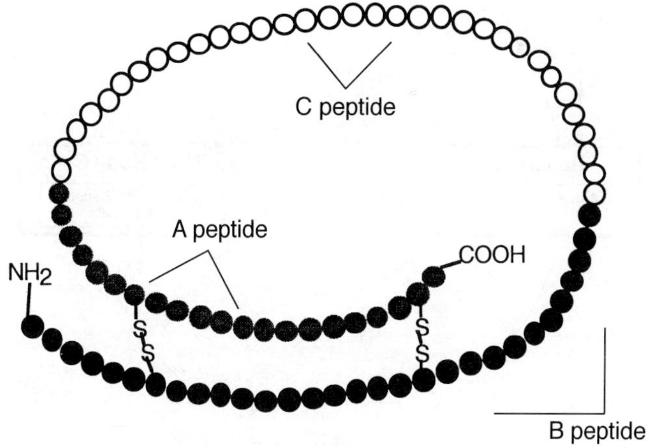

Figure 17-1. Proinsulin molecule.

the number of glucose-transporter molecules present on the outside of the cell membrane. The glucose-transporter molecules, called glut-4 glucose transporters, are necessary for the facilitated diffusion of glucose into most cells. Once transported inside the cells, glucose can be used for immediate energy production through the Krebs cycle, or it can be stored in the cell as glycogen, a glucose metabolite. When glucose is carried into the cell, it results in decreased blood levels of glucose, reducing the further stimulation of insulin release. This is an example of negative feedback as shown in Figure 17-2.

Insulin release is also stimulated by amino acids and the hormones of digestion (i.e., CCK, secretin, and glucose-dependent insulinotropic peptide [GIP]; see Chapter 16). The autonomic nervous system also stimulates insulin release by means of parasympathetic nerves to the pancreas. Both the release of GIP and the activation of the autonomic nervous system occur with the onset of eating a meal; this results in a release of insulin at the beginning a meal, even before glucose is absorbed. Sympathetic stimulation to the pancreas decreases insulin release.

Insulin is the major anabolic (building) hormone of the body and has a variety of other effects besides stimulating glucose transport. It also increases amino acid transport into cells, stimulates protein

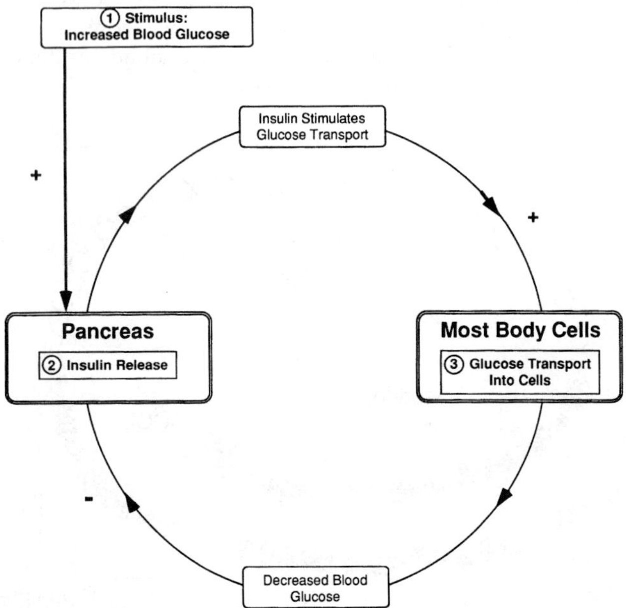

Figure 17-2. Feedback cycle demonstrating the effect of decreased blood glucose on insulin release.

synthesis, and inhibits the breakdown of fat, protein, and glycogen stores. Insulin also inhibits **gluconeogenesis**, the new synthesis of glucose, by the liver. In summary, insulin serves to provide glucose to our cells, build protein, and maintain low plasma glucose levels.

THE BRAIN, GLUCOSE, AND INSULIN

Unlike most other cells, brain cells do not require insulin for glucose entry. Also unlike other cells that may use free fatty acids or amino acids for energy, brain cells must use only glucose or glycogen to meet their energy demands and drive their cellular functions. In other words, brain cells are obligate users of glucose and glycogen. This means that gluconeogenesis by the liver is important: If glucose were not produced between meals by the liver, the brain would have no usable energy source during that time.

SECRETION OF GLUCAGON

Glucagon is a protein hormone released from the *alpha cells* of the islets of Langerhans in response to *low* blood glucose levels and increased plasma amino acids. Glucagon is primarily a hormone of the **postabsorptive stage** of digestion that occurs during fasting periods in between meals. Its functions are mainly catabolic (breaking down). In most respects, glucagon works the opposite of insulin. For example, glucagon acts as an insulin antagonist by inhibiting glucose movement into cells. Glucagon also stimulates liver gluconeogenesis and causes the breakdown of stored glycogen to be used as an energy source instead of glucose. Glucagon stimulates the breakdown of fats and the release of free fatty acids into the bloodstream so they may be used as an energy source instead of glucose. These functions serve to increase blood glucose levels. The release of glucagon by the pancreas is stimulated by sympathetic nerves.

SECRETION OF SOMATOSTATIN

Somatostatin is secreted by *delta cells* of the islets of Langerhans. Somatostatin is also called growth hormone–inhibiting hormone and is released as well by the hypothalamus. Somatostatin from the hypothalamus inhibits the release of growth hormone from the anterior pituitary. Somatostatin from the pancreas appears to have a minimal effect on the release of growth hormone from the pituitary. Rather, it acts to control metabolism by inhibiting the secretion of insulin and glucagon. Its exact function is otherwise unclear.

TESTS OF PANCREATIC FUNCTION

Fasting Plasma Glucose

Measurement of plasma glucose above 126 mg/100 mL on more than one occasion is diagnostic of diabetes mellitus. Levels of greater than 110 mg/100 mL indicate insulin resistance. Nonfasting plasma glucose of greater than 200 mg/100 mL with symptoms of polyurea, polydipsia, and polyphagia is also diagnostic.

Urine Glucose Tests

Glucose in the urine may or may not be indicative of diabetes. Likewise, the absence of glucose in the urine cannot be used to discount diabetes. Under most conditions, however, glucose is not spilled in the urine of healthy, nonpregnant individuals.

Glycosylated Hemoglobin

Throughout the 120-day life span of the red blood cell, hemoglobin slowly and irreversibly becomes glycosylated (glucose bound). Normally, approximately 4 to 6% of red blood cell hemoglobin is glycosylated. If there is chronic hyperglycemia, the level of glycosylated hemoglobin increases. Poorly controlled diabetics show the highest level of glycosylated hemoglobin, which may be greater than 10%. The particular hemoglobin most often measured and reported is glycohemoglobin A1c ($HbA_{1c.}$). Measurement of $HbA_{1c.}$ is important because it offers an indication of how well controlled the blood glucose has been over the previous 2 to 4 months.

Serum Amylase

Amylase is a pancreatic enzyme. Its increased concentration in the serum suggests pancreatic pathology.

PATHOPHYSIOLOGIC CONCEPTS

Hypoglycemia

Hypoglycemia is a blood glucose level less than 50 mg/l00 mL of blood. Hypoglycemia can be caused by fasting or, especially, fasting coupled with exercise, because exercise increases the usage of glucose by skeletal muscle. Most commonly, hypoglycemia is caused by an insulin overdose in an insulin-dependent diabetic.

Because the brain relies on blood glucose as its main energy source, hypoglycemia results in many symptoms of altered central nervous system (CNS) functioning, including confusion, irritability, seizure, and coma. Hypoglycemia can cause headache, as a result of alteration of cerebral blood flow, and changes in water balance. Systemically, hypoglycemia causes activation of the sympathetic nervous system, stimulating hunger, nervousness, sweating, and tachycardia.

Hyperglycemia

Hyperglycemia is defined as blood glucose higher than the normal, fasting range of 126 mg/100 mL of blood. Hyperglycemia is usually caused by insulin deficiency, as seen in type 1 diabetes, or as a result of decreased cellular responsiveness to insulin, as seen in type 2 diabetes. Hypercortisolemia, which occurs in Cushing's syndrome and in response to chronic stress, can cause hyperglycemia by stimulation of liver gluconeogenesis. Acute conditions of elevated thyroid hormone, prolactin, and growth hormone all increase blood glucose as well. Prolonged high levels of these hormones, especially growth hormone, are considered diabetogenic (producing diabetes) because they overstimulate insulin release by beta cells of the pancreas, leading to an eventual decrease in the cellular response to insulin.

CONDITIONS OF DISEASE OR INJURY

Diabetes Mellitus

"Diabetes" is a Greek word that means to siphon or to pass through. "Mellitus" is a Latin word for honey or sweet. The disease diabetes mellitus is one in which an individual siphons large volumes of sweet urine. It is a disease of hyperglycemia characterized by the absolute lack of insulin or a cellular insensitivity to insulin. New diagnostic criteria put forth by the American Diabetes Association in 1997 have lowered the standard by which diabetes is diagnosed to a fasting plasma glucose greater than 126 mg/100 mL on two separate occasions. In addition, fasting plasma glucose levels greater than 110 mg/100 mL of blood are now considered indicative of insulin resistance and are a risk factor for diabetic complications such as coronary artery disease and hypertension. They also indicate a likely progression to frank diabetes. Lowering the diagnostic criteria for diagnosis and suspicion of risk allows for earlier intervention and prevention of serious complications. This is extremely important because at the time of diagnosis of type 2 diabetes, 20% of patients already have retinal damage, 8% renal dysfunction, and 9% neurologic symptoms.

TYPES OF DIABETES MELLITUS

In the 1997 consensus paper put forth by The Expert Committee on the Diagnosis and Classification of Diabetes Mellitus, the American Diabetes Association outlined a new classification system for diabetes mellitus. In this system, four major categories of diabetes are described, with types given Arabic rather than the Roman numerals of the past. These four types include: type 1, characterized by absolute lack of insulin; type 2, characterized by insulin resistance with an insulin secretory defect; type 3, other specific types; and type 4, gestational diabetes (Table 17-1). Types 1, 2, and 4 are discussed in the following section. Other specific types of diabetes (type 3) include pancreatic trauma, neoplasm, or diseases characterized by other endocrine disorders, for example Cushing's disease (Chapter 10).

Table 17-1. Diabetes Mellitus: A Revised Classification Scheme

TYPE	CHARACTERISTICS	1° ETIOLOGY	TREATMENT
Type 1	Absolute lack of insulin	Autoimmune	Insulin
Type 2	Insulin insensitivity and insulin secreting deficiency	Obesity, Genetics	Diet Exercise Hypoglycemic agents Transporter-stimulating drugs
Type 3	Other specific causes	Depends	Depends on cause
Type 4	Gestational diabetes	Increased metabolic demands	Diet Hypoglycemic agents

Type 1 Diabetes Mellitus

Hyperglycemia caused by an absolute lack of insulin is known as type 1 diabetes mellitus. Previously, this type of diabetes has been referred to as insulin-dependent diabetes mellitus (IDDM) because individuals who have this disease must receive insulin replacement. Type 1 diabetes is usually seen in nonobese individuals less than 30 years old and occurs in a slightly higher proportion of males than females. Because the incidence of type 1 diabetes peaks in the early teens, it also has been referred to as juvenile diabetes. However, type 1 diabetes mellitus can occur at any age.

Causes of Type 1 Diabetes Type 1 diabetes results from autoimmune destruction of the beta cells of the islets of Langerhans. It is likely that individuals who have a genetic tendency to develop this disease (see the following section) experience an environmental trigger that initiates the autoimmune process. Examples of possible triggers include viral infections such as mumps, rubella, or chronic cytomegalovirus (CMV). It also has been suggested that exposure to certain drugs or toxins (for instance, nitrosamines present in preserved meats) may somehow trigger an attack. Because type 1 diabetes develops over several years, there is often no identified stimulating event. Antibodies to the islet cells are present in most individuals at the time of diagnosis of type I diabetes.

Why an individual develops antibodies against the islet cells in response to a triggering event is unknown. One mechanism may be that the environmental agent antigenically changes the islet cells in such a way as to stimulate the production of autoantibodies. It is also possible that individuals who develop type 1 diabetes mellitus share antigenic similarities between their pancreatic beta cells and certain triggering viruses or drugs. In the course of responding to the virus or drug, the immune system may fail to distinguish the pancreatic cells as "self."

Genetic Tendency for Type 1 Diabetes Mellitus There appears to be a genetic tendency for individuals to develop type 1 diabetes mellitus. Certain individuals appear to have "diabetogenic genes," meaning a genetic profile that predisposes them to type 1 diabetes (or possibly any autoimmune disease). Genetic loci that pass an inherited tendency for type 1 diabetes appear to be part of the histocompatibility complex genes (see Chapter 3). The histocompatibility complex controls the recognition of self antigens by the immune system; loss of self-tolerance is core to developing autoantibodies. The histocompatibility genes are primarily coded for on chromosome 6. Another specific insulin-related gene on chromosome 11 has been implicated in the development of type 1 diabetes through its effects on beta-cell development and replication. Siblings of individuals who have type 1 diabetes and children of a parent who has type 1 diabetes have an increased risk of developing the disease compared with those without an affected first-degree relative. In clinical studies, nonsymptomatic siblings show a higher incidence (2–4%) of antibodies against pancreatic beta cells than those who do not have a first-degree relative who has diabetes; the earlier onset of antibodies and the higher the level, the worse the prognosis for those siblings developing the disease later in life.

Characteristics of Type 1 Diabetes Individuals who have type 1 diabetes show normal glucose handling before disease onset. In the past it was believed that there was a sudden onset of type 1 disease with little warning. Currently, however, it is believed that type 1 diabetes in most cases develops slowly over the course of many years, with the presence of autoantibodies against the beta cells and their steady destruction occurring well in advance of diagnosis.

By the time type 1 diabetes is diagnosed, there is usually little or no insulin being secreted from the pancreas, and more than 80% of the pancreatic beta cells have been destroyed. Blood glucose levels increase because glucose cannot enter most cells of the body without insulin. At the same time, the liver begins to undertake gluconeogenesis (new glucose synthesis) using the available substrates of amino acids, fatty acids, and glycogen. These substrates are present in high concentrations in the circulation because the catabolic action of glucagon is unopposed by insulin. This results in functional cell starvation in the face of high glucose levels. Only the brain and red blood cells are spared from glucose deprivation because they do not require insulin for glucose entry.

All other cells switch to the use of free fatty acids for energy. Metabolism of free fatty acids in the Krebs cycle (Chapter 1) supplies cells with the adenosine triphosphate (ATP) necessary to run cell functions. Extensive reliance on fatty acids for energy production increases production of various ketones by the liver. Ketones are acids, which cause plasma pH to decrease.

Type 2 Diabetes Mellitus

Hyperglycemia caused by cellular insensitivity to insulin is called type 2 diabetes mellitus. In addition, there is a corresponding insulin secretory defect that results in the pancreas being incapable of secreting enough insulin to maintain normal plasma glucose. Although insulin levels may be only slightly reduced or even within the normal range, they are inappropriately low, considering the elevated level of plasma glucose. Because insulin is still produced by the pancreatic beta cells, type 2 diabetes mellitus was previously called noninsulin-dependent diabetes mellitus (NIDDM), a misnomer because many individuals who have type 2 are treated with insulin. Women are overrepresented compared with men. There is a strong genetic predisposition and obvious environmental factors.

Causes of Type 2 Diabetes The number one risk factor for type 2 diabetes mellitus for most Americans is obesity. In addition, the genetic tendency to develop the disease is strong. It is possible that an unidentified genetic trait causes the pancreas to secrete an altered insulin or causes the insulin receptors or second messengers to fail to respond to insulin adequately. It is also possible that a genetic link is associated with obesity and prolonged stimulation of the insulin receptors. Prolonged stimulation of receptors may lead to a decrease in the number of receptors for insulin present on body cells. This is called **downregulation**. It is also possible that individuals who develop type 2 diabetes produce insulin autoantibodies that bind to the insulin receptor, blocking insulin's access to the receptor, but do not stimulate carrier activity. Other studies suggest that a deficit in the production of the hormone leptin in genetically susceptible individuals may be responsible for type 2 diabetes. Lack of the gene to produce leptin, called the obesity gene, has been identified in some animal studies as causing insulin insensitivity. Without leptin, animals, perhaps including humans, are more likely to become obese.

Although obesity is the main risk factor for type 2 diabetes, there are certain individuals who develop type 2 diabetes at a young age and are thin or of normal weight. One example of this type of disease is maturity-onset diabetes of the young (MODY), a condition related to a genetic defect in the pancreatic beta cell such that it is unable to produce insulin. In this circumstance and a few others, there appears to be an even stronger genetic link than in most types of type 2 diabetes.

Pediatric Consideration

Type 2 diabetes mellitus typically occurs in individuals older than 30 years of age and in the past has been referred to as adult-onset diabetes. Unfortunately, this distinction is becoming less and less true as more teenagers and preteens are developing insulin resistance, most likely related to the increasing prevalence of obesity in childhood. Several studies suggest that over 20% of American children are obese; this finding has enormous implications for health and health care costs as these children reach adulthood and experience the complications of long-term hyperglycemia.

Characteristics of Type 2 Diabetes An individual who has type 2 diabetes still secretes insulin. However, there is often a delay in the initial secretion and a lessening of the total amount released. This trend worsens as a person ages. In addition, the cells of the body, especially muscle and adipose tissue cells, show a resistance to the insulin that does circulate. As a result, the glucose carrier (the glut-4 glucose transporter) is inadequately present on cells and blood glucose levels increase. Once again, the liver initiates gluconeogenesis, and triglycerides, proteins, and glycogen stores are broken down to provide alternative sources of fuel. Only the brain and red blood cells continue to use glucose as an effective energy source. Because there is some insulin, individuals who have type 2 diabetes seldom rely totally on fatty acids for energy production and so are not ketosis prone.

Gestational Diabetes

Type 4 diabetes mellitus, or gestational diabetes, occurs in a previously nondiabetic woman during pregnancy. Approximately 50% of affected women revert to the nondiabetic state after the pregnancy is over. However, the risk of developing type 2 diabetes at a later time is higher than normal.

Causes of Gestational Diabetes The increased energy demands during pregnancy and the continually high levels of estrogen and growth hormone are believed to be the causes of gestational diabetes. Growth hormone and estrogen stimulate insulin release and may result in a type 2 diabetic picture of oversecretion of insulin, leading to decreased cellular responsiveness. Growth hormone has some anti-insulin effects as well, for example, the stimulation of glyconeogenesis (the breakdown of glycogen) and the breakdown of adipose tissue. All these factors may contribute to the hyperglycemia seen in gestational diabetes. Women who develop gestational diabetes may have subclinical problems with glucose control even before diabetes develops.

Results of Gestational Diabetes Gestational diabetes can negatively affect the pregnancy by increasing the risk of congenital malformations, stillbirths, and large-for-date babies, which can result in problems during delivery. Gestational diabetes is routinely tested for during prenatal medical examinations. Women who have gestational diabetes are treated with diet, insulin, or both, if necessary.

THE ROLE OF GLUCAGON

The role of glucagon in the development of diabetes mellitus must be addressed. Although glucagon is not considered a cause of diabetes mellitus, slightly elevated or normal glucagon levels in the face of high blood glucose and fatty acids suggest that the regulation of glucagon release is amiss. The presence and catabolic effects of glucagon, and its stimulation of gluconeogenesis when blood glucose is already high, offer an interesting focus for research on the cause of diabetes mellitus.

CLINICAL MANIFESTATIONS OF DIABETES MELLITUS

- Polyuria (increased urine output) as water follows glucose loss in the urine.
- Polydipsia (increased thirst) caused by the high urine volume and loss of water, leading to extracellular dehydration. Intracellular dehydration follows extracellular dehydration because intracellular water diffuses out of cells, down its concentration gradient, and into the hypertonic (highly concentrated) plasma. Intracellular dehydration stimulates antidiuretic hormone (ADH) release and causes thirst.
- Fatigue and muscle weakness caused by catabolism of muscle protein and the inability of most cells to use glucose for energy. Poor blood flow seen in long-term diabetics also contributes to fatigue.
- Polyphagia (increased hunger) caused by the chronic catabolism of fat and protein, and relative cellular starvation. Weight loss frequently occurs.
- Type 1 diabetics may present with nausea and severe vomiting.

Although both type 1 and 2 diabetics may show the clinical manifestations outlined above, individuals who have type 2 diabetes frequently present with more nonspecific symptoms, including

- Increased rate of infections because of increased glucose concentration in mucus secretions, poor immune function, and reduced blood flow in long-term diabetics.
- Visual changes related to changes in water balance or, in more severe cases, retinal damage.
- Parathesias, or changes in sensation.
- Vaginal candidiasis (yeast infection), resulting from increased glucose levels in vaginal secretions and urine, and poor immune function may lead to vaginal itching and discharge. Vaginal infections are a common presenting condition in women.
- Infants born to mothers who have gestational diabetes may experience hypoglycemia and be large for gestational age.

DIAGNOSTIC TOOLS

- In most cases, the suspicion of type 1 diabetes arises clearly with a history of polyurea, polydipsia, polyphagia, and weight loss. It is confirmed by plasma glucose testing.
- Suspicion and testing for type 2 diabetes may be delayed, because

symptomology is often nonspecific. Type 2 diabetes is also confirmed by plasma glucose testing.

- Throughout pregnancy, women are tested for gestational diabetes by being screened for urine glucose, and at 28 weeks' gestation, their fasting plasma glucose or plasma glucose level after a glucose load ("glucose tolerance test") is measured. Women who do not receive prenatal care will not be tested for gestational diabetes.
- Fasting plasma glucose levels greater than 126 mg/100 mL on two separate occasions are diagnostic of diabetes mellitus. Fasting glucose is elevated because most cells cannot move glucose intracellularly without insulin and gluconeogenesis is stimulated. Postprandial (after eating) glucose levels are elevated as well.
- Glucose present in the urine is suggestive of diabetes. Glucose handling in the kidney depends on carrier-mediated transport. As described in Chapter 14, glucose is freely filterable across the renal glomerular capillaries. In nondiabetics, all glucose that is filtered into the urine is actively transported back into the blood. Normal urine glucose is zero. When glucose levels are greater than approximately 180 mg/100 mL of blood, as can occur with moderate or severe diabetes mellitus, the renal carriers that move glucose out of the urine and back into the blood become saturated. Therefore, they can no longer carry glucose. Any glucose more than 180 mg/100 mL of blood is lost in the urine (Figure 17-3). Long-term diabetics may have a slightly higher renal threshold for glucose excretion, as much as 200 mg/100 mL of blood, because the tubules tend to adapt and reabsorb glucose more efficiently. This puts a

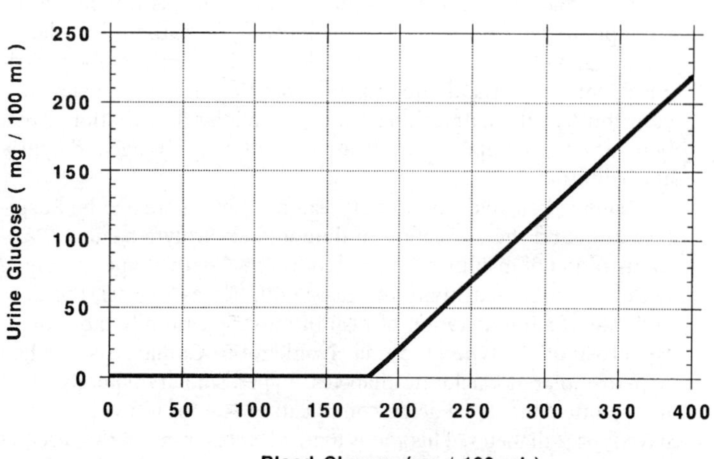

Figure 17-3. Urine glucose concentration as affected by blood glucose concentration. Note that no urine glucose is found until the blood glucose concentration exceeds a threshold value of 180 mg/10mL.

strain on the kidneys of an individual who has long-term diabetes. Because glucose is osmotically active in the urine filtrate, water stays in the filtrate and is excreted in the urine with glucose, resulting in polyuria, a frequent symptom of diabetes. Absence of urine glucose does not rule out diabetes.

- Ketones may be present in the urine. This is especially true for individuals who have poorly controlled type 1 diabetes.
- Elevated levels of glycosylated hemoglobin indicate poorly controlled diabetes. $HbA_{1c.}$ levels maintained below 8% appear to be sufficient for the avoidance of most complications of diabetes. Levels less than 6% are considered in the normal range.

ACUTE COMPLICATIONS

- **Diabetic Ketoacidosis:** Almost always seen in type 1 diabetics, diabetic ketoacidosis is an acute complication characterized by a drastic worsening of all symptoms of diabetes. Diabetic ketoacidosis may occur after physical stress such as pregnancy or an acute illness or trauma. Sometimes it is the presenting symptom of type 1 diabetes.

  With diabetic ketoacidosis, blood glucose levels rise rapidly as a result of gluconeogenesis and a progressive increase in fat breakdown. Polyuria and dehydration follow. Ketone levels also rise (ketosis) as a result of the nearly total use of fatty acids to produce ATP. The ketones spill into the urine (ketonuria) and cause a recognizable fruity smell to the breath. With ketosis, pH decreases below 7.3. The low pH causes metabolic acidosis and stimulates hyperventilation, called Kussmaul's respirations, as the individual attempts to reduce the acidosis by blowing off carbon dioxide.

  An individual who has diabetic ketoacidosis frequently experiences nausea and abdominal pain. Vomiting may occur and may contribute to the extracellular and intracellular dehydration. Total body levels of potassium fall as a result of prolonged polyuria and vomiting.

  Diabetic ketoacidosis is life-threatening and is treated by hospitalization and the correction of fluid and electrolyte balances. Administration of insulin is required for reversal of the hyperglycemia. Because insulin sensitivity increases with decreasing pH, the dose and rate of administration of insulin must be carefully monitored.
- **Hyperosmolar Hyperglycemia Nonketotic Coma:** Also called hyperosmolar nonacidotic diabetes, hyperosmolar hyperglycemia nonketotic coma is an acute complication seen in individuals who have type 2 diabetes. This too is a drastic worsening of the disease. Although not ketosis prone, type 2 diabetics may develop severe hyperglycemia with blood glucose levels well in excess of over 300 mg/100 mL. This causes plasma osmolality, normally tightly controlled at 275 to 295 mOsm/L, to increase to more than 310 mOsm/L. This situation results in liters of lost urine, massive thirst,

severe potassium deficit, and, in approximately 15 to 20% of patients, coma and death. Treatment is geared toward fluid and electrolyte replacement. Hyperglycemic, hyperosmotic, nonketotic coma is usually seen in elderly diabetics after consumption of a high-carbohydrate meal.

- **Somogyi Effect:** The Somogyi effect is an acute complication characterized by a unique decrease in blood glucose levels during the night, followed by a rebound increase in the morning. The cause of the nighttime hypoglycemia is most likely related to the evening insulin injection. The hypoglycemia in turn, causes a reflex increase in glucagon, catecholamines, cortisol, and growth hormone. These hormones stimulate gluconeogenesis, leading to the morning hyperglycemia. Treatment of the Somogyi effect is aimed at manipulation of the evening insulin injection so as not to initiate hypoglycemia. Dietary interventions can also reduce the Somogyi effect. The Somogyi effect is most common in children.
- **Dawn Phenomenon:** Because this complication is an early-morning (between 5 AM and 9 AM) hyperglycemia that appears because of a circadian increase in glucose levels in the morning, it is known as the dawn phenomenon. It can be seen in type 1 or 2 diabetics. Hormones that show circadian variation in the morning include cortisol and growth hormone, both of which stimulate gluconeogenesis. In type 2 diabetics, a decrease in insulin sensitivity might also occur in the morning, either as a normal circadian variation or in response to growth hormone or cortisol.
- **Hypoglycemia:** Usually type 1 diabetics experience the complication of hypoglycemia after an insulin injection. Symptoms may be light-headedness or loss of consciousness. Coma may develop if hypoglycemia is severe. Tightly controlled type 1 patients, that is, patients who perform multiple insulin injections throughout the day and maintain HbA_{1c} levels equal to or less than 7%, are at increased risk of experiencing hypoglycemic events. For some, the benefits of excellent HbA_{1c} levels must be balanced by the risks of hypoglycemia.

LONG-TERM COMPLICATIONS

Diabetes mellitus has many long-term complications. Most seem directly caused by high blood glucose concentration. All contribute to the morbidity and mortality of the disease. These complications affect almost all body organs.

- **Cardiovascular System:** Long-term diabetes mellitus has a drastic effect on the cardiovascular system. Microvascular damage occurs to the small arterioles, the capillaries, and the venules. Macrovascular damage occurs to the large and medium arteries. All organs and tissues of the body suffer as a result of these microvascular and macrovascular injuries.

  Microvascular complications arise from a thickening of the basement membrane of the small vessels. The cause of the thickening is unknown, but seems directly related to high blood glucose levels. Microvascular thickening leads to ischemia and a decreased passage of oxygen and nutrients to the tissues. In addition, glycosylated hemoglobin has an increased affinity for oxygen, resulting in the hemoglobin molecule binding more tightly to oxygen, making it less available to meet tissue needs. Acidosis causes a decrease in red blood cell 2,3-diphosphoglycerate (2,3-DPG), which also increases hemoglobin's affinity for oxygen, making it less likely that tissues will be adequately oxygenated.

Resulting chronic hypoxia can directly damage or destroy cells. Chronic hypoxia can lead to the development of hypertension by causing the heart to increase its cardiac output in an attempt to deliver more oxygen to ischemic tissues. The kidneys, retina, and peripheral nervous system, including both somatic motor and sensory neurons and the peripheral autonomic nerves, are severely affected by diabetic microvascular disease. Poor microvascular circulation impairs the immune and the inflammatory reactions because these depend on good tissue perfusion for delivery of immune cells and inflammatory mediators.

Macrovascular complications primarily arise from development of atherosclerosis. Macrovascular complications contribute to poor blood flow, long-term complications, and high mortality. Macrovascular damage can occur even without the presence of overt diabetes mellitus (plasma glucose > 126 mg/100 mL).

Damage to the endothelial layer of the arteries occurs in diabetes. Damage may result directly from the high circulating levels of blood glucose, a glucose metabolite, or high levels of circulating fatty acids commonly seen in individuals who have diabetes. With injury, endothelial cell permeability increases, and lipid-laden molecules enter the artery. Damage to the endothelial cells initiates an immune and inflammatory reaction, leading to deposition of platelets, macrophages, and fibrous tissue. Smooth muscle cells proliferate. The thickened arterial wall leads to hypertension, which further damages the endothelial lining of the arteries by exerting shear forces on the cells. Refer to Chapter 12 for a full discussion of atherosclerosis. Vascular effects of long-term diabetes include coronary artery disease, stroke, and peripheral vascular disease. Diabetic patients who suffer a myocardial infarct have a poorer prognosis than do nondiabetics who suffer an infarct. Coronary artery disease is a main cause of morbidity and mortality in the diabetic population.

Stroke, or a cerebral vascular accident, also is a common outcome of diabetes. This is especially true for type 2 diabetes as a result of atherosclerosis of the cerebral vessels and by hypertension, which weakens and may ultimately burst the vessels.

Peripheral vascular disease also occurs from severe atherosclerosis. It contributes to the amputations and impotence often seen in long-term diabetics.

- **Vision Loss:** A common long-term complication of diabetes is vision loss. The most serious threat to vision is retinopathy, or damage to the retina resulting from the lack of oxygen. The retina is highly active metabolically, and with chronic hypoxia, it progressively demonstrates breakdown in capillary structure, microaneurysm formation, and spots of hemorrhage. Areas of infarcts (dead tissue) develop; neovascularization (new vessel formation) and sprouting of old vessels occurs. Unfortunately, the new vessels and sproutings are thin walled, and frequently hemorrhage. This leads to activation of the inflammatory system and to scarring of the retina. Interstitial edema occurs and intraocular pressure rises, leading to the collapse of the capillaries and the remaining nerves, and blindness may ensue. Diabetes is the number one cause of blindness in the United States. It is also associated with the frequent development of cataracts and glaucoma.
- **Renal Damage:** Long-term diabetes resulting in renal damage is extremely common, causing diabetic nephropathy to be the number one cause of kidney failure in the United States and in other Western nations. In the kidney, damage to the glomerular capillaries from hypertension and high plasma glucose, causes thickening of the basement membrane and glomerular enlargement. Nodular, sclerotic lesions, called Kimmelstie-Wilson nodules, develop among the glomeruli, blocking blood flow and further damaging the nephron.

  With glomerular enlargement, worsened by hypertension, patients who have diabetes, especially type 1, begin to spill protein into the urine. Although the initial amount of protein lost in the urine may be small (microproteinuria), the damage continues, and progresses in a positive-feedback cycle; protein leakage across the glomeruli further damages the nephron, leading to more protein leakage. Eventually, frank proteinuria develops. This occurrence is associated with a predictable decrease in kidney function and life expectancy.

  The loss of plasma proteins in the urine also causes a decrease in capillary osmotic pressure, leading to a decrease in the reabsorption of fluid from the interstitial space. With net filtration of plasma into the interstitial space, generalized edema, called **anasarca**, occurs. This leads to compression of small capillaries and nerves and to further tissue hypoxia and nerve damage throughout the body, including in the kidney. The kidneys begin to deteriorate rapidly, and fluid overload and severe hypertension develop. With kidney deterioration, the ability to secrete hydrogen ions into the urine decreases, causing metabolic acidosis. Decreased renal production of vitamin D leads to bone breakdown. Decreased renal production of erythropoietin leads to red blood cell deficiency and anemia. Glomerular filtration decreases progressively, and renal failure may develop. Diabetics account for over 30% of renal dialysis transplant patients in the United States. For a full description of renal failure, see Chapter 14.

- **Peripheral Nervous System:** Diabetes mellitus damages the peripheral nervous system, including sensory and motor components of both the somatic and autonomic divisions. Neural disease related to diabetes mellitus is called **diabetic neuropathy**. Diabetic neuropathy is caused by chronic hypoxia of the nerve cells as well as by the effects of hyperglycemia, including hyperglycosylation of proteins involved in neural function. It also appears that nerve support cells—the Schwann cells—begin to use alternative methods to handle the chronically high glucose load, which eventually results in segmental demyelination of the peripheral nerves. Some components of diabetic neuropathy are reversible or preventable with good glucose control; others are not. This suggests that unknown mechanisms of injury in diabetes besides those related to high blood glucose also occur. Recently, C peptide, the protein fragment that is part of the proinsulin molecule, has been implicated in the neuropathy of diabetes.

  Demyelination causes slowing of nerve conduction and loss of feeling. Loss of temperature and pain sensation predisposes an individual to severe and often unnoticed injury. Such injuries, coupled with poor blood flow and an impaired immune system, are responsible for the fact that the number one cause of foot amputations in the United States, other than trauma, is diabetes mellitus.

  Damage to the peripheral autonomic nerves can lead to postural hypotension; changes in gastrointestinal function; impaired bladder emptying, with resultant urinary tract infection; and, in men, impotence.

TREATMENT

- The most important goal of those who study or treat diabetes mellitus is prevention. Although there is no known mechanism to prevent type 1 diabetes, attempts are underway to identify individuals at high risk of developing type 1 (e.g., siblings of affected individuals) by monitoring for anti-beta-cell antibodies and to devise interventions. Different experimental protocols (e.g., providing insulin injections before the demonstration of any symptoms of type 1 with the expectation that antibody development against the beta cells may be prevented) are being tried with this population. For type 2 diabetes, prevention of obesity, especially childhood obesity, is imperative for reducing the incidence of the disease. For those who have gestational diabetes, early identification of risk factors and prompt dietary intervention or other treatments can minimize infant and maternal morbidity and mortality.
- If diabetes mellitus does occur, the goal of treatment becomes consistent normalization of blood glucose levels with minimum day-to-day, hour-to-hour variability. Recent studies demonstrate that keeping blood glucose levels as normal as possible as often as

possible can successfully reduce the morbidity and mortality of diabetes mellitus. This goal is accomplished by different means, each suited precisely to the individual and the type of diabetes he or she has.

- **Insulin:** Type 1 diabetics require insulin therapy. Different types of insulin with different origins and purity are available. Today, human insulin is most commonly used and is associated with the fewest side effects and complications. Insulin preparations vary in terms of time to onset of action, peak time of action, and duration of action. Insulin injections are typically given subcutaneously 1 to 4 times a day after baseline blood glucose levels are measured. With studies showing the definite advantage of more frequent insulin injections, it is recommended that individuals test their plasma glucose levels frequently and use at least 3 to 4 injections per day. More frequent testing is required if there is a change in activity or if an individual becomes ill. Other means of administration include subcutaneous insulin pumps that can be programmed to release a given amount of insulin at given times of the day. More or less than a usual amount of insulin may be programmed to be released if changes in routine (activity or diet) are planned or during times of illness. Insulin pumps have the advantage that injections need not be administered, an important consideration for all diabetics and especially children. Disadvantages to the pump involve mistakes in programming, which can cause hypoglycemia or hyperglycemia, and pump failures, which can result in death. In addition, infection is a danger with the implant, especially given the poor blood flow and compromised immune system of most diabetics. In addition, the pumps are expensive.
- The first stage of treatment for type 2 diabetics is usually the improvement of insulin sensitivity and secretion by diet, weight loss, and exercise. Studies have shown that with modification of diet and the initiation of an exercise program, many type 2 diabetics can normalize their blood sugar. If glucose normalization cannot be achieved by diet and exercise alone, or if patients cannot follow the regimen required, many type 2 diabetics benefit from oral hypoglycemic drugs. These drugs, include the sulfonylureas, which work by stimulating the beta cells of the pancreas to increase insulin secretion. They also appear to increase the sensitivity of cells to insulin. For this type of drug to work, there must be some residual insulin secretion by the pancreas. Another class of hypoglycemic drug is the biguanides, of which metformin is the most common. Metformin appears to act by inhibiting liver gluconeogenesis and by increasing insulin sensitivity. Newer drugs for type 2 diabetes work on stimulating the production of the glut-4 glucose transporters directly. By increasing the glucose transporters, these agents increase the cellular response to insulin. Specific oral hypoglycemic drugs differ in time to onset of action, time to peak onset, and

duration of action. Some are contraindicated in individuals who have renal disease. Often combinations of different types of drugs are more effective than a single drug alone.

- Type 2 diabetics, although considered noninsulin dependent, also may benefit from insulin therapy. In type 2 diabetes, release of insulin may be deficient or the insulin produced may be subtly altered to be less effective than normal. When provided with exogenous insulin, type 2 diabetics may have a more efficacious insulin than that which they naturally produce. Some studies suggest that with provision of insulin exogenously, the course of type 2 diabetes may be slowed because of the elimination of stress on the pancreatic beta cells.
- **Dietary Plans:** Dietary regimens are individually calculated, depending on growth needs, weight-loss goals (usually for type 2 diabetics), and activity levels. Distribution of calories is generally 50 to 60% from complex carbohydrates, 20% from protein, and 30% from fat. Fiber, vitamins, and minerals are included. It is especially important for children who have type 1 diabetes to ingest adequate calories and minerals to ensure optimum growth.
- **Exercise:** An exercise program coupled with weight loss has been shown to increase insulin sensitivity and to reduce the need for pharmacologic intervention. For both types of diabetes, exercise has been demonstrated to increase cellular glucose utilization, thereby reducing blood glucose levels.

  Type 1 diabetics must be careful while exercising because the exercise-induced decrease in blood glucose may precipitate hypoglycemia. This is especially true if insulin administration is not matched to the exercise regime.
- **Prevention:** For diabetic ketoacidosis, the most important aspect of care is prevention. This consists of careful monitoring of blood glucose levels and diet, especially in times of added stress or during a viral illness. If diabetic ketoacidosis occurs, it is treated with carefully administered insulin and interventions to balance fluid and electrolytes.
- **Fluid Replacement:** Hyperosmolar hyperglycemia nonketotic coma is treated with large volumes of fluid replacement and slow correction of potassium deficits. It can be prevented with good dietary control.
- **Other Pharmacologic Interventions:** Antihypertensive medications are among the pharmacologic interventions to be considered for diabetics. Antihypertensives, especially the angiotensin II converting enzyme inhibitors (ACE inhibitors), have been shown to reduce hypertension in diabetics and to delay the onset of renal disease. Even patients who do not have clinical hypertension appear to have less renal pathology when placed on ACE inhibitors.
- Pancreatic transplantation has the potential to normalize glucose homeostasis. It also appears to reverse some of the established

complications of diabetes, including improving diabetic neuropathy (but not diabetic retinopathy). Although clearly of benefit in normalizing plasma glucose levels, pancreatic transplantation carries with it the risks of surgery, the risks of rejection, and the necessity for lifelong immunosuppression.

- Recent advances in pancreatic islet cell replacement techniques have resulted in several thousand individuals worldwide treated with islet cell transplantations. This treatment offers a significant hope for a diabetes cure in the future. At present, however, only 20% or so of patients become insulin-free, and immunosuppression is required. This approach is less invasive than pancreatic transplantation.
- Preliminary experiments designed to allow for the insertion of the gene for insulin in individuals who have type I diabetes are also underway. This procedure would offer a future cure for diabetes rather than drug therapy.

Pediatric Consideration

Common childhood illnesses, especially viral infection, may precipitate ketoacidosis in a child with type 1 diabetes. A child is sometimes diagnosed for the first time as diabetic when he or she presents critically ill with ketoacidosis. Diabetic ketoacidosis, hypoglycemia, and the Somogyi effect are more common in children than adults because of especially labile glucose levels.

Treatment of a toddler or young child who has diabetes is extremely demanding and difficult for parents. Encouragement, and often counseling for the entire family, are needed. Older children and teens may rebel against strict carbohydrate control and frequent insulin injections as expressions of normal developmental stages of independence and autonomy. Providers and parents who encourage and allow the older child and teen to make as many decisions as possible regarding his or her care may be able to diffuse some of these demonstrations of independence.

Acute Pancreatitis

Acute pancreatitis is an inflammation of the pancreas characterized by autodigestion of the pancreas by pancreatic enzymes. Pancreatic cells are injured or killed, leading to areas of cell necrosis and hemorrhage. Stimulation of the immune and inflammatory systems contributes to the swelling and edema of the organ.

CAUSES OF PANCREATITIS

Pancreatitis may occur as a result of blockage of the pancreatic duct, usually caused by a gallstone in the common bile duct. Hyperlipidemia is a risk factor for the development of pancreatitis. Hyperlipidemia may overstimulate the release of pancreatic enzymes, or it may contribute to the development of gallstones. Chronic alcoholism is associated with pancreatitis, perhaps because of stimulation of pancreatic enzyme release or because of damage caused to the sphincter of Oddi at the opening of the small intestine from the common bile duct.

CLINICAL MANIFESTATIONS

- Pain, often in the epigastric area and radiating to the back, after a large meal or excess alcohol consumption is the usual presenting symptom. Pain is caused by the swelling and stretching of the pancreatic duct. Pain may be severe.
- Vomiting and nausea may accompany an attack of pancreatitis. The patient appears ill.

DIAGNOSTIC TOOLS

- Blood analysis typically demonstrates elevated levels of serum amylase and lipase.
- Hyperglycemia and hyperlipidemia are common during an acute attack.
- Increased white blood cell count occurs with the inflammation and rises further with infection.

COMPLICATIONS

- Decreased blood pressure and cardiovascular shock may develop with a severe attack as a result of the systemic release of inflammatory mediators.
- A pancreatic abscess may occur if the pancreas becomes infected. Necrosis of the tissue may be widespread. Hemorrhage, circulatory collapse, and sepsis may follow.

TREATMENT

- Withholding of food and fluids reduces pancreatic secretions.
- Fluids are given intravenously to maintain blood volume and pressure.
- Narcotics, usually meperidine (Demerol), are administered to relieve pain. Morphine, which may cause spasm of the sphincter of Oddi, is not used.

Pancreatic Cancer

Pancreatic cancer is a common cancer in the United States. The cause of pancreatic cancer is unknown, but it may develop from either exocrine or endocrine cells. Cancers of the exocrine cells of the small pancreatic ducts are most common and lead to blockage of the ducts.

These tumors frequently penetrate the pancreas and invade surrounding tissue. Metastasis via the portal vein or lymphatics is common and rapid.

CLINICAL MANIFESTATIONS

- Pancreatic cancer may be asymptomatic (until advanced) or may be associated with vague complaints of aversion to food. Pain may be an early complaint or may occur only with advanced disease.
- Advanced disease is associated with jaundice, severe pain, and pronounced weight loss. Metastases to the brain and lung are common. Mortality is nearly 100% within less than 5 years.

DIAGNOSTIC TOOLS

- Laparotomy (penetration of the abdomen with a fiber-optic tool for visualization and sampling) can confirm the diagnosis.
- Ultrasound and computed tomography (CT scan) may be used.

TREATMENT

- Surgery to relieve pain may include bypass of the blocked ducts.

Selected Bibliography

Barbosa, J., Steffes, M., Sutherland, D. E. R., et al. (1994). Effect of glycemic control on early diabetic renal lesions. *New England Journal of Medicine* 272, 600–606.

World Health Organization, DIAMOND Project Group on Epidemics (1992). Childhood Diabetes, Epidemics, and Epidemiology: An Approach for Controlling Diabetes. *American Journal of Epidemiology* 135, 803–816.

Dornhorst, A. & Rossi, M. (1998). Risk and prevention of type 2 diabetes in women with gestational diabetes. Diabetes Care, 21 Supp, B43–B49.

Estacio, R. O., Jeffers, B. W., Hiatt, W. R., et al. (1998). The effect of nisoldipine as compared with enalapril on cardiovascular events in patients with non-insulin dependent diabetes and hypertension. *New England Journal of Medicine* 338, 645–652.

Guyton, A. C. & Hall, J. (1997). *Textbook of medical physiology (9th ed.)*. Philadelphia: W.B. Saunders.

Linder, B. (1997). Improving diabetic control with a new insulin analog. *Contemporary Pediatrics* 14, 52–73.

Peters, A. L. & Schriger, D. L. (1998). The new diagnostic criteria for diabetes: the impact on management of diabetes and macrovascular risk factors. *American Journal of Medicine* 105 (1A), 15S–19S.

Peters, S. (1998). Diabetic foot ulcers. *ADVANCE for Nurse Practitioners* 6, 59–62.

Polonsky, K. S., Sturis, J., & Bell, G. I. (1996). Non-insulin-dependent diabetes mellitus—a genetically programmed failure of the beta cell to compensate for insulin resistance. *New England Journal of Medicine* 334, 777–784.

Porth, C. M. (1998). *Pathophysiology concepts of altered health states (5th ed.)*. Philadelphia: J.B. Lippincott Company.

Seaquist, E. R. (1998). Microvascular complications of diabetes. *Postgraduate Medicine* 103, 61–68.

The Expert Committee on the Diagnosis and Classification of Diabetes Mellitus. (1997). Report of the Expert Committee on the Diagnosis and Classification of Diabetes Mellitus. *Diabetes Care* 20, 1183–1197.

Thomas, P. K. (1997). Clinical features and investigation of diabetic somatic peripheral neuropathy. *Clinical Neuroscience* 4, 341–345.

Viberti, G. (1995). A glycemic threshold for diabetic complications? *New England Journal of Medicine* 332, 1293–1294.

Resources

American Diabetes Association, 1660 Duke St., Alexandria, VA 22314. Phone: (800) 232-3472.

18 THE LIVER

The liver lies in the upper right quadrant of the abdominal cavity and is the largest organ in the body. The many diverse and essential functions it performs depend on its unique blood flow system and specialized cells (Table 18-1).

● ● ●

PHYSIOLOGIC CONCEPTS

Structure

The liver is encased in a fibroelastic capsule called **Glisson's capsule** and is grossly separated into **right** and **left lobes**. Glisson's capsule contains blood vessels, lymph vessels, and nerves. The two liver lobes consist of many smaller units called **lobules**. The lobules contain the liver cells (**hepatocytes**) that line up together in plates. The hepatocytes are the functional units of the liver. Liver cells are capable of cell division and so readily reproduce when needed to replace damaged tissue.

Hepatic Blood Flow

The liver receives its blood supply from two different sources. Most liver blood flow, approximately 1000 mL/min, is venous blood draining

Table 18-1. Functions of the Liver

METABOLIC	
Absorptive Period	Converts glucose to glycogen and triglycerides, stores glycogen. Converts amino acids to fatty acids or stores amino acids. Makes lipoprotein from triglycerides and cholesterol.
Postabsorptive Period	Produces glucose from glycogen (glycogenolysis) and fatty acids and amino acids (glyconogenesis). Converts fats to ketones (accelerated if fasting). Produces urea from protein catabolism.
IMMUNOLOGIC	Macrophages filter blood.
METABOLIC TRANSFORMATION	Detoxifies or conjugates waste products, hormones, drugs.
CLOTTING FUNCTIONS	Produces several essential clotting factors.
PLASMA PROTEINS	Synthesizes albumin and other plasma proteins.
EXOCRINE FUNCTIONS	Synthesizes bile salts.
ENDOCRINE FUNCTIONS	Involved in activation of vitamin D. Produces angiotensinogen. Secretes insulin-like growth factors (somatomedin).

from the stomach, the small and large intestines, the pancreas, and the spleen. This blood comes to the liver via the portal vein. Because this is venous blood, it is poorly oxygenated, but it has a rich supply of nutrients. It may also contain intestinal bacteria and toxins. The other source of blood for the liver enters via the hepatic artery at a flow rate of approximately 500 mL/min. This is arterial blood and is highly saturated with oxygen. Both blood sources drain into the liver capillaries, called **sinusoids**. From the sinusoids, blood drains into a central vein in each lobule and from there into the hepatic vein. The hepatic vein empties into the inferior vena cava.

Hepatic Blood Pressure

In healthy individuals, there is virtually no resistance to the flow of blood in the portal vein. As a result, blood pressure in the portal venous system is low, approximately 3 mm Hg. Blood flows easily out of the liver into the vena cava as well, where pressure is nearly 0 mm Hg.

Metabolic Functions of the Liver

Metabolism refers to the cellular processes that occur when basic food molecules (sugars, amino acids, and fatty acids) are built into cell structures or energy stores, and then are broken down again later to run cell functions. The buildup of cell structures and energy stores is called **anabolism**; the breakdown is called **catabolism**. The cells of the liver are key components in the interplay between anabolism and catabolism.

GLUCOSE HANDLING BY THE LIVER

After glucose is digested and absorbed into the bloodstream, it is delivered to all cells of the body to be used as an energy source. As discussed in Chapter 17, insulin is required for glucose to gain entry to most cells. If glucose is unnecessary for immediate energy, it can be stored in cells as glycogen. The liver is especially capable of storing large amounts of glucose as glycogen. Because the liver can store glycogen, it acts as a glucose buffer for the blood. When glucose levels rise in the blood, the liver's conversion of glucose to glycogen and the storage of glycogen, increase. Glycogen formation is called **glycogenesis**. Glycogenesis occurs in the **absorptive phase of digestion**, which is the period soon after a meal when glucose levels are high. Glycogenesis is insulin dependent. By increasing the conversion and storage of glucose in times of excess, the liver returns plasma glucose levels toward normal.

In times of fasting or between meals, the breakdown of glucagon to glucose occurs in the liver, again serving to normalize circulating levels of glucose. The breakdown of glycogen is called **glycogenolysis**. In addition, when glucose levels decrease between meals, the liver initiates **gluconeogenesis** (the new formation of glucose) to keep blood glucose levels constant. Gluconeogenesis is accomplished in the liver by conversion of amino acids to glucose after deamination (removal of the amino group) and by conversion of glycerol from fatty acid breakdown to glucose. The breakdown of glycogen and the formation of glucose occur in the **postabsorptive phase of digestion**; the time between meals when external food sources are not readily available. The postabsorptive stage of digestion is under the control of the pancreatic hormone glucagon.

AMINO ACID HANDLING BY THE LIVER

After digestion, amino acids enter all cells and are converted to proteins to be used by the cells to make either enzymes or structural components such as ribosomes, collagen, muscle contractile proteins, and nuclear DNA or RNA. Although a variety of organs (including the kidney and intestinal mucosa) participate in the storage of extra amino acids as proteins, the liver is the major storage tissue for protein. When amino acids are needed, the breakdown of stored protein occurs, and free amino acids are liberated. A decrease in plasma amino acids below a certain level triggers the breakdown of stored proteins.

All cells, including liver cells, have limits on how much protein they can store. When no further amino acids can be stored as protein, the liver deaminates the extra amino acids and either uses the products as energy or changes them into glucose, glycogen, or fatty acids. These substances can be stored in the liver: glucose as glycogen and fatty acids as triglycerides (fat). Fatty acids can also be stored in other cells of the body, especially adipose tissue.

During deamination of amino acids, ammonia is released. It is almost entirely converted in the liver to urea, which is then excreted by the kidneys.

FATTY ACID HANDLING BY THE LIVER

Nearly all digested fats are absorbed into the lymphatic circulation as **chylomicrons**—conglomerates of triglycerides, phospholipids, cholesterol, and lipoprotein. The chylomicrons are delivered by the lymph to the thoracic duct where they join the systemic circulation. Triglycerides are subsequently changed back into fatty acids and glycerol by enzymes in the walls of all capillaries, especially the capillaries that serve the liver and the adipose tissue. From the capillaries, fatty acids and glycerol can diffuse into most cells.

Once inside the liver and other cells, fatty acids and glycerol again form triglycerides. Triglycerides are stored until needed during the postabsorptive stage. At this time they may be metabolized to glycerol and free fatty acids. Glycerol and fatty acids can enter the Krebs cycle to produce ATP so that cells are provided with energy. Elevations in the hormones glucagon, cortisol, growth hormone, and the catecholamines signal cells to break down stored triglycerides into free fatty acids and glycerol.

Instead of directly entering the Krebs cycle, some glycerol and free fatty acids may be used by the liver to produce new glucose. This may result in the production of ketones when triglyceride breakdown is excessive. The brain itself cannot use free fatty acids directly for energy production. Therefore, the liver's conversion of fats to glucose (gluconeogenesis) is essential for supporting the energy needs of the brain when glucose levels are low.

CHOLESTEROL HANDLING BY THE LIVER

Cholesterol is a lipid substance produced by the liver and used in the digestion of fat. During digestion, cholesterol is packaged with bile salts, phospholipids, and the triglycerides (fats) into small suspensions called micelles. Once the triglycerides are suspended as micelles, they can be digested by pancreatic enzymes and absorbed into the bloodstream. The cholesterol from the micelles is recirculated to the liver. The liver metabolizes some of the cholesterol and recycles it to be used again in digestion. The remainder is complexed with phospholipids and released into the bloodstream as **lipoproteins**. As lipoproteins, the cholesterol is carried to body cells to be used for the production of cell membranes, intracellular structures, and steroid hormones. High levels of two types of lipoproteins, low-density lipoprotein (LDL) and very low-density lipoprotein (VLDL), suggest that the liver is handling high amounts of cholesterol. These types of lipoproteins may injure cells, including the endothelial cells lining the arteries, by releasing free radicals or high-energy electrons during their metabolism. High-density lipoprotein (HDL) carries cholesterol away from cells to the liver and protects against arterial disease.

Bile Secretion

Bile is made by all hepatocytes and consists of water, bile salts, bilirubin, cholesterol, fatty acids, lecithin, and electrolytes. Except for water, the most abundant substance in bile is bile salt. Bile salts are synthesized in the liver from cholesterol that either has been delivered to the liver from the small intestines or is synthesized directly by the liver in the process of fat metabolism. All hepatic cells participate in making bile and each secretes bile into the small bile **canaliculi** that surround all liver cells. The canaliculi empty into progressively larger ducts that ultimately join into the **hepatic duct** and **common bile duct**. These ducts deliver bile either to the gallbladder for storage or into the intestine directly. Bile salts function in the digestion of fat (Chapter 16) and are normally recycled after use in the small intestine. Without bile, as much as 40% of fats in the diet would not be absorbed across the intestine and so would be lost in the stool. Fat-soluble vitamin absorption across the small intestine would be similarly affected. For example, a vitamin K deficit would occur and be apparent in less than a week. Without adequate vitamin K, blood coagulation would be impaired.

Another liver function is the handling of another component of bile, bilirubin. Bilirubin is formed as an end product of hemoglobin breakdown and must be metabolized by the liver for it to be excreted.

Metabolic Biotransformation

The liver has an important role in transforming biologic substances that may be toxic at high levels or that cannot be excreted from the body without transformation. Substances acted upon in this manner by the liver may include both those an individual ingests as well as those produced by the body itself. Examples of substances that are transformed by the liver include bilirubin, various hormones, drugs, and toxins. Metabolic biotransformation is also referred to as metabolic detoxification.

BILIRUBIN BIOTRANSFORMATION

Bilirubin is a product of red blood cell breakdown. When a red blood cell has lived out its 120-day life span, the cell membrane becomes fragile and ruptures. Hemoglobin is released and is acted upon by circulating phagocytic cells to form free bilirubin. Free bilirubin binds to plasma albumin and circulates in the bloodstream to the liver.

Free bilirubin is considered unconjugated in that, although it is bound to albumin, the binding is reversible. Once in the liver, bilirubin releases from albumin and, because free bilirubin is lipid soluble, moves easily into the hepatocytes. Once inside the hepatocytes, bilirubin is rapidly bound to another substance, usually glucuronic acid, and is now considered conjugated. Conjugated bilirubin is water soluble, not lipid soluble.

Most conjugated bilirubin is actively transported into the bile canaliculi. From there it is delivered along with the other components of bile to the gallbladder or small intestine. A small amount of conjugated bilirubin does not go to the intestine as a bile component, however, but rather is absorbed back into the bloodstream. Therefore, in the bloodstream, there is always a small amount of conjugated bilirubin present, along with unconjugated bilirubin on its way to the liver.

Once in the intestine, conjugated bilirubin is acted upon by bacteria and changed into urobilinogen. Some urobilinogen is excreted in the stool, most is excreted by the kidneys in the urine, and some is recycled back to the liver in the enterohepatic (intestinal to liver) circulation. The steps involved in the conjugation and excretion of bilirubin are shown in Figure 18-1.

The conjugation of bilirubin is essential for its excretion. Without conjugation, bilirubin cannot be excreted by either the kidneys or the intestines. The handling of bilirubin by the liver is a form of metabolic

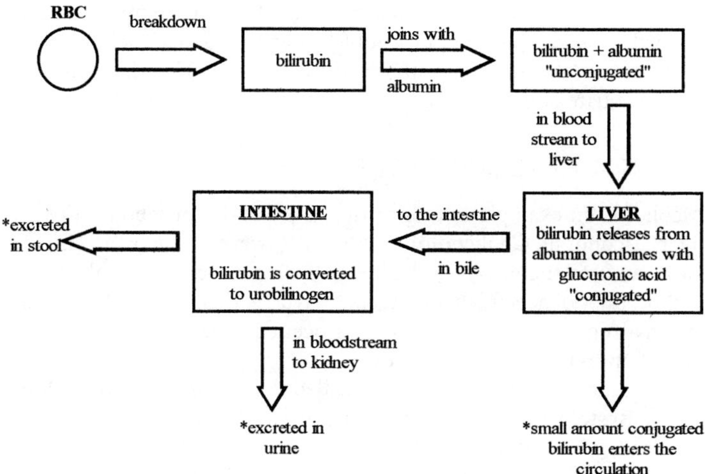

Figure 18-1. Conjugation of bilirubin.

detoxification. Without conjugation, unconjugated bilirubin would build up in the bloodstream to toxic levels.

HORMONE BIOTRANSFORMATION

The liver inactivates or modifies many hormones of the body. The liver acts on steroid hormones, including cortisol, estrogen, testosterone, progesterone, and aldosterone, to make them water soluble rather than lipid soluble, allowing them to be excreted. If this biotransformation does not occur, these hormones tend to concentrate in the body and build up in tissues, especially adipose tissue.

Other hormones such as insulin, glucagon, and antidiuretic hormone (ADH) are inactivated or deaminated by liver proteases. Thyroxine is deiodinated and inactivated. These actions allow the hormones to be excreted from the body.

AMMONIA BIOTRANSFORMATION

Ammonia is a byproduct of protein breakdown. It is transformed into urea in the liver and excreted in the urine. Without this liver function, ammonia levels build up in the blood and cause neurologic dysfunction and possibly coma and death.

DRUG AND TOXIN METABOLISM

Drugs and toxins are modified by the liver to be either inactivated or made water soluble by conjugation with another chemical compound. By these processes, the liver permits the body to excrete these substances. Without good liver function, many drugs and toxins accumulate in the body. Moreover, many of the chemical compounds used by the liver to conjugate lipid-soluble drugs and toxins, such as plasma proteins, are themselves synthesized by the liver. Therefore, they are in inadequate supply in the case of a poorly functioning liver.

ALCOHOL HANDLING BY THE LIVER

Alcohol is an example of a drug that is primarily metabolized by the liver. Alcohol metabolism follows two pathways in the liver. The first pathway uses the enzyme, alcohol dehydrogenase, and results in the end product of acetaldehyde. Acetaldehyde is then changed to acetate and hydrogen ions. These reactions occur in the cytoplasm and the mitochondria of the hepatocyte.

The second metabolic pathway, called the **microsomal ethanol oxidizing system** (MEOS) pathway, named after the specific enzymes involved, occurs in the endoplasmic reticulum of the hepatocyte and is primarily used in the liver of individuals who have a long history of alcohol abuse. This pathway results in the production of acetaldehyde and free radicals. The free radicals and the acetaldehyde produced by either metabloic pathway are highly damaging to liver cells.

The MEOS pathway is also damaging to an individual because one of the enzymes required for running this pathway, cytochrome P-450, is essential in the liver's transformation of many other toxins and drugs and excess fat-soluble vitamins. If this enzyme is preferentially used to detoxify alcohol, it is unavailable for its other roles. Thus, long-term alcohol abusers are susceptible to damage from many different toxins and drugs, and to the toxic effects of some vitamins.

Another coenzyme in alcohol metabolism is **nicotinamide adenine dinucleotide** (NAD). This coenzyme is also required for many other metabolic processes, including running the Krebs cycle to metabolize nutrients, making ATP, and allowing the liver to perform gluconeogenesis. Without NAD, hypoglycemia and lactic acid accumulation may develop. Hypoglycemia is a significant problem for many long-term alcohol abusers who typically have poor diets. Lactic acid accumulation can contribute to gout because increased lactic acid decreases the renal excretion of uric acid.

Blood Storage in the Liver

The liver is a storage organ for blood. If blood volume decreases, for example, during a hemorrhage, the liver can release blood to the circulation. Likewise, the liver can increase its blood storage if volume is significantly increased or if blood backs up in the peripheral circulation in response to a failing right heart. The amount of blood stored at any one time varies depending on an array of cardiovascular indices, but it may be as much as 400 to 500 mL.

Plasma Protein Synthesis

The liver is responsible for synthesizing plasma proteins, including albumin. The albumin concentration in the plasma is the main source of plasma osmotic pressure, the primary force causing reabsorption of fluid from the interstitial space into the capillary. If the liver is incapable of making adequate amounts of plasma proteins, osmotic pressure in the capillary will be low, and plasma filtered out at the start of the capillary will not flow back in by the time the capillary reforms to a venule. Therefore, swelling and edema of the interstitial space occurs.

Clotting Factor Synthesis

The liver functions in the production of several clotting factors, including factors I (fibrinogen), II (prothrombin), and VII (proconvertin). Without adequate production of these substances, blood clotting is impaired and bleeding may be extensive. In addition, vitamin K is a fat-soluble vitamin required for the formation of these and other clotting factors. Because bile salts are required for across-the-gut absorption of all fat-soluble vitamins, liver dysfunction resulting in decreased synthesis or supply of bile to the intestine can also lead to bleeding problems.

Immunologic Function

The many capillaries of the liver are called sinusoids. Blood flow in the sinusoids is a mixture of venous blood from the portal vein and arterial blood from the hepatic artery. The sinusoids are lined with phagocytic macrophage cells called **Kupffer's cells**. These cells remove bacteria, dead cells, and other foreign substances from the blood, especially the portal blood, perfusing the liver from the intestines.

Storage of Vitamins and Minerals

The liver has the capability to store vitamins B_{12}, D, and A. Iron is stored in the liver as ferritin. The vitamins and iron can be released to the body from the liver when circulating levels decrease.

Tests of Liver Function

Tests of liver function are frequently performed. Some of the most common ones include:

- Measurement of total bilirubin, as well as separate levels of conjugated and unconjugated bilirubin. Levels increase in various combinations with liver disease.

- Measurement of liver enzymes, including serum glutamic pyruvic transaminase (SGPT), serum glutamic oxaloacetic transaminase (SGOT), and alkaline phosphatase. Levels increase with liver disease.
- Measurement of plasma protein concentration. Levels decrease with liver disease.
- Measurement of prothrombin time (a test of coagulation). Because coagulation depends on adequate liver production of coagulation factors, prothrombin time increases with liver disease.
- Ultrasound, computed tomography (CT) scan, and magnetic resonance imaging (MRI) can indicate structural defects or stones in the bile duct or gallbladder.
- Liver biopsy allows tissues to be observed directly for signs of infection, fat or fibrosis, and cancer.

PATHOPHYSIOLOGIC CONCEPTS

Portal Hypertension

Portal hypertension is excessively high pressure in the portal vein. Normal portal venous pressure is approximately 3 mm Hg. Pressure greater then 9 to 10 mm Hg in the portal vein is considered portal hypertension. Portal hypertension develops when the resistance to blood flow into or through the liver is high.

With the development of portal hypertension, blood, which normally goes into the liver via the portal vein, begins to bypass the liver in search of alternative routes that offer less resistance to flow. This can result in collateral vessels opening from the portal vein to other lower-resistance vessels. When blood bypasses the liver, the hepatocytes cannot maintain their essential functions of biologic transformation, detoxification, and metabolism of foodstuffs. In addition, the opened collateral circulations frequently cannot handle the increased blood flow, and third spacing results (see "Third Spacing" below).

CAUSES OF PORTAL HYPERTENSION

Portal hypertension may develop if there is obstruction to flow through or out of the liver. Obstruction to flow through the liver can occur as a result of fibrosis and scarring of the liver, conditions that occur with repeated infections, or long-term liver disease such as cirrhosis. Obstruction to flow through the liver can also result from acute or chronic inflammation, because swelling and edema in the interstitial space—which occurs as part of the processes of inflammation—provide resistance to blood flow. Hepatitis is an infection of the liver that is associated with acute or chronic inflammation. Likewise, a thrombus in the portal vein itself can block blood flow through the liver. If blood flow through the liver is impeded by any cause, portal pressure increases and portal hypertension can develop.

Obstruction to flow out of the liver can occur if there is a thrombus (arterial buildup) or an embolis (blood clot) in the hepatic vein, draining the liver. Likewise, anything that blocks flow through the vena cava or into or out of the right side of the heart, including right-heart failure, cardiac myopathy, and pericarditis, can cause blood to back up into the liver, increasing the pressure in the portal venous system.

Third Spacing

Third spacing refers to fluid, primarily water, filtered from the plasma. This fluid accumulates in areas of the body other than inside cells or in the vascular system.

TYPES OF THIRD SPACING

There are two types of third spacing that occur with liver pathology: **ascites** and **interstitial edema**. Ascites is the accumulation of serous (serumlike) fluid in the peritoneal cavity. The peritoneal cavity includes the abdominal cavity and the pelvic region up to the underside of the diaphragm, excluding the kidneys. It is lined by a thin membrane called the peritoneum.

Ascites usually occurs as a result of portal hypertension. With high resistance to blood flow through the liver, blood flow is diverted to mesenteric (abdominal-peritoneal) vessels. The increased flow causes increased capillary pressure in these vessels of the abdominal cavity, resulting in net filtration of fluid out of the vessels and into the peritoneal cavity. In addition, high pressure in the liver itself causes fluid to ooze across the liver into the peritoneal cavity. This fluid is a plasma filtrate with a high concentration of albumin. The loss of albumin in ascites contributes to the depletion of plasma proteins seen with advanced liver disease. It also contributes to the decrease in plasma osmotic pressure, leading to the development of interstitial edema.

Interstitial edema occurs throughout the body with advanced liver disease. It occurs as a direct result of the loss of serum albumin in ascites and from impaired protein synthesis. If plasma protein concentration is reduced, the force favoring reabsorption of fluid into all capillaries from the interstitial space is reduced, and edema of the interstitial compartment occurs (Chapter 12).

EFFECT OF THIRD SPACING ON BLOOD PRESSURE

As a result of the accumulation of fluid in the peritoneal cavity and in the interstitial compartment throughout the body, circulating blood volume decreases. A significant decrease in blood volume can result in decreased blood pressure. When blood pressure decreases, the carotid and the aortic baroreceptors are activated (Chapter 12), leading to various reflex responses aimed at returning pressure toward normal. One of these reflex responses (Chapters 12 and 14) is an increase in the release of the hormone renin from the juxtaglomerular cells of the kidney.

REFLEX RESPONSES TO THIRD SPACING

As described in previous chapters, increased renin ultimately results in an increase in the production of the hormone angiotensin II. Angiotensin II causes constriction of arterioles throughout the body, increasing total peripheral resistance and blood pressure. Increased angiotensin II also causes increased release of the hormone aldosterone from the adrenal cortex. Aldosterone increases the reabsorption of sodium ions across the kidney tubules and back into the blood. Because ADH from the posterior pituitary is also released with a decrease in blood pressure, water follows the sodium ions back into the blood, expanding blood volume and increasing blood pressure. In fact, levels of ADH and aldosterone can become highly increased with liver disease because a poorly functioning liver is less able to inactivate these and other hormones.

With increased plasma volume, more fluid moves into the peritoneal cavity and the interstitial space, causing the ascites, swelling, and edema to increase. Eventually, hydrostatic (water) pressure in the peritoneal cavity and the interstitial space increases enough so that further filtration is opposed, and a new equilibrium of fluid pressures inside and outside of the capillaries is reached.

Portal-Systemic Venous Shunts

When portal hypertension reduces blood flow through the liver, collateral vessels, or **shunts**, open between the portal vein and the systemic veins that drain the abdominal wall, esophagus, and rectum. The shunts divert blood flow, bypassing the liver. Unfortunately, these thin-walled vessels are poorly equipped to handle such high blood flow and begin to develop into varices (distorted, swollen veins). The varices are subject to rupture and, especially in the esophagus, significant bleeding may occur. Variceal rupture can lead to a fatal hemorrhage if shunt flow is high. Rectal varices can cause painful hemorrhoids. Complicating and worsening any hemorrhage is the fact that production of many coagulation factors is decreased with liver pathology, prolonging bleeding time.

Splenomegaly

Splenomegaly is enlargement of the spleen. With portal hypertension, blood flow is diverted to the spleen via the splenic vein. Some extra blood (as much as a few hundred milliliters in an adult) can be stored in the spleen, leading to its enlargement. Because the blood stored in the spleen is unavailable to the general circulation, anemia (decreased red blood cells), thrombocytopenia (decreased platelets), and leukopenia (decreased white blood cells) can occur.

Jaundice

Jaundice is the yellowish discoloration of the skin and sclera of the eyes seen as a result of excess bilirubin in the blood (greater than 1.2 mg/dL). Bilirubin is a product of red blood cell breakdown. Jaundice is also referred to as **icterus**. There are three main types of jaundice: hemolytic jaundice, intrahepatic jaundice, and extrahepatic obstructive jaundice.

HEMOLYTIC JAUNDICE

Caused by excessive red blood cell lysis (breakdown), hemolytic jaundice is a prehepatic cause of jaundice because it occurs as a result of factors not necessarily related to the liver. Hemolytic jaundice can occur anytime red blood cell destruction is excessive and the liver cannot conjugate (and so the body cannot excrete) all the released bilirubin. It is seen with transfusion reactions and with red-cell lysis associated with faulty hemoglobin (e.g., sickle cell anemia and thalassemia). Autoimmune destruction of red cells can also lead to hemolytic jaundice.

In hemolytic jaundice of any cause, some bilirubin is conjugated. Therefore, urine and stool color are normal. Unconjugated bilirubin levels (called free bilirubin or indirect hyperbilirubinemia) are elevated.

INTRAHEPATIC JAUNDICE

Decreased hepatic uptake, conjugation, and excretion of bilirubin due to dysfunction of the hepatocytes or obstruction of the bile canaliculi are triggers of intrahepatic jaundice. Liver dysfunction can occur if the hepatocytes are infected by a virus, for instance, in hepatitis, or if the cells of the liver are damaged by cancer or cirrhosis. Some congenital disorders also affect the liver's ability to handle bilirubin. Certain drugs, including steroid hormones, some antibiotics, and the anesthetic halothane, can impair liver cell function. When the liver cannot conjugate bilirubin, unconjugated levels increase, leading to jaundice.

Intrahepatic jaundice caused by obstruction of the small bile canaliculi can occur with a hepatic tumor or stone, or it may result from widespread inflammation. Although the hepatocytes do conjugate bilirubin, obstruction in the canaliculi reduces the passage of the conjugated bilirubin into the bile duct. This obstruction results in an increase in the amount of conjugated bilirubin that enters the bloodstream. Depending on the degree of obstruction, stools may be pale or nearly normal in color. The urine is dark and frothy because large amounts of bilirubin are excreted by way of this route.

EXTRAHEPATIC OBSTRUCTIVE JAUNDICE

Blockage of bile flow through the bile duct also leads to obstructive jaundice. Extrahepatic obstruction can occur if the bile duct is blocked by gallstones or by a tumor. In this case, the liver continues to conjugate bilirubin, but the bilirubin cannot reach the small intestine. The result is reduced or absent stool excretion of urobilinogen, causing clay-colored stools. The conjugated bilirubin enters the bloodstream and much is excreted by the kidneys, giving the urine a dark, frothy appearance. If the obstruction is unrelieved, the bile canaliculi in the liver eventually become congested and rupture, spilling the bile into the lymph and the bloodstream.

Cirrhosis

Diffuse liver scarring and fibrosis characterize cirrhosis. Normal liver tissue is replaced by hard fibrous nodules and constrictive, fibrous bands encircle the hepatocytes. Normal liver architecture and function are disrupted.

Cirrhosis occurs in the liver in response to repeated incidents of cellular injury and the resultant inflammatory reactions. Causes of cirrhosis include infections, such as hepatitis; bile duct obstruction, leading to bile buildup in the canaliculi, and the subsequent rupture of the canaliculi; and toxin-induced injury to the hepatocytes. Alcohol is the toxin most often implicated in causing injury and inflammation in the liver.

Hepatitis

Hepatitis is the inflammation of the liver. It can be caused by an infection or by toxins, including alcohol, and is seen with hepatic cancer. Signs and symptoms for each type of hepatitis are similar. Modes of transmission, if the cause is viral, and eventual outcomes may be different.

CONDITIONS OF DISEASE OR INJURY

Physiologic Jaundice

A significant example of hemolytic jaundice is jaundice seen in the newborn, called physiologic jaundice. This condition is especially prevalent in premature infants. It occurs because of the increased breakdown of fetal hemoglobin in the first few days after birth and the immaturity of the liver at birth (especially in premature infants). Levels of unconjugated bilirubin build up in the blood, and because unconjugated bilirubin cannot be excreted in the urine, jaundice develops. It is more common in breast-fed infants, and indeed, jaundice caused by breast-feeding may be a normal occurrence in the healthy infant.

CLINICAL MANIFESTATIONS

Development of jaundice, which peaks approximately 4 days after birth. Unconjugated bilirubin levels usually subside on their own within 1 week. Jaundice caused only by breast-feeding may occur 3 to 4 weeks after birth.

DIAGNOSTIC TOOLS

- Peak bilirubin levels may reach 12 mg/dL, compared with normal levels of approximately 0.5 mg/dL.

COMPLICATIONS

- Brain damage from even higher levels of unconjugated bilirubin, called **kernicterus**, may rarely occur (see below in "Hemolytic Disease of the Newborn").

TREATMENT

- Infants who have hyperbilirubinemia are treated with phototherapy if the condition is mild. Phototherapy involves exposing an infant to fluorescent light in the visible spectrum (between 420- and 470-nm wavelength) for extended periods (usually 1–3 days). This wavelength of light causes unconjugated bilirubin to be converted to a more water-soluble form which, like conjugated bilirubin, can be excreted in the urine and feces.
- Breast-feeding jaundice need not be treated.

Hemolytic Disease of the Newborn

Hemolytic disease of the newborn is a more serious type of jaundice that appears at birth. This disease may result from either red blood cell ABO or Rh incompatibility between the infant and the mother; ABO incompatibility is more common; Rh factor incompatibiity is more serious. In Rh incompatibility, a mother who does not possess the Rh antigen (Rh-negative) on her red blood cells makes antibodies against that antigen after being exposed to it, usually after repeated pregnancies. An Rh-negative woman could be exposed to the Rh antigen if the father of her children were Rh-positive and her fetuses carried that trait. With significant maternal antibody produced against fetal red blood cells, excessive lysis of the fetal cells can occur. Lysis of red blood cells leads to the release of bilirubin as well as agglutination (clumping) of the cells. This can occur before or during birth, overloading the already reduced capacity of the infant's liver to conjugate bilirubin (see Chapter 6).

CLINICAL MANIFESTATIONS

- Hemolytic disease of the newborn may be mild or severe, depending on the degree of maternal antibodies and the extent of infant red-cell lysis. If the disease is mild, the skin is moderately pale and the liver may be slightly enlarged.

- With severe disease, obvious jaundice, hepatomegaly, and splenomegaly are present. In addition, the classic symptoms of anemia, including increased heart rate and respiratory rates, are present.

DIAGNOSTIC TOOLS

- With pronounced disease, blood analysis demonstrates severe anemia and high levels of unconjugated bilirubin.
- An indirect Coombs' test measuring maternal antibodies to the Rh antigen is positive, demonstrating the mother has been exposed to the antigen.
- A direct Coombs' test measuring maternal antibodies actually bound to fetal or newborn red cells confirms hemolytic disease.

COMPLICATIONS

- If unconjugated bilirubin levels reach 25 to 30 mg/dL, infants may develop **kernicterus**. Kernicterus is a complex of neurologic symptoms related to high levels of unconjugated bilirubin crossing the neonatal blood-brain barrier and gaining access to the infant's central nervous system. Neurologic symptoms include behavioral changes and lethargy. If the condition persists or worsens, tremors, hearing loss, seizures, and death can occur. Even survivors, if severely affected, may be mentally retarded, deaf, or seizure prone.
- With high levels of maternal antibodies, the fetus may die *in utero* of a condition called **hydrops fetalis**. Hydrops fetalis is characterized by gross edema of the entire fetus.

TREATMENT

- For mild cases, phototherapy may successfully treat the disease.
- In cases of moderate or severe hyperbilirubinemia, infants are treated with exchange blood transfusions. Exchange blood transfusions involve transfusing the infant with Rh-positive blood containing no Rh antibody. Transfusions are continued until twice the baby's blood volume has been replaced and the bilirubin levels are decreased. This treatment also resolves the anemia. Some Rh-positive fetuses at risk of dying *in utero* may be treated before birth with transfusions of red blood cells.
- The most important aspect of treatment of hemolytic disease of the newborn is prevention of the disease by identification of mothers at risk of developing Rh antibodies. These are Rh-negative women who are carrying a child by an Rh-positive father. It is now possible to administer a concentrated form of Rh-positive antibody, called Rh immune globulin, or RhoGAM, to women at risk. RhoGAM binds any Rh-positive antigen that gains entrance to the mother's bloodstream, thereby taking the antigen out of circulation before the mother develops her own permanent antibodies against it. Administration of RhoGAM produces a temporary, passive immunity to the Rh antigen in the mother. RhoGAM is typically given to

women at 7 months' gestation if Rh incompatibility is suspected. Within 72 hours of delivery of an Rh-positive infant to an Rh-negative mother, RhoGAM is again administered to the mother to protect future pregnancies. RhoGAM cannot remove antibodies to the Rh antigens if the mother has already produced them in previously untreated pregnancies (including miscarriages and abortions), but it might reduce the extent of new antibody production.

Alcoholic Cirrhosis

Also called Laënnec's cirrhosis, alcoholic cirrhosis occurs after years of alcohol abuse. The end products of alcohol digestion, especially the end products produced in the liver of a chronic alcohol abuser, are toxic to hepatocytes. Poor nutrition, commonly seen in this type of patient as well, also contributes to liver damage, perhaps by overstimulating the liver to undergo gluconeogenesis and protein metabolism. Alcoholic cirrhosis has three stages.

Fatty liver disease is the first stage. It is a reversible condition characterized by triglyceride accumulation in the hepatocytes. Alcohol may cause triglycerides to accumulate in the liver by acting as fuel for energy production such that cells use alcohol and fatty acids are no longer needed. Alcohol end products, especially acetaldehyde, also interfere with the oxidative phosphorylation of fatty acids by the hepatocyte mitochondria, causing trapping of fatty acids inside the hepatocytes. In this first stage of cirrhosis, fatty infiltration of the liver is reversible if alcohol ingestion stops.

Alcoholic hepatitis is the second stage of alcoholic cirrhosis. Hepatitis is the inflammation of liver cells. Inflammation and subsequent necrosis of some cells usually occurs after a serious increase in alcohol intake in long-term alcohol abusers. Damage to the hepatocytes probably occurs as a result of the cellular toxicity of the end products of alcohol metabolism, especially acetaldehyde and hydrogen ion. This stage also may be reversible if alcohol intake stops.

Cirrhosis itself is the final, irreversible stage of alcoholic cirrhosis. In this stage, dead liver cells are replaced by scar tissue. Fibrous bands develop from the chronic activation of inflammatory responses and encircle and entwine between the remaining hepatocytes. The chronic inflammation results in substantial interstitial swelling and edema, which can collapse small blood vessels and cause increased resistance to blood flow through the liver, resulting in portal hypertension and ascites. Esophageal, rectal, and abdominal varices are common, and hepatocellular jaundice is apparent. Resistance to flow through the liver progressively increases and liver function further deteriorates.

CLINICAL MANIFESTATIONS

- Early stages of cirrhosis may cause no specific symptoms, but hepatomegaly may be present.

- With continued progression, vague abdominal discomfort, anorexia, and nausea may occur. Fatigue is common. Edema, ascites, and jaundice begin.
- With advanced cirrhosis, manifestations of liver failure may appear.

DIAGNOSTIC TOOLS

- Liver function tests are altered with all stages of alcoholic cirrhosis except fatty liver.
- Elevated bilirubin levels are present.
- Prolonged prothrombin time as a result of decreased coagulation factors.
- Liver biopsy verifies cirrhosis.

COMPLICATONS

- Liver failure may develop.

TREATMENT

- A diet with adequate nutrition is recommended to reduce the metabolic load on the liver.
- Cessation of alcohol ingestion is essential.
- Rest is recommended.
- Management of complications of liver failure if required.

Viral Hepatitis

The viruses that cause hepatitis can lead to hepatocyte injury and death by directly killing the cells as well as by stimulating inflammatory and immune reactions that secondarily injure or destroy the hepatocytes. The inflammatory reactions involve mast-cell degranulation and histamine release, cytokine production, complement activation, lysis of infected and neighboring cells, and edema and swelling of the interstitium. A later-occurring immune response supports the inflammatory responses. Further stimulation of complement and cell lysis and direct antibody attack against the viral antigens cause destruction of infected cells. The liver becomes edematous, collapsing capillaries and decreasing blood flow, leading to tissue hypoxia. Scarring and fibrosis of the liver can result.

TYPES OF HEPATITIS

Several viruses have been identified that are known to infect hepatocytes. Those most common include hepatitis A, B, C, D, and E (Table 18-2). Other hepatitis viruses also have been identified, with new strains likely to become recognized in the future.

Hepatitis A (HAV) was formerly called infectious hepatitis. It is primarily passed by oral-fecal contamination resulting from poor hygiene or contaminated food. Individuals living in close quarters where

Table 18-2. Currently Identified Hepatitis Viruses

TYPE	TRANSMISSION	PROGNOSIS	DIAGNOSIS
Hepatitis A	Oral or fecal.	Usually self-limiting.	Hepatitis-A antibody; IgM (early), IgG (later)
Hepatitis B	Bloodborne, especially maternal to child. Also sexual transmission.	Usually self-limiting. 10% may become chronic or fulminating.	Hepatitis-B surface antigen (HbsAg) and core antigen (HBeAg) followed by antibody against hepatitis B surface (HbsAb) and core (HbeAb) antigens.
Hepatitis C	Bloodborne (low rate sexual transmission).	50% may become chronic infection.	Hepatitis-C antibody.
Hepatitis D	Bloodborne. Coinfects with Hepatitis B only.	Increases the likelihood of Hepatitis B progression.	Hepatitis-D antigen, Hepatitis-D antibody.
Hepatitis E	Contaminated water, oral or fecal.	Usually self-limiting, but high mortality in pregnant women.	Measurement of Hepatitis-E virus.

hygiene may be inadequate, such as day care centers, mental institutions, prisons, and homeless shelters, are at risk of developing the disease. The virus may occasionally be passed in the blood. In some countries, HAV infection is endemic.

The time between exposure and onset of symptoms (incubation period) for HAV is between 4 and 6 weeks. Individuals who have the disease may be contagious for as long as 2 weeks before symptoms appear. Antibodies against the hepatitis A virus are present with the onset of symptoms. The disease usually runs its course within approximately 4 months after exposure. No carrier state in which an individual remains contagious for an extended period after the acute illness develops, nor does a fulminating condition occur after the acute illness. Acute HAV infection in patients who have chronic hepatitis C (HCV) may worsen the progression of that disease.

Hepatitis B (HBV) is sometimes called serum hepatitis. It is a serious disease throughout the world, with over 300 million people suffering from chronic infection. In some countries, notably Southeast Asia, China, and Africa, HBV is endemic, with more than one-half of the population infected at some point in their lives, and more than 8% chronic carriers of the virus. In countries with high rates of HBV, transmission usually occurs either by way of mother to infant before or during birth or from one child to another in early childhood. In countries with low levels of infection, including the United States, transmission is usually through sexual transmission or blood exposure in young adults. Infants are less commonly infected in countries such as the United States because of widespread vaccination of all newborn infants, as described in "Pediatric Consideration" below. Others at high risk of developing HBV are injection drug users, health care workers, and non-monogomous sexually active heterosexuals and homosexuals. Teenagers are demonstrating high rates of HBV, frequently contracted through sexual exposure. A public health campaign to immunize teens and school-aged children in the United States is underway. Transmission during tattooing and body piercing may also occur.

HBV has a long incubation period, between 1 and 7 months with average onset of 1 to 2 months. The acute stage of an active infection may last up to 2 months. Approximately 5 to 10% of adults with HBV develop chronic hepatitis and continue to experience hepatic inflammation for longer than 6 months. Chronic hepatitis may be slowly progressive or may be fulminant, leading to hepatic necrosis, cirrhosis, liver failure, and death. An individual infected with HBV might also develop a persistent carrier state, causing him or her to be contagious without demonstrating symptoms. Especially likely to become chronic carriers are those infected during infancy and those who are immunosuppressed.

The HBV virus is a double-stranded DNA virus, called a Dane particle. It has a number of well-described surface and viral core antigens that can be identified in the labortory from a blood sample. The antigen that is usually produced first by infected hepatocytes is a surface antigen on the viral coat labeled HBsAg. Identification of this antigen or the hepatitis DNA itself in the serum is diagnostic of active infection with HBV. Blood donations are routinely screened for the presence of HBV antigens.

In response to the different viral antigens, several different antibodies develop in individuals in a predictable sequence, beginning from the acute stage of illness until the beginning of recovery. Some forms of antibody to HBV last throughout the lifetime of an individual who has recovered from the disease. If one continues to harbor the HBV as shown by continual expression of HBsAg, the person is likely suffering from chronic hepatitis. With chronic hepatitis, no antibody to HBsAg is detectable.

HCV, previously called non-A, non-B hepatitis, was identified in 1989. This RNA virus is passed in the same manner as HBV and has especially entered the United States population through blood transfusions before screening was available. In addition, soldiers and other personnel who served in the Vietnam War have an increased incidence of infection compared with those who did not serve in Southeast Asia. Many of those infected at that time are only now finding out they have the disease. Others who have confirmed infection have no knowledge of infection and no medical or social history indicative of high risk. On the other hand, although the virus is present in semen and vaginal secretions, it is uncommon for long-term sexual partners of HCV carriers to become infected with the virus, although individuals who have multiple sexual partners or who engage in high risk behaviors may be more likely to become infected. Although antibody to HCV now can be measured in donated blood, it is difficult to eliminate HCV totally from the commercial blood supply because there is a considerable time lapse between when an individual who has the disease is contagious and when he or she begins to express antibodies.

Hepatitis D (HDV) is called the delta hepatitis agent and is actually a defective virus that cannot on its own infect the hepatocyte to cause hepatitis. Instead, it coinfects with HBV, leading to a worsening of the HBV infection. Infection with HDV might also develop later in an individual who has mild chronic HBV. The delta agent increases the risk of developing fulminating hepatitis, liver failure, and death. HDV is passed similarly to HBV. HDV antigen and antibodies can be tested in blood donations.

Hepatitis E (HEV) was identified in 1990. It is an RNA virus primarily transmitted by ingestion of contaminated water. Most reported cases have been in developing countries. It neither results in a carrier state nor causes chronic hepatitis. However, fulminating disease leading to liver failure and death have occurred. Currently, there is no test for HEV.

CLINICAL MANIFESTATIONS

Clinical manifestations of viral hepatitis can range from asymptomatic to profound illness, hepatic failure, and death. There are three stages of illness for all types of hepatitis: the prodromal stage, the icterus (jaundice) stage, and the convalescent (recovery) period.

The prodromal stage, called the preicterus period, begins after the viral incubation period end and the person begins to have signs of illness. This stage is preicterus because jaundice (icterus) has not yet developed. An individual is highly infectious at this time. Antibodies to the virus are not usually present. This stage lasts 1 to 2 weeks. It is characterized by

- general malaise
- fatigue
- symptoms of upper respiratory tract infection
- myalgia (muscle pain)
- an aversion to most foods

The icterus or jaundice stage is the second stage of viral hepatitis, and it may last 2 to 3 weeks or much longer. It is characterized in most people, as its name suggests, with the development of jaundice. Other manifestations include

- worsening of all symptoms present during the prodromal stage
- hepatic tenderness and enlargement
- splenomegaly
- possible itchiness (pruritis) of the skin

The recovery stage is the third stage of viral hepatitis and usually happens within 4 months for HBV and HCV and within 2 to 3 months for HAV. During this period

- symptoms subside, including jaundice,
- appetite returns.

DIAGNOSTIC TOOLS

- Liver enzymes are abnormal, beginning in the prodromal stage.
- Antibodies to the virus are elevated, starting in the icterus stage. Some antibody levels subside during the recovery stage; others remain elevated for years.

COMPLICATIONS

- A complication of hepatitis is the development of chronic hepatitis that occurs when individuals continue to report symptoms and viral antigens persist for more than 6 months. Symptoms of chronic active or fulminating hepatitis may include those of liver failure, with death occurring anywhere from 1 week to several years later.

Individuals who are immunocompromised have poorer outcomes.
- Individuals infected with HBV and HCV are at increased risk of developing cirrhosis, liver cancer, and death.

TREATMENT

- Treatment for viral hepatitis is mainly supportive and includes rest as needed.
- Patients who have hepatitis should avoid consumption of alcohol. Alcohol worsens the degree and accelerates the progression of HBV and especially, HCV. Alcohol use in patients who have HCV increases the risk of hepatocellular carcinoma and decreases the response to treatment.
- Individuals with hepatitis should be educated concerning modes of transmission to sexual partners and family members.
- Injections of interferon alpha, a potent cytokine, have been used to treat both HBV and HBC. The efficacy of interferon alpha for either disease is variable. Even in individuals who do show improvement in liver profile with treatment, it is still questionable as to whether the relief is permanent or temporary, with sustained disappearance of HCV occurring in only 10 to 15% of patients. Combination therapy with other antiviral medications, including ribavirin, may increase the sustained response to treatment. The optimum dosing schedule for interferon alpha is unclear at present and dose-limiting side effects restrict its use. Other drug therapies are currently under investigation as well.
- Relatives of individuals diagnosed with hepatitis are offered a purified gamma globulin specific against HAV or HBV, which may offer passive immunity against infection. This is a temporary immunity.
- A vaccine against HAV is available. This vaccine is made from inactivated hepatitis virus. Studies have shown that it is 96% effective after one dose.
- A vaccine against HBV is also available. Given the highly contagious nature of the virus and its potentially deadly effects, it is strongly recommended that all individuals in high-risk categories, including all health care workers or others exposed to blood products, be vaccinated. It is also recommended that other individuals at high risk for becoming infected by the virus, including homosexuals and heterosexuals sexually active with more than one partner and injection drug users, be vaccinated as well. Recently, concerns have arisen that HBV vaccination of adults may increase the risk of certain collagen disorders, including systemic lupus erythematous (SLE) and rheumatoid arthritis. Research is ongoing in this area, but it may be prudent to individualize risk of disease before vaccinating adults.
- For infants, there does not appear to be any adverse effects of vaccination, and in many countries, a series of three HBV vaccinations is begun soon after birth. This has resulted in a drastic decrease in the

transmission of virus from mother to child and a corresponding decrease in chronic HBV infection and worldwide liver cancer in children.

- Vaccination against HBV is produced by way of recombinant DNA administered intramuscularly three times at predetermined intervals. The first and second doses are given 1 month apart, and the third dose is given 2 to 6 months after the second. It is 85% effective in producing immunity. Individuals who do not show immunity after three doses, as evidenced by negative HBV antibody titers, are revaccinated. After a third or fourth vaccination, most individuals respond.

Pediatric Consideration

Especially at risk of developing HAV are toddlers and children who have poor toilet hygiene and children who are cared for by individuals (in day care centers or at home) who do not follow rigorous handwashing practices after diaper changing.

Especially at risk of developing HBV are infants born to mothers who have HBV. The virus responsible for HBV may pass from mother to fetus through the placenta if the mother becomes infected in the third trimester of pregnancy or suffers from chronic HBV infection. Exposure of an infant to infected blood before or during birth may also result in the infant developing the disease. There is a 90% risk of chronic hepatitis developing in infants infected with HBV before or during birth, making it a serious neonatal infection. Therefore, all infants, regardless of the known HBV status of the mother, are recommended to receive vaccination against HBV within 7 days of birth. Those born to mothers known to be infected are also recommended to receive the HBV immunoglobulin (gamma globulin).

Liver Failure

Liver failure is the ultimate outcome of any severe, unrelenting liver disease. Liver failure may follow years of low-grade HCV infection or may occur suddenly with the onset of fulminating HBV. Acute liver failure also may follow an overdose of acetaminophen, taken either during a suicide attempt or in inadvertently high doses by individuals using the drug for pain relief. Liver failure is a complex syndrome characterized by the impairment of many different organs and body functions. Two conditions of liver failure are hepatic encephalopathy and hepatorenal syndrome.

HEPATIC ENCEPHALOPATHY

Hepatic encephalopathy is a complex of central nervous system disorders seen in individuals suffering from liver failure. It is characterized by memory lapses and personality changes. A flapping tremor can develop. Other jerking movements and poor balance may also be present. An individual suffering from hepatic encephalopathy may ultimately lapse into a coma and die.

Hepatic encepahlopathy most likely results from the accumulation of toxins in the blood, which occurs when the liver fails to transform or detoxify adequately. A failing liver is not only unable to detoxify the blood because of poor hepatocyte function, but it receives less blood to detoxify than usual because much of the portal flow is diverted by high resistance and portal hypertension.

One of the main toxins that accumulates and is implicated in causing many of the symptoms of hepatic encephalopathy is ammonia. Ammonia is a byproduct of protein metabolism and intestinal bacterial action. An important function of the liver is to transform ammonia to urea. Unlike ammonia, urea is easily excreted by the kidneys. When the ammonia is not transformed into urea, blood levels increase and ammonia is delivered to the brain. Other substances such as hormones, drugs, and gastrointestinal toxins also accumulate in the blood with advanced liver disease and undoubtably contribute to hepatic encephalopathy.

HEPATORENAL SYNDROME

Hepatorenal syndrome refers to the occurrence of renal failure seen in association with advanced liver disease. The kidneys of individuals who have advanced liver disease frequently cease producing urine and fail to function, although the kidneys appear to be physically capable of functioning. The oliguria (decreased production of urine) usually occurs suddenly and is most commonly seen in individuals suffering from alcoholic cirrhosis or fulminating hepatitis. With hepatorenal syndrome, blood volume expands, hydrogen ion accumulates, and electrolyte balance is disturbed.

Suspected causes of functional renal failure associated with liver disease include significant variceal hemorrhage, leading to vascular collapse and shock. Shock of any type leads to a decrease in renal blood flow, which can irreversibly damage the kidney (Chapter 14). Decreased blood flow to the kidneys might also occur as a result of the peripheral vasoconstriction that occurs in response to ascites and the interstitial accumulation of fluid. Finally, the accumulation of toxins specifically damaging to the kidneys increases because the failing liver is unlikely to be performing biotransformation or detoxification adequately.

CLINICAL MANIFESTATIONS

Clinical manifestations of liver failure may be initially subtle but may become extreme as liver failure progresses:

- Jaundice from impaired ability to conjugate bilirubin.
- Abdominal pain or tenderness from inflamed liver.
- Nausea and anorexia with a profound distaste for certain foods.
- Fatigue and weight loss from deficiencies in the performance of many of the liver functions of metabolism.

- Splenomegaly.
- Ascites.
- Peripheral edema caused by a decrease in the forces favoring reabsorption of fluid into the capillary from the interstitial space, which results from a decrease in plasma protein production and a loss of albumin in ascites.
- Varices of the esophagus, rectum, and abdominal wall resulting from portal hypertension.
- Bleeding tendencies caused by thrombocytopenia (decreased levels of platelets) resulting from blood accumulation in the spleen and prolonged prothrombin time caused by impaired production of several coagulation factors.
- Petechia (small hemorrhagic spots on the skin) caused by thrombocytopenia.
- Amenorrhea in women, caused by alterations in steroid hormone production and metabolism.
- Gynecomastia (breast enlargement) in males caused by estrogen buildup as the liver fails to perform its biotransformation functions. Testosterone levels usually decrease in men, accompanied by impotence and loss of libido (sex drive).

DIAGNOSTIC TOOLS

- Altered liver function tests.
- Blood analysis demonstrates anemia owing to various small and large bleeds, sequestration of red blood cells in the spleen, and impaired production of red blood cells.
- Bleeding and clotting studies are abnormal.
- Hypoglycemia may occur because gluconeogenesis is impaired.

COMPLICATIONS

- Hepatic encephalopathy.
- Hepatorenal syndrome.
- Variceal bleeding.
- Coma and death may result.

TREATMENT

Although there is no cure for liver failure short of liver transplant, individual symptoms and clinical manifestations can be treated. Treatments are specific for various manifestations.

Ascites is treated as follows:

- Dietary restriction of salt and a potassium-sparing diuretic to increase water excretion.
- Potassium supplementation may be necessary to reverse the effects of high aldosterone.
- Measures to remove ascitic fluid to relieve discomfort may be per-

formed and include placing a shunt between the peritoneal cavity and the vena cava, or paracentesis-aspiration drainage of fluid out of the peritoneal cavity with a large-bone needle. Both of these measures increase the risk of infection, and paracentesis can cause hypotension. Neither treatment is a cure for the ascites, which returns as long as liver disease continues.

Portal hypertension is treated as follows:

- A connection or shunt between the portal vein and another systemic vein can be made to relieve the diversion of blood to the esophagus and other collateral vessels. This maneuver does not restore liver function, but it may reduce collateral flow and the complication of variceal bleeding.

Variceal bleeding is treated as follows:

- A vasoconstrictor drug may be given to decrease flow. Balloon tamponade—the insertion of a balloon catheter into the esophagus to exert pressure on the bleeding varix—may be performed. Surgical treatment to tie off the collateral vessels sprouting from the portal vein may be attempted. Vitamin K supplementation can help control bleeding.

Hepatic encephalopathy treatments are as follows:

- Ventilation and sedation to protect the airway and to reduce psychomotor agitation, and bolus injections of mannitol to reduce cerebral edema are administered. Blood glucose is closely monitored because hypoglycemia may occur with liver failure.
- Liver transplants are becoming more common for the treatment of advanced liver disease. There is variable success for this procedure, depending on the cause of liver failure and the individual patient.
- Most dietary advice is concerned with restriction of dietary protein and inclusion of high-carbohydrate sources.
- Prevention of infections and rapid treatment is important.

Liver Cancer

Primary liver cancer is uncommon in the United States. When it does occur, it is usually seen in individuals who have a history of HBV or HCV infection or who have chronic liver disease, for example, cirrhosis. Others known to be at high risk for developing liver cancer include those exposed to high levels of known carcinogens, including aflatoxins found on moldy corn or peanuts. Primary liver cancers may be of the hepatocytes themselves (hepatocellular carcinoma) or of the bile ducts (cholangiocarcinoma).

Secondary liver cancer is the result of a metastasis of cancers from areas of the body (e.g., the intestine or the pancreas) that drain into the liver through the portal vein. Both primary and secondary liver cancers themselves frequently metastasize outside the liver, especially to the heart and lungs, because hepatic drainage encounters these organs first. All types of liver cancer have poor prognoses, with only approximately 1% of afflicted individuals surviving for longer than 5 years.

CLINICAL MANIFESTATIONS

- Dull abdominal pain.
- A feeling of abdominal fullness.
- Nausea and vomiting.
- Jaundice.
- Anorexia (decreased appetite) and aversion to certain foods.
- If the tumor obstructs the bile duct, portal hypertension and ascites may develop. Jaundice worsens, and colicky pain may develop.
- Hepatomegaly.

DIAGNOSTIC TOOLS

- Elevated liver enzymes
- Elevated levels of a protein normally not present in adult serum, alpha-fetoprotein

TREATMENT

- Surgery for some tumors is possible.
- Chemotherapy.

Selected Bibliography

Agnes, S., Avolio, A. W., Foco, M., et al. (1993). Liver transplantation for fulminant liver failure: a dilemma in therapeutic approach. *Transplantation Proceedings* 25, 1867–1871.

Gross, J. B., Jr. (1998). Clinicians guide to hepatitis C. *Mayo Clinic Proceedings* 73, 355–360.

Guyton, A. C. & Hall, J. (1997). *Textbook of medical physiology (9th ed.)*. Philadelphia: W.B. Saunders.

Hoofnagle, J. H. & Di Bisceglie, A. M. (1997). The treatment of chronic viral hepatitis. *New England Journal of Medicine* 336, 347–356.

Lee, W. M. (1997). Hepatitis B virus infection. *New England Journal of Medicine* 337, 1733–1745.

Marsano, L.S. & Pena, L. R. (1998). The interaction of alcoholic liver disease and hepatitis C. *Hepato-Gastroenterology* 45, 331–339.

Porth, C. M. (1998). *Pathophysiology concepts of altered health states (5th ed.)*. Philadelphia: J.B. Lippincott Company.

Possle, M., Haag, K., Ochs, A., et al. (1994). The transjugular intrahepatic portosystemic stent-shunt procedure for variceal bleeding. *New England Journal of Medicine* 330, 165–171.

Riordan, S. M. & Williams, R. (1997). Treatment of hepatic encephalopathy. *New England Journal of Medicine* 337, 473–478.

Schiodt, F. V., Rochling, F. A., Casey, D. L., & Lee, W. M. (1997). Acetaminophen toxicity in an urban county hospital. *New England Journal of Medicine* 337, 1112–1117.

Trevilyan, J. & Carroll, P. J. (1997). Management of portal hypertension and esophageal varices in alcoholic cirrhosis. *American Family Physician* 55, 1851–1858.

Van Thiel, D. H., De Maria, N., Colantoni, A., & Idilman, R. (1998). Current and future therapies for HCV infection. What should the end point for treatment be? *Hepato-Gastroenterology* 45, 308–320.

Vento, S., Garofano, T., Rensini, C., et al. (1998). Fulminant hepatitis associated with hepatitis A virus superinfection in patients with chronic Hepatitis C. *New England Journal of Medicine* 338, 286–290.

19 THE INTEGUMENT

The integument is the skin: the largest mass of tissue in the body. The skin functions to protect and insulate underlying structures and serves as a calorie reserve. The skin mirrors our emotions and stresses, and affects how others perceive and treat us. In a lifetime, the skin may be cut, bitten, irritated, burned, or infected. The skin has enormous resilience and capacity for recovery.

• • •

PHYSIOLOGIC CONCEPTS

Structure and Function of the Skin

The skin is composed of three layers, each consisting of different cell types and serving different functions. The three layers are the **epidermis**, **dermis**, and **subcutaneous** layer. A diagram of the skin is shown in Figure 19-1.

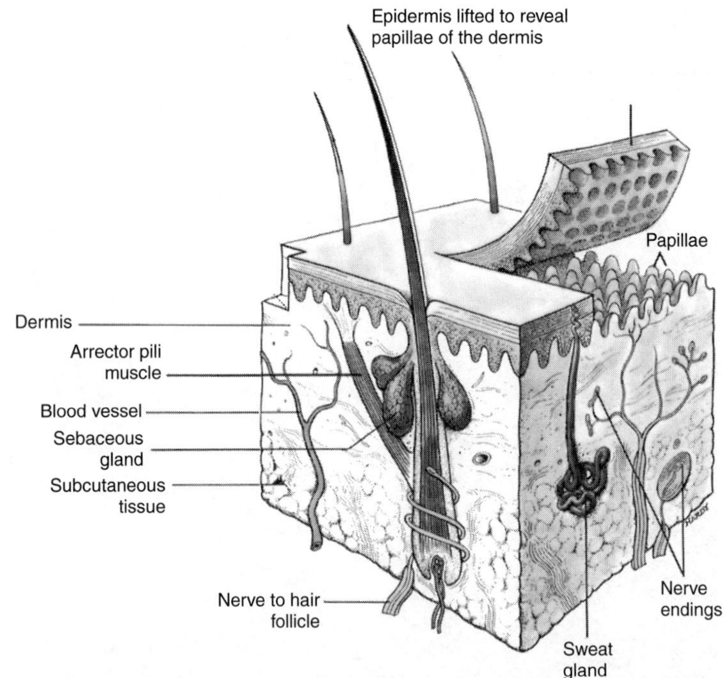

Figure 19-1. Three-dimensional view of the skin (from Porth, 1994).

EPIDERMIS

The outermost layer of the skin is the epidermis. The cells of the epidermis continually undergo mitosis and are replaced approximately every 30 days. The epidermis contains sensory receptors for touch, temperature, vibration, and pain.

The main component of the epidermis is the protein keratin, produced by cells called **keratinocytes**. Keratin is an extremely durable, tough substance that is insoluble in water. Keratin prevents loss of body water and protects the epidermis from irritants or microorganisms that cause infection. Keratin is the main component of the skin appendages: the nails and the hair.

Melanocyte cells are present at the base of the epidermis. Melanocytes synthesize and secrete melanin in response to stimulation by the anterior pituitary hormone, melanocyte-stimulating hormone. Melanin is a black pigment that disperses throughout the epidermis to protect cells from ultraviolet radiation.

Immune cells, called **Langerhans' cells**, are present throughout the epidermis. Langerhans' cells recognize foreign particles or microorganisms that enter the skin, and initiate an immune attack. Langerhans' cells may be responsible for recognizing and eliminating dysplastic or neoplastic skin cells. Langerhans' cells are physically associated with sympathetic nerves, suggesting a relation between the nervous system and the ability of the skin to fight off infection or prevent skin cancer. Stress may affect the functioning of Langerhans' cells by increasing sympathetic stimulation. Ultraviolet radiation may damage Langerhans' cells, reducing their ability to prevent cancer.

DERMIS

Lying immediately under the epidermis, the dermis is considered loose connective tissue and is composed of fibroblast cells that secrete the proteins collagen and elastin. The collagen and the elastin fibers are arranged haphazardly, giving the dermis distensibility and resilience. A gellike substance, hyaluronic acid, is secreted by the connective tissue cells. It surrounds the proteins and gives the skin elasticity and turgor (tension). Throughout the dermis are blood vessels, sensory and sympathetic nerves, lymphatic vessels, hair follicles, and sweat and sebaceous glands. Mast cells, which release histamine during injury or inflammation, and macrophages, which phagocytize dead cells and microorganisms, are also present.

Blood vessels in the dermis supply the dermis and epidermis with nutrients and oxygen and remove waste products. Dermal blood flow offers a means for the body to control its temperature. With a decrease in body temperature, sympathetic nerves to the blood vessels increase the release of norepinephrine. The release of norepinephrine causes constriction of the vessels, resulting in a conservation of body heat. If body temperature is too high, sympathetic stimulation of the dermal blood vessels is reduced, dilating the vessels and allowing for the transfer of body heat to the environment. Arteriovenous (AV) connections, called anastomoses, are present on some blood vessels. AV anastomoses facilitate skin temperature regulation by allowing blood to bypass the upper layers of the dermis in times of severe cold. Sympathetic nerves to the dermis also innervate sweat glands, sebacious (oil) glands, and hair follicles.

SUBCUTANEOUS LAYER

Lying beneath the dermis, the subcutaneous layer of the skin is composed of fat and connective tissue and acts as both a shock absorber and a heat insulator. The subcutaneous layer is a calorie reserve station as well, in that stored fat may be broken down for energy when needed.

Hair and Nails

The nails are keratinized plates that extend from the fingers and the toes. The nails protect the fingertips and most likely evolved with an original purpose of defense. The hair is hardened keratin that grows at variable rates on different parts of the body. Hair grows as a follicle shaft in a canal, beginning deep in the dermis. In addition to a hair follicle, each canal contains a sebaceous gland and a smooth muscle fiber, called an erector pili muscle. When this muscle cell is stimulated by a neuron of the sympathetic nervous system, it causes the hair to stand on end. Hair on the head may protect against sunburn.

Sebaceous Glands

The sebaceous glands accompany the hair follicles. They secrete an oily substance called sebum into the surrounding canal. Sebaceous glands are present all over the body, especially on the face, chest, and back. Testosterone increases the size of the sebaceous glands and the production of sebum. Testosterone levels increase in males and females during puberty.

Sweat Glands

There are two types of sweat glands: eccrine and apocrine. Eccrine sweat glands open directly onto the surface of the skin and are distributed over the entire body. Eccrine glands function mainly in cooling the body by means of evaporative heat loss. They are especially concentrated on the hands, feet, and forehead. Aprocrine glands are mainly located in the axillae (armpits) and in the pubic and the anal areas. Apocrine glands secrete sweat into the canals of the hair follicles. When acted upon by surface bacteria, the secretions of the apocrine glands cause the characteristic odor of perspiration.

Geriatric Consideration

As an individual ages, all three layers of the skin change. The epidermis loses its elasticity and turgor and has a reduced capacity to produce and distribute melanin. Age spots (concentrated deposits of melanin) appear. The hair and nails become thin and brittle. The hair grays as melanocytes are lost. The number of Langerhans' cells decreases, further increasing the skin's susceptibility to solar damage. Poor blood flow and decreased Langerhans' cell function increase the risk of infection. Sensory receptors are reduced in number, contributing to an increased risk of injury. Wound healing is delayed because of poor blood flow and reduced immune function. Decreased sebaceous and sweat gland functioning cause drying and wrinkling of the skin. The ability of the body to cool itself with sweating or vasodilatation or to conserve heat with vasoconstriction, is reduced. This reduced cooling ability increases the risk of hyperthermia in elderly adults exposed to prolonged elevations in temperature and of hypothermia if they are exposed to severe cold.

Vitamin D

Involved in the maintenance of serum calcium, vitamin D is a hormone obtained in the diet in an inactive form. For it to function, it must be activated by the body. The first step in vitamin D activation occurs in the skin as a result of ultraviolet radiation, after which it is further acted upon by the kidney and the liver. Vitamin D activation is increased in response to a decrease in serum calcium and results in an increased absorption of calcium across the gut and a decreased renal excretion of calcium. Because vitamin D acts as a hormone, the skin may be considered an endocrine gland.

● PATHOPHYSIOLOGIC CONCEPTS

Many different lesions occur on the skin. They are described on the basis of size, depth, color, and consistency.

Bulla

With a measurement larger than 1.0 cm and filled with watery fluid, a bulla is a large, raised area on the skin. Large blisters are bulla that can occur after a burn.

Crust

A crust is the accumulation of dried serous (serumlike) or seropurulent (pus) exudate on the skin (e.g., the crust seen on an impetigo or herpes lesion). It is usually golden in color.

Erosion

An erosion is an area on the body characterized by the loss of superficial epidermis. Typically the area is moist, but it does not bleed (e.g., the skin after bursting of a blister or vesicle).

Excoriation

An excoriation is a scratch on the skin (e.g., a skinned knee). There may be slight bleeding.

Fissure

A fissure is a linear crack in the skin, for example, that seen with athlete's foot. The fissure may be pink or red, but there is usually no bleeding.

Keloid

Defined as a scar formation on the skin that is out of proportion to the injury, a keloid is raised, red, and firm. Development of keloids is especially common in African Americans. An individual prone to keloid formation should alert a health care provider when a skin injury occurs. Removal of a keloid may worsen the scarring.

Lichenification

Thickened, roughened skin that may occur with constant irritation is known as lichenification. This condition is seen, for example, in skin with atopic dermatitis.

Macule

A macule is a flattened area of the skin, characterized by a change in color. A macule (e.g., a freckle or a flat mole [nevus]) is typically smaller than 1.0 cm in diameter.

Nodule

A nodule is a solid, elevated mass with a measurement between 1.0 cm and 2.0 cm in diameter. It is firmer in consistency than a papule and deeper in the dermis (e.g., a cyst).

Papule

A papule is a solid, elevated mass, smaller than 1.0 cm in diameter. Example of papules are an elevated mole or a wart.

Petechia

A deep red spot of pinpoint hemorrhage under the skin is called petechia. Petechiae may signify a bleeding disorder or fragility of the capillaries and may accompany serious infections as well.

Plaque

A plaque is a flat, raised surface with a measurement larger than 1.0 cm. Examples of plaque are several papules grouped together or the lesions seen with psoriasis.

Pruritus

Pruritus refers to itching of the skin. Pruritus may occur as a primary response to a surface irritant or inflammation, for example, after a mosquito bite, or with dry skin. Primary pruritus results from release of histamine during inflammation. Pruritus may occur secondarily to a systemic disease, such as liver or kidney failure. With systemic disease, metabolic toxins may accumulate in the interstitial fluid under the skin.

Purpura

A purpuric lesion is a large patch of purple discoloration under the skin associated with hemorrhage. It may result from a variety of causes, including thrombocytopenia (decreased platelets), trauma (a "black and blue mark"), or an allergic response. A purpuric lesion occurring without trauma may signal bleeding elsewhere in the body, including the brain.

Pustule

A pustule is an elevated vesicle filled with pus. Examples of this are the lesions of impetigo or acne.

Scale

A scale is a flake of epidermis. Examples of scaling are seen in dandruff or dried skin.

Scar

A scar is an area of the body where the skin has been replaced by fibrous tissue, (e.g., a burn scar). It may be thin or thick.

Tumor

A tumor is a large, solid mass that is elevated and larger than 1.0 to 2.0 cm. Tumors may be neoplastic or benign, for example, a breast cancer versus a lipoma.

Ulcer

An ulcer is an area with loss of epidermal and deeper layers of the skin, which may bleed and scar. An example of an ulcer is a decubitus ulcer (pressure sore).

Urticaria

Urticaria, also known as hives, consists of raised edematous plaques (wheals) associated with intense itching (pruritis). Urticaria results from the release of histamine during an inflammatory response to an allergen to which the individual has become sensitized. Chronic urticaria may accompany systemic disorders such as hepatitis, some cancers, or thyroid abnormality.

Vesicle

A vesicle is a small, raised area on the skin with a measurement of smaller than 1.0 cm. It is formed by the presence of serous fluid within the skin layers (e.g., a chickenpox blister).

Wheal

A wheal is a raised area of skin edema that exists only temporarily and itches (e.g., the area surrounding a mosquito bite or the skin during an occurrence of urticaria [hives]). The center of a wheal is pink or red, with a surrounding circle of paler skin.

Geriatric Consideration

The elderly frequently present with purpura and petechia, especially on the legs. Petechia and purpura in the elderly usually indicate fragility of the blood vessels or a platelet disorder. However, in some cases, they may be caused by a fall or an episode of violence. Idiopathic purpura may occur in young women.

CONDITIONS OF DISEASE OR INJURY

Contact Dermatitis

Contact dermatitis is an acute or chronic inflammation of the skin caused by exposure to an irritant (irritant dermatitis) or allergen (allergic dermatitis). The location on the skin of the dermatitis corresponds to the site of exposure. Allergic contact dermatitis occurs when Langerhans' cells process and present an allergen to nearby T cells. The T cells respond with a type IV hypersensitivity response against the allergen. The response is delayed in that it takes hours to days to be evident. In contrast, irritant dermatitis does not involve the immune system. The response is only inflammatory.

Common causes of allergic dermatitis include poison ivy or poison oak and chemicals found in jewelry. Common causes of irritant dermatitis include soaps, detergents, household cleaners, insecticides, and dusts. Some foods and spices may also cause contact dermatitis.

CLINICAL MANIFESTATIONS

- Both types of dermatitis present acutely with localized papules, erythema (redness), and oozing vesicles in an area of contact. The vesicles burst and crust. Pruritis may be intense.
- Allergic dermatitis typically presents 1 to 2 days after exposure.

DIAGNOSIS

- Dermatitis usually follows a pattern of exposure—for example, poison ivy typically travels vertically up the legs or may be present only on areas of the skin that were bare. A circle of lesions around the wrist may indicate allergy to a bracelet or watch, whereas lesions below the umbilicus may indicate an allergy to the metal of a zipper. Reddened, irritated hands may indicate an inflammatory response to dishwashing. A good history accompanying the physical pattern is the key to diagnosis.
- Allergy skin testing may be indicated.

COMPLICATIONS

- Chronic conditions may cause lichenification, fissures, and scales.
- An infection of the skin may result from repeated scratching.
- A severe response to poison ivy or another potent allergen may result in drastic reddening and swelling of the face. The eyes may be closed because of edema.

TREATMENT

- Identifying the cause of the dermatitis and avoiding exposure prevents recurrence.
- Cool compresses reduce inflammation. Oatmeal soaks or baths in other soothing chemicals may provide relief. Antihistamines may be used to reduce itching.
- Short-term topical anti-inflammatory, steroidal therapy may be used to interrupt the inflammation. For severe attacks involving the eyes and face, a burst of systemic corticosteroids often is used.

Atopic Dermatitis

Atopic dermatitis is an inflammation of the skin involving overstimulation of T lymphocytes and mast cells. Histamine from the mast cells causes itching and erythema. Scratching can cause skin breakdown. Atopic dermatitis is frequently seen in infants and children, but it may persist into adulthood. There appears to be a genetic tendency toward the disease. In addition, it is frequently seen in families with a high rate of other inflammatory disorders such as asthma or allergy.

CLINICAL MANIFESTATIONS

- Erythema with crusted or oozing lesions. In infants, lesions often appear on face and buttocks. In older children and teens, the lesions

appear more commonly on the hands and feet, behind the knees, and in the bends of the elbows.
- Pruritis is intense and leads to a continual cycle of inflammation and lesion formation.

DIAGNOSIS

- Usually accomplished by a good history and physical examination.

COMPLICATIONS

- Infection of the skin with common surface bacteria, especially *Staphylococcus aureus,* or with viruses such as herpes simplex may develop. Individuals should avoid inoculation with live, attenuated viruses.

TREATMENT

- Avoidance of known irritants or allergens.
- Antihistamines to help control itching.
- Cool compresses to reduce inflammation.
- Topical low-dose steroids to reduce inflammation and allow healing.

Acne

Acne is a common inflammatory disease of a sebaceous gland associated with a hair follicle, called the **pilosebaceous unit**. There are two types of acne: inflammatory and noninflammatory. Both types of acne are characterized by excessive sebum production. The excess sebum accumulates in the follicle, causing the follicle to swell.

In inflammatory acne, the follicle becomes blocked by the sebum and bacteria proliferate in the canal. Eventually, the follicle ruptures and the sebum and bacteria are released into the dermis, causing inflammation of the dermal tissue. In noninflammatory acne the follicle does not burst, but remains dilated. The sebum either moves to the skin surface (a blackhead) or the canal remains blocked (a whitehead).

Acne is commonly seen in teenagers and young adults, beginning with the onset of puberty. Although both boys and girls suffer from acne, it is especially severe and common in boys. Adults, especially women, may have a recurrence of acne.

CAUSES OF ACNE

Sebum production is stimulated by androgens, especially testosterone. The sharp increase in androgens seen in both girls and boys during puberty is responsible for the onset and severity of acne. Bacterial infection of the obstructed follicle can be worsened by poor hygeine, poor nutrition, and stress. Some individuals may be genetically prone to develop acne, which may be related to oversensitivity of the sebacous glands to androgen. Estrogen opposes the action of androgen on the sebacious gland and reduces the development of acne. In adult women, the development of acne may be related to other systemic conditions or may occur as the ratio of testosterone to estrogen begins to rise in the early perimenopausal years.

Acne rosacea is a condition of the skin that develops in middle-aged adults of both sexes and is characterized by redness (erythema), papules, and pustules, especially on the forehead, nose, cheeks, and chin. Although no specific cause of acne rosacea has been identified, it is associated with heightened sensitivity to the sun. The condition may come and go and is typically exacerbated by hot drinks and alcohol. It may result in hypertrophy of the sebaceous glands, with thickening of the nose (*rhinophyma*)—a permanent development. Eye irritation, including conjunctivitis, may be present.

CLINICAL MANIFESTATIONS

- Acne may present with a variety of lesions on one individual. Lesions can include blackheads, whiteheads, nodules, pustules, cysts, and scars. Lesions are commonly over the face, back, and shoulders.
- In women, acne may increase before or during the menstrual period when estrogen levels are lowest.
- With rosacea, the face may turn bright red with even limited sun exposure or alcohol, and papules and pustules may develop.

COMPLICATIONS

- Scarring may occur in severe cases of acne. Self-esteem may be affected even with less severe conditions.
- Rhinophyma may occur with rosacea.

TREATMENT

- Topical agents such as benzoyl peroxide and retinoic acid (vitamin A, Retin A) are used to dry and to peel the skin. This opens the follicles and facilitates the movement of sebum to the skin. Retin A may lead to drying and redness of the skin, and individuals using Retin A must avoid unprotected sun exposure.
- Antibacterial soap may reduce bacterial contamination of the skin.
- Topical gels combining benzoyl peroxide with an antibiotic may be prescribed for use twice a day. Treatment with this regimen typically takes at least 4 weeks to induce notable improvement.
- Oral antibiotic therapy (e.g., tetracycline) may be administered to reduce bacterial proliferation in the follicle. Antibiotic therapy requires several weeks to be effective. Tetracycline damages developing teeth, so is contraindicated in pregnant women or women planning to get pregnant. Tetracycline is also the drug of choice for rosacea.

- Birth-control pills containing estrogen can suppress sebum production. They may be used to treat acne in girls and women.
- Systemic 13-cis-retinoic acid (isotretinoin) may be administered for severe nodular cystic acne. This drug can cause severe birth defects and should not be used by young women who are or may get pregnant.

Psoriasis

Psoriasis is a chronic skin disease characterized by rapid turnover of epidermal cells, leading to abnormal proliferation of the epidermis and the dermis. Normal epidermal cell turnover is approximately 28–30 days. With psoriasis, the epidermis in affected areas may shed every 3–4 days. Rapid cell turnover results in increased metabolic rate and increased blood flow to the cells to support the metabolism. High blood flow causes erythema. The rapid turnover and proliferation lead to poorly developed and immature cells. Small trauma to the skin results in exaggerated inflammation, causing epidermis thickening and plaque formation. Psoriasis typically is established by the late 20s but may occur earlier.

CAUSES OF PSORIASIS

There appears to be a genetic tendency for the development of psoriasis, with an increased incidence among family members. Immune factors may be involved because severe disease may occur in immunocompromised individuals.

CLINICAL MANIFESTATIONS

- Well-demarcated (clear borders) erythematous plaques covered with silvery white scales, especially over knees, elbows, scalp, and in skin folds.
- Lesions typically develop insidiously, with just one or two lesions later coalescing into many. Lesions also may develop after any trauma to the skin.
- Nail pitting or separation of the nail is common.

DIAGNOSIS

- Diagnosis is made based on history and physical examination. A family history of the disease may be recalled.

COMPLICATIONS

- Severe infections of the lesions may develop.
- A deforming arthritis similar to rheumatoid arthritis, called psoriatic arthritis, occurs in approximately 5% of individuals.

TREATMENT

- Mild disease may be treated with emolients or topical steroids.
- Moderate disease may be treated with applications of tar or other drugs with or without ultraviolet light or with an antimetabolite such as methotrexate.

- Severe disease may require hospitalization and systemic steroids.
- Psoralen with ultraviolet radiation (**PUVA**) is a treatment regimen that has been available for a number of years and is highly effective. Long-term use, however, is associated with an increase in the development of squamous cell carcinoma and should be avoided in those who have a history of exposure to ionizing radiation or arsenic, which are other potentially carcinogenic agents sometimes used to treat psoriasis. Individuals using PUVA should be screened regularly for skin cancer.
- The use of vitamin D_3 analogs has recently been approved for psoriasis. Vitamin D_3 analogs appear to inhibit various aspects of cutaneous inflammation and epidermal proliferation. Treatment also leads to more normal keritinization of the skin. Vitamin D_3 analogs are frequently used as adjunct therapy with topical corticosteroids, PUVA, or other medications.

Geriatric Consideration

The prevalence of psoriasis increases with age, making it a common disorder of the elderly. Because of the changes in renal and hepatic clearance rates in the elderly, there is an increased risk of adverse drug side effects in this population. Many elderly patients are also on other medications, increasing the risk of drug interactions as well.

Viral Rashes

A variety of viral infections may present with a skin rash. Many of these rashes are most common during childhood (Table 19-1) but may occur at any time.

RUBEOLA

Rubeola, also called 10-day or red measles, is an upper respiratory tract infection caused by the paramyxovirus. Rubeola is usually seen in children and is passed person to person by way of inspired droplets. It has a 7 to 12–day asymptomatic incubation period before signs of the disease appear and is highly contagious. Active disease is characterized by early symptoms (prodromal) followed by a rash.

CLINICAL MANIFESTATIONS

- Prodromal symptoms include high fever, barking cough, runny nose, and enlargement of lymph nodes.
- Active infection is characterized by Koplik's spots over the buccal (cheek) mucosa. Koplik's spots are pinpoint white spots surrounded by a red ring.
- A maculopapular rash with erythema, beginning on approximately day 3 or 4, is another manifestation. The rash starts on the face, spreads to the trunk, and finally the extremities. The rash lasts approximately 4 days.

Table 19-1. Common Childhood Rashes

INFECTION	CAUSATIVE AGENT	CHARACTERISTIC OF THE RASH	COMPLICATIONS
Rubella (3-day measles)	Rubella virus	Diffuse, red pink macular rash beginning on face and trunk, spreading to extremities.	Congenital rubella syndrome, if contacted by mother during pregnancy.
Rubeola (10-day measles)	Paramyxovirus	Erythematous macular-papular rash, beginning on face, moving to trunk and extremities; Koplick's spots (pinpoint white) in mouth 1–3 days before rash.	Measles encephalitis; secondary bacterial infection, including otitis and pneumonia.
Roseola	Herpes virus-6	High fever followed approximately 3 days later by a erythematous, macular rash, especially on the trunk.	Unusual
Chicken Pox	Herpes varicella-zoster	Macules, vesicles, and scabbings present at the same time. Intense itching.	Varicella pneumonia, secondary bacterial infection, joint pain. Mothers infected during first trimester of pregnancy may suffer loss or congenital deformity of the fetus. Newborns infected at birth may have serious morbidity or mortality. Adults infected may become severely ill.
Scarlet Fever	Type A beta hemolytic streptococcus	Sandpaperlike erythematous macular-papular rash	Poststreptococcal glomerularnephritis, rheumatic fever.

DIAGNOSIS

- Diagnosis is usually made by history and physical examination.

COMPLICATIONS

- Measles encephalitis is a common complication of rubeola. It may be caused by the measles virus, or it may be a secondary bacterial infection. Recovery is usually complete, but lasting brain damage and death might occur.
- Pneumonia may occur after measles.

TREATMENT

- Primary treatment is prevention by vaccination with a live attenuated virus at 15 months after birth. A booster is usually administered at 4 to 5 years, and sometimes in the teen years.
- Treatment of measles infection is supportive and may involve antibiotics if a secondary bacterial infection develops.

RUBELLA

Rubella, also called German or 3-day measles, is a viral infection of the respiratory tract caused by the rubella virus. There is a 14 to 21–day incubation period after infection, followed by prodromal symptoms lasting 1 to 4 days. A rash then develops. Rubella is very contagious during the prodromal stage, but it may not be contagious once a rash develops.

CLINICAL MANIFESTATIONS

- Prodromal stage is characterized by low-grade fever, malaise, lymph node enlargement (especially postauricular), sore throat, and headache.
- Active infection is characterized by a diffuse maculopapular rash, which begins on the trunk and spreads to the extremities. The rash lasts for approximately 2 to 3 days.

DIAGNOSIS

- Diagnosis is made by history and physical examination.

COMPLICATIONS

- Infection in a pregnant woman, especially during the first trimester, may cause severe birth defects in her infant.

TREATMENT

- Primary treatment is prevention by vaccination with a live, attenuated virus at 15 months, 4 to 5 years, and sometimes in the teen years. The vaccine is a combination vaccine for rubeola, rubella, and mumps.

- All women of childbearing age should be tested for the presence of antibodies against rubella (a rubella titer test). A woman who is antibody negative (has never had rubella or been adequately vaccinated against it) should be vaccinated against the virus. After vaccination, a woman is advised to wait at least 3 months before becoming pregnant.
- Treatment of rubella infection is supportive.

Pediatric Consideration

Rubella is a strong teratrogenic agent (one that causes birth defects) and is most highly contagious before an individual develops obvious signs of infection. To protect pregnant women from infection and subsequent injury to a developing fetus, it is imperative that all children be vaccinated against the virus during early childhood. This protects any pregnant woman with whom they may come in contact.

ROSEOLA INFANTUM

Roseola is a common infection of infants between the ages of 6 months and 2 years, although children as old as 4 years may also develop the infection. Roseola is presumably viral in origin and is characterized by a sudden onset of high fever (38.9°C to 40.5°C), in an otherwise well child, lasting 3 to 5 days. After this time, a rash develops, especially over the trunk.

CLINICAL MANIFESTATIONS

- Sudden, high fever in an otherwise apparently well child, followed 3 to 5 days later by a red, lacy, macular rash over the trunk and neck.

DIAGNOSIS

- Diagnosis is made by history and physical examination. Typically, there is no lymph node enlargement (adenopathy).

TREATMENT

- Reassurance is usually the only treatment required. Fever medication may be used.

HERPES SIMPLEX 1 AND 2

The herpesviruses include herpes simplex 1 and 2. Herpesviruses cause characteristic skin and mucous membrane lesions and are passed by viral shedding from the lesions. The incubation period for both viruses is approximately 2 to 24 days after infection. A prodromal period often precedes the appearance of lesions. During the prodromal period and the time of open lesions, the virus is contagious. This may include a 2- to 6-week period. After an initial infection, the virus may lay dormant in the sensory nerve tract innervating the primary lesion. The dormant virus may become active again at any time, causing the reappearance of lesions. Reactivation of a latent herpes infection may occur with illness, stress, excessive sun exposure, or at certain times of the menstrual cycle.

Herpes simplex 2 is typically a genital or anal infection, whereas herpes simplex 1 is usually responsible for cold sores on the face. Either virus, however, is capable of infecting any site on the body. Herpes simplex 2 is considered a sexually transmitted disease.

CLINICAL MANIFESTATIONS

- Symptoms during the prodromal stage may include low-grade fever, malaise, and a burning or itching on mouth or genitals.
- With active infection, clusters of painful vesicles erupt on lips, face, skin, nose, oral mucosa, genitalia, or anus. The vesicles may burn and itch. The vesicles rupture within 3 to 4 days and crust over. They usually disappear within the next week.

DIAGNOSIS

- Diagnosis is made by history and physical examination, although a culture of the cells may be used to confirm a suspected outbreak.

COMPLICATIONS

- Secondary bacterial infection of the vesicles may develop.
- Herpes simplex 1 may infect the eye, causing blindness (keratoconjunctivitis).
- A primary herpes simplex 2 infection during pregnancy may cause damage to the fetal central nervous system, including blindness and mental retardation. Risk to the fetus is especially high if the pregnant woman is exposed to the virus for the first time late in her pregnancy.
- Neonatal infection by the virus may occur with an ascending vaginal or cervical infection during the pregnancy or during passage of the newborn through an infected birth canal.

TREATMENT

- Oral or topical treatment with an antiviral drug (acyclovir, zamcyclovir), may reduce the frequency, duration, and intensity of the lesions.
- Cesarean section is performed if active genital herpes infection is present or if there is suspicion that the pregnant woman is in the prodromal stage.

CHICKENPOX AND SHINGLES

Chickenpox (**varicella**) and shingles (**zoster**) are infections caused by another herpesvirus, the varicella-zoster virus. Infection by the varicella-zoster virus causes the development of pruritic, fluid-filled vesicles on the skin.

Chickenpox is the primary infection by the virus. Chickenpox is highly contagious and is passed person to person by way of respiratory droplets. Chickenpox is usually an illness of childhood, but adults exposed to the virus for the first time may develop the disease. The varicella virus has an incubation period of 7 to 21 days and is contagious during a brief prodromal period (approximately 24 hours before lesions appear) and until all lesions are crusted over. The disease is usually self-limiting and resolves within 7 to 14 days.

Shingles usually occurs years after a chickenpox infection. Shingles is caused by varicella virus that has remained latent in a sensory nerve tract after recovery from chickenpox. When the virus is expressed again, it is called zoster. Zoster typically occurs along the dermatome (skin region) innervated by the infected nerve. Zoster often is seen in the elderly or in an individual who has a reduced immune system caused by illness or stress. Zoster appears to spread by direct contact with the lesion.

CLINICAL MANIFESTATIONS

- Low-grade fever and malaise may be present 24 hours before vesicles appear.
- The rash of chickenpox begins as red macules, usually first appearing on the trunk and spreading to the face and extremities. Within a few hours, the macules become fluid-filled vesicles, with more macules developing in the mouth, axillia, labia, and vagina. These too soon become fluid-filled vesicles. The vesicles burst after a few days and crust over.
- Numerous macules, vesicles, and scabs at different stages in formation may be present at any one time.
- The vesicles of shingles typically present on the skin, unilaterally along the infected dermatome (one side of the body). Frequent sites of eruptions are the face, neck, and thoracic areas. The lesions may be small or large and few or many in number.

DIAGNOSIS

- Diagnosis is made by history and physical examination.
- The key diagnostic tool for shingles is the unilateral location and pain.

COMPLICATIONS

- Secondary bacterial infection of the vesicles may develop.
- Pneumonia, encephalitis, or joint inflammation and pain may follow chickenpox infection.

- Reye's syndrome may develop in children given aspirin during a chickenpox infection.
- Adults who have chickenpox may have a particularly severe disease course and are at higher risk of developing pneumonia or other complications.
- Chickenpox and shingles may spread internally in immunocompromised individuals, leading to increased morbidity and mortality.
- Postherpetic neuralgia (pain) may occur in a large percentage (between 10% to 70%) of individuals suffering from shingles. Postherpetic neuralgia refers to pain that persists for longer than 1 month after the acute onset of shingles. It is most common in elderly patients and is difficult to relieve once it becomes established.

TREATMENT

- Prevention of chickenpox is possible with the varicella vaccine. This vaccine can be given to children or adults, and is highly successful in preventing infection. Some individuals (approximately 10%) may develop a few vesicles 10 to 20 days after immunization and may be contagious to others at that time. It is hoped that by preventing varicella, the incidence of shingles will also decline, although this has not as yet been documented.
- Treatment of active chickenpox infection is mainly supportive and is geared at preventing the development of secondary skin infections. Oatmeal baths, calamine lotion, and antihistamines may be used to reduce itching. In children, the nails may be cut, or mittens may be worn to reduce scratching.
- Antiviral drugs (acyclovir, vidarabine, sorivudine) may be prescribed after exposure or at the earliest sign of chickenpox infection in adults or in immunocompromised children to limit the degree of infection. The use of antiviral drugs in healthy children who have chickenpox may also be considered to reduce lesion number and length of infection.
- Treatment of shingles includes analgesics for pain and antiviral drugs to limit viral replication. Systemic corticosteroids may be provided to reduce the risk of developing postherpatic neuralgia. Individuals who do develop postherpatic neuralgia may be treated with topical anesthetic agents and tricyclic antidepressants for pain relief. Better outcomes are achieved when treatment is instituted early.

WARTS

In humans, warts are caused by infection with the human papillomavirus (HPV). Warts (verrucae) are benign papules that can occur anywhere on the skin. There are many different strains of HPV. Some preferentially infect the genital or anal region, causing genital warts, whereas others colonize the fingers and hands, causing simple warts. Plantar warts are warts on the bottom of the feet that grow in rather than out from the skin. Warts are passed by skin-to-skin contact. Genital warts are considered a sexually transmitted disease.

Some studies suggest that over 40% of young women using university health care centers for their gynecologic care have genital warts. Certain strains of genital warts have been identified as causing cervical cancer; other strains are unlikely to progress to cancer. The risk of developing cervical cancer is especially high in women who have genital warts and who smoke. This is most likely because cervical mucus concentrates tobacco toxins, which may then act synergistically with HPV to produce cancer.

CLINICAL MANIFESTATIONS

- Skin warts may be flat or round, large or small.
- Genital warts have a cauliflower-type appearance. They may be seen on the head or shaft of the penis, on the labia, in the vagina, or surrounding the anus.

DIAGNOSIS

- Diagnosis is made by history and physical examination.
- Occasionally, a biopsy of the lesion may be taken for histologic confirmation of HPV. Typing of the lesion may be performed at that time as well.

COMPLICATIONS

- Cervical cancer in women can be considered a sexually transmitted disease that results from infection with certain strains of HPV.
- Infrequently, a newborn exposed to genital warts during the birth process may develop esophageal warts.
- Low self-esteem and feelings of guilt and shame may occur. Individuals who have HPV may be reluctant to establish new relationships.

TREATMENT

- Warts go away on their own when the immune system is stimulated to recognize their presence. This typically happens with vascularization or bleeding of the wart.
- Irritation of a skin or plantar wart by the application of salicylic acid, formaldehyde, podophyllum, or other skin irritants may stimulate an immune reaction against the wart. All types of warts frequently reappear after treatment.
- Liquid nitrogen, cryosurgery, or laser may be used to remove stubborn or unsightly warts, or warts on the genital or esophageal regions.

Bacterial Infections of the Skin

IMPETIGO

A superficial skin infection, usually caused by staphylococcus or group A streptococcal infection, is known as impetigo. There are two types of impetigo: vesicular and bullous.

Vesicular impetigo most commonly occurs in children, presenting as pustules on the skin filled with a honey-colored fluid. The pustules burst and crust over. Vesicular impetigo is highly contagious, and easily passes from one area of the body to another and from person to person with contact.

Neonates may develop bullous impetigo, as a result of contagion in the nursery. This type of impetigo is caused by *Staphylococcus aureus* and is also highly contagious. Bullous impetigo is characterized by vesicles that burst and crust. Any area of the body may be infected.

CLINICAL MANIFESTATIONS

- Localized pustules, which burst and crust, anywhere on the body. Crusts and fluid are honey-colored.
- Lesions often spread.

DIAGNOSIS

- Diagnosis is made by history and physical examination.
- Bacterial culture and drug sensitivity testing is recommended.

COMPLICATIONS

- Acute poststreptococcal glomerulonephritis (inflammation of the kidney nephron) may occur from antibody-antigen complexes depositing in the kidney (type III hypersensitivity response).
- Widespread infections in infants is possible.

TREATMENT

- Systemic antibiotics may be administered after culture and identification of the organism. Topical antibiotics may be adequate if the lesion is small.
- Sterilization of towels and frequent handwashing must be used to prevent spread on the body and to family members.

Pediatric Consideration

Impetigo is a common childhood skin infection. It is highly contagious in crowded environments, such as schools and day care centers, especially if sanitary practices are poor.

CELLULITIS

Cellulitis is a bacterial infection of the dermis or subcutaneous layer of the skin. Cellulitis typically occurs after a surface wound, bite, or untreated carbuncle or furuncle.

CLINICAL MANIFESTATIONS

- The skin appears swollen and red. It is tender and warm to the touch. There may be present an exudate of serous or purulent fluid.
- Fever may be present.

DIAGNOSIS

- Diagnosis is made by history and physical examination.

TREATMENT

- Warm soaks in an antibacterial medium or Burow's solution may be used.
- Systemic antibiotics are necessary.

FOLLICULITIS

Infection of a hair follicle, usually by the bacterium *Staphylococcus aureus* is known as folliculitis. Inflammation occurs in the follicle. Risk factor include trauma to the skin and poor hygiene.

CLINICAL MANIFESTATIONS

- Surface pustules characterized by redness, pain, and swelling.

DIAGNOSIS

- Diagnosis is made by history and physical examination.

COMPLICATIONS

- A boil, also called a **furuncle**, may develop if the inflamed follicle bursts and spreads the bacteria into the dermis. Pain and inflammation worsen. Oozing of pus and cellulitis may develop.

TREATMENT

- Soap and water and topical antibiotics.
- Warm compresses and incision of the lesion may be required.
- Systemic antibiotics may be required.

CARBUNCLE

A carbuncle is a collection of hair follicles infected in the subcutaneous and dermal layers. An abscess may develop as immune cells encircle the infection.

CLINICAL MANIFESTATIONS

- A hard, firm mass under the skin that is painful and may drain purulent material.
- Systemic signs of infection, including chills, fever, and malaise may develop.

DIAGNOSIS

- Diagnosis is made by history and physical examination.

TREATMENT

- Warm compresses and topical or systemic antibiotics.
- An abscess may require lancing and drainage.

SCARLET FEVER

Although not itself a bacterial infection, scarlet fever is a skin rash caused by toxins released during infection with group A β-hemolytic streptococci. Scarlet fever, also called scarlatina, is usually associated with a pharyngeal strep infection.

CLINICAL MANIFESTATIONS

- The rash of scarlet fever is usually pink, mainly over the neck, trunk, and groin, with a feeling akin to fine sandpaper. It is typically accompanied by other signs of a pharyngeal streptococcal infection: sore throat, fever, headache, and nausea.

DIAGNOSTIC TOOLS

- A throat culture is usually positive for group A b-hemolytic streptococci. This coupled with a good history and physical examination usually confirms scarlet fever.

COMPLICATIONS

- Poststreptococcal glomerulonephritis, rheumatic fever, and peritonsillar abscess may all follow a strep infection.

TREATMENT

- Treatment is with penicillin, or if the individual is allergic to penicillin, erythromycin or another macrolide.

Fungal Infections of the Skin

Fungal infections of the skin are considered superficial infections and are typically described based on the site of infection. The infections of the skin are called tinea (mistakenly referring to a worm). **Tinea**

pedis is an infection of the foot (e.g., athlete's foot); **tinea corporis** (ringworm), an infection of the body; **tinea barbae**, an infection of the beard; and **tinea capitis**, an infection of the scalp. **Tinea versicolor** is a fungal infection of the body that may result in patches of discoloration, that are worsened by exposure to sunlight.

Fungal infections of the mouth (thrush), gastrointestinal (GI) tract, and vagina usually are a result of the yeastlike fungus Candida albicans and are called **candidiasis**. Candida albicans is part of the normal human flora that, under some conditions, may multiply excessively and cause symptoms.

Deep fungal infections of the respiratory tract or brain usually occur only in immunocompromised individuals and are considered opportunistic infections. Histoplasmosis is a fungal infection of the respiratory tract that may develop in normal individuals as well.

CAUSES OF FUNGAL INFECTIONS

Fungal infections occur in individuals who are somehow predisposed to their development. Predisposition may develop in people for no obvious reason, but often individuals are predisposed as a result of certain behaviors, such as frequent participation in athletic events associated with perspiration and frequent showering where the fungus may be present (i.e., locker rooms). A predisposition is also present in individuals suffering from decreased immune function (e.g., diabetics, pregnant women, and young infants). Those who have severe immunodeficiency, including those suffering from acquired immunodeficiency syndrome (AIDS), are at special risk of chronic, debilitating fungal infections. In fact, vaginal or oral yeast infections are frequently the first opportunistic infections seen in individuals infected with the human immunodeficiency virus (HIV). Persons who have chronic fungal infections should be evaluated for diabetes mellitus and HIV-AIDS.

Treatment with antibiotics for a bacterial infection may kill normal vaginal bacteria that usually exist in balance with vaginal yeast. This may predispose women or girls so treated to a vaginal yeast infection.

CLINICAL MANIFESTATIONS

- Skin infections cause inflammation with erythema and itching.
- Ringworm may present as a ring of erythema with a pale interior. Scaling of the edges may be present.
- Yeast infections may appear as inflamed pustules that itch and are painful. Vaginal infections are associated with a cheesy white discharge. Oral infections present with multiple white ulcerations surrounded by erythema, which may be extremely painful.

DIAGNOSIS

- Fungal infections are diagnosed by history and physical examination as well as with a microscopic examination of skin scrapings prepared with potassium hydroxide to identify hyphae (characteristic spores and filaments of fungi) under the microscope.

- Viewing the affected area using an ultraviolet light (Wood lamp) may also allow for recognition of fungal infections as the spores fluoresce blue-green under this condition. If hyphae or spores cannot be seen, scrapings may be sent for culture to confirm or refute diagnosis. Sometimes, cultures are sent even if hyphae or spores are seen.

COMPLICATIONS

- Surface infections may become secondarily infected by bacteria.
- Deep fungal infections (internal) may cause significant morbidity and mortality.
- Scarring of the skin or, with tinea capitis, alopecia (hair loss) may occur.
- Side effects of oral medication used to treat tinea pedis or stubborn skin or scalp infections may occur.
- Painful oral lesions that interfere with eating may contribute to the wasting seen in individuals suffering from AIDS.

TREATMENT

- Skin infections are treated with type-specific antifungal medications applied topically or occasionally given systemically. Scalp and foot infections are often treated with systemic agents.
- Candidiasis is treated with antifungal cream or suppositories.
- Partners may be treated in women with chronic vaginal yeast infection.
- Deep fungal infections may require extensive, specific antifungal therapy and hospitalization.

Pediatric Consideration

Infants who have oral thrush may be asymptomatic or may nurse poorly. If a breastfeeding infant is diagnosed with thrush, both infant and mother should be treated because infection can pass back and forth from the mouth to the nipple.

Scleroderma

Scleroderma is a connective tissue disease. It may only involve the skin, or may occur systematically and involve the kidneys, lungs, and gut. The disorder appears to be an autoimmune condition, and affects women more commonly than men.

Scleroderma is characterized by massive deposits of collagen under the skin or in internal organs, resulting in inflammation and fibrosis. Skin deposits are in the dermis and subdermal tissue. Calcium deposits accumulate under the skin. The disease may cause Raynaud's phenomenon, characterized by spasm of the arterioles of the fingers. The nails and fingertips may fall off.

CLINICAL MANIFESTATIONS

- The skin appears tight, shiny, and often red from inflammation.
- Fingertips and nails may be narrow or missing.
- Hard, calcium nodules under the skin may be visible and palpable.
- Muscular atrophy, pain, and deformity may develop.

DIAGNOSIS

- Often made by excluding other connective tissue disease and from the history and physical examination.

COMPLICATIONS

- An approximately 50% mortality rate if the disease progresses to involve internal organs.

TREATMENT

- There is no specific treatment for scleroderma. It is recommended that patients avoid exposure to cold temperature and smoking, both of which cause vasoconstriction and worsen symptoms.
- Steroidal anti-inflammatory medication may be used to slow the autoimmune response.

Burns

Burns may result from exposure of the skin to high temperature, electrical shock, or chemicals. Burns are classified according to tissue depth of the burn and extent of the burned body surface area.

DEPTH OF A BURN

A burn may be classified as first-degree, second-degree superficial, second-degree deep partial thickness, or third-degree full thickness. Severe electrical burns may cause major internal charring and searing of tissue and are classified as fourth-degree burns.

First-degree burns (e.g., sunburn) are limited to the epidermis. There is erythema and pain but no immediate blistering. Healing is spontaneous and occurs within 3 to 4 days. The burn does not scar. There are usually no complications.

Second-degree, superficial, partial-thickness burns extend through the epidermis and into the dermal layer. The burn is extremely painful and blisters within minutes. The burn usually heals without scarring, although certain individuals, especially African Americans, may scar after this type of burn. Healing usually requires as long as a month.

Complications are uncommon, although secondary infection of the wound may occur.

Second-degree, deep, partial-thickness burns extend through the entire dermis. The hair follicles remain intact and regrow. This type of burn is only partially sensitive to pain because of extensive destruction of the sensory neurons. However, surrounding areas usually have painful second-degree, superficial burns.

Healing of a second-degree, deep, partial-thickness burn takes several weeks and includes surgical debridement (cleaning) to remove dead tissue. Grafting is usually required. Scar formation always occurs with this burn.

Third-degree burns extend through the epidermis and the dermis and into the subcutaneous tissue layer. Capillaries and veins may be singed, and blood flow to the area may be reduced. Nerves are destroyed, so the burn is without pain. However, surrounding areas typically demonstrate extremely painful second-degree burns. A third-degree burn may require months to heal, and surgical debridement and grafting are necessary. A third-degree burn scars, and the tissue appears leathery and hard. Fourth-degree burns extend through muscle, bone, and internal tissues.

EXTENT OF A BURN

The extent of a burn refers to the percentage of an individual's body that has second-degree or deeper burns. To determine the extent of a burn, the body is divided into percentages of surface area. One method of determining the percentage of a burn is called "**The Rule of Nines**." With this method, an arm (front and back) is considered 9% of the body surface area, whereas a leg is considered 18% of the body surface area. The percentages of the body burned are added to give a total percent that is burned. Major burns are defined as those involving between 25% and 40% of the body surface area of an adult and between 15% and 25% of the surface area of a child. Burns of greater than 40% in adults or 25% in children are associated with significant mortality. The overall health of the individual must be taken into consideration when predicting survival from any burn. Children and the elderly have increased mortality compared with middle-aged and young adults. An individual suffering from a severe burn should be transferred to a burn care facility as soon as possible.

EFFECTS OF A MAJOR BURN

A major burn affects the metabolism and function of every body cell. All systems are compromised, especially the cardiovascular system. Given the dependence of every organ on adequate blood flow, alteration in cardiovascular function has wide-ranging implications for survival and recovery. Cellular changes also occur.

CARDIOVASCULAR RESPONSE TO A MAJOR BURN

Within hours of a major burn, the ability of the capillary to act as a barrier to diffusion is lost, and fluid drains out of the vascular system. A plasma filtrate accumulates in the interstitial space between cells, leading to widespread interstitial edema and a drastic decrease in blood pressure. Irreversible shock may develop. The loss of capillary integrity is described as **a loss of capillary seal**. The mechanisms responsible for the loss of capillary seal are not well understood, although research suggests that the release of several mediators of inflammation, including histamine and prostaglandin, are involved. Histamine and some of the prostaglandins are potent vasodilators.

During the period of capillary leak, red and white blood cells do not pass through the capillaries. This increases blood viscosity and causes sluggish blood flow. Individuals are at increased risk of clot formation. Cardiac contractility lessens, which further decreases blood flow and blood pressure. Irreversible shock may develop. With a weakly beating heart, blood accumulates in the lungs, causing pulmonary congestion and increasing the risk of embolus formation. Decreased blood flow to the kidneys causes renal hypoxia and a significant decrease in urine output. The renin-angiotensin system is stimulated, resulting in increased salt and water retention. Because the capillaries do not contain the increased volume, additional edema develops, further increasing the risk of pulmonary congestion and pneumonia. Hypoxia of the gut causes injury to the mucus-producing cells, leading to gastric and deuodenal ulcers (*Curling's ulcer*). Within approximately 24 to 48 hours after a burn, the capillaries reseal and fluid is slowly reabsorbed back into the circulation. However, the effects of the loss of seal remain, and the risk of morbidity and mortality continues to be high.

CELLULAR RESPONSE TO A BURN

In response to a major burn, cells become leaky to electrolytes, sodium accumulates intracellularly, and swelling develops. Potassium leaves the cell and enters the extracellular fluid. Magnesium and phosphate leak from the cells. These changes affect the membrane potential of all cells and can lead to cardiac dysrhythmias and alterations in central nervous system function.

Immune function is inhibited by a major burn. Loss of immune function, combined with the loss of the barrier function of the skin, puts the individual at a high risk for infection. Decreased immune function appears to result from the release of hormones, including but not limited to the glucocorticoids, especially cortisol. Cortisol is released with stress and is immunosuppressant at high concentrations.

Metabolic rate is drastically increased after a major burn. Hypermetabolism may result from activation of the sympathetic nervous system and the stress response, as well as from attempts to balance the heat loss that occurs when the insulatory function of the skin is lost. Healing of the burn also requires huge amounts of energy. The temperature control center in the hypothalamus is affected by the response to a major burn, leading to an increase in hypothalamic set-point. This may result from cytokines and other peptides released during the widespread inflammatory response. The hypermetabolism, as well as the increase in cortisol and epinephrine (hormones of the post-absorptive state) and changes in insulin sensitivity, lead to tissue breakdown and protein and fat wasting. Protein breakdown especially leads to severe muscle wasting.

CLINICAL MANIFESTATIONS

- A first-degree burn is characterized by redness and pain. Blisters may develop after 24 hours, and the skin may later peel.
- A second-degree, superficial burn is characterized by rapid blister formation and intense pain.
- A second-degree, deep, partial-thickness burn is characterized by blisters or thin dry tissue covering the wound, which peels off. The wound may not be painful.
- A third-degree burn appears flat, thin, and dry. Coagulated blood vessels may be seen. The skin may be white, red, or black and leathery.
- Electrical burns may appear similar to thermal burns, or may appear as silver, raised areas. Electrical burns usually occur at points of electrical contact. The internal damage caused by an electical burn may be much more severe than is apparent from the external wound.

DIAGNOSTIC TOOLS

- The Rule of Nines is used to evaluate the percentage of body surface burned.
- Urine output is followed closely during the period of burn shock and after resealing of the capillaries. This is essential for evaluating the success of volume replacement during burn shock. When urine output returns to normal, the capillaries are said to have "resealed."

COMPLICATIONS

- Any burn may become infected, causing further disability or death. Methicillin-resistant *Staphylococcus aureus* is an especially frequent cause of hospital-acquired (nosocomial) infection in burn patients.
- Sluggish blood flow may lead to the development of a blood clot, causing a cerebral vascular accident, a myocardial infarct, or a pulmonary embolus.
- Lung damage may occur from smoke inhalation or embolus formation. Pulmonary congestion may result from left-heart failure or a myocardial infarct. Adult respiratory distress syndrome may develop.

- Electrolyte disturbance may lead to a cardiac dysrhythmia and cardiac arrest.
- Burn shock may irreversibly damage the kidneys, leading to renal failure within the first week or two after the burn. Renal failure also may develop as a result of renal hypoxia or rhabdomyolysis (myoglobin obstruction of the kidney tubules secondary to widespread muscle necrosis).
- Decreased blood flow to the gut may result in hypoxia of the mucus-producing cells, leading to peptic ulcer disease.
- Disseminated intravascular coagulation (DIC) may occur with widespread tissue destruction.
- With a major or disfiguring burn, psychologic trauma may lead to depression, family breakup, and thoughts of suicide. Pscyhologic symptoms may occur any time after a burn. Symptoms may come and go repeatedly over a lifetime.
- The financial burden to the family of an individual who has a severe burn is enormous. Not only are wages lost if the individual is an adult, but care is continuing and costly.

TREATMENT

- Individuals experiencing a burn should immediately be removed from the burning agent and the burned area of the skin should be immediately immersed under cool water to stop further tissue destruction. The application of ice should be avoided because ice decreases blood flow to the area and may worsen the degree of the burn. Clothes should not be removed from a serious burn, because removing clothes may also remove skin.
- Individuals who have a severe burn must receive medical treatment. Infants, young children, and the elderly who suffer anything other than a minor burn, should be evaluated by a medical provider, as should those who have any chronic illness or condition. Burns to the hands, face, and genitals should be evaluated by medical personnel.
- First-degree burns usually require only prolonged exposure to large amounts of cool water or the application of cool compresses and anti-inflammatory medication.
- First-degree chemical burns should be flushed with cool water for several minutes.
- Burns deeper than first-degree require antimicrobial therapy and should be evaluated by medical personnel.
- Major burns require quick intravenous fluid replacement to combat the loss of capillary seal. To maintain blood pressure and prevent irreversible shock, infusions in an adult may reach the staggering amount of 30L in 24 hours. The high rate of fluid replacement also flushes the kidney and reduces the risk of renal failure.
- Early and continued nutritional support is required for severely burned individuals. Because of the hypermetabolic response to a severe burn, calories and protein must be in adequate supply to

prevent muscle catabolism and wasting. Enteral feeding is optimal for those who suffer severe burns, both because of its ability to provide adequate calories for healing and because it appears to protect the gut mucosa, reducing damage to the gut barrier.

- Second-degree, total-thickness and third-degree burns require surgical cleaning of the wound and grafting. If possible, grafting should be from nondamaged skin of the burn patient (autograft). Other grafting sources are from a human donor, alive or dead (homograft), or a nonhuman donor, usually a pig (heterograft). Cultured autografts and artificial skin grafts are being studied and used experimentally.
- Tissue expansion techniques have been used to improve the chances for successful skin grafting. These techniques appear to work by stimulating a stretch-induced signal transduction pathway whereby stretch increases the growth of keratinocytes and stimulates protein synthesis in skin to be used for autografts.
- Pain control is a major goal of burn therapy. Burns themselves can be excruciatingly painful, as can the treatments used to help a burn to heal. Alleviating pain as much as possible reduces stress, which may improve immune function and healing. Adequate pain relief also may relieve the psychologic trauma associated with burns, some of which continues long after the burn is physically healed.

Pediatric Consideration

Burns are a major cause of morbidity and mortality in children. Most burns to children are preventable. Frequent sources of burns include scalds from kitchen stove spills, or hot water exposure. Because children have skin that is much thinner than an adult's, even brief exposure (less than a second) to hot water can scald a child. Fire injury from being unable to escape a burning home or car and electrical burn injuries from electrical sockets or cords also account for a substantial number of childhood burns. Children may be burned purposefully in situations of *abuse*. Signs of this type of burn are delays in seeking medical attention, contact burns to parts of the body such as the backs of hands or genitals, and burns on the buttocks and legs indicative of forced immersion in hot water. Any burn in a child is a frightening, painful experience, and all possible steps should be taken to prevent a burn from occurring.

Decubitus Ulcers

Decubitus ulcers, also called pressure sores or bed sores, are lesions on the skin that occur after the breakdown of the epidermis, the dermis, and, occasionally, the subcutaneous tissue and underlying bone. Decubitus ulcers are usually seen in individuals who are bedridden or have decreased mobility. Even if mobility is normal, those suffering a reduced sensation to pain (e.g., individuals who have diabetes mellitus or stroke) may develop an ulcer. The severity of an ulcer is based on the depth of erosion into the tissue. Even ulcers that look small on the surface of the skin may be associated with significant injury under the skin.

There are four forces that together produce a decubitus ulcer: pressure, shearing, friction, and moisture. A decubitus ulcer usually forms on an area of the skin overlying a bony process. It develops when the **pressure** in that area is unrelieved for a long period, causing collapse of the supplying blood vessels. This leads to tissue hypoxia and cellular death. Decubitus ulcers are common on skin areas exposed to sliding or **shear** forces, where there is a high degree of **friction** between the skin and the surface, and on skin exposed for prolonged periods to the **moisture** of **urine or feces**, which further breaks down the skin and makes it susceptible to infection.

CLINICAL MANIFESTATIONS

- A sign of early injury is an area of redness that does not disappear with fingertip pressure (nonblanching).
- An ulcer on the skin is seen with more severe injury. A visible skin lesion may be partial or full thickness, extending through the dermis or even through the subcutaneous tissue. A full-thickness injury may damage the bone.
- Pain and systemic signs of inflammation, including fever and increased white blood cell count, may develop.

DIAGNOSIS

- Decubitus ulcers are diagnosed with a good history and physical examination. Those at high risk should be checked frequently for an early stage of development. Such an early stage is suggested by skin that remains blanched with pressure for more than a brief period.

COMPLICATIONS

- Infection leading to prolonged disability and hospitalization may occur with even small ulcers.

TREATMENT

- Prevention of a decubitus ulcer is essential and involves turning bedridden individuals frequently (at least every 2 hours). Caloric intake should be kept high to assist in immune function and maintain overall general good health.
- If a pressure sore does develop, relief of the pressure on the skin and the placement of a clean, flat, nonbulky dressing is required.
- Deep sores may require surgical debridement.

Skin Cancer

Skin cancer is common in the United States. The incidence of skin cancer varies geographically, peaking at high altitude and sunny re-

Table 19-2. Skin Cancer

TYPE	CHARACTERISTICS	TREATMENT
Basal cell	Flesh-colored or pink nodule, often depressed in the center, enlarges over time. Shiny/waxy most frequently seen on sun-exposed areas, often the ear, face, or hand.	Excision.
Squamous cell	Scaly, slightly elevated lesion, with central area of ulceration. Irregular borders may be crusted in later stages. Most frequently seen on sun-exposed areas, often the face, or on scarred areas.	Excision may require radiation therapy.
Malignant melanoma	Rapidly growing lesion arising *de novo* or from a preexisting mole. Usually raised, black or brown, or sometimes varied in color. The borders are irregular and asymmetrical; they may bleed. Most frequently seen on sun-exposed areas, but may develop anywhere. Related to burning sun exposures.	Excision, surgical removal of surrounding tissue, lymph node biopsy. Radiation, chemotherapy, or immune therapy may be used.

gions of the country. Skin cancer is more common in light-skinned individuals compared with dark-skinned individuals, although individuals from all races are at risk. There are three types of skin cancer: basal cell, squamous cell, and malignant melanoma (Table 19-2). All types of skin cancer are increasing in incidence in the United States and other countries and are being seen in individuals at younger ages. This is most likely because of the increase in recreational sun exposure seen in the last several decades.

BASAL CELL CARCINOMA

Basal cell carcinoma is a superficial cancer of immature epithelial cells. The tumors typically are slow growing and seldom metastasize, although they can cause localized tissue destruction. They are caused by cumulative exposure to sunlight and are usually seen in the elderly. Genetic factors are likely involved as well. Basal cell carcinoma is the most common type of skin cancer.

SQUAMOUS CELL CARCINOMA

Squamous cell carcinoma is a cancer of the epidermal cells, which may spread horizontally over the skin or vertically into the dermis. Spread may be slow or aggressive. Squamous cell carcinoma may metastasize to other sites of the body. Squamous cell cancer is most common in the elderly and develops after prolonged exposure to the sun. It frequently develops on areas of the skin demonstrating precancerous lesions or irregularities, such as keratosis (a horny growth), actinic dermatitis, or areas of previous discoloration. Squamous cell carcinoma not uncommonly develops at the site of a previous scar (e.g., a burn scar).

MALIGNANT MELANOMA

Malignant melanoma is an aggressive tumor of the melanin-producing cells at the base of the epidermis. Malignant melanoma may develop at the site of a preexisting nevus (mole), or may might develop spontaneously on the skin. This type of skin cancer often occurs during middle age and appears to result from intense burns with blistering during the first or second decades of life. Other risk factors include light skin, freckles, and fair-colored hair. Research suggests melanoma occurs from a radiation-induced decrease in the functioning of immune cells of the skin, Langerhans' cells. A genetic predisposition for melanoma is likely with gene studies underway. Metastasis is common. The incidence of melanoma is increasing, especially among the young.

CLINICAL MANIFESTATIONS

- Basal cell carcinoma usually appears on sun-exposed areas of the body, including the face, arms, and chest. Lesions appear as dome-shaped papules or nodules, well circumscribed, with a pearly white color. They are painless.

- Squamous cell carcinoma usually occurs on sun-exposed areas of the body or on scarred tissue. The lesions appear as scaly red plaques or raised nodules with central necrosis.
- Malignant melanoma may appear as a multicolored nodule growing vertically or as a circular spread of pigmentation larger than 1 cm. Borders of either lesion are irregular and often asymmetric and bleeding may occur. Melanoma may develop on sun-exposed areas, or on the palms of the hands, the soles of the feet, or the oral or vaginal mucosa.

DIAGNOSIS

- Skin cancer diagnosis is made as a result of a physical examination followed by the excision and biopsy of a suspicious lesion. Any lesion should be considered suspicious if it demonstrates one of the "ABCDs" of skin cancer: **A**symmetry, irregular **B**order, a change in **C**olor, or an increasing **D**iameter such that the lesion is greater than 0.5 cm (approximately the size of a pencil eraser).

COMPLICATIONS

- Local invasion and destruction of tissue may occur with any type of skin cancer.
- Metastasis to regional lymph nodes and throughout the body may occur, especially with malignant melanoma.

TREATMENT

- Prevention of basal and squamous cell carcinoma is possible with rigorous protection from the sun, including avoidance of the sun at peak hours and the use of hats, protective clothing, and broad-spectrum sunscreen.
- Individuals can reduce the incidence of malignant melanoma by avoiding sun exposure and by wearing protective clothing. Sunscreen may not protect against the development of malignant melanoma.
- Basal cell carcinoma is surgically excised. Prognosis is good.
- Squamous cell carcinoma is surgically excised and radiation therapy may be required. Prognosis is good, especially if metastasis has not occurred.
- Malignant melanoma is surgically excised, along with a margin of surrounding tissue. Lymph node biopsy is performed to determine if metastasis has occurred. Sentinal lymph-node biopsy, that is, biopsy of the node closest to the malignancy, has been shown to be an effective predictor of metastasis and a means of directing therapy.
- Chemotherapy and immunotherapy both may be required in addi-

tion to surgery for malignant melanoma and sometimes squamous cell carcinoma.

- Tumor vaccines active against specific antigens in malignant melanoma are being used in selected patients. Gene therapy for malignant melanoma is also being studied.
- Currently, the prognosis for malignant melanoma depends on the size of the lesion and the outcome of the lymph- node biopsy. Nodular growth has a worse prognosis.

Selected Bibliography

Arblaster, G. (1998). Pressure sore incidence: strategy for reduction. *Nursing Standard* 12, 49–52.

Bardolph, E. & Ashton, R. (1998). Psoriasis: a review of present and future management. *Nursing Standard* 12, 43–47.

Bates, B. (1998). *A guide to physical examination (7th ed.)*. Philadelphia: J. B. Lippincott Company.

Bonfanti, C., Carducci, M. Mussi, A., & D'Auria, L. (1998). Recognition and treatment of psoriasis. Special consideration in elderly patients. *Drugs and Aging* 12, 177–190.

Bullock, B. L. & Rosendahl, P. P. (1992). Pathophysiology: adaptations and alterations in function (3rd ed.). Philadelphia: J.B. Lippincott Company.

Cohen, G. L.& Falkson, C. I. (1998). Current treatment options for malignant melanoma. *Drugs* 55, 791–799.

Cook, N. (1998). Methicillin-resistant *Staphylococcus aureas* versus the burn patient. *Burns* 24, 91–96.

Cortiella, J. & Marvin, J. A. (1997). Management of the pediatric burn patient. *Nursing Clinics of North America* 32, 311, 329.

Friedlander, S. F. (1998). Contact dermatitis. *Pediatrics in Review* 19, 166–171.

Friedmann, P. S. (1998). Contact and atopic eczema. *BMJ* 316, 1226–1229.

Guyton, A. C. & Hall, J. (1997). *Textbook of medical physiology (9th ed.)*. Philadelphia: W. B. Saunders.

Hansbrough, J. F. (1998). Enteral nutritional support in burn patients. *Gastrointestinal Endoscopy Clinics of North America* 8, 645–667.

Mackensen, A. (1994). Direct evidence to support the immuno-surveillance concept in a human regressive melanoma. *Journal of Clinical Investigation* 93, 1397–1402.

Momtaz, K. & Fitzpatrick, T. B. (1998). The benefits and risks of long-term PUVA photochemotherapy. *Dermatologic Clinics* 16, 227–234.

Ollila, D. W., Kelley, M. C., Gammon, G., & Morton, D. L. (1998). Overview of melanoma vaccines: active specific immunotherapy for melanoma patients. *Seminars in Surgical Oncology* 14, 328–336.

Pal, K. K., Cortiella, J., & Herndon, D. (1997). Adjunctive methods of pain control in burns. *Burns* 23, 404–412.

Porth, C. M. (1998). *Pathophysiology concepts of altered health states* (5th ed.). Philadelphia: J. B. Lippincott Company.

Reintgen, D., Balch, C.M., Kirkwood, J., & Ross, M. (1997). Recent advances in the care of the patient with malignant melanoma. *Annals of Surgery* 225, 1–14.

Takei, T., Mills, I., Arai, K., & Sumpio, B.E. (1998). Molecular basis for tissue expansion: clinical implications for the surgeon. *Plastic and Reconstructive Surgery* 101, 247–258.

Van de Kerkhof, P. C. (1998). An update on vitamin D3 analogues in the treatment of psoriasis. *Skin Pharmacology and Applied Skin Physiology* 11, 2–10.

20 THE SENSES

Our senses link us to each other and to the world. Each sense allows us to respond to subtle and not so subtle stimuli with precision and recognition. Because of the way our senses bring the external environment to us, the day-to-day implications of losing a sense are enormous. The senses include sight, hearing, taste, smell, and touch.

● ● ●

PHYSIOLOGIC CONCEPTS

Sight

Activation of light-sensitive receptors in the eye, called photoreceptors, results in sight. The stimuli received by the photoreceptors is transmitted to the brain by way of electrical signaling passed through several levels of increasingly complex cell networks. Once the signals reach the brain, they are interpreted as a particular visual image based on the complexity of firing patterns, the rate of firing frequency, and the coding of color. Therefore, to have the sense of sight, one needs a functioning eye to receive a stimulus, cells capable of coding it electrically, intact neural pathways to transmit the electrical code, and a cerebral cortex capable of interpreting the signal into a meaningful image.

STRUCTURE OF THE EYE

A diagrammatic representation of the eye is presented in Figure 20-1. The outermost (anterior portion) of the eye consists of a tough white membrane covering the eyeball, called the **sclera**. At the center of the eye, the sclera becomes a transparent membrane, the **cornea**. Light rays enter the eye through the cornea. By way of its natural curvature, the cornea bends the rays, causing the light to become less scattered and more focused on the underlying tissue. The image projected through the cornea is upside down and reversed right to left where it strikes the back of the eye.

The **choroid**, a pigmented membrane lying under the sclera, helps reduce light scatter. Directly under the cornea, the choroid becomes the **iris**. The iris is a colored membrane that gives the eye its tint. At the center of the eye is the **pupil**. The cornea focuses the light rays on the pupil. The diameter of the pupil is controlled by smooth muscles that innervate the iris. These muscles cause the pupil to contract in the light and to dilate in the dark. Variations in pupil diameter control the amount of light that passes deeper into the eye.

Posterior to the iris and pupil is the **lens**. The lens is a curved transparent structure that further bends the light rays. By passage

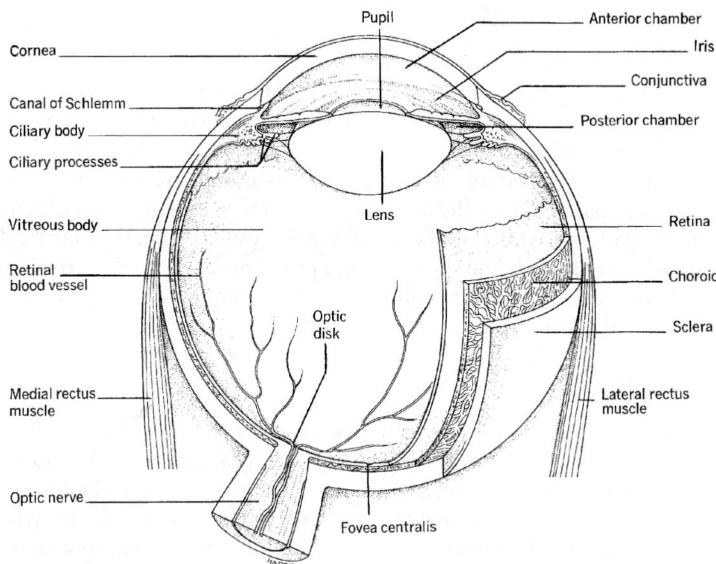

Figure 20-1. Transverse section of the eyeball (from Porth, 1993 p. 1120).

through the lens, light rays are focused exactly on the most posterior and sensitive portion of the eye, the **retina**. The shape of the lens is controlled by a muscle that allows the lens to focus both distant and close objects precisely on the retina. The retina contains the photoreceptors of the eye, the **rods** and **cones** that change light rays into electrical messages the brain interprets as vision. In the center of the retina is the **macula**, the site of the most acute and finely detailed vision. The retina also contains the cells that join together to form the **optic nerve**—the pathway by which the visual signal travels to the brain. The **fovea centralis** is a depression in the macula corresponding to the point of central vision. Between the lens and the retina, the eyeball is filled with blood vessels and a gelatinous fluid, called **vitreous fluid**.

Geriatric Consideration

The center of the lens receives no direct capillary supply. Therefore, as a person ages, the cells at the center of the lens are the oldest and least oxygenated. When the cells in the center of the lens die, they are not replaced. This tends to make the lens stiff and less transparent. The lens becomes less able to change its shape to focus an object on the retina, which causes the object to appear out of focus. Visual quality is often reduced in the elderly. The lens may also become opaque with age, a condition known as cataracts. Cataracts further limit visual quality.

Cells of the Retina

The structures of the eye anterior to the retina function primarily to focus the light rays scattered by a particular image exactly on the retina. Once the light rays strike the retina, the cells there have the job of changing the light signal into an electrical signal and then passing the signal to the brain. The cells of the retina that receive and transform the signal are the photoreceptors: the **rods** and the **cones.** The second class of cells in the pathway is the **bipolar cells**; bipolar cells receive the electrical signal from the rods and the cones and pass that signal to the third class of cells in the retina: the **ganglion cells**. The axons of the ganglion cells travel to the central nervous system as the optic nerve.

Rods

Rod-shaped photoreceptors are heavily concentrated on the periphery of the retina. Each rod is connected by way of a chemical synapse to a bipolar cell. The rods contain the photosensitive chemical rhodopsin, which is one of the four photopigments present in the retina (the other three are found in the cones). Rhodopsin decomposes when struck by light. When decomposed, sodium permeability in the rod is reduced. This leads to a hyperpolarization of the rod (the inside becomes more negative). Hyperpolarization *decreases* the firing rate of the rod on the bipolar cell. Normally, the rod inhibits the firing of the bipolar cell. When the rod is hyperpolarized by light, bipolar cell inhibition is removed, and the bipolar cell depolarizes. Depolarization of the bipolar cell causes an action potential to fire in the next cell, the ganglion cell. Action potentials produced by the ganglion cells are sent to the brain via the optic nerve. Rods fire even with low levels of light and so function to provide night vision.

Cones

Cone photoreceptors are heavily concentrated in the center of the eye. They are the only photoreceptors present at the center of the macula, an area called the fovea. Each cone cell contains one of the other three photopigments that, like rhodopsin, decomposes when struck by light. Also, like the rod cells, decomposition of the photopigment in the cone cell hyperpolarizes the cone cell, removing its inhibitory influence from the bipolar cell and causing an action potential to fire in the bipolar cells. As before, the bipolar cells transmit this action potential to a ganglion cell that sends the signal to the brain via the optic nerve. Unlike the rods, the cones are insensitive to faint light and so contribute little to night vision. Vitamin A is an important component of photopigments—both rhodopsin of the rods and the photopigments of the cones.

Reactivation of the Photopigments Immediately after decomposition, the original structure of the photopigments is returned. The rods and cones again inhibit the firing of the bipolar cells and are ready to respond to another light signal.

Differences Between the Rods and Cones: Rods are capable of responding to low levels of light; therefore, they provide limited vision in the dark. Many rods usually converge on one bipolar cell. This reduces the acuity, but increases the sensitivity, of rod vision. Rods are not color sensitive. Therefore, all stimulation is perceived in shades of gray. Cones stimulation requires higher levels of light and so cones do not fire in the dark or in near dark. Because few cones converge on one bipolar cell, there is increased acuity of cone vision.

Color Vision: The different photopigments of the cones allow for color vision because of their sensitivity to the colors red, blue, and green. The ratio of red, blue, and green cones activated at any one time results in color vision. Which cones are stimulated determine which bipolar cells depolarize and which ganglion cells fire action potentials. Ganglion cells may receive information from several different bipolar cells activated by one color-specific or a few different color-specific cones. Ganglion cells may be activated by one color, but inactivated by a second color. The result of these variations and levels of stimuli is fine discrimination of many shades of color.

Lateral Neurons

Two types of neurons, the horizontal cells and the amacrine cells, lay laterally (sideways) in the retina and fire in such a way that they modify and control the message being passed from the rods and cones to the bipolar cells or from the bipolar cells to the ganglion cells. Horizontal cells connect rods and cones to each other and to bipolar cells. Horizontal cells fine-tune the transmission of signals to the bipolar cells, thereby refining visual acuity. The amacrine cells fine-tune signals between the ganglion cells, apparently functioning to sharpen transient responses. Given the large number of lateral neurons in the retina, their importance in fine visual discrimination must be great indeed, although their exact mechanism of action is poorly understood.

Optic Nerve

Ganglion cell axons join together to form the eye's optic nerve (cranial nerve II). The optic nerve leaves the eye as a bundle through an area of the retina called the **optic disk**. The optic disk is without rods or cones; therefore, it does not participate in the response to light (i.e., a "blind spot"). The central artery of the retina enters the eye through the optic disk. An area called the physiologic cup is at the center of the optic disk.

When the optic nerve reaches the brainstem, some fibers from the left eye cross and project to the right side of the brain. At the same time, some fibers from the right eye cross and project to the left side of the brain. This allows both cerebral hemispheres access to information from each eye. Other fibers do not cross sides. The optic nerves terminate in the thalamus, in an area called the dorsal lateral geniculate nucleus, and there, activate other neurons that then project to the occipital lobe. It is in the occipital lobe—the area of the brain that interprets the electrical signals as a meaningful visual image—that the visual cortex of the brain resides (Fig. 20-2). The integrity of the image from the dorsal lateral geniculate to the occipital lobe is ensured because each cell in the dorsal lateral geniculate passes the information in the same exact spatial arrangement to the visual cortex. The pathway of vision is shown in Figure 20-3.

Descending Inhibition to the Dorsal Lateral Geniculate Nucleus Descending fibers from higher brain centers can influence the transmission of signals from the dorsal lateral geniculate nucleus to the visual cortex. These inhibitory and excitatory fibers come from the visual cortex itself and from areas of the brainstem. Descending stimulation can limit or accentuate what visual information is allowed to pass into consciousness.

Integration of the Visual Pathways Integration of the pathways of vision occurs at each level of the retina: between the rods and the cones, at the horizontal cells, at the amacrine cells, at the bipolar cells,

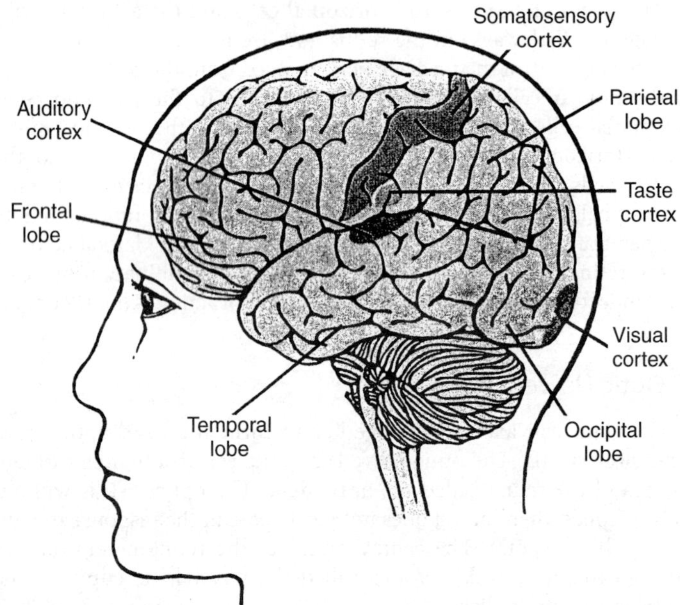

Figure 20-2. Primary sensory areas of the cerebral cortex (used with permission from Vander, A. J., Sherman, J. & Luciano, D. (1998). *Human physiology (7th ed)*. Boston: McGraw-Hill.

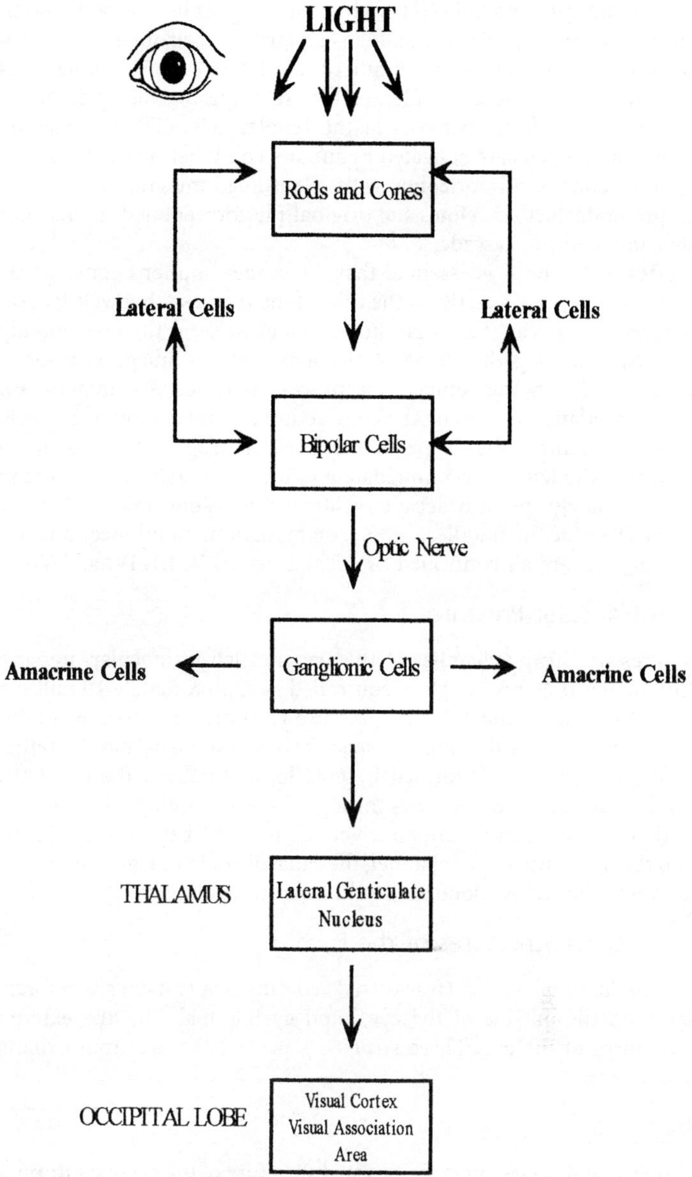

Figure 20-3. Pathway of vision.

and at the ganglion cells. At each level, some cells fire with certain stimuli, such as specific on-off fields or various horizontal and vertical patterns, while the same stimuli turn off the firing of other cells. Ganglion cells have a complex pattern of firing that depends on the various on-off firing patterns of the bipolar cells and the amacrine cells. Bipolar cells are activated by unique combinations of the firings of rods, cones, and horizontal cells. Continued integration of signals in the brain further refines the original photoreceptor decompositon that initiated the cascade.

Optics of Vision It is essential that the cornea and lens converge the light rays to strike exactly on the cells of the retina so that well-focused images can appear. Although the cornea must bend the rays initially, it is by changing the shape of the lens that the image is made to land exactly on the retina. This process is called **accommodation**. Accommodation occurs by the contraction and relaxation of the muscles that control the shape of the lens. A progressive loss in the ability of the lens to accommodate and focus the light rays occurs by approximately the fifth decade of life and is responsible for the loss of near vision in middle age. Accommodation, pupil size, and eye movements are all controlled by cranial nerves II, III, IV, and VI.

Intraocular Pressure

Pressure in the chamber of the eye is called intraocular pressure. Intraocular pressure is tightly controlled at approximately 15 millimeters of mercury (mmHg). The pressure is determined by the amount of aqueous humor that fills the space between the lens and the retina.

Aqueous humor is formed by cilia located behind the iris. Once formed, aqueous humor flows through the eye, bathing all structures. It then exits the eye through a venous channel between the cornea and the iris. This venous channel, the canal of Schlemm, joins extraocular veins that carry blood and fluid away from the eye.

External Structures of the Eye

The lacrimal glands (tear ducts), conjunctiva (mucous membrane layer on the outside of the eye), and eyelids make up the external structures of the eye. These structures protect the eye from irritants and injury.

Hearing

When sound waves enter the external structure of the ear, pass through the middle ear to the inner ear, and stimulate specific receptor cells in the inner ear that then fire action potentials, hearing occurs. The action potentials are transmitted via the coclear nerve (part of cranial nerve VIII) to the auditory cortex, a structure located in the temporal lobe of the brain (Fig. 20-2), where they are interpreted as sounds. A diagrammatic representation of the ear is presented in Figure 20-4.

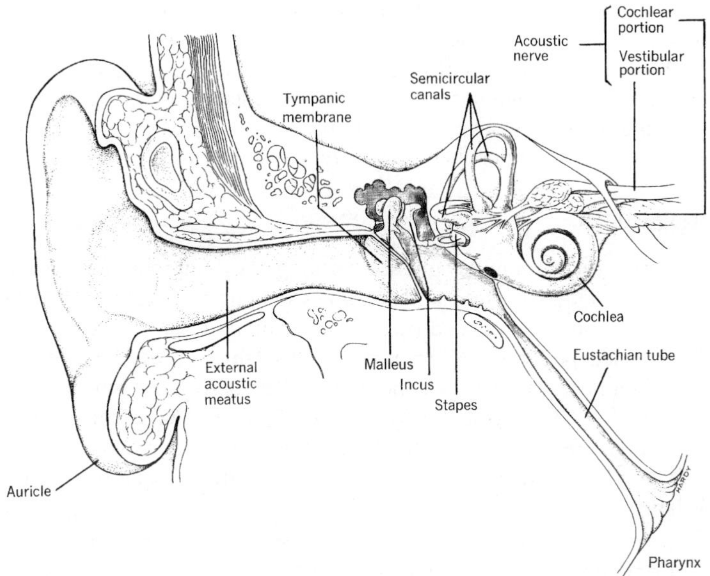

Figure 20-4. External, middle, and internal subdivisions of the ear (from Porth, 1993).

EXTERNAL EAR

The external ear consists of the **auricle** (outside cartilage) and the **external ear canal**. The auricle gathers the sound waves and projects them into the external canal. The external ear canal is a tube through which the sound waves travel to the middle ear. Separating the external ear from the middle ear is the **tympanic membrane**, also called the eardrum. A part of the temporal bone, the mastoid process, lies behind and below the external canal.

MIDDLE EAR

The tympanic membrane is stretched tightly across the end of the external canal. When sound waves strike the eardrum, it is pushed in, or bowed, toward the middle ear. The degree of bowing of the eardrum depends on the loudness of the sound. After one sound wave, the eardrum returns to its previous position. It can be pushed in again and again if the sound waves continue, causing the drum to vibrate. The frequency with which the eardrum vibrates depends on the frequency of the sound waves.

The middle ear has three bony processes, which are connected in series to the eardrum: the **malleus**, the **incus**, and the **stapes**. Vibrations of the eardrum are transmitted from one small bone to the next, eventually striking the **oval window**. The oval window is a small membrane at the entrance to the inner ear.

The middle ear is connected to the nose and throat via the **eustachian tube**. Although normally closed, the eustachian tube opens with yawning or swallowing. This allows the pressure in the middle ear to remain equal to atmospheric pressure.

INNER EAR

The inner ear is a complex organ consisting of two mazelike structures: the outer **bony labyrinth** and the inner **membranous labyrinth**. The bony labyrinth is separated from the membranous labyrinth by thick fluid called perilymph. The membranous labyrinth is filled with a slightly different fluid called endolymph. The bony labyrinth contains the **cochlea**, the **vestibule**, and the **semicircular canals**. The cochlea is the organ responsible for changing sound waves to action potentials. The vestibule and the semicircular canals maintain equilibrium and balance.

Cochlea

The cochlea is a shell-shaped organ, filled with perilymph. The cochlea is separated down the middle by a structure called the **basilar membrane**. On the basilar membrane is a blanket of hair cells that together with the basilar membrane, compose the **organ of Corti**. The hair cells on the basilar membrane depolarize when deformed or bent. Each hair cell synapses upon an afferent neuron, the axons of which make up the acoustic nerve. Depolarization of a hair cell initiates a receptor potential, which, if large enough, stimulates an action potential in the afferent neuron. The hair cells are covered by an overhanging membrane, called the **tectorial membrane**. It is against the tectorial membrane that the hair cells bend when a sound wave is passed into the inner ear.

Sound Wave Transmission

When a sound wave strikes the oval window, a pressure wave is generated in the fluid-filled inner ear. The pressure wave causes a wavelike displacement of the basilar membrane against the overhanging tectorial membrane. As the hair cells rub against the tectorial membrane, they are bent. This leads to the depolarization of the hair cell and the production of a receptor potential. With significant deformation, the afferent nerves synapsed by the hair cells are stimulated to fire action potentials and the signal is transmitted to the auditory cortex. The pathway of hearing is shown in Figure 20-5.

The frequency of the pressure wave determines which hair cells are displaced and consequently which afferent neurons fire action

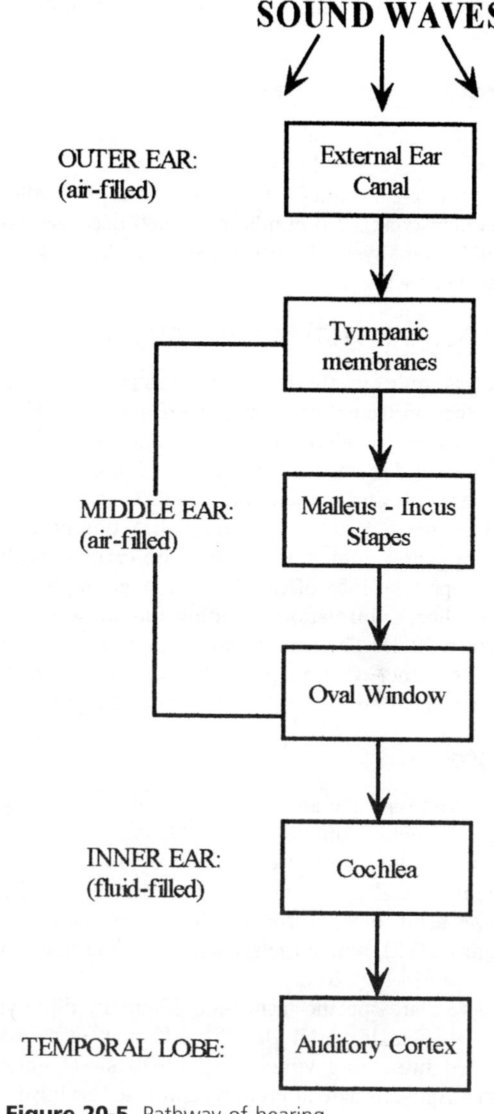

Figure 20-5. Pathway of hearing.

potentials. For instance, the hair cells lying on the part of the basilar membrane nearest the oval window are most displaced by high-frequency sounds, whereas the hair cells lying on the basilar membrane farthest from the oval window are most displaced by low-frequency sounds. The brain interprets the pitch of a sound by which neurons are activated. The brain interprets the intensity of a sound by the frequency of neuronal impulses and the number of afferent neurons firing.

Geriatric Consideration

Hearing acuity generally decreases with age. Causes include atherosclerosis and poor blood flow to the of structures of the ear, stiffening of the middle-ear bones, and loss of receptor cells in the inner ear. Cerumen (wax) also builds up, which decreases sound transmission. Concomitant systemic disease, such as diabetes mellitus, may reduce hearing as well.

VESTIBULAR SYSTEM AND EQUILIBRIUM

The vestibule and the semicircular canals also contain hair cell receptors that are sensitive to movement and position. When the head is turned, the hair cells are bent as they pass through the thick endolymph surrounding them. As in the organ of Corti, bending of a hair cell in the vestibule and semicircular canals causes depolarization of the cell and the firing of an action potential. Action potentials initiated in the vestibule and semicircular canals are carried via the vestibular nerve to the parietal lobe of the brain, converging near the somatosensory area where information on joint and muscle position is integrated (Figure 20-2). The semicircular canals and the vestibular apparatus work together with other tactile and visual systems to determine the current position of the body and any change in motion or direction.

Taste

Receptors for taste are called **taste buds**. Taste buds are located in a pattern on the tongue and are depolarized in response to specific chemical stimulation. Depolarization of the taste buds leads to action potentials and the firing of cranial nerves V, VII, IX, and X. These nerves send their information to the taste cortex in the parietal lobe (Figure 20-2), where the sensation is identified. The pathway of taste is shown in Fig. 20-6.

There are specific taste buds for many different taste sensations, some of which are unidentified. Known taste receptors are usually divided into those which respond to sweet, bitter, salty, and sour tastes. Activation of different receptors to varying degrees by substances found in food allows for a wide range of tastes. The sense of taste initiates digestion and provides a stimulus to eat. There can be adaptation (decreased firing) of the taste buds if exposure to a chemical stimulus is prolonged.

Olfaction

The sense of smell is provided by receptor cells called **olfactory cells** that line the membranes of the nasal mucosa. The olfactory cells contain

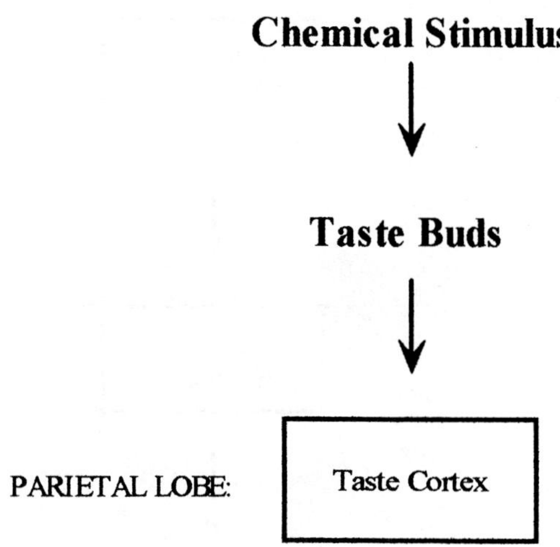

Figure 20-6. Pathway of taste.

cilia that depolarize when bound by certain chemicals corresponding to specific odors in the air. A few types of cilia hyperpolarize in response to a specific odor. Significant depolarization or hyperpolarization of the cilia leads to the firing of action potentials in the neurons of the olfactory nerve (cranial nerve I) that terminate in the olfactory bulbs of the frontal lobe. From there, the signal is passed to the olfactory cortex in the limbic system of the brain (Figure 20-2). The olfactory receptor cells adapt rapidly to a continuing smell. The pathway of smell is shown in Figure 20-7.

Geriatric Consideration

Loss of taste and smell acuity occur with normal aging. Concomitant disease, including Alzheimer's disease, and certain medications taken by the elderly worsen the normal loss of taste and smell. Reduced taste and smell may contribute to the poor appetite seen in some elderly individuals and may partially explain why the elderly often oversalt their food. Interestingly, the perception of sweet taste does not disappear with age, which may contribute to the weight gain seen in some individuals.

Touch

Tactile sensations include the body's recognition of touch, pressure, and vibration. It appears that each of these sensations is mediated by receptors that vary only in location; touch receptors are located in or near the skin, whereas pressure receptors are found deeper in the tis-

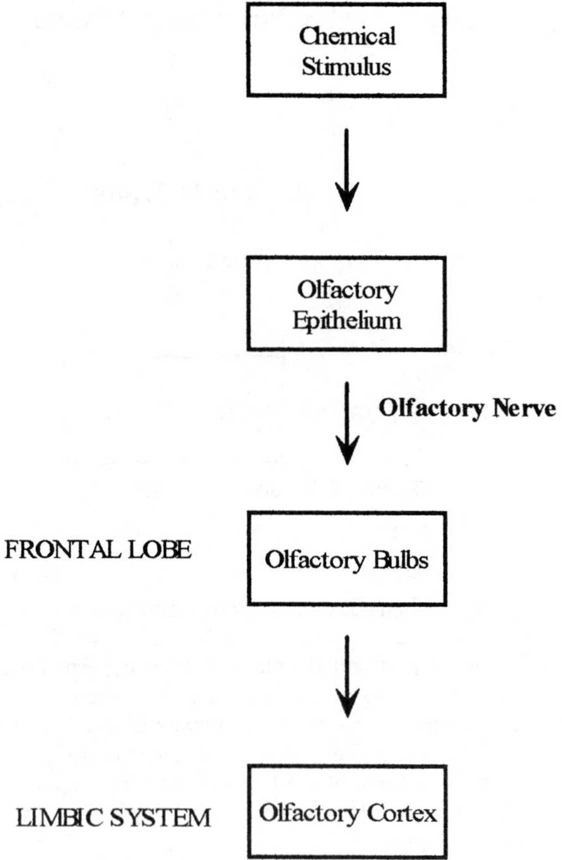

Figure 20-7. Pathway of smell.

sues. Vibration is sensed as rapidly repeating stimuli activating both touch and pressure receptors.

TACTILE RECEPTORS

There are several types of tactile receptors spread over the body. Tactile receptors are **mechanoreceptors**. Mechanoreceptors respond to physical deformation and compression with depolarization, causing a receptor potential. If the depolarization is great enough, the nerve fiber attached to the receptor fires an action potential and transmits the information to the spinal cord and the brain. Different tactile receptors vary in sensitivity and in the velocity with which they send their impulses. Receptors vary as to which type of nerve fiber transmits their signal to the spinal cord and the brain.

PERIPHERAL NERVE FIBERS THAT TRANSMIT TACTILE INFORMATION

Tactile sensation is carried to the spinal cord by one of three types of sensory neurons: large type A beta (β) fibers, smaller type A delta (δ) fibers, and small type C fibers. Both types of A fibers are myelinated, transmitting action potentials rapidly; the larger fibers transmit faster than the smaller fibers. Tactile information carried in the A fibers is typically well localized and pinpoint. The small C fibers are unmyelinated, transmitting action potentials to the spinal cord much more slowly than the A fibers. Tactile information carried in the C fibers is poorly localized.

TRANSMISSION OF TACTILE INFORMATION IN THE SPINAL CORD

Virtually all information on touch, pressure, and vibration enters the spinal cord via the dorsal roots of the corresponding spinal nerve. After synapsing in the spine, highly localized information carried in the fast-firing A fibers (both β and δ) is sent to the brain by way of the dorsal column-lemniscal system. Nerve fibers in this system cross over left to right in the brainstem and travel through the thalamus before synapsing in the somatosensory cortex (Figure 20-2). Information on temperature and poorly localized touch is carried to the spinal cord by way of the slow-firing C fibers. This information is sent to the reticular area of the brainstem and then to higher centers via fibers carried in the anterolateral system. Pain and some sexual sensations are transmitted in the anterolateral tracts.

TYPES OF TACTILE RECEPTORS

There are six basic types of tactile receptors: free nerve endings, Meissner's corpuscles, expanded-tip tactile receptors, hair end-organ receptors, Ruffini's end-organ receptors, and pacinian corpuscles. These are discussed individually in the following sections.

Free Nerve Endings

Receptors that respond to touch are found all over the skin and are called free nerve endings. Most of these receptors send their information to the spinal cord via the small type A δ fibers. From the spinal cord, information from the free nerve endings is sent through the thalamus to the somatosensory area (parietal lobe) of the cortex. Some free nerve endings send their information to the cord via the slow type C fibers. Free nerve endings respond to stimuli perceived as painful.

Meissner's Corpuscles

Touch receptors found on areas of the body not covered with hair, especially the fingertips and lips, are called Meissner's corpuscles.

These receptors allow for precise discrimination concerning the location of a touch. Information from Meissner's corpuscles is carried to the spinal cord via fast-firing type A β nerve fibers. From the spinal cord, information from Meissner's corpuscles is sent through the thalamus to the somatosensory area of the cortex.

Expanded-Tip Tactile Receptors

The expanded-tip tactile receptors are present in association with Meissner's corpuscles and also on areas of the body that do have hair. These receptors provide information on continuous touch, responding with a strong signal when a touch is initiated and continuing with a weak signal for as long as the touch remains. These receptors send their information to the spinal cord via the type A β fibers, allowing for fine discrimination concerning the location and the quality of the touch. From the spinal cord, information is delivered through the thalamus to the somatosensory area of the cortex.

Hair End-Organ Receptors

Each hair follicle on the body has a nerve fiber at its base that acts as a touch receptor. When a hair is bent, the nerve fires an action potential. The hair receptors send their information to the spinal cord via type A β fibers and then on through the thalamus to the somatosensory area of the cortex.

Ruffini's End Organs

Nerve fibers located deep in the skin and underlying tissues are known as Ruffini's end organs. These receptors fire continuously in response to deformation. Ruffini's end organs are present in the joints and provide information on joint position and movement. They send their information to the spinal cord via type A β fibers and then on through the thalamus to the somatosensory area of the cortex.

Pacinian Corpuscles

Rapidly adapting fibers under the skin and in other body tissues such as the penis, clitoris, and nipples are called Pacinian corpuscles. They fire quickly with the onset of a touch, especially one involving deep pressure or high-frequency vibration, and then adapt. They send information to the spinal cord via type A β fibers and then on through the thalamus to the somatosensory area of the cortex. The pathways of touch are shown in Figure 20-8.

TEMPERATURE SENSATION

Temperature is sensed by specific warm and cold receptors located immediately under the skin. There are more cold receptors than warm receptors. Pain receptors also participate in temperature sensation.

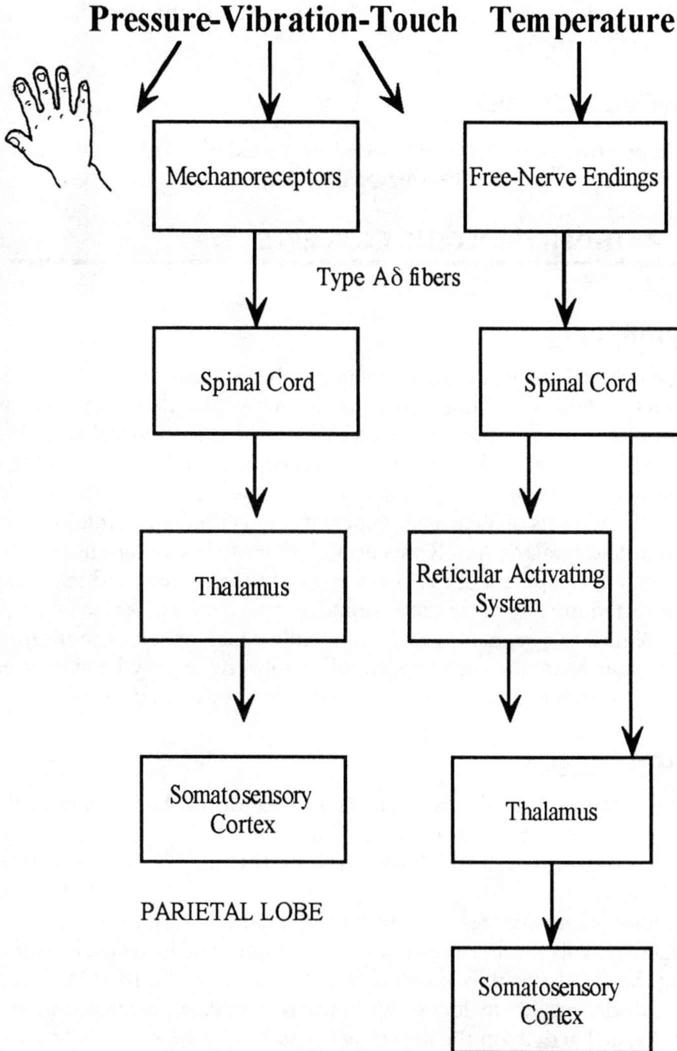

Figure 20-8. Pathway of touch.

Warm receptors are poorly understood but appear to be free nerve endings that depolarize with a warm stimulus. Cold receptors have been identified as free nerve endings of the small type A δ fibers. From the spinal cord, nerves carrying information on temperature pass through the reticular-activating system on their way to the thalamus. A few fibers continue to the somatosensory area of the cortex. Temperature receptors are not mechanoreceptors. They are activated chemically by substances produced by cells after temperature-induced changes in metabolic activity.

Geriatric Consideration

Temperature sensation is decreased in the elderly. This may result in accidental burns from heating pads or hot baths.

PATHOPHYSIOLOGIC CONCEPTS

Amblyopia

The reduction in visual acuity in an eye that appears to be structurally intact is known as amblyopia. With amblyopia, there develops an inability of the central nervous system to identify a visual stimulus; that is, the signal is sent but not recognized in the brain. Often, amblyopia develops from the disuse of one eye ("lazy eye") that results from conditions of abnormal binocular interaction (e.g., strabismus or infantile cataracts). Amblyopia occurs under these conditions because normal development of the visual areas of the thalamus and the visual cortex require binocular visual stimuli during a critical period of development (0 to 5 years of age). Occasionally, amblyopia may result from ingestion of toxins such as alcohol or tobacco or may be associated with a systemic disease such as renal failure or diabetes mellitus.

Strabismus

The condition called strabismus is a deviation in the position of the eyes relative to each other. With strabismus, the eyes may appear to be crossed. An individual who has strabismus often complains of double vision.

Strabismus may result from a congenital inability to use the eyes together. This is called nonparalytic strabismus and is treated by patching the eye that can fix on an object ("the good eye"). Patching forces the deviating eye to focus. Without treatment, ambylopia develops and visual activity in the deviating eye is lost by approximately age 6.

Paralytic strabismus usually occurs later in life after paralysis of one or more of the muscles controlling eye movement. Tumor, injury, or infection may cause paralytic strabismus.

Nystagmus

The involuntary, rhythmic movement of one or both eyes is called nystagmus. The movement may be jerking, rotating, or pendular. Causes of nystagmus include damage to the vestibular system; injury of cranial nerves III, IV, or VI; cerebellar disturbance; or drug intoxication. Rotating nystagmus is frequently associated with dizziness and nausea. Miners exposed to years of working in the dark may develop pendular nystagmus.

Myopia

Also called nearsightedness, myopia, occurs when the eye is unable to accommodate sufficiently to far objects. Myopia may result from developmental elongation of the eyeball. This causes the image to be focused in front of the retina. Myopia appears to have a genetic predisposition and frequently develops in late childhood. It is especially common in children who read extensively, perhaps as a result of changes in the length of the eyeball after prolonged focusing on near objects. Myopia is treated with a concave lens in eyeglasses or contact lenses.

Hyperopia

The condition of hyperopia, also called farsightedness, occurs when the eye is unable to accommodate sufficiently to close objects. Hyperopia typically develops after the fourth decade of life (presbyopia) and is caused by inflexibilty of the aging lens. This causes the image to be focused past the retina. Hyperopia is treated by providing a convex lens to eyeglasses or contact lenses.

Astigmatism

In astigmatism, light rays are scattered rather than focused on the retina because of an unsymmetric curvature of the cornea. The image is distorted or blurred. Astigmatism may occur with myopia or hyperopia. Specially constructed lenses are required.

Color Blindness

Color blindness is usually a sex-linked genetic disorder caused by a deficiency in one of the three photopigments. Color-blind individuals see colors only formed by the activity of the other two types of cones. Color blindness is passed on the X chromosome; therefore, it usually affects males. In extreme cases, more than one color cone can be deficient.

Geriatric Consideration

With age, most people experience a decline in color vision caused by yellowing of the lens. This may interfere with visual cues and contribute to falls.

Papilledema

Papilledema is the swelling of the optic disk where the optic nerve leaves the eye and enters the brain. Because the optic disk is in communication with the brain, papilledema can occur in any condition that causes severely increased intracranial pressure. Such conditions may include brain tumor, infection, or injury. Papilledema is often an important diagnostic clue in severe brain pathology.

Conductive Hearing Loss

Conductive hearing loss is a decrease in hearing caused by a blockage in the conduction of sound waves in the external or middle ear. Conductive hearing loss may occur if a foreign object is present in the ear or if there is an excessive wax or fluid buildup in the external or middle ear. Middle-ear infections (otitis media) may cause conductive hearing loss. A hearing aid may offer improvement.

Pediatric Consideration

A child who suffers repeated episodes of otitis media may develop a speech deficiency if hearing is reduced during critical periods of language development. Repeated episodes of middle-ear infections may cause scarring of the eardrum and permanent loss of hearing.

Sensorineural Hearing Loss

Sensorineural hearing loss is a decrease in hearing caused by dysfunction of the organ of Corti, the auditory nerve, or the brain. The organ of Corti may become damaged from prolonged exposure to high levels of noise or after the use of ototoxic (damaging to the ears) drugs. Ototoxic drugs include aminoglycoside antibiotics (gentamicin, neomycin, and streptomycin), analgesics (aspirin), tobacco, and alcohol. Systemic diseases, including diabetes mellitus and syphilis, may also cause sensorineural hearing loss.

Pediatric Consideration

Congenital sensorineural hearing loss may occur after fetal exposure to rubella or maternal drug exposure (including to the aminoglycosides). Congenital sensorineural hearing loss may also be inherited.

Geriatric Consideration

The basilar membrane of the cochlea stiffens with age, resulting in sensorineural hearing loss, called **presbycusis**. Receptor hair cells die and are not replaced. Loss of receptors in the high-frequency range is especially common. Because of these changes, the elderly person is better able to hear deep voices compared with higher-pitched voices.

Tinnitus

Described as a ringing in one or both ears, tinnitus may accompany ear wax buildup or presbycusis. Aspirin overdose or other drugs may induce tinnitus. Middle-ear infection, Menière's disease, or otosclerosis (irregular ossification of middle-ear bones) may also cause tinnitus.

Vertigo

The sensation of motion or spinning, often described as a feeling of being off balance, is called vertigo. Vertigo is sometimes accompanied by nausea, weakness, and mental confusion. Inner-ear inflammation, especially of the semicircular canals, is the most common cause of vertigo. Cranial nerve disorders may also cause vertigo.

Hyposmia

A decrease in the sensation of smell is called hyposmia. Hyposmia may be bilateral or unilateral. If all smells are affected, congestion of the nasal passages is the most common cause. Hyposmia of a specific smell suggests nerve tract damage. Individuals who suffer a frontal-lobe injury often suffer hyposmia.

Hypogeusia

A decrease in taste sensation is called hypogeusia. Loss of taste sensation may be of a specific taste or of all tastes. It may indicate damage to one of the cranial nerves innervating either the tongue or the palate. Sometimes tastes previously enjoyed are suddenly perceived as distasteful. This phenomenon is called parageusia and may occur with drug therapy, including chemotherapeutic drugs, or with liver dysfunction. In the elderly, hypogeusia sometimes occurs spontaneously.

CONDITIONS OF DISEASE OR INJURY

Conjunctivitis

Inflammation of the conjunctiva of the eye caused by an infectious process, physical irritation, or an allergic response is known as conjunctivitis. With inflammation, the conjunctiva becomes red, swollen, and tender. Conjunctivitis because of a bacterial infection is sometimes called pink eye. It may be an infection only of the eye, or it may coexist with an ear infection. Viral conjunctivitis is often caused by adenovirus infection. Bacterial and viral conjunctivitis are highly contagious. Allergic conjunctivitis occurs as part of the inflammatory reaction to an environmental allergen. Physical stimulation by a foreign object in the eye irritates the conjunctiva, causing inflammation and pain.

CLINICAL MANIFESTATIONS

- Red, swollen conjunctiva. With infectious or allergic conjunctivitis, both eyes are usually affected.

- Photophobia (an aversion to light).
- A purulent discharge is characteristic of bacterial conjunctivitis. Infection and discharge often begin in one eye and spread to the other. The eyes may be matted shut by a greenish crust.
- A clear, watery discharge is characteristic of viral conjunctivitis. Viral conjunctivitis frequently accompanies an upper respiratory tract infection.
- Burning and itching of the eyes is characteristic of allergic conjunctivitis.
- Conjunctivitis due to a foreign object is associated with discomfort and a feeling of sand or grit in the eye. Usually with a foreign object, only one eye is affected.

DIAGNOSIS

- Diagnosis follows history and physical examination. Cultures may be required in some circumstances.
- A foreign object in the eye should be visualized with the use of a speical lamp, called a Wood's lamp.

COMPLICATIONS

- Certain bacterial infections (gonorrorhea, some types of chlamydial conjunctivitis) and severe viral infections may cause permanent damage to the eye if untreated.
- A foreign body in the eye may lead to corneal abrasion and scarring.
- Conjunctivitis may be an early symptom of the severe systemic disease **Kawasaki's disease**. This disease is one of widespread vasculitis that affects many organs of the body, including the heart, brain, joints, liver, and eyes. It begins acutely with a high fever, followed shortly by bilateral conjunctivitis that is notable for its lack of discharge and its prolonged course. A rash and swelling of hands and feet accompany these early symptoms. Early diagnosis is important to prevent damage to the coronary arteries. Treatment for Kawasaki's disease involves the use of aspirin and gamma globulin.

TREATMENT

- Bacterial conjunctivitis is usually treated with antibiotic eye drops or cream, but it often resolves on its own within approximately 2 weeks without treatment. Because it is highly contagious among family members and schoolmates, excellent handwashing techniques and separate towels for infected individuals are required. Family members should not share bed linens or pillows.
- Conjunctivitis co-associated with otitis media is treated with systemic antibiotics. Warm compresses placed on the eyes may remove the discharge.

- Viral conjunctivitis is usually treated with warm compresses. Excellent handwashing techniques are required to prevent transmission.
- Allergic conjunctivitis is treated by avoidance of the allergen if possible. Antihistamines or steroid-containing eyedrops are used to reduce itching and inflammation.
- Conjunctivitis caused by an irritant is treated by removal of any foreign object, and the use of antibacterial medication.

Pediatric Consideration

Newborns may develop conjunctivitis during birth. The causative microorganism is often chlamydia, which may colonize in the mother's cervix, or gonorrhea. Both of these diseases are sexually transmitted. Pregnant women with confirmed sexually transmitted disease should be treated with antibiotics before giving birth.

Cataracts

A cataract is a progressive loss in the transparency of the lens. The lens becomes cloudy or gray-white in color, and visual acuity is reduced. Cataracts occur when proteins in the normally transparent lens break down and coagulate on the lens.

CAUSES OF CATARACTS

Most cataracts, called senile cataracts, develop as a result of degenerative changes associated with aging. Lifelong exposure to sunlight and a hereditary predisposition contribute to the development of senile cataracts.

Cataracts also may occur at any age after either trauma to the lens or eye infection, or they may occur as a result of exposure to radiation or certain drugs. Fetal exposure to the rubella virus may cause cataract formation. Individuals who have long-term diabetes mellitus frequently develop cataracts, most likely caused by poor blood flow to the eye and by the altered handling and metabolism of glucose.

CLINICAL MANIFESTATIONS

- Progressively decreased visual acuity.
- Blurring of vision, glaring, and loss of color perception occur.

DIAGNOSIS

- Cataracts are diagnosed following a history and physical examination, during which whitish opacities on the lens may be seen.
- In infants, there may be an absence of the red reflex on eye examination.

COMPLICATIONS

- Loss of vision may occur if untreated.

TREATMENT

- Treatment may involve excision of the entire lens and replacement with an artificial lens, or it may involve fragmentation of the lens by ultrasound or laser, followed by aspiration of the fragments and lens replacement.

Glaucoma

Glaucoma is a condition of the eye caused by an abnormal increase in intraocular pressure (to greater than 20 mm Hg). The high pressures, sometimes reaching 60 to 70 mm Hg, cause compression of the optic nerve as it leaves the eyeball, leading to death of the nerve fibers. Loss of peripheral vision occurs first, followed by loss of central vision. Glaucoma is one of the main causes of blindness in the United States. Blindness caused by glaucoma usually develops gradually, but it may occur within a few days if intraocular pressures suddenly become high.

CAUSES OF GLAUCOMA

Glaucoma is usually caused by an obstruction of aqueous humor flow. Obstruction to flow out of the angle between the cornea and the iris (acute angle closure) may occur suddenly with infection or injury. Age-related fibrosis of the angle or other channels involved in the flow of aqueous humor may gradually increase intraocular pressure. Occasionally, an increase in the production of aqueous humor also may lead to increased intraocular pressure.

CLINICAL MANIFESTATIONS

- Acute glaucoma is characterized by severe eye pain and sudden blurring of vision. The pupil remains dilated and unresponsive to light.
- Chronic glaucoma is characterized by a slow decrease in visual acuity and blurring, beginning with peripheral vision. Headache and eye pain may develop as the condition worsens.

DIAGNOSIS

- Glaucoma can be diagnosed from history and physical examination. Intraocular pressure readings are high, and close inspection of the optic nerve shows characteristic color changes and cupping of the retinal rim.
- It is essential to diagnose glaucoma early to reduce the risk of blindness.

COMPLICATIONS

- Blindness may develop with any type of glaucoma. Acute angle closure glaucoma is a medical emergency.
- Topical agents used to treat glaucoma may have adverse systemic effects, especially in the elderly. These effects may include worsening of cardiac, respiratory, or neurologic conditions.

TREATMENT

- Eyedrops are applied to decrease intraocular pressure. These drops work by reducing the secretion or increasing the absorption of aqueous humor.
- With acute angle closure, diuretics may be used to decrease intraocular pressure. Surgery may be required. Intraocular pressures should be monitored annually in individuals older than age 40 or anyone who has an increased risk of the disorder.

Otitis

Otitis is an inflammation of the ear. **Otitis media** refers to inflammation of the middle ear. Otitis media often results from a bacterial infection, usually by *Streptococcus pneumoniae, Haemophilus influenza,* or *Staphylococcus aureus*. Otitis media may also result from a viral infection. **Serous otitis media** is the accumulation of fluid in the middle ear that often results from an allergy. There may be an associated infection. Middle-ear inflammation occurs when the eustachian tubes that normally drain middle-ear secretions to the throat become blocked. This causes middle-ear secretions and fluid to accumulate. When the tubes reopen, pressure in the congested ear can draw contaminated nasal secretions through the eustachian tubes into the middle ear, leading to infection. **Otitis externa** refers to inflammation of the external ear canal.

CLINICAL MANIFESTATIONS

- Pain in the affected ear, especially with an infectious cause, is the most common symptom of otitis media.
- Fever, fussing, and pulling on the ear, in an infant or toddler may signify otitis.
- Anorexia, vomiting, and diarrhea sometimes accompany a middle-ear infection.
- An uncomfortable feeling of fullness in the ear is common with allergic (serous) otitis media.
- Pain with manipulation of the external structures of the ear suggests otitis externa.

DIAGNOSTIC TOOLS

- Otoscopic examination of the ear provides information on the eardrum that can be used to diagnose otitis media. Infectious (acute)

otitis media appears as a reddened bulging eardrum when examined otoscopically. Bony landmarks and the light reflex may be obscured. Serous otitis media may appear as a gray eardrum, either bulging or depressed inward. Otitis externa is diagnosed by the observance of a reddened, inflamed external canal.
- The use of a pneumonic device with the otoscope further assists diagnosis of otitis media. By squeezing an air-filled bulb connected to the otoscope, a small bolus of air can be injected into the external ear. The mobility of the tympanic membrane can be observed by the examiner through the otoscope. With otitis media and serous otitis media, tympanic mobility is reduced.
- A tympanogram, a test that involves placing a small probe in the external ear and measuring the movement of the tympanic membrane (eardrum) after the presentation of a fixed tone, can also be used to evaluate tympanic mobility. With otitis media and serous otitis media, the mobility of the eardrum is reduced.
- Audiologic testing may show a hearing deficit. This deficit is an indication of fluid buildup (infectious or allergic).

COMPLICATIONS

- Repeated or untreated otitis media may cause scarring of the eardrum and permanent reduction in hearing acuity.
- Meningitis or infection of the mastoid bone may develop from an untreated ear infection.

TREATMENT

- Infectious otitis media is usually treated with antibiotics.
- Serous otitis media may be treated with antihistamines or decongestants, with or without antibiotics.
- Otitis externa is treated with anti-inflammatory drops, antimicrobial drops, or both.

Pediatric Consideration

Infants and young children are most susceptible to middle-ear infections because of their short, straight eustachian tubes compared with older children and adults. Prevention of otitis media in infants includes not putting a baby to bed with a bottle and feeding an infant with the head raised. Young children who have repeated ear infections may have reduced hearing acuity or experience language delays. To prevent this, tubes may be placed in the ear to assist drainage.

Ménière's Disease

A chronic disorder of the semicircular canals and labyrinths of the inner ear is called Ménière's disease. This disease is associated with severe attacks of vertigo. The cause of Ménière's disease is unknown, but it appears related to an overproduction of endolymph in the inner ear. Occurrences of Ménière's disease may follow middle-ear infection or head trauma or may be associated with systemic illness such as thyroid disease. The condition may also show a genetic predisposition. Typically, the disorder is unilateral (only one ear affected).

CLINICAL MANIFESTATIONS

- Ménière's disease is characterized by extreme vertigo, lasting several minutes to a few hours. The episodes come and go, often with several months between attacks.
- Fluctuating tinnitus and hearing loss accompany the attacks.
- Nausea, vomiting, hypotension, and sweating often occur with attacks.

DIAGNOSIS

- Ménière's disease can be diagnosed from history and physical examination. Tests of vestibular function, including balance testing and tests of nystagmus eye movements may help confirm the diagnosis.

COMPLICATIONS

- Ménière's disease may progress to unilateral nerve deafness.

TREATMENT

- Symptoms may decrease if the patient lies down or sits still, making no sudden movements.
- Treatments to reduce fluid volume, including diuretics and a low-salt diet, are suggested. Antihistamines and steroid hormones may be used as well with varying degrees of success.
- Medications are available that can reduce nausea.
- Surgical placement of a shunt to drain excess endolymph may be performed.

Pain

Pain is a subjective sensation of unpleasantness usually associated with actual or potential tissue damage. Pain can be protective, in that it causes an individual to back away from a dangerous stimulus, or it can serve no function, as is the case of chronic pain. Pain is sensed when specific pain receptors are activated. Description of pain is subjective and objective, based on the duration, the speed of sensation, and the location.

RECEPTORS FOR PAIN

Pain receptors are called **nociceptors**. Nociceptors include the free nerve endings that respond to many stimuli, including mechanical pressure, deformation, temperature extremes, and various chemicals. With intense stimuli, other receptors such as the Pacini's corpuscles and Meissner's corpuscles also send information perceived as painful. Chemicals that cause or worsen pain include histamine, bradykinin, serotonin, several prostaglandins, potassium ion, and hydrogen ion. Each of these substances accumulates at sites of cellular injury, hypoxia, or death, alerting the individual to these happenings. Although all pain receptors are capable of responding to any type of tactile stimuli, each receptor appears to respond most readily to one type of stimulation compared with another.

DURATION OF PAIN

Pain is separated into acute (lasting less than 6 months) and chronic (lasting longer than 6 months). Acute pain can be beneficial, serving to alert the individual to danger. Chronic pain is never beneficial.

SPEED OF SENSATION

Fast pain is sensed less than 1 second (usually much less) after the application of a painful stimulus (e.g., touching a hot burner). Fast pain is well localized to the site and is frequently described as pricking or sharp. Fast pain is usually felt on or near the surface of the body. It is transmitted to the spinal cord by the A δ fibers.

Slow pain is felt 1 second or more after the application of a painful stimulus (e.g., pain that continues after a bump to the head). Slow pain is frequently described as dull, throbbing, or burning. It can intensify over the course of several minutes and may occur on the skin or in any deep tissue of the body. Slow pain can become chronic pain and lead to great disability. Slow pain is transmitted to the spinal cord by the slow C fibers. The C fibers are believed to release the neurotransmitter substance P when they synapse in the spinal cord. The neurotransmitter released by the A δ fibers is unknown. The pathways of pain are shown in Figure 20-9.

LOCATION

Cutaneous pain is pain felt on the skin or in subcutaneous tissues (e.g., pain felt with a pinprick or a skinned knee). It is well localized over a dermatome (an area of the skin innervated by a certain spinal cord segment) and is transmitted rapidly. **Deep somatic** pain is pain arising from bones and joints, tendons, skeletal muscles, blood vessels, and deep nerve pressure. The pain of a headache is considered deep somatic pain. Deep somatic pain is slow pain, which may radiate along a nerve route. **Visceral** pain is pain in the abdominal or thoracic cavity. Visceral pain is typically severe and may be well localized at one spot, but it may also be referred to different parts of the body. Visceral pain localizes over embryonic dermatomes and is caused by stimulation of several pain receptors.

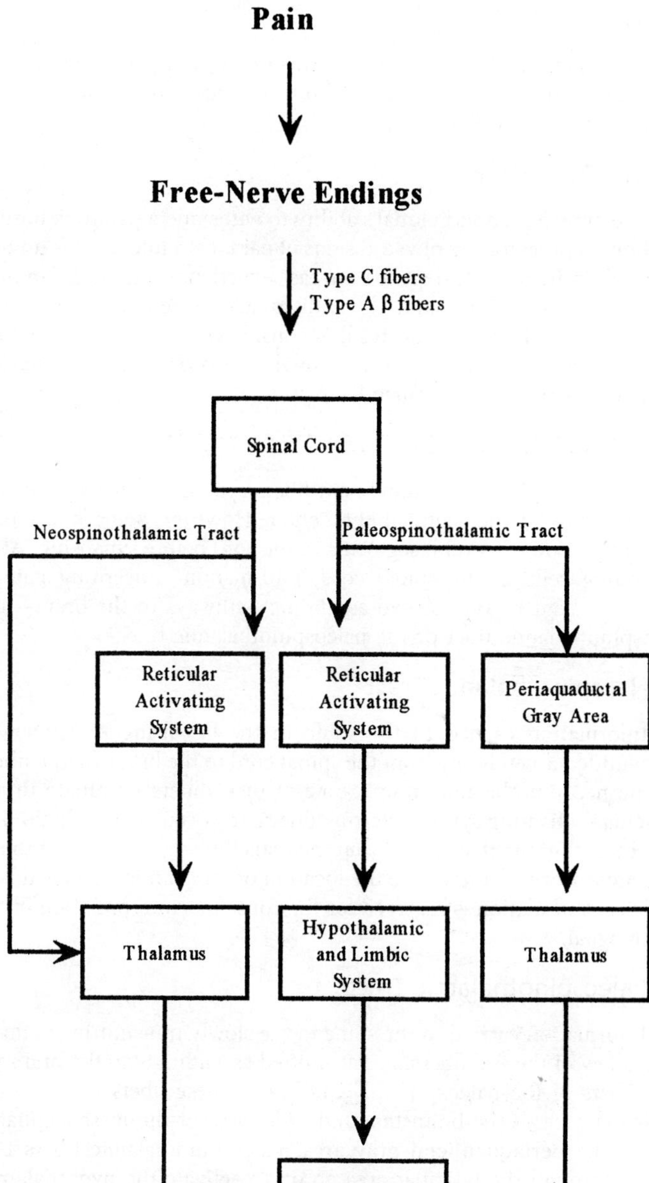

Figure 20-9. Pathway of pain.

PAIN THRESHOLD

Pain threshold is the level of a stimulus that is first perceived as pain. In general, humans have similar pain thresholds. An individual's pain threshold varies little over time.

PAIN TOLERANCE

Pain tolerance is an individual's ability to withstand a painful stimulus without demonstrating physical signs of pain. Pain tolerance is unique for each individual. It depends on past experience; cultural, familial, and role expectations; and the individual's current emotional and physical state. In some cultures it is considered weak to "show pain," so pain tolerance is high. An individual who is depressed or anxious may have a reduced tolerance for pain.

CENTRAL NERVOUS SYSTEM PATHWAYS FOR PAIN

Once in the spinal cord, most pain fibers synapse on neurons in the dorsal horns of the segment they enter. However, some fibers may travel up or down several segments in the cord before synapsing. After activating cells in the spinal cord, information concerning painful stimuli is sent by one of two ascending pathways to the brain—the neospinothalamic tract or the paleospinothalamic tract.

Neospinothalamic Tract

Information carried to the spine in the fast-firing A δ fibers is transmitted ascendingly from the spinal cord to the brain via the fibers of the neospinothalamic tract. Some of these fibers terminate in the reticular-activating system, alerting one to the occurrence of pain, but most travel to the thalamus. From the thalamus, signals are sent to the somatosensory cortex where the location of the pain is well localized. Cortical stimulation is required for the conscious interpretation of the pain signal.

Paleospinothalamic Tract

Information carried to the spine in the slowly transmitting C fibers and a few of the A δ fibers, is transmitted ascendingly to the brain via the fibers of the paleospinothalamic tract. These fibers travel to the reticular area of the brainstem and to an area of the mesencephalon called the **periaqueductal gray area**. Paleospinothalamic fibers that travel through the reticular area go on to activate the hypothalamus and the limbic system, influencing the function of these emotion-controlling areas. The periaqueductal gray area is an important integrating center for pain; the perception of pain is highly modified in this area. Pain carried in the paleospinothalamic tract is poorly localized and is responsible for causing the emotional distress associated with pain.

GATING OF PAIN IN THE SPINAL CORD AND THE BRAIN

Experimental evidence suggests that the likelihood of transmitting painful stimuli from the spinal cord to the brain can be influenced by descending neurons firing on the cells of the spinal cord. Descending input to the spine may increase the transmission of a painful stimulus, or it might decrease the likelihood that a stimulus is perceived as painful. Reduced passage of a painful stimulus is called **analgesia**.

Descending neurons that affect pain transmission come from the cerebral cortex, the hypothalamus, the limbic system, and, especially, the periaqueductal gray area. The ability of upper brain areas to influence transmission of pain in the spinal cord is called **gating**. Gating occurs at each level of pain transmission (across both the neospinothalamic and the paleospinothalamic tracts) and in the brain as well. Fibers from the periaqueductal gray area that diffusely innervate the cerebral cortex, the limbic system, the hypothalamus, and the reticular formation are especially important in influencing pain transmission in the brain.

Interpretation of the Gate Theory

The gate theory of pain offers an explanation of how cultural and personal expectations, mood, and fear can influence an individual's perception of pain and pain tolerance. By emphasizing the ability of descending pathways to influence pain perception, the gate theory of pain explains how distraction or relaxation techniques may reduce pain, whereas focusing on a painful stimulus may increase the likelihood of the stimulus being passed into consciousness.

The gate theory of pain also explains how gating can occur with peripheral nervous stimulation to the spinal cord. Data suggest that when the large A β neurons carrying skin tactile information are stimulated at the same time that the A δ and C fibers are transmitting painful stimuli, spinal activation of both the neospinothalamic and the paleospinothalamic tracts is reduced. This appears to be because of lateral inhibition of the cells in the dorsal spine by the large A β neurons. Rubbing the head or skin after an injury stimulates the large A β fibers and produces some degree of analgesia. This is an example of gating the passage of a painful stimulus.

Endorphins, Enkephalins, and Serotonin

Some of the analgesic responses described above appear to result from the central nervous system production and release of the endogenous opiates: the endorphins and the enkephalins. Serotonin, another neurotransmitter, is also involved in producing analgesia.

Enkephalin is a small peptide released in the spinal cord from neurons descending from the periaqueductal gray area. Enkephalin causes presynaptic inhibition of types C and A δ fibers in the spine. This reduces the passage of a painful stimulus beyond the spinal cord. Enkephalin is also present in the limbic system and the hypothalamus.

The endorphins and serotonin act as neurotransmitters in the brain to reduce the passage or perception of pain. Endorphin is released by the pituitary in response to intense exercise and during painful experiences such as labor and delivery. Endorphins also affect mood. Prolonged pain has been shown to deplete endorphin levels, perhaps contributing to the despair and anguish seen in individuals who have chronic pain. Serotonin is produced in the brain and is released from descending fibers synapsing in the spinal cord. Drugs that increase brain serotonin levels, such as the tricyclic antidepressants, reduce pain perception.

Pediatric Consideration

Infants and children acutely feel pain and should never be exposed to painful therapies without pain medication. Infants may express pain differently from older children and adults.

CLINICAL MANIFESTATIONS

- Acute pain is characterized by increased heart rate, increased respiratory rate, facial grimacing, withdrawal, and crying. Dilated pupils and sweating occur. Usually, a person suffering acute pain highly focuses on the pain.
- Chronic pain is associated with a return of heart and respiratory rate to normal. An individual who has chronic pain may appear quiet and subdued. Depression and despair may develop.

DIAGNOSTIC TOOLS

- Rating scales from 1 to 10 allow an individual to evaluate pain and may help a clinician recognize the intensity of a person's pain.
- Recognizing the subtle cues an individual who is in pain may show is important for responding to pain when cultural, linguistic, or age barriers to communication exist.

COMPLICATIONS

- Pain stimulates the stress response. Stress can reduce the functioning of the immune and inflammatory systems, and thus healing is delayed.
- Acute, severe pain may lead to cardiovascular collapse and shock.

TREATMENT

- Application of cool compresses may reduce pain associated with inflammation.
- Comfort measures such as a back rub may reduce pain by stimulat-

ing the large A β fibers and by activating descending pathways stimulated by distraction.

- Behavioral techniques, including distraction and imaging, may stimulate descending pathways that block the transmission of painful stimuli to the brain. The Lamaze method of breathing during labor works on this principle.
- Transcutaneous electric nerve stimulation (electrodes on the skin) may relieve pain by stimulating the large type A β nerve fibers. Acupuncture may stimulate these fibers and reduce pain as well.
- Analgesics such as aspirin or acetaminophen can relieve mild pain.
- Nonsteroidal anti-inflammatory drugs, such as ibuprofen, or steroids may be used for moderate pain.
- Narcotics, such as morphine, can reduce intense pain.
- Nerve block by injection of drugs or surgery may occasionally be used to treat severe pain.

Selected Bibliography

Bates, B. (1998). *A guide to physical examination (7th ed.)*. Philadelphia: J.B. Lippincott.

Daw, N. W. (1998). Critical periods and ambylopia. *Archives of Opthalmology* 116, 502–504.

Grievink, E. H. (1993). The effects of early bilateral otitis media with effusion on language ability: a prospective cohort study. *Journal of Speech and Hearing Research* 36, 1004–1012.

Guyton, A. C. & Hall, J. (1997). *Textbook of medical physiology (9th ed.)*. Philadelphia: W.B. Saunders.

Hodges, C. (1998). Easing children's pain. *Nursing Times* 94, 55–56.

Howie, V. M. (1993). Otitis media. *Pediatric Review* 8, 320–323.

Montauk, S. L. & Martin, J. (1997). Treating chronic pain. *American Family Physician* 55, 1151–1160.

Paparella, M. M. (1993). Pathogenesis and pathophysiology of Meniere's disease. *Acta Otolaryngology Supplement (Stockholm)* 485, 26–35.

Podolsky, M. M. (1998). Exposing glaucoma. Primary care physicians are instrumental in early detection. *Postgraduate Medicine* 103, 131–136.

Porth, C. M. (1998). *Pathophysiology concepts of altered health states (5th ed.)*. Philadelphia: J.B. Lippincott.

Schiffman, S. S. (1997). Taste and smell losses in normal aging and disease. *JAMA* 278, 1357–1362.

Schuknecht, H. F. (1993). *Pathology of the ear (2nd ed.)*. Philadelphia: Lea & Febiger.

Shea, J. J., Jr. (1993). Classification of Meniere's disease. *American Journal of Otology* 14, 224–229.

Stewart, R. E., DeSimone, J. A., & Hill, D. L. (1997). New perspectives in a gustatory physiology: transduction, development, and plasticity. *American Journal of Physiology* 272 (1 Pt 1)C1–C26.

Vander, A. J., Sherman, J., & Luciano, D. (1998). *Human physiology (7th ed.)*. Boston: McGraw-Hill.

Whitaker, R., Jr. & Whitaker, V. B. (1998). Glaucoma: what the nurse practitioner should know. *Nurse Practitioner Forum* 9, 7–12.

Wu, S. M. (1994). Synaptic transmission in the outer retina. *Annual Review of Physiology* 56, 141–168.

21 THE REPRODUCTIVE SYSTEM

The goal of evolution is for members of a species to pass on their genes to viable offspring. Most species, including humans, have elaborate mating rituals and reproductive systems that have evolved to further this goal. Some philosophers and scientists have argued that all the magnificence of the human body exists only to make us successful producers, carriers, and deliverers of egg and sperm. Even those who believe humans are more than vessels of reproduction acknowledge the essential importance of reproduction for the species. Pathology of the reproductive system can interfere with an individual's ability to contribute to the genetic pool.

● ● ●

PHYSIOLOGIC CONCEPTS

Male Reproductive Anatomy

The reproductive role of the human male is to produce and deliver sperm to impregnate a female. To carry out these functions, a male has internal and external sexual organs and secondary sex characteristics. Internal and external structures include the testes, several tubules that carry sperm out of the testes, various glands, and the penis (see Fig. 21-1).

THE TESTES

The **testes** are the gonads of the male. The testes develop during gestation in response to the production of androgenic hormones by the male embryo. The primary androgen is testosterone, the synthesis of which begins at approximately 8 weeks' gestation.

During early gestation, the fetal testes are located in the abdominal cavity. At approximately 6 months' gestation, the testes descend from the abdominal cavity through the inguinal canal into an external sac, called the **scrotum**. Associated blood vessels, nerves, and a supporting cord descend from the abdominal cavity simultaneously. After descent, the abdominal opening of the canal closes. The scrotum sits dorsal to the **penis**, the male sexual organ and structure for urination. Because of their location outside the body, the testes remain at a lower-than-body temperature. This provides optimal conditions for sperm formation.

SEMINIFEROUS TUBULES

Each testis is filled with hundreds of long, coiled tubules, called **seminiferous tubules**. Immature sperm arise from stem cells present in the tubular walls and then migrate into the tubule lumen. The seminiferous tubules include two types of cells: **Sertoli cells**, which line the inside

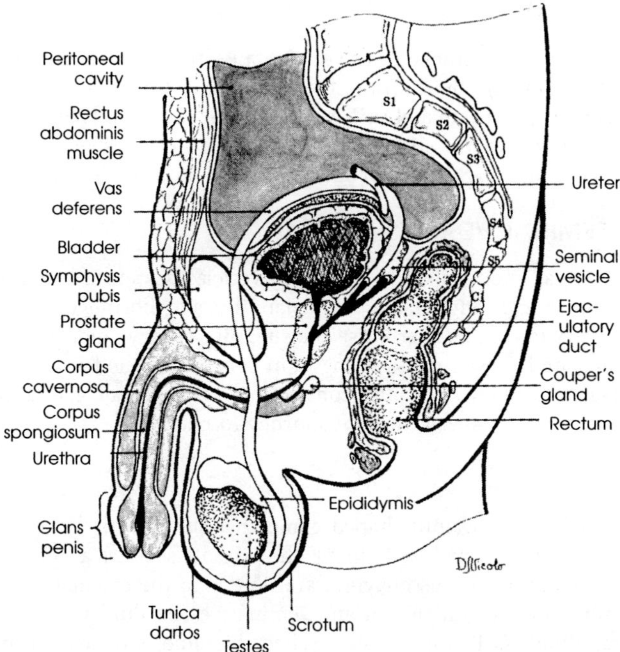

Figure 21-1. Side view of male genitourinary anatomy (from Bullock and Rosendahl, 1992).

of the tubules, and **Leydig interstitial cells**, which surround the outside of the tubules. The developing sperm receive essential support and nourishment from the Sertoli cells during their long maturation. The Leydig interstitial cells synthesize and secrete testosterone during gestation and after puberty. Testosterone affects both sperm maturation and Sertoli cell function.

THE EPIDIDYMIS, VAS DEFERENS, AND URETHRA

From the seminiferous tubules, sperm journey into another long tubule, the **epididymis**. The epididymis curves around the posterior side of the testes and ascends toward the peritoneal cavity. The epididymis leads into the **vas deferens**. The vas deferens enter the peritoneal cavity and widens to form a space called the **ampulla**, which has a glandular, convoluted structure called a **seminal vesicle** on each side.

At the ampulla, the vas deferens forms the **ejaculatory duct**. The ejaculatory duct passes through the **prostate gland** and joins with the **internal urethra** below the **bladder**. The internal urethra enters the penis and forms the **urethra**. Mucus-secreting glands line the urethra.

Sperm Maturation

Sperm at the entrance to the epididymis are immature and unable to fertilize an egg. By the time the sperm have traveled through the vas deferens (approximately a 2-week trip), the sperm will have become fully mature. Mature sperm can be stored in the vas deferens and ampulla, remaining viable for more than a month.

THE SEMINAL VESICLES

With sexual excitement, the seminal vesicles secrete a mucus-like substance containing sugar, prostaglandins, and fibrinogen into the ejaculatory duct. The sperm use the sugar for energy, and the prostaglandins are believed to assist sperm in penetrating the female cervix. Prostaglandins may also cause contractions of the female genital tract, which propel the sperm in their journey to reach the egg.

THE PROSTATE

The prostate is a walnut-shaped gland that sits directly beneath the bladder. During sexual excitement, the prostate secretes a thin, milky fluid containing various enzymes and ions into the ejaculatory duct. This fluid adds to the sperm and seminal vesicle fluid volume. The prostate fluid is alkaline (basic). When this fluid is deposited in the vagina of the female, it neutralizes the acidic vaginal secretions; this is important because sperm have poor motility in low pH.

NEURAL INNERVATION OF THE MALE REPRODUCTIVE SYSTEM

Afferent sensory neurons and efferent parasympathetic and sympathetic fibers are found throughout the male genitalia. Afferent sensory fibers are activated in response to tactile stimulation and send their information to the spinal cord. Parasympathetic nerves exit the spine at the level of the sacral area and innervate the arteries and arterioles of the penis. Parasympathetic fibers release the neurotransmitter acetylcholine, causing dilation of the blood vessels. Sympathetic nerves exit the spine from the upper lumbar areas and innervate the smooth muscle of the vas deferens and ampulla. Sympathetic fibers release the neurotransmitter norepinephrine, which causes smooth muscle contraction. Sympathetic fibers also innervate and cause contraction of the prostate and the seminal vesicles. Descending neurons from the cerebral cortex influence the firing of the parasympathetic and sympathetic fibers.

The Male Sexual Act

Physical manipulation of the penis or sexual thoughts activate the parasympathetic and sympathetic nerves, causing sexual excitement.

There are four stages of the male sexual act: erection, emission, ejaculation, and resolution. All stages can occur as simple spinal reflexes initiated by sensory stimulation. They do not require central nervous system involvement. Normally, however, mental and physical stimuli contribute to sexual excitement. Inhibitory cerebral stimulation may interrupt the spinal reflexes at any point.

Erection

The penis hardens and becomes elongated during sexual excitement. An erection occurs following activation of the parasympathetic fibers to the penis, resulting in vasodilatation and increased blood flow. As the arteries and arterioles of the penis fill up with blood, the veins draining the penis become compressed and occluded. Venous occlusion causes the spongy tissue in the shaft of the penis, the **corpus cavernosum** and **corpus spongiosum**, to become engorged. Engorgement of these tissues results in an erection. Parasympathetic stimulation also causes glands lining the urethra to secrete mucus. Mucus lubricates the glans (head) of the penis, This facilitates and increases the pleasure associated with penetration of the female. During this stage, heart rate and respiratory rate increase.

Emission

When sexual excitement reaches a critical level, activation of the sympathetic nerves to the penis causes contraction of the vas deferens and ampulla. This results in **emission**—the propulsion of the sperm out of the vas deferens and ampulla through the ejaculatory duct and into the internal urethra. During emission, sympathetic stimulation to the prostate and seminal vesicles causes release of prostate and seminal vesicle secretions into the ejaculatory duct. The combination of sperm, prostate secretions, and seminal vesicle secretions is called **semen.**

Ejaculation

With the addition of semen in the internal urethra, a feeling of fullness occurs. Sensory fibers traveling to the spinal cord transmit this feeling, resulting in further activation of the sympathetic fibers and smooth muscle contraction of the ducts. Motor neurons to skeletal muscles at the base of the penis are also activated, leading to contraction of these muscles. The culminating responses are wavelike, rhythmic contractions associated with intense pleasure. During these contractions, semen is forcefully propelled through the urethra and out the urethral opening. Emission and ejaculation comprise the male **orgasm**. Heart rate and respiratory rate reach a maximum at this time.

Resolution

After experiencing an orgasm, a male shows a reversal of sexual excitement, including disappearance of the erection and a return of heart rate and breathing patterns to normal.

Spermatogenesis

Spermatogenesis (the formation of sperm) begins during puberty and continues throughout the lifetime of a male. Undifferentiated germ cells lining the seminiferous tubules undergo a programmed number of mitotic cell divisions, resulting in the production of the **primary spermatocytes** (immature sperm), which ultimately develop into the **spermatozoon** (mature sperm). Spermatogenesis requires approximately 2 months. From each primary spermatocyte, four viable sperm (each with 23 chromosomes) are produced. Spermatogenesis occurs in the seminiferous tubule under the control of two pituitary hormones, follicle-stimulating hormone (FSH) and luteinizing hormone (LH), and the sex hormones, testosterone and estrogen.

FOLLICLE-STIMULATING HORMONE

FSH is a protein hormone released from the anterior pituitary in response to a stimulating hormone from the hypothalamus: gonadotropin-releasing hormone (GnRH) (Chapter 8). FSH binds to receptors present on the membranes of the Sertoli cells that line the seminiferous tubules, and activates a cyclic adenosine monophosphate (cAMP) second messenger system. The final effect of FSH is to cause Sertoli cells to proliferate and to secrete various nutrients, ions, and proteins into the tubule that stimulate the continued proliferation and differentiation of the immature sperm.

Sertoli cells exert feedback on the hypothalamus and pituitary to control the further release of FSH by secreting the hormone **inhibin**. Inhibin levels rise with increased cell activity and inhibit the further release of FSH.

LUTEINIZING HORMONE

LH is the second protein hormone released from the anterior pituitary in response to stimulation by GnRH. LH binds to the Leydig cells that surround the tubule, and again through the activation of a cAMP second messenger system, stimulates the synthesis of the steroid hormone testosterone. Testosterone diffuses into the seminiferous tubules and binds to the Sertoli cells, stimulating them to continue to secrete the proteins, ions, and nutrients required to maintain proliferation and differentiation of the sperm. One protein that is manufactured by the Sertoli cells, androgen-binding protein, ensures that levels of testosterone remain high in the lumen of the seminiferous tubule. Mature Leydig cells usually develop at approximately 10 years of age in a boy.

Testosterone feeds back on the hypothalamus, and to a lesser extent on the anterior pituitary, to inhibit the further release of GnRH and LH. This keeps the levels of circulating testosterone relatively constant. Besides being required for the successful formation of sperm, testosterone is also essential for the production of the male secondary sexual characteristics and the maintenance of the male libido (sex drive).

STIMULI CONTROLLING GnRH RELEASE

GnRH is released in small pulses throughout the day, resulting in relatively constant day-to-day levels. Increases or decreases in GnRH release may occur seasonally and with different physical and psychological conditions—for example, anxiety or depression. Changes in the secretion of GnRH may affect sperm formation by affecting LH and FSH and may alter libido.

Male Secondary Sexual Characteristics

Male secondary sexual characteristics are under the control of the male androgens, especially testosterone. The effects of testosterone are described fully in Chapter 8. The male secondary sexual characteristics include the following:

- Increased protein anabolism and muscle mass.
- Increased bone growth and strength.
- Male pattern of hair on the face, axillary, and pubic regions. Hair growth thickens on most areas of the body.
- Male pattern baldness, typically beginning with a bald spot on the top of the head. A genetic tendency influences male pattern baldness.
- Increased metabolic rate, probably as a result of increased protein anabolism (buildup) and muscle mass formation. This raises the caloric needs of males, beginning at puberty, compared to females.
- Proliferation and activation of sebaceous glands in the skin, which produce sebum. This can result in acne, especially during the teenage years.
- A deepening voice, as a result of hypertrophy of the larynx.

Female Reproductive Anatomy

The reproductive roles of the female include the monthly development and secretion of an ovum (egg), the provision of an appropriate internal environment if the ovum is fertilized by a sperm, and the carriage and nourishment of an embryo and fetus until survival outside the womb is possible. Internal reproductive structures that make these roles possible include the **ovaries**, **fallopian tubes**, **uterus**, and **vagina**. After the birth of an infant occurs, the female's role continues as she nourishes the infant with milk produced in her **breasts**. The breasts are usually considered accessory reproductive organs. The **clitoris** is erectile tissue located at the anterior portion of the female external genitalia. Although not essential for reproduction, the clitoris is important in providing a woman's pleasure during the sexual act. The external genitalia consist of fatty tissue called the **mons pubis** and **outer** and **inner** folds of tissue, called the **labia majora** and **labia minora**, respectively. The opening of the urethra is located between the vagina and the clitoris. Internal female reproductive anatomy is shown in Figure 21-2.

THE OVARIES

A female is born with two ovaries located bilaterally in the lower abdominal cavity beside the uterus. The ovaries are the gonads of the female and contain the female sex cells—the ova (singular term is ovum). At birth, the female infant has approximately 1 million ova that have undergone numerous mitotic, but no meiotic, divisions. The ova remain latent in the ovary until a girl enters puberty between approximately 11 and 16 years of age.

THE FOLLICLE

Each individual ovum is surrounded in the ovary by a group of supporting cells, called **granulosa** cells. The ovum plus its surrounding granulosa cells is called a **follicle**. In childhood, the immature follicle, called a **primordial follicle**, consists of an ovum and a single layer of granulosa cells surrounding it. When a female enters puberty, the entire ovary and many of the primordial follicles enlarge. This includes increasing layers of granulosa cells and an increase in the size of each ovum. The enlarged follicle is called a **primary follicle.** Each month during a woman's reproductive life, one of the primary follicles responds to hormonal stimulation with **ovulation**—the release of a mature ovum from the ovary.

THE FALLOPIAN TUBES

The fallopian tubes, also called the oviducts, are smooth muscle passageways that open at one end into the body of the uterus and at the other end into the peritoneal cavity. The opening into the peritoneal cavity has fingerlike projections, called **fimbriae**, that surround the ovary. These projections are covered with **cilia**. The cilia wave toward the fallopian tube, drawing an ovum released from the ovary into the fallopian tube. The movement of the fimbriae is so effective that an ovum released by one ovary can enter the fallopian tube on the opposite side if the same-side tube is blocked or absent.

Once in the fallopian tube, the ovum travels a short distance to enter a widened area called the **ampulla**. Fertilization of the ovum by a sperm typically occurs in the fallopian tube at the ampulla. From

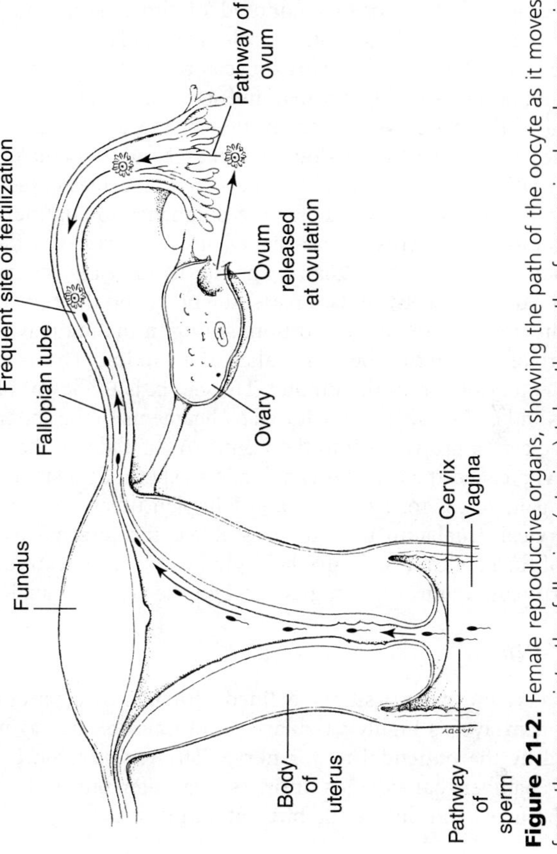

Figure 21-2. Female reproductive organs, showing the path of the oocyte as it moves from the ovary into the fallopian (uterine) tube; the path of sperm is also shown, as is the usual site of fertilization (from Porth, 1994).

the ampulla, the ovum travels over the next 3 to 4 days to the uterus. If the ovum has been fertilized by a sperm, the newly fertilized egg is called a **zygote**. Cell division of the zygote occurs during transit through the fallopian tube to the uterus. By the time it reaches the uterus, the fertilized egg will consist of approximately 100 cells; at this point, the fertilized egg is called a **blastocyst**.

THE UTERUS

The uterus is a hollow organ composed of three layers: an inner endometrial layer, a middle smooth muscle layer, and an outer connective tissue layer. During the menstrual cycle, the endometrium hypertrophies and becomes highly vascular and secretory in preparation for the arrival of the blastocyst. If fertilization of the ovum has not occurred, the endometrial layer is sloughed off each month in the process of **menstruation**. If fertilization has occurred, the blastocyst must implant in the wall of the uterus for the pregnancy to continue.

The nonpregnant uterus is pear-shaped and approximately the size of a woman's fist. During pregnancy the uterus increases severalfold in size. The uterus consists of two parts: the **body** and the **cervix**. The body of the uterus is the upper portion, sitting in the midpelvis. The upper part of the uterine body is called the **fundus**. The fallopian tubes are extensions from the fundus. The cervix is the lower part of the uterus and is the only part anchored by ligaments to the abdominal cavity. The cervix protrudes into the vagina. A canal down the center of the cervix, called the **cervical canal**, allows sperm deposited in the vagina to gain access to the uterus and fallopian tubes. The opening of the cervical canal into the uterus is called the **internal os**. The opening of the cervical canal into the vagina is called the **external os**. A newborn passes out of the uterus through the cervical canal.

THE VAGINA

The vagina is a muscular passageway lined with mucus-secreting cells. The muscular layer is highly vascularized. Muscles of the vagina are innervated by the **pudendal motor nerve**. The vagina is normally a collapsed chamber that expands during sexual intercourse to accommodate the penis and during the birth of an infant.

THE FEMALE BREAST

The breast is the mammary gland. Under appropriate hormonal influence, the breast is capable of secreting milk after the birth of an infant. The breasts are located on the upper anterior portion of the chest and consist of 15 to 30 lobes of glandular tissue. Each lobe drains into a lactiferous (milk) duct, which opens at the tip of the nipple.

Before puberty, a girl's breasts are small and undeveloped. The nipple is flat against the chest. With onset of puberty, and under the influence of estrogen, the breasts increase in size, fatty deposits, and ductal structure. During pregnancy, under the influence of pregnancy hormones, the ductal system develops further, and the glandular cells become capable of producing milk.

The Menstrual Cycle

The menstrual cycle is the cyclic maturation and release of an ovum. It involves the growth of a follicle, ovulation of the ovum, and characteristic changes in the endometrial lining of the uterus. For a point of reference, the first day of the menstrual cycle is considered the first day of menstruation (bleeding). Each menstrual cycle is approximately 28 days in length. There are two distinct phases of the menstrual cycle: the **follicular phase** and the **luteal phase**. These two phases are separated by **ovulation**. (See Fig. 21-3, discussed in the following). During the follicular phase, the follicle develops and secretes estrogen. The uterine endometrial cells reproduce and grow. During the luteal phase, progesterone is secreted by the remaining cells of the follicle while the lining of the uterus becomes highly vascularized and secretory. Hormones from the hypothalamus, anterior pituitary, and ovary work together in an intricate balance to control the menstrual cycle.

THE FOLLICULAR PHASE OF THE MENSTRUAL CYCLE

The development of the follicle depends on the release of FSH and LH from the anterior pituitary. FSH begins to increase slightly in the first few days after the start of menstruation. LH levels show a moderate rise. Under the influence of FSH, and to a lesser extent LH, 6 to 12 primary follicles begin to develop during the first week of the menstrual cycle.

By the beginning of the second week, the growth of one of the primary follicles dominates and the others begin to deteriorate in a process called **atresia.** The granulosa cells of the dominant follicle respond to FSH and LH with secretion of **estrogen**. A second class of follicular cells, called **thecal cells**, grow to surround the granulosa layers. The estrogen secretions accumulate in the follicle, causing an **antrum** (cavity) to form. Increasing levels of estrogen act locally to increase the number of FSH receptors on the follicle, furthering the secretion of estrogen and initiating a positive feedback cycle. Toward the end of the second week of the menstrual cycle, the ovum inside the follicle completes its first meiotic division. As a result of the first meiotic division, one daughter cell becomes a mature ovum, which contains 23 chromosomes.

OVULATION

On approximately day 12 of the menstrual cycle, there is a dramatic rise (6 to 10–fold) in the release of LH from the anterior pituitary.

This is called a preovulatory LH surge. FSH increases to a lesser degree. These two hormones initiate a profound, final growth of the follicle, which begins to swell with its accumulated secretions. At this time, LH begins to convert the thecal cells from estrogen-secreting cells to mostly progesterone secreting cells. By day 13, estrogen levels have fallen and progesterone levels begin to rise. On day 14, swelling of the follicle causes it to ooze secretions. The follicle ruptures, releasing the ovum into the abdominal cavity. Some granulosa cells are released as well, and they continue to surround the ejected ovum.

THE LUTEAL STAGE OF THE MENSTRUAL CYCLE

After ovulation, the granulosa and thecal cells remaining in the follicle, enlarge and undergo the process of **luteinization**, changing to yellowish, lipid-laden cells. The complex of granulosa and thecal cells left behind in the ruptured follicle is known as the **corpus luteum**. The corpus luteum continues to secrete large amounts of progesterone and estrogen that act in a negative feedback manner on the hypothalamus to reduce the further secretion of LH and FSH. Progesterone and estrogen production by the corpus luteum, however, appears to be partially dependent on the remaining, but falling, levels of LH. Within approximately 10 days, LH and FSH levels are very low, and if fertilization of the ovum has not occurred, the corpus luteum degenerates. With degeneration of the corpus luteum, progesterone and estrogen levels rapidly fall and reach their lowest point on the last day (day 28) of the menstrual cycle. A lack of progesterone initiates menstruation.

If the ovum is successfully penetrated by a sperm, a second meiotic division occurs in the ovum. Only one daughter cell, containing 23 chromosomes, is produced at the end of the second meiotic division (not four, as with sperm formation). Fusion of the chromosomes present in the egg and sperm results in the formation of a 46-chromosome cell, the zygote. This first cell divides rapidly and early embryogenesis begins.

UTERINE CHANGES DURING THE MENSTRUAL CYCLE

During the follicular stage of the menstrual cycle, estrogen causes **proliferation** (reproduction and growth) of the endometrial and smooth muscle cells of the uterus, to prepare the uterus in case an egg is fertilized later in the cycle. Estrogen also causes the mucus-secreting cells of the cervix to secrete a large amount of clear, thin fluid that facilitates easy passage of sperm through the cervix.

After ovulation, progesterone effects on the uterus dominate. The endometrial cells that proliferated earlier in the cycle begin to **secrete** glycogen-rich fluid and various enzymes. The myometrial (smooth muscle) cells become highly vascularized and engorged with blood as the uterus continues to prepare for the arrival of a fertilized ovum. Cervical mucus secretions become thick and plug the cervical openings, to prevent the ascent of anything that might disrupt fertilization or implantation of an embryo.

If fertilization of an egg does not occur, progesterone and estrogen levels fall toward the end of the cycle, causing the swelled blood vessels to constrict, and depriving the uterine cells of oxygen and nutrients. This causes the uterine lining to disintegrate and menstrual flow to begin. Within 2 to 3 days of the onset of menstruation, the cycle starts over as FSH and LH rise, initiating a new follicular phase. If fertilization does occur, the uterine lining remains well oxygenated and well nourished, and menstruation will not occur. The hormonal and uterine profiles seen during a menstrual cycle are shown in Figure 21-3.

CONTROL OF THE LH SURGE

The cause of the preovulatory LH surge is not completely understood. It has been hypothesized that positive feedback stimulation on the hypothalamus or pituitary hormones occurs when estrogen levels get very high. The very high levels of estrogen that develop by day 12 of the menstrual cycle are believed to be responsible for the burst of LH.

HYPOTHALAMIC CONTROL OF THE MENSTRUAL CYCLE

The hypothalamus controls the release of the FSH and LH by the secretion of GnRH. GnRH levels have not been precisely measured during a menstrual cycle. It is likely that GnRH levels undergo fluctuations during the month that precede the fluctuations in FSH and LH levels, including the LH surge. GnRH secretion increases at puberty. Inhibition of GnRH release can occur with physical or emotional stress.

Implantation of the Blastocyte

If the ovum is fertilized and conception occurs, the fertilized egg travels through the fallopian tubes and, as the blastocyte, implants in the uterine lining that has been prepared for its arrival. Implantation happens as a result of the development of special enzyme-secreting **trophoblast cells** on the surface of the blastocyst. The secreted enzymes break down the lining of the uterus, allowing the early embryo entrance to the endometrial layer. Cells of the endometrium swell to nourish the embryo, becoming specialized cells, called **decidual cells** (the decidua). The decidua nourishes the growing embryo for the next 8 weeks.

The Placenta

The trophoblast cells that attach to the uterus form the placenta, an organ consisting of fetal and maternal tissue. With implantation, invading trophoblasts begin to secrete the placental hormone, human chorionic gonadotropin (hCG). hCG prolongs the life of the corpus

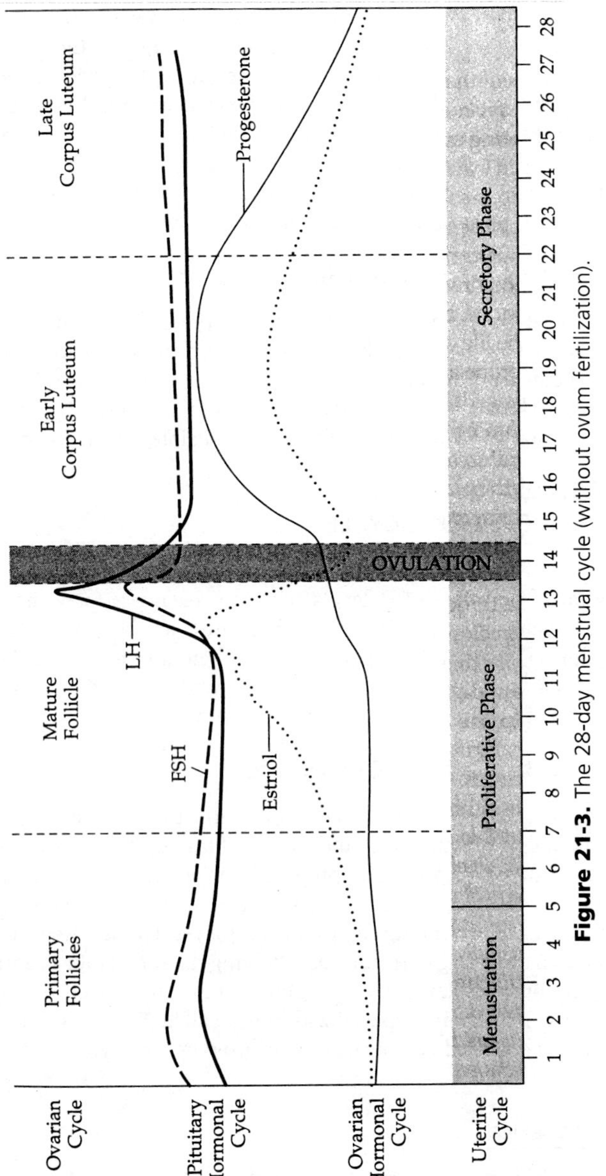

Figure 21-3. The 28-day menstrual cycle (without ovum fertilization).

luteum, continuing the secretion of progesterone and estrogen required for maintenance of the uterine lining. Placental secretion of hCG is measurable in the serum within 24 hours of implantation and remains elevated for the duration of pregnancy. By approximately the third month of pregnancy, the placenta has taken over all hormonal roles of the corpus luteum, and the corpus luteum disintegrates.

In addition to functioning as an endocrine organ, the placenta functions in **gas and nutrient exchange** between the fetal and maternal circulations. In the placenta, blood flows through fetal arteries to a fetal capillary network, which lies in close approximation to a maternal capillary network. Across this capillary interface, oxygen and nutrients are delivered from the mother to the fetus, and fetal waste products are removed to the maternal circulation. The fetal capillaries regroup to form veins, and the oxygen-rich and nutrient-rich blood returns to the fetal heart. Maternal capillaries reform to veins that deliver fetal waste to the mother's lungs and kidneys. The fetus grows and develops in this nourishing and protective environment for approximately 38 to 42 weeks.

Parturition

Parturition is the delivery of the infant at the end of pregnancy. At this time, the placenta is also delivered. Parturition occurs when a combination of factors increases the excitability of the uterus, initiating contractions of the smooth muscle. The contractions increase in frequency and intensity, resulting in softening and widening of the cervix to allow for delivery of the infant. The factors involved in exciting the uterus include an increasing ratio of estrogen to progesterone, starting at approximately the seventh month of pregnancy. Estrogen excites uterine smooth muscle whereas progesterone relaxes uterine and other smooth muscle. An increase in the ratio of estrogen to progesterone will therefore increase uterine contractility. In addition, as the fetus grows, the uterus and cervix stretch. This causes the smooth muscle of the uterus to contract in response, with the contractions becoming more forceful as the fetal size increases. Maternal release of the posterior pituitary hormone oxytocin near the end of pregnancy also stimulates uterine smooth muscle contraction. The release of fetal hormones, especially the prostaglandins and oxytocin, also appear to stimulate the uterus to contract. The factors that stimulate parturition are outlined in Figure 21-4.

Lactation

Lactation is the secretion of milk from the breast. Under the influence of estrogen, progesterone, and prolactin during pregnancy, the breasts increase in size and undergo growth and branching of the breast ductal system. Once the ducts are fully developed, secretory cells in the breasts prepare to produce milk. Estrogen and progesterone, although

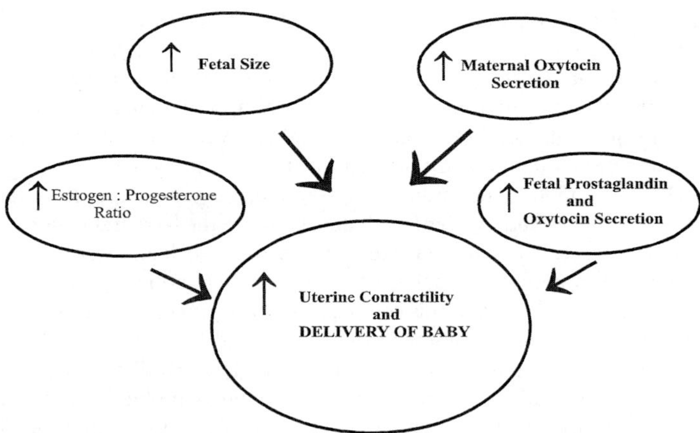

Figure 21-4. Factors that stimulate parturition.

essential in preparing the breasts to lactate, inhibit actual milk production. Prolactin, a hormone from the anterior pituitary, is stimulatory for both breast development and milk production. This hormonal interplay means that milk production does not occur to any significant degree until pregnancy is over and the source of estrogen and progesterone (the placenta) is removed. This leaves the lactogenic (milk-producing) effects of prolactin unopposed. Prolactin levels increase in the woman each time she nurses her baby, for as long as she continues to breast-feed. Release of prolactin is under the control of two opposing hypothalamic hormones: prolactin-inhibitory hormone (PIH) and prolactin-stimulatory hormone. PIH is believed to be the neurotransmitter dopamine. Release of both PIH and prolactin-stimulatory hormone can be influenced by emotional and physical factors. Prolactin inhibits the release of LH and FSH from the pituitary. This reduces the likelihood that a lactating woman will release another egg and become pregnant. This scenario does not always hold true, however, especially if the infant is bottle-fed as well as breast-fed, and many nursing women do become pregnant.

Ejection of the milk from the nipples occurs as a result of the release of oxytocin from the posterior pituitary in response to sucking on the nipple of a prolactin-primed breast. Oxytocin stimulates contraction of the smooth muscle of the breast ducts and causes expulsion of milk. Oxytocin is under hypothalamic control and is influenced by emotional and physical factors.

Female Sexual Response

The female sexual response includes excitement, orgasm, and resolution. It involves physical and psychological responses.

Excitement

Excitement occurs when physical manipulation of the genitalia or sexual thoughts activate the parasympathetic nerves supplying the region. The clitoris is especially sensitive to physical manipulation. Activation of the parasympathetic nerves causes dilation of the blood vessels, leading to engorgement of erectile tissue in the vagina and clitoris. Mucus-secreting cells of the vagina are stimulated to secrete mucus, lubricating the vagina. For women, higher brain centers usually play a major role in facilitating parasympathetic activation. Heart rate and respiratory rate increase.

Orgasm

When sexual excitement reaches a very high level, muscles of the vagina and perineal area (posterior to the vagina) begin to contract rhythmically. Uterine and fallopian smooth muscles also appear to undergo waves of contraction. Intensely pleasurable sensations accompany the muscle contractions. Vaginal and uterine contractions may help propel sperm toward the fallopian tubes.

Resolution

After orgasm, the period of resolution occurs. This period is characterized by a reduction in genital blood flow and a return of heart rate and respirations to normal.

Female Secondary Sexual Characteristics

The female secondary and associated sexual characteristics are under the control of estrogen and, to a lesser extent, progesterone (Chapter 8). These effects include the following:

- The development of the breast.
- The female pattern distribution of pubic hair. The growth of pubic and axillary hair in women is not estrogen dependent, but it occurs as a result of adrenal gland androgen release.
- Bone growth and closure of the epiphyseal plates.

Puberty

Puberty is the beginning of sexual maturation. Puberty typically occurs at a younger age in girls than boys. It begins in girls between 8 and 14 years of age, and in boys between 10 and 16 years of age. The menstrual cycle is the culmination of puberty in girls. In boys, puberty culminates in the ability to ejaculate mature sperm.

Puberty is initiated when the hypothalamus begins to secrete GnRH. It appears that the hypothalamus responds to cues concerning body mass index and maturation of other brain areas, including the limbic system. Prior to puberty, the anterior pituitary and the gonads are capable of responding to hormonal stimulation, making hypothalamic activation the pivotal event.

Menopause

Menopause occurs in a women when her ovaries no longer respond to LH and FSH with estrogen and progesterone production. Menopause usually occurs between the ages of 40 and 50 years, and can be an 8- to 10-year process. During the long process of menopause, fluctuations in the timing and duration of the menstrual cycle occur, ultimately resulting in cessation of the menses.

Symptoms of menopause are caused by the absence of estrogen. Symptoms may include episodes of flushing of the skin (hot flashes), sensations of dyspnea (difficulty in breathing), fatigue, and occasional irritability or overemotionality. Vaginal atrophy and drying occur, which may make intercourse painful. Lack of estrogen causes the skin to lose its elasticity and become dry and loose. Decreases in bone mass may result in osteoporosis, thereby increasing the risk of bone fracture. In addition, estrogen protection against coronary artery disease is lost after the menopause, contributing to a dramatically increased risk of myocardial infarct. Estrogen also influences cognitive functioning, and its lack may play a role in the development of forgetfulness and even Alzheimer's disease.

Because of the many changes that occur in the body after the loss of estrogen, especially the increased risk of developing osteoporosis and coronary artery disease, it has been recommended that most women in the United States be encouraged to consider hormone replacement therapy (HRT) during and after menopause. Most studies suggest that HRT increases life expectancy and quality of life for the majority of women. Many women, however, decide against HRT, for a variety of reasons, including lack of education as to its benefits, disinclination to use drugs, and a wish to avoid side effects such as vaginal spotting or periods. In addition, women with a strong family or a personal history of breast cancer or who have experienced blood clot formation are discouraged from receiving hormone replacement. Sometimes, just the fear of breast cancer, even in women without high risk, causes women to choose not to use hormone replacement, despite its many benefits.

PATHOPHYSIOLOGIC CONCEPTS

Impotence

Impotence is the inability of a male to achieve or maintain an erection. Impotence can occur infrequently, frequently, or every time a man attempts to have sexual intercourse. It may be caused by physical or, less commonly, psychological factors.

PHYSICAL CAUSES OF IMPOTENCE

One of the main physical causes of impotence is atherosclerosis of the penile arteries. With atherosclerosis, blood flow to the penis is reduced and there is an inability of the penile arteries to dilate during sexual excitement. Other physical causes of impotence include systemic diseases (such as hypothyroidism), acromegaly, and most commonly, diabetes mellitus. Diabetes in particular is associated with atherosclerosis as well as changes in sensory transmission. Many drugs are known to interfere with a man's ability to achieve orgasm as well, including some antihypertensive and psychotropic medications. Impotence may occur following surgery in the genital region, for example, after treatment for prostate cancer. Fatigue may also cause impotence.

There are numerous treatments available for physical causes of impotence, including mechanical aides and pumps and penile injections that cause local vasodilation. In addition, in 1998, pharmaceutical advances resulted in the production and marketing of the highly effective oral anti-impotence medication, sildenafil (trade name, Viagra). Viagra acts as a phosphodiesterase inhibitor, preventing the inactivation of second messengers required for smooth relaxation of the erectile tissue. By preventing relaxation, the penis more fully fills with blood, and erection is achieved. Viagra is usually taken 1 hour before intercourse, and it enhances the normal sexual response. Side effects such as headache, facial flushing, and visual abnormalities may occur. It is contraindicated for men with certain types of heart disease. For causes of impotence related to prescribed medications, reevaluation of drug dosage or drug choice may reduce symptoms. Impotence associated with systemic disease or fatigue must be addressed directly.

PSYCHOLOGICAL CAUSES OF IMPOTENCE

Psychological impotence may occur as a result of descending inhibitory impulses originating in the cerebral cortex. Psychological conditions associated with impotence include stress, anger, worry, and depression. Psychological impotence may be relieved by relaxation techniques, counseling, or sexual therapy.

Infertility

Infertility is the inability or reduced ability to produce offspring. Infertility in a couple may result from female factors (30–40%), male factors (30–40%), or a combination (20%). Infertility in a couple may occur from the start of the relationship (primary infertility) or after the couple has already produced one or more offspring (secondary infertility).

FEMALE FACTORS

Female factors causing infertility can include problems with follicular growth, anovulation (failure to ovulate), or ovulatory irregularities. Structural abnormalities, vaginal or uterine infection, or inappropriately thick cervical mucus may cause infertility. Blockage of the fallopian tubes following pelvic infection or uterine abnormalities that prevent implantation may be involved. Immune responses may destroy the implanted embryo if the woman is either hyperimmune to the embryo or fails to develop tolerance to it. Miscarriages later in gestation may occur if the placenta is poorly placed or poorly perfused with blood, or if the cervix cannot support the weight of the growing fetus.

Treatment of female infertility is specific to the cause. Drugs to induce ovulation or superovulation (more than one ovum) may be administered. Harvesting of eggs from the woman for in vitro fertilization (outside of the body) may be attempted. Eggs fertilized outside the body may be implanted into the fallopian tube or uterus. For some women, eggs from a donor may be fertilized in vitro and then implanted into the infertile woman's uterus and carried there to term.

MALE FACTORS

Male factors causing infertility may include defects in spermatogenesis, which result in poorly formed sperm or sperm too few in number to allow for successful penetration of the ovum. Sperm motility (movement) may be impaired. Male infertility may occur following infection and scarring of the testicles, epididymis, vas deferens, or urethra. Systemic infections, such as mumps, may cause swelling of the testicles and destruction of the seminiferous tubules. Obstruction of the blood vessels supplying the testes can cause hypoxia and a failure of the sperm to develop or survive. Autoantibodies produced against sperm will reduce sperm number and quality. Exposure of the testicles to high temperature may reduce spermatogenesis. Erection, emission, or ejaculation may be dysfunctional with nerve damage, atherosclerosis, or psychological disturbance. Congenital anomalies may affect the ability of the penis to deliver sperm inside the vagina.

Treatment of male factors of infertility are specific to the cause. Sperm may be obtained from a male with a low sperm count. The sperm will be introduced artificially into his partner after techniques to increase the concentration of the highest-quality sperm have been performed. This process is called artificial insemination.

Gynecomastia

Gynecomastia is the enlargement of breast tissue in males. Gynecomastia can result from excess production of estrogen in the male or the liver's inability to break down normal male estrogen secretions. Gynecomastia is frequently seen during early puberty in some males, and may be a normal development, or may be related to excess body weight or a hormonal imbalance.

Dysmenorrhea

Dysmenorrhea is painful menstruation that occurs without evidence of pelvic infection or disease. Dysmenorrhea is usually caused by excessive release of a specific prostaglandin, prostaglandin F_{2a}, from the uterine endometrial cells. Prostaglandin F_{2a} is a potent stimulator of myometrial smooth muscle contraction and uterine blood vessel constriction. It worsens the uterine hypoxia normally associated with menstruation, causing significant pain. For most women, prostaglandin inhibitors, such as ibuprofen, can effectively reduce cramping; acetaminophen is less helpful. Prostaglandin inhibitors should be used at the first sign of pain, or for some women, at the first sign of menstrual flow. Because forceful menstrual cramping may contribute to the development of endometriosis (painful growth of uterine tissue outside of the uterus), complaints of dysmenorrhea should always be taken seriously, and attempts should be made to reduce its incidence.

Amenorrhea

Amenorrhea is the absence of a menstrual cycle. Amenorrhea exists naturally before puberty and after menopause. Amenorrhea also occurs during pregnancy, after parturition, and may occur during lactation. Emotional disturbances, physical stress, and low body mass index (such as experienced by female athletes) may also cause amenorrhea. Endocrine disorders, especially involving the ovaries, pituitary, thyroid, or adrenal glands, can cause amenorrhea as well.

CONDITIONS OF DISEASE OR INJURY

Precocious Puberty

Precocious puberty is the occurrence of puberty in a girl younger than 8 years of age or a boy less than 9 years of age. Premature development of sexual characteristics appropriate to the sex of the child is called **isosexual precocious puberty**. Development of sexual characteristics appropriate to the opposite sex is called **heterosexual precocious puberty**. Heterosexual precocious puberty is rare, and usually is caused either by a disorder in the fetal adrenal gland or decreased sensitivity of a genetically male fetus to androgens, which reverses during puberty (see Chapter 8). Signs of early sexual development, although not really precocious puberty, may be present at birth as a result of an oversensitivity of the fetus to sex hormones produced by the mother. In this case, after birth and the removal from maternal hormones, the early signs of sexual development disappear.

CAUSES OF ISOSEXUAL PRECOCIOUS PUBERTY

True isosexual precocious puberty is more common and usually occurs when the hypothalamus prematurely begins to secrete GnRH. The anterior pituitary responds to GnRH with the secretion of FSH and LH. FSH and LH cause the gonads to secrete the sex hormones and signs of puberty appear. Hypothalamic prematurity may occur idiopathically (for no known cause), especially in girls, or may result from a central nervous system tumor or disease. Ectopic production of a gonadotropin and a hormone-secreting tumor of the gonads are other causes of precocious puberty.

CLINICAL MANIFESTATIONS OF ISOSEXUAL PRECOCIOUS PUBERTY

- Premature development of breasts (thelarche), pubic or axillary hair (adrenarche), or menses (menarche) in girls.
- Premature growth of the penis, scrotum, beard, or pubic hair in boys. A deepening of the voice may occur.

DIAGNOSTIC TOOLS

- A physical examination and hormonal profile is used for diagnosis of precocious puberty.
- Imaging techniques, including computed tomography (CT scans), ultrasound, and magnetic resonance imaging (MRI) are used to identify tumors.
- DNA testing may be used to establish gender in certain cases.

COMPLICATIONS

- Estrogen and testosterone can cause premature growth of the skeleton and early closure of the epiphyseal bone plates, leading to short height in adulthood.
- Psychosocial stress may occur for children and their families.

TREATMENT

- If a tumor is identified, surgical resection, radiation, or chemotherapy may be used.
- For precocious puberty of idiopathic origin, treatment may consist of administration of a long-lasting GnRH agonist. This results in decreased pituitary responsiveness to endogenous GnRH, and LH and FSH levels fall, shutting off the pubertal sequence.
- Some children will not be treated. Appropriate counseling for the family and child is important.

Cryptorchidism

Cryptorchidism is the failure of one or both testicles to descend into the scrotum of a male infant. Cryptorchidism is present at birth and is especially common in premature infants. For most infants born with this condition, the testes will descend on their own within the first year of birth. If descent does not occur, the testes will remain at a higher temperature than optimal for spermatogenesis. This may affect sperm quantity and quality, leading to infertility later in life. Cryptorchidism is associated with a high risk of other congenital reproductive disorders that may independently affect fertility. Male sexual function and secondary sexual characteristics are normal. The cause of cryptorchidism is not known, but may involve developmental delay or mechanical barriers to descent.

CLINICAL MANIFESTATIONS

- One or both testes will not be palpable in the scrotum at birth.

DIAGNOSTIC TOOLS

- Physical examination is used to diagnose the condition. Ultrasound or other imaging techniques may be used.

COMPLICATIONS

- Infertility in the adult if the descent does not occur.
- Increased risk of testicular cancer exists in individuals with cryptorchidism, even after surgical repair.

TREATMENT

- Most cases of cryptorchidism will reverse spontaneously within 1 year. If spontaneous descent does not occur, treatment with hCG may stimulate descent.
- If hormonal therapy is ineffective, surgery is required to locate and move the testes into the scrotum. Surgery should be performed by 2 years of age.
- Testicular self-examination and regular examinations by a health care provider are important to detect testicular cancer early.

Varicocele

A varicocele is an abnormal dilation of a vein in the spermatic cord, usually supplying the left testicle. Varicoceles typically appear after puberty. A left-side varicocele usually develops as a result of valvular incompetence, associated with backflow and accumulation of blood in the vein. A right-side varicocele may indicate obstruction of the inferior vena cava. A sudden occurrence of a varicocele in an older man may indicate an advanced renal tumor.

CLINICAL MANIFESTATIONS

- A varicocele may be asymptomatic or associated with a vague feeling of discomfort and testicular heaviness.
- Tortuous, dilated veins may be palpable.

DIAGNOSTIC TOOLS

- Physical examination is used to diagnose the condition. Ultrasound may be used.

COMPLICATIONS

- Poor blood flow to the testes may cause infertility.

TREATMENT

- A support for the testicles is worn to relieve discomfort.
- To maintain fertility, surgical ligation of the vein may be performed.

Hydrocele

A hydrocele is the collection of a plasma filtrate in the scrotum, outside the testes. This results in scrotal swelling and can reduce blood flow to the testes. A hydrocele may be a congenital problem or may be caused by trauma to the genitals. A testicular tumor may cause formation of a hydrocele. Idiopathic development may also occur.

CLINICAL MANIFESTATIONS

- A hydrocele may be asymptomatic or associated with palpable or visible swelling and discomfort.

DIAGNOSTIC TOOLS

- Diagnosis is based on physical examination, usually with the use of enhanced imaging techniques including ultrasound. Visual inspection using a light focused on the testicle may be able to identify fluid.

TREATMENT

- Identification of the cause and drainage of the fluid.

Benign Prostatic Hyperplasia

Benign prostatic hyperplasia (BPH) is the noncancerous enlargement of the prostate gland. BPH is seen in more than 50% of men older than 60 years of age. BPH may cause compression of the urethra as it passes through the prostate, making urination difficult, reducing force of the flow of the urine stream, or causing dribbling of urine to occur. The cause of BPH is unclear but it appears related to an imbalance between estrogen and testosterone in the prostate.

CLINICAL MANIFESTATIONS

- Increased frequency of urination, with delay in initiating urination and a reduction in the force of the urine stream.
- As the condition progresses, the bladder may not empty completely, causing dribbling or overflow of urine. The time required to urinate increases.

DIAGNOSTIC TOOLS

- Diagnosis involves a good history and physical examination coupled with the use of imaging techniques. Biopsy of the prostate may be required to rule out neoplasia.

COMPLICATIONS

- With advanced BPH, urinary tract obstruction may occur as urine is unable to pass through the prostate. This can lead to urinary tract infections and, if unrelieved, renal failure.

TREATMENT

- Mild prostate enlargement may not be treated or may be treated with drugs to shrink the size of the prostate or relax the muscles of the bladder and prostate. This improves urine flow.
- Surgery may be required to remove the hyperplastic tissue in order to ensure adequate passage of urine.
- A permanent catheter might be placed in individuals unwilling or unable to tolerate surgery.
- Annual digital rectal examinations and screening for prostate-specific antigen (PSA) are encouraged to identify a malignancy that may arise from the hyperplastic cells.

Inflammatory Disorders of the Male Reproductive Tract

Inflammation of the male genital tract can occur anywhere between the testes and the urethral opening. Inflammation is usually due to a sexually transmitted disease or a urinary tract infection and is most commonly seen in sexually active men. Other causes of inflammation include systemic disease such as mumps, or trauma. Inflammation of the prostate may occur in older men with benign prostatic hyperplasia. Common inflammatory conditions of the genitalia in men include the following.

URETHRITIS is an inflammation of the urethra. Urethritis is usually caused by a sexually transmitted microorganism, commonly *Neisseria gonorrhoeae* or *Chlamydia trachomatis*.

EPIDIDYMITIS is an inflammation of the epididymis. Epididymitis is usually caused by a sexually transmitted microorganism, commonly *N. Gonorrhoeae* or *C. Trachomatis*. Epididymitis usually occurs from ascending urethral infection.

ORCHITIS is an acute inflammation of the testes. Orchitis usually develops following epididymitis or a systemic disease such as mumps.

PROSTATITIS is an inflammation of the prostate gland. Prostatitis is especially common in older men. It is often caused by an acute or chronic infection, usually ascending from the urethra. Prostatitis may be noninfectious and idiopathic in origin.

CLINICAL MANIFESTATIONS

- Urethritis may present with pain and burning on urination. A discharge from the penis may be present.
- Epididymitis may present with acute scrotal or inguinal pain. Flank pain may be present. The scrotum may be inflamed and tender on the affected side.
- Orchitis usually presents acutely with a very high fever (104°F) and swelling and redness of the testicle and scrotum. The individual appears very ill, and malaise is obvious.
- Prostatitis from an ascending urinary tract infection usually presents with painful and frequent urination. Interrupted or slow urine stream and nocturia (urination at night) may be present. Fever and malaise are common. Low back or perineal pain is common, especially when standing. Digital examination reveals a very tender and enlarged prostate.

DIAGNOSTIC TOOLS

- Diagnosis involves a thorough history and physical examination. Blood and urine cultures for the identification of an infectious organism may be required.

COMPLICATIONS

- Epididymitis and orchitis may cause infertility, related to poor testicular blood flow, and infarct of the testicular cells.

TREATMENT

- Antibiotic therapy is required for all bacterial or chlamydial infections.
- Orchitis is treated with bed rest, analgesics for pain, and elevation

of the testicles to increase venous drainage. Cold compresses may reduce initial inflammation. If a testicular abscess occurs, surgical removal of the testicle may be necessary.

Pelvic Inflammatory Disease

Pelvic inflammatory disease is the infectious inflammation of any of the organs of the upper genital tract in women, including the uterus, fallopian tubes (salpingitis), or ovaries (oophoritis). The infectious agent is usually bacterial and is often acquired during sexual intercourse. A variety of microbial agents may be implicated, including *Neisseria gonorrhoeae, Chlamydia trachomatis*, and *Escherichia coli*. In severe cases, the entire peritoneal cavity may be affected.

CLINICAL MANIFESTATIONS

- Although occasionally a woman will be asymptomatic, she usually presents with a high fever and bilateral, severe abdominal pain.
- Bleeding between periods may occur.
- Abdominal pain worsens with intercourse and physical activity.

DIAGNOSTIC TOOLS

- The cervix is tender to the touch and extremely painful when moved on bimanual examination.
- Purulent discharge at the external os may be apparent on inspection.
- Culture of the cervical discharge may indicate the infecting microorganism.
- White blood cell count and cell sedimentation rate are usually elevated.
- Visualization of the inflamed pelvis by laparoscopy, the insertion of a fiberoptic probe, can be used to confirm the diagnosis of PID.

COMPLICATIONS

- PID may lead to scarring and adhesions of the uterus or fallopian tubes, predisposing the woman to infertility.
- Pelvic adhesions and scarring increase the risk of a subsequent **ectopic pregnancy.** In an ectopic pregnancy, the embryo implants and grows at a site other than the uterus, usually the fallopian tube. Rupture of the fallopian tube may occur, leading to internal hemorrhage and maternal death.
- Approximately 5 to 10% of women with PID die, usually from septic shock.

TREATMENT

- Antibiotic therapy at home or in the hospital is required.
- Avoidance of sexual intercourse until the inflammation has subsided allows healing to occur and reduces the risk of reinfection.
- Education on the use of barrier methods of contraception (condom,

diaphragm with foam or jelly) to prevent future occurrences of sexually transmitted disease is important. Birth control pills may reduce PID by increasing the production of cervical mucus, but do not replace the need for a condom.

- The sexual partner(s) of an affected woman should be treated with antibiotics to prevent reinfection.
- Appendicitis must be ruled out as the cause of abdominal pain.

Endometriosis

Endometriosis is the presence of uterine endometrial cells outside the uterus, anywhere in the pelvic or abdominal region. The endometrial cells respond to estrogen and progesterone with proliferation, secretion, and bleeding during the menstrual cycle. This can cause inflammation and severe pain. The inflammation may lead to scarring of pelvic or abdominal organs and infertility.

Retrograde menstruation is the main risk factor for endometriosis. Retrograde menstruation is the movement of some menstrual discharge *up* the fallopian tubes into the peritoneal cavity during menstruation, rather than down and out the vagina. However, retrograde menstruation occurs in most women without causing symptoms of endometriosis. A genetic predisposition and a depressed immune system that allows the debris to seed the peritoneal cavity may increase a woman's risk of endometriosis. Exposure to environmental toxins may contribute to the development of endometriosis in some women.

CLINICAL MANIFESTATIONS

- Menstrual cramping and pain, ranging from mild to severe, before and/or during menstruation is the most common symptom of endometriosis. The intensity of the pain is not proportional to the absolute amount of endometrial tissue in extrauterine sites (i.e., women may have severe pain with little endometriosis visible during surgical inspection or may have only minor pain with significant spread).
- Changes in bowel movements, either diarrhea or constipation, may occur around the time of menstruation.
- Pain on intercourse (dyspareunia)—or on defecation if rectal tissue is involved—may occur. The pain is usually worst during menstruation, but in severe cases, pain may be constant.

DIAGNOSTIC TOOLS

- Visualization of the peritoneal cavity using laparoscopic techniques can diagnose endometriosis and assign a stage to the disease.

COMPLICATIONS

- Infertility is a common (30–40%) complication of endometriosis. Endometriosis may cause infertility by causing scarring and obstruc-

tion of the fallopian tubes or by initiating a maintained state of inflammation. Hormonal disturbances may occur.
- Emotional distress, family and marital discord, and low self-esteem may develop in some women, especially if infertility is a concern.

TREATMENT

- Treatment is based on the stage and severity of the disorder and is aimed at pain management, reducing the disease progress, and preventing or reversing infertility. The following treatments contribute to these goals:
  - Medications to interrupt the menstrual cycle and stop the proliferation and secretion of extrauterine cells are frequently used to treat endometriosis. Medications include birth control pills that reduce menstrual flow and cramping, nonsteroidal anti-inflammatory drugs such as aspirin or ibuprofen, to reduce cramping, and gonadotropin-releasing hormone agonists or androgen agonists to block the release of LH and FSH thereby preventing ovulation and menstruation. These treatments are all aimed at providing time for the extra uterine tissue to regress and inflammation to subside. After several months, a woman may discontinue therapy, and after a recommended period, she may attempt to become pregnant if desired.
  - Conservative surgical treatments, including laser surgery, may be used to remove visible endometrial implants.
  - Radical surgical interventions, including removal of the uterus (hysterectomy), fallopian tubes, and ovaries may be required if the pain is unbearable or significantly interfering with a woman's life. This would cause irreversible infertility.

Polycystic Ovarian Syndrome

Polycystic ovarian syndrome is the presence of cysts in the ovaries. These cysts consist of preovulatory follicles that have undergone atresia (degeneration). In polycystic ovarian syndrome, the ovaries are intact and responsive to FSH and LH, but ovulation of an ovum does not occur. FSH levels are less than normal throughout the follicular stage of the cycle. LH levels are higher than normal but do not show a surge. The consistently high LH increases androgen and estrogen production by the follicle and the adrenal gland. The anovulatory follicles degenerate and form cysts, giving the condition its name.

CLINICAL MANIFESTATIONS

- Amenorrhea or dysfunctional uterine bleeding.
- The development of male secondary sexual characteristics (hirsutism), including a deepening of the voice, facial hair, and clitoral enlargement in response to high androgen levels, is common.

DIAGNOSTIC TOOLS

- Blood hormonal assay will show excess androgen and estrogen levels with low FSH and no LH surge.

COMPLICATIONS

- Infertility may be present due to lack of ovulation.
- There is an increased risk of developing estrogen-dependent tumors of the breast and endometrium.

TREATMENT

- Antiestrogen drugs (e.g., clomiphene citrate) are provided to lower estrogen levels, causing FSH and LH to rise, and stimulating ovulation. Other drugs may be used to stimulate ovulation.
- Oral contraceptives, containing low-dose estrogen and progesterone, can limit cyst development.
- Surgical resection of the ovaries, or drug therapy to suppress ovarian function, may be required.

Fibrocystic Disease of the Breast

Fibrocystic disease of the breast is also called benign breast disease. It is characterized by palpable lumps in the breasts that change in size and tenderness during the different stages of the menstrual cycle. The swellings are very common among normal, healthy women. The incidence of fibrocystic disease increases with advancing age until menopause occurs. Although the exact cause of the disease is unknown, it appears that estrogen is at least partially responsible. Although most lumps that vary through the menstrual cycle are benign, some of the lesions may proliferate and show atypical cellular growth. Women with repeated and large cyst development may be at a higher risk for breast cancer and should be screened regularly.

CLINICAL MANIFESTATIONS

- Tenderness in the breasts, especially near menstruation is the main symptom.
- Palpable lumps that increase in size during the menstrual cycle are common.

DIAGNOSTIC TOOLS

- Biopsies of the lumps may be performed to rule out carcinoma and to identify precancerous conditions.
- Mammography or ultrasound may be able to distinguish the fluid-filled cyst from a solid tumor. A biopsy may be necessary.

COMPLICATIONS

- Lesions that are proliferative and show atypical cells may progress to cancer. This is especially a risk for women with a personal or family history of breast cancer.

TREATMENT

- Pain may be relieved by changing dietary habits. For some women, eliminating caffeine from the diet reduces symptoms. Support bras, especially when the breasts are most sensitive, may reduce pain.
- Cysts may be drained in cases of severe pain.
- A synthetic androgen (e.g., danazol) may be prescribed in cases of severe pain.

Cancer of the Male Reproductive Tract

Cancer of the male reproductive tract may include cancer of the penis, testes, or prostate.

PENILE CANCER

Primary cancer of the penis is rare in the United States. It usually occurs in noncircumcised men, possibly related to accumulations of smegma (thick secretions) under the foreskin. It occurs between 40 and 80 years of age and is more common in African Americans than Caucasians. Secondary penile cancer may occur from metastasis of bladder, rectal, or prostate cancer.

TESTICULAR CANCER

Testicular cancers are rare, mostly occurring in young men between the ages of 15 and 35. Testicular cancer is usually a germ cell (gamete) cancer but may develop from Leydig or Sertoli cells. The cause of testicular cancer is unknown, but there appears to be a genetic factor. Testicular cancer is more common in Caucasians and occurs more frequently in men with a history of cryptorchidism. Trauma and prenatal exposure to the synthetic estrogen, diethylstilbestrol (DES), may increase risk.

PROSTATE CANCER

Prostate cancer is the number one cancer identified in American males and the second-leading cause of death due to cancer in that population (the first is lung cancer). Prostate cancer is usually diagnosed in men older than 65 years of age; however, it is being more frequently diagnosed in younger men, perhaps as a result of more aggressive screening. Autopsy studies show that approximately 50% of men older than 50 years of age have some cancerous prostate cells, which is causing significant debate over recommended treatment, especially for elderly men with slow-growing, early-stage tumors. A recently developed inexpensive blood test can detect proteins released from even microscopic prostate tumors, thereby allowing diagnosis of the condition at an earlier stage than in the past.

The cause of prostate cancer is unknown although both genetic and environmental factors are believed to play a role. The risk of prostate cancer is increased in men who have a first-degree relative with the disease, in African American men, and in men exposed to certain environmental or occupational toxins, such as cadmium. Prostate cancer appears to be related to lifelong levels of testosterone. Prostate cancers are testosterone-dependent until late in the course of the disease.

Using clinical and biopsy results, prostate tumors are staged from A to D. **Stage A** tumors are well differentiated (A1) or moderately/poorly differentiated (A2) but restricted to the prostate gland. These tumors are asymptomatic and their presence is reported in more than 80% of men older than 80 years of age. Stage A tumors cannot be felt on digital examination. **Stage B** tumors include a single nodule (B1) or a group of discreet nodules (B2) palpable on digital examination and confined to the prostate. **Stage C** tumors are large masses that fill the entire prostate gland (C1) and may extend beyond the edges of the gland (C2). **Stage D** tumors are metastatic, with cancerous cells found in the lymph nodes draining the pelvis (D1) and in other sites (D2), often the bone.

CLINICAL MANIFESTATIONS

- Penile cancer is characterized by an ulcerative lesion on the shaft of the penis that may or may not be painful.
- Testicular cancer is characterized by the development of a mass in the testis, which may become painful as it grows. Testicular heaviness or aching may occur. Gynecomastia may develop.
- Prostate cancer may be asymptomatic or associated with increased frequency and urgency of urination, and a decrease in the force of the urine stream. Blood may be passed in the ejaculate, and in advanced disease, back pain may be present.

DIAGNOSTIC TOOLS

- Biopsy of cells of the penis can diagnose and stage penile cancer.
- Transillumination of the testes, ultrasound, and MRI may identify a testicular mass and support clinical findings of a testicular cancer.
- A digital rectal examination may reveal a fixed, firm mass in the prostate, suggestive of a tumor. The mass is often painless with irregular borders and results in asymmetry of the prostate gland. Ultrasound may be used to pinpoint the location of a prostate tumor. A biopsy of prostate cells taken via a transurethral resection can confirm the diagnosis of prostate cancer.

- A blood test that measures the level of a glycoprotein released by the prostate gland, prostate-specific antigen (PSA), can be used to identify the presence of early-stage prostate cancer. Current recommendations are to perform a biopsy if the PSA level is greater than 4 nanograms per milliliter (ng/mL) of blood; levels greater than 10 ng/ml suggest cancer. However, PSA elevation may occur with noncancerous conditions such as prostatitis or benign prostatic hyperplasia. Likewise, in approximately 25% of men, PSA measurements may be in the normal range even when cancer is present. The need to treat stage A cancers detected by PSA assay is controversial, especially in elderly men.

  A recently suggested strategy to address the issue of false-negative and false-positive PSA readings is to evaluate PSA levels on a sliding scale, depending on if the male is young (younger than 50 years) or older. For young men, a PSA of even 2.6 ng/mL may be considered significant, especially if a previous lower baseline measurement is available. In older men, a moderately elevated level may not call for aggressive follow-up. In addition, measuring free versus protein-bound PSA may allow for better discrimination of cancer versus benign source, with a lower ratio of free-to-bound expected in men with cancer.

COMPLICATIONS

- Untreated, progressive penile cancer has an extremely high mortality rate (>90%).
- Testicular cancer may metastasize to the lungs, lymph nodes, or central nervous system.
- Survival with prostate cancer depends on the stage at diagnosis. Most men diagnosed with stage D cancer die within 3 to 5 years.
- Impotence and incontinence may develop as a result of any of the male reproductive cancers. Impotence and urinary incontinence may develop following treatment of the cancers as well.

TREATMENT

- Surgical excision of the penile cancer, with or without radiation and chemotherapy, is required.
- For testicular cancer, surgery to remove the affected testis is performed. Radiation and chemotherapy are provided.
- A chest radiograph and a lymph node biopsy are performed on men with testicular cancer to rule out metastasis.
- Watchful waiting may be adequate for some elderly men with stage A prostate cancer.
- Radical prostatectomy (surgical removal of the prostate) or radiation therapy is usually used to treat all stage B and C prostate tumors and all stage A tumors in young men. Treatment options can include external-beam radiation, implanted radiation seeds, and cryother-

apy. Stage D tumors are treated with hormonal therapy to slow the spread of the disease and palliative measures to reduce pain. Hormonal therapy includes antiandrogen drugs, estrogen therapy, and drugs that block the release of the hypothalamic gonadotropin-releasing hormone (leuprolide). Orchiectomy (removal of the testes) may accompany hormonal therapy.

Cancer of the Female Reproductive Tract

Cancer of the female reproductive tract may develop in the vagina, uterus, or ovaries.

VAGINAL CANCER

Vaginal cancer is rare in the United States, usually occurring in women older than 60 years of age. The vaginal squamous cells are most often involved. Frequently, the cancer is a secondary metastasis. The risk of developing vaginal cancer increases in women who were exposed prenatally to DES or in those who have had previous cervical cancer.

UTERINE CANCER

Uterine cancer includes cancer of the cervix and endometrium. **Cervical cancer** is often a result of a sexually transmitted disease of the cervix caused by certain strains of the human papillomavirus (HPV). Cervical cancer is most common in women who have had multiple sexual partners or whose sexual partners have had many partners. Women who are infected with HPV during their teenage years are especially at risk of developing cervical cancer, possibly related to the high rate of cell division occurring in the cervix during those years when exposed to the virus. Because of the ability of cervical mucus to concentrate carcinogens present in cigarette smoke, smoking is considered a cofactor in the development of cervical cancer. Premalignant changes in the cervix usually precede cervical cancer by many years. The premalignant changes, called dysplasia, can be identified and staged during cytologic studies of a cervical smear (the Papanicolaou smear, or Pap smear).

Endometrial cancer is the most common female reproductive cancer and is usually an adenocarcinoma (from the epithelial cells). Endometrial cancer is related to lifetime exposure to estrogen and typically presents in postmenopausal women. Lifetime estrogen exposure increases in women who are obese (estrogen concentrates in adipose tissue), who have never been pregnant, or who experience early menarche and late menopause. Women with a high-fat diet are at increased risk, apparently related to associated obesity. Other risks include hormonal exposure in the diet and reduced intake of fruits and vegetables. Oral contraceptives reduce the risk of developing endometrial cancer by reducing lifetime estrogen exposure. Exposure to estrogen replacement therapy increases the risk of endometrial cancer in postmenopausal women; this risk is eliminated by the coadministration of progesterone in combined hormone replacement therapy (HRT). Therefore, the use of estrogen alone is contraindicated in women with an intact uterus.

OVARIAN CANCER

Although relatively rare, ovarian cancer causes death more often than any other female reproductive cancer. Ovarian cancer is usually of the epithelial cells and is related to lifelong estrogen exposure. In children or adolescents, ovarian cancer may develop in the germ cells (ova) and is associated with a genetic predisposition. Ovarian cancer is highest among women who have had a first-degree relative with ovarian cancer. High-fat diet, obesity, and lack of childbearing increase the risk of ovarian cancer. Oral contraceptives and, in some studies, tubal ligation (severing of the fallopian tubes) seem to protect against ovarian cancer. Moderate exercise, which is related to lower estrogen levels, may decrease the risk of ovarian cancer.

CLINICAL MANIFESTATIONS

- Vaginal cancer may be asymptomatic or associated with bleeding, discharge, or pain.
- Cervical cancer may be asymptomatic, or associated with bleeding after intercourse or spotting between menstrual periods. A vaginal discharge with odor may be present.
- Endometrial cancer may be asymptomatic or associated with abnormal bleeding.
- Ovarian cancer is usually asymptomatic until the disease is advanced. Late symptoms include abdominal swelling and pain. Gastrointestinal obstruction may cause vomiting, constipation, or small-volume diarrhea.

DIAGNOSTIC TOOLS

- The Pap smear can identify cervical and endometrial cancer.
- Direct cytologic sampling of the vagina and endometrium can diagnose vaginal and endometrial cancer.
- Ovarian cancer can be identified by use of ultrasound or MRI. Surgery is required to stage the disease and identify metastases. Increased level of an ovarian tumor cell antigen, CA-125, in a symptomatic woman or a woman with a family history of ovarian or breast cancer can be an early indication of disease.

COMPLICATIONS

- Death may occur with any of the reproductive cancers. Survival rates are highest (75–95%) with endometrial cancer and lowest

(25–30%) with ovarian cancer. Early detection can improve survival rate significantly. This is especially true for cervical cancer with a survival rate near 100% if identified in situ (before it has spread).

TREATMENT

- Surgery, with or without chemotherapy, is the treatment of choice for all the reproductive cancers. Laser surgery or cryosurgery (freezing) may be used for vaginal or cervical cancers.

Breast Cancer

Breast cancer is a relatively common cancer among women in the United States, and it is the leading cause of death in women between 45 and 64 years of age. Breast cancer may be discovered while in situ (localized), or it may be discovered as a malignant (spreading) neoplasm. Breast cancer is usually an adenocarcinoma found in the milk ducts.

The risk that a woman in the United States will develop breast cancer at some time in her life is approximately one in eight. Breast cancer incidence increases with age and is influenced by genetic, hormonal, and environmental factors. Men may develop breast cancer although the incidence is low.

RISK FACTORS FOR BREAST CANCER

A strong risk factor for breast cancer is a history of the disease in one or more first-degree relative (sisters or mother). Genetic studies have identified a variety of genes, including BRCA1 and BRCA2, that contribute to familial breast cancer. Mutations in these two genes are associated with an increased lifetime risk of breast cancer, ovarian cancer, or both. Women who inherit a gene for breast cancer typically develop the disease at an earlier age than women who do not have a family history of the disease. The genes for breast cancer can be carried and passed by either parent, in an apparently autosomal-dominant manner. Other common cancer genes, including mutated myc- or p53-genes, also are seen in breast tumors.

Lifetime estrogen exposure also is related to the development of breast cancer. Women who experience early menarche and late menopause are at increased risk. Ages of menarche and menopause are genetically influenced. Lack of or delayed childbearing also increases the risk of breast cancer, as may estrogen replacement therapy in some women. Fibrocystic disease of the breast characterized by epithelial hyperplasia is associated with increased risk. A high-fat diet and in some studies but not others, alcohol consumption have also been linked to breast cancer. Protection against breast cancer is possible by consuming a diet rich in fruits and vegetables, exercising throughout one's lifetime, and controlling one's weight.

CLINICAL MANIFESTATIONS

- A painless lump or mass in the breast. Most cancers occur in the upper outer quadrant of the breast (50%) or in the center of the breast (20%). The lump is usually fixed (nonmobile) with irregular borders. It is unilateral and does not usually show variation in size with the menstrual cycle.
- Retraction of the nipple, nipple discharge, or puckering of the breast tissue may signal an underlying tumor.
- Lymph node swelling, either axillary or clavicular, may indicate metastasis.

DIAGNOSTIC TOOLS

- Breast self-examination (BSE) performed on a regular (monthly) basis is important for early detection of a tumor. BSE should be performed by all women older than 20 years of age.
- Mammography, a radiograph of the breast, is an important screening tool to identify breast cancer before a lump can be felt. Annual or biannual mammography is recommended for all women older than 40 years of age and for younger women with a family history of the disease or other risk factors.
- Biopsy of a suspected lump will confirm the diagnosis. Determination of tumor size, tumor characteristics, and examination of surrounding lymph nodes allows for staging and histologic classification of the tumor. Staging is from I to IV and is important in determining treatment and in estimating prognosis.
- Measurement of estrogen receptors on the tumor cells indicates the estrogen sensitivity of the tumor. A high level of estrogen receptors indicates the tumor may respond well to hormonal therapy.

COMPLICATIONS

- Widespread metastases may occur. Sites of metastasis include the brain, lungs, bone, liver, and ovaries. Survival rates depend on staging: stage I (tumor <2 cm, no metastases), 80%; stage II (tumor 2–5 cm, axillary node metastasis), 65%; stage III (tumor >5 cm, axillary node metastasis and spread to skin or chest wall), 40%; stage IV (widespread metastases), 10%.

TREATMENT

- Mastectomy or lumpectomy, with dissection of the axillary nodes is indicated in most cases.

- Adding radiotherapy or chemotherapy in conjunction with surgery improves survival and reduce the likelihood of recurrence.
- Antiestrogens or estrogens specifically designed to interfere with the growth of breast tissue, have been used for several years to treat breast tumors positive for estrogen receptors. These same drugs, including tamoxifen, are now being used to treat breast tumors that do not appear to be specifically estrogen sensitive (Chapter 5). These drugs, often called "designer estrogens" or "selective estrogen receptor modulators," appear to improve survival and reduce the likelihood of recurrence.
- Breast reconstruction may be performed following surgery to improve appearance.
- Counseling and support for the woman, her partner, and her family is essential.

Sexually Transmitted Disease

Sexually transmitted disease (STD) may develop in anyone having sexual contact with multiple partners or with one partner who has had sexual contact with others. Microorganisms capable of causing an STD include the bacteria *Neisseria gonorrhoeae*, responsible for causing gonorrhea, and *Treponema pallidum*, responsible for causing syphilis. Chlamydia, the most common STD in the United States, is caused by the intracellular bacterium *Chlamydia trachomatis*. The herpes simplex virus, human papillomavirus (HPV), hepatitis B virus, and human immunodeficiency virus (HIV) are also sexually transmitted. *Trichomonas vaginalis* is a protozoan responsible for causing trichomoniasis. An STD may be passed via semen or vaginal secretions or by skin-to-skin contact. Clinical manifestations of an STD depend on the agent responsible, host characteristics, and the stage of infection. Treatments are specific to the causative agent. Herpes simplex, hepatitis B, HPV, and HIV infection are discussed elsewhere in this text.

CLINICAL MANIFESTATIONS

- Gonorrhea may be asymptomatic or may present with purulent discharge from the urethra or vagina and burning on urination. Some individuals, including infants born to infected mothers, may develop conjunctivitis or pharyngitis.
- Primary syphilis is characterized by the presence of a painless genital ulcer (chancre) that spontaneously regresses. Secondary syphilis develops weeks to months later and is characterized by a temporary skin rash, typically located on the palms of the hands and the soles of the feet. Tertiary syphilis may develop decades after the initial infection and is characterized by sensory loss, muscle weakness, and heart defects.
- Chlamydia may be asymptomatic or may present with urethritis or cervicitis characterized by discharge, itching, and burning on

urination. In women, spotting between periods or after intercourse may occur.
- Trichomoniasis may be asymptomatic or may present with greenish discharge and itching. Pain with intercourse is common. Men are seldom symptomatic.

DIAGNOSTIC TOOLS

- Smears of vaginal or urethral discharge observed under the light microscope may indicate the presence of *N. gonorrhoeae* and *C. trachomatis*. Diagnosis may also be based on pH, odor, color, and the presence of white blood cells. The protozoan *T. vaginalis* may be visible with a light microscope.
- Vaginal or urethral cultures can identify the presence of *N. gonorrhoeae* and *C. trachomatis*.
- *T. pallidum* is identified in a blood test (VDRL or RPR).

COMPLICATIONS

- **Untreated gonorrhea** may cause female sterility or pelvic inflammatory disease, and increases the risk of ectopic pregnancy. Both men and women may develop disseminated infection with arthritis, endocarditis, or conjunctivitis leading to blindness. If passed to a newborn during birth, blindness may result.
- **Untreated syphilis** may cause heart failure and neurologic deterioration. If passed to a fetus during pregnancy, fetal death or neonatal infection may occur.
- **Chlamydial** infection may cause infertility in men and women, and epididymitis in males. Pelvic inflammatory disease and ectopic pregnancy may occur in infected women. If passed to a newborn, conjunctivitis may occur.

TREATMENT

- Because of the prevalence of penicillin-resistant gonorrhea, gonorrhea is currently treated with a single intramuscular dose of ceftriaxone.
- Syphilis is treated with intramuscular penicillin. If pregnant, erythromycin or ceftriaxone is used. If allergic to penicillin, but nonpregnant, doxycycline or tetracycline is recommended.
- Chlamydial infection may be treated with a macrolide (clarithromycin, azithromycin, or erythromycin; the latter during pregnancy), doxycycline, or tetracycline. Since gonorrhea frequently occurs with chlamydia, individuals suspected of having either disease are usually treated with both ceftriaxone and a second drug. A large dose (1 g) of azithromycin may be given in the office for a one-dose treatment.
- Trichomoniasis is treated with metronidazole (Flagyl), or topical clotrimazole during pregnancy.

Selected Bibliography

Bates, Barbara (1998). *A guide to physical examination (7th ed.)*. Philadelphia: J.B. Lippincott.

Becker, T.B. (1994). Sexually transmitted diseases and other risk factors for cervical dysplasia among southwestern Hispanics and non-Hispanic white women. *Journal of the American Medical Association* 271, 1181-1188.

Braunstein, G.D. (1993). Diagnosis and treatment of gynecomastia. *Hospital Practice* 28, 37-47.

Burnett, A.L. (1998). New options for erectile dysfunction. *Clinician Reviews (Supp, June)* 3-7.

Catalona, W.J., D.S. Smith & D.K. Ornsten. (1997). Prostate cancer detection in men with serum PSA concentrations of 2.6 to 4.0 ng/ml and benign prostate examination: enhancement of specificity with free PSA measurements. *JAMA* 277, 1452-1455.

Col, N.F., M.H. Eckman, R.H. Kares, S.G. Parker, R.J. Goldberg, et. al. (1997). Patient-specific decisions about hormone replacement therapy in postmenopausal women. *JAMA* 277, 1140-1147.

Cunningham, F.G., et al. (1993). *Williams obstetrics (19th ed.)*. Norwalk, CT: Appleton Lange.

Garnick, M.B. & W.R. Fair. (1998). Combating prostate cancer. *Scientific American* 279, 74-83.

Goolsby, M.J. (1998). Screening, diagnosis, and management of prostate cancer: improving primary care outcomes. *The Nurse Practitioner* 23, 11-41.

Guyton, A.C. & Hall, J.E. (1998). *Textbook of medical physiology (8th ed.)*. Philadelphia: W.B. Saunders.

Hatcher, R.A. (1998). *Contraceptive technology*. New York: Irvington Publishers Inc.

Healy, D.L., A.O. Trounson, A.N. Andersen (1994). Female infertility: causes and treatment. *Lancet* 343, 1539-1544.

Hortobagyi, G.N. (1998). Treatment of breast cancer. *New England Journal of Medicine* 339, 974-984.

Kampen, D.L. (1994). Estrogen and verbal memory in healthy post-menopausal women. *Obstetrics and Gynecology* 83, 979-983.

Keltz, M.D., and D.L. Olive (1993). Diagnostic and therapeutic options in endometriosis. *Hospital Practice* 28, 15-49.

Kritz-Silverstein, D., E. Barrett-Connor (1993). Early menopause, number of reproductive years, and bone mineral density in post-menopausal women. *American Journal of Public Health* 83, 983-988.

Limauzin-Lamothe, M.A., N. Mairon, C.R.B. Joyce & M. Le Gal. (1994). Quality of life after the meonopause: influence of hormonal replacement therapy. *American Journal of Obstetrics and Gynecology* 170, 618-624.

McGregor, J.A., and H.A. Hammill (1993). Contraception and sexually transmitted diseases: interactions and opportunities. *American Journal of Obstetrics* 168, 2033-2041.

Moen, M.H. (1993). The familial risk of endometriosis. *Acta Obstetrics and Gynecology Scandinavia* 172, 560-564.

Overgaard, M., Hansen, P.S., Overgaard, J., Rose, C., et.al., for the Danish Breast Cancer Cooperative Group. (1997). Postoperative radiotherapy in high-risk premenopausal women with breast cancer who receive adjuvant chemotherapy. New England Journal of Medicine, 337, 949-955. *New England Journal of Medicine* 337, 949-955.

Porth, C.M. (1998). *Pathophysiology concepts of altered health states (5th ed.)*. Philadelphia: J.B. Lippincott Company.

Postmenopausal Estrogen/Progestin Interventions (PEPI) Trial (1994). Effects of estrogen or estrogen/progestin regimens on heart disease risk factors in postmenopausal women. *Journal of the American Medical Association* 273, 199-208.

Sobel, J.D. (1997). Vaginitis. *New England Journal of Medicine* 337, 1896-1903.

Special Issue: Benign prostatic hyperplasia/obstruction. (1993). *Journal of Urology* 150, 1587-1750.

Special Medical Report (1994): NIH develops consensus statement on ovarian cancer. *American Family Physician* 50, 213-216.

INDEX

Note: Page numbers in *italics* indicate illustrations; those followed by t indicate tables.